IMMUNOLOGY

Second Edition

The Benjamin/Cummings Series in the Life Sciences

F. J. Ayala
Population and Evolutionary Genetics: A Primer
(1982)

F. J. Ayala and J. A. Kiger, Jr.
Modern Genetics, second edition (1984)

F. J. Ayala and J. W. Valentine
Evolving: The Theory and Processes of Organic Evolution (1979)

M. G. Barbour, J. H. Burk, and W. D. Pitts
Terrestrial Plant Ecology (1980)

C. L. Case and T. R. Johnson
Laboratory Experiments in Microbiology (1984)

L. L. Cavalli-Sforza
Elements of Human Genetics, second edition
(1977)

R. E. Dickerson and I. Geis
Hemoglobin (1983)

P. B. Hackett, J. A. Fuchs, and J. W. Messing
An Introduction to Recombinant DNA Techniques: Basic Experiments in Gene Manipulation
(1984)

L. E. Hood, I. L. Weissman, W. B. Wood, and
J. H. Wilson
Immunology, second edition (1984)

L. E. Hood, J. H. Wilson, and W. B. Wood
Molecular Biology of Eucaryotic Cells (1975)

J. B. Jenkins
Human Genetics (1983)

K. D. Johnson, D. L. Rayle, and H. L. Wedberg
Biology: An Introduction (1984)

R. J. Lederer
Ecology and Field Biology (1984)

A. L. Lehninger
Bioenergetics: The Molecular Basis of Biological Energy Transformations, second edition (1971)

S. E. Luria, S. J. Gould, and S. Singer
A View of Life (1981)

E. N. Marieb
Human Anatomy and Physiology Lab Manual: Brief Edition (1983)

E. N. Marieb
Human Anatomy and Physiology Lab Manual: Cat and Fetal Pig Versions (1981)

E. B. Mason
Human Physiology (1983)

A. P. Spence
Basic Human Anatomy (1982)

A. P. Spence and E. B. Mason
Human Anatomy and Physiology, second edition (1983)

G. J. Tortora, B. R. Funke, and C. L. Case
Microbiology: An Introduction (1982)

J. D. Watson, N. Hopkins, J. Roberts, J. Steitz, and A. Weiner
Molecular Biology of the Gene, fourth edition (1985)

I. L. Weissman, L. E. Hood, and W. B. Wood
Essential Concepts in Immunology (1978)

N. K. Wessells
Tissue Interactions and Development (1977)

W. B. Wood, J. H. Wilson, R. M. Benbow, and
L. E. Hood
Biochemistry: A Problems Approach, second edition (1981)

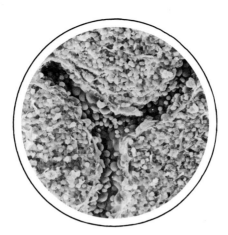

IMMUNOLOGY

Second Edition

Leroy E. Hood

California Institute of Technology

Irving L. Weissman

Stanford University

William B. Wood

University of Colorado, Boulder

John H. Wilson

Baylor College of Medicine

THE BENJAMIN/CUMMINGS PUBLISHING COMPANY, INC.

Menlo Park, California • Reading, Massachusetts
London • Amsterdam • Don Mills, Ontario • Sydney

Front Cover:

Natural transplantation in Tunicates

Among some nonvertebrates, such as tunicates, individuals can fuse to form a multi-individual colony. *Colonial tunicates* form colonies by a complex recognition system involving fusion or rejection of extracorporeal blood vessels between two individuals or two colonies. When fused, the two colonies share blood cells. On the cover a colony bearing orange pigment cells (lower right) has fused with a colony bearing purple pigment cells (upper left), resulting in a mixing of the blood cells. Fusion or rejection is genetically controlled in this species by a single gene locus which has many alleles; two individuals must share the same allele to fuse. The same locus (or a closely linked locus) also controls *fertilization* (sperm-egg fusion) between two individuals; in this case sperm and egg must *not* share alleles to fuse.

This type of genetic control of "transplantation" extends into all vertebrates, where a genetic region called the *major histocompatibility complex* (MHC) encodes transplantation antigens (cell-surface glycoproteins) which prevent the acceptance of the type of unnatural transplants tried by transplantation biologists and physicians. The products of the MHC are also used as signals for intercellular communications between immunity cells within an individual, and through these signals control our susceptibility to infections. Because the biology and molecular genetics of the MHC are recurring themes throughout this book, we have chosen this cover to illustrate an example of the unity of important biological principles, including the possibility that tunicate fusion/rejection genes may be forerunners of the vertebrate MHC. (Photo courtesy of Virginia Scofield and Irving Weissman).

Back Cover:

Structure of an Antibody Molecule

This computer graphic representation by Arthur J. Olson illustrates the protein backbone of the human myeloma IgG Dob. This representation is based on the X-ray crystal studies of M. Navia, E. Silverton, V. R. Sarma, G. H. Cohen, and D. R. Davies. The image was produced using software developed by Olson, T. J. O'Donnell, and Michael L. Connolly.

Sponsoring Editor: *Jane Reece Gillen*
Production: *Mary Forkner*
Manuscript Editor: *Ruth Cottrell*
Cover Designer: *Rick Chafian*
Text Designer: *John Edeen*
Illustrations: *Georgeann Waggeman and Barbara Norris*

Library of Congress Cataloging in Publication Data

Main entry under title:

Immunology.

Rev. ed. of: Immunology/ Leroy E. Hood, Irving L. Weissman, William B. Wood. c1978.
Includes bibliographies and index.
1. Immunology. I. Hood, Leroy E. II. Hood, Leroy E. Immunology. [DNLM: 1. Allergy and immunology. QW 504 I3636]
QR181.I426 1984   616.07'9   84-6227
ISBN 0-8053-4407-1

CDEFGHIJ--HA--8987654

Second Printing

The Benjamin/Cummings Publishing Company, Inc.
2727 Sand Hill Road
Menlo Park, California 94025

Preface

Scope and Purposes of the Book

Although the study of the immune system began in the nineteenth century, immunology remained largely a descriptive science until the early 1960s. During the last 15 years, however, the tools of modern biochemistry, genetics, cell biology, and molecular biology have transformed immunology into a discipline with a dual nature, partly descriptive and partly molecular. Aspects such as the structure of antibody molecules and genes are understood at the molecular level, whereas others, including much of cellular immunology, are still in a descriptive stage. In this book we attempt to describe both aspects clearly and, where possible, to integrate phenomena with the detailed molecular picture that is now emerging. Indeed, since the publication of the first edition of *Immunology*, important insights into the molecular biology of antibody genes and genes of the major histocompatibility complex have been gained. One striking new feature of this edition is the detailed molecular description of these two systems in Chapters 4 and 6.

In this second edition, we have organized the subject matter of immunology into thirteen chapters. Chapter 1, The Immune System, provides a general introduction for this subject. Chapter 2, Antibodies, considers the structure and function of immunoglobulins. Chapter 3, Detection and Application of Antigen-Antibody Reactions, considers the discipline of immunochemistry, with emphasis on important techniques for immunoassay and immunodiagnosis. Chapter 4, Expression of Antibody Genes, analyzes the fascinating story of antibody gene structure, organization, rearrangements, and diversification. Chapter 5, Molecular Recognition at Cell Surfaces, deals with the general structure and function of the plasma membrane and the characteristics of some simple metazoan cellular recognition systems. Chapter 6, Genes and Proteins of the Major Histocompatibility Complex, deals with the general problem of self-nonself recognition, with particular emphasis on genes and proteins encoded by the major histocompatibility complex. Chapter 7, Development of the Immune System, moves into cellular immunology, with a consideration of the architecture and developmental biology of the immune system. Chapter 8, The Immune Response, surveys the cellular biology and cell-cell interactions of the vertebrate immune response. Chapter 9, Effector Mechanisms of the Immune System, deals with a variety of the effector mechanisms utilized by the vertebrate immune system, with special reference to their role in immunity to infection. Chapter 10, Tolerance and the Regulation of Immunity, analyzes the regulation of immunity by suppressor T-cell circuits and by idiotype-antiidiotype networks and considers in detail the development of immunological tolerance. Chapter 11, Tissue Transplantation, considers the immunogenetics of transplantation antigens, the effector functions mediating transplantation rejection, and the current status of clinical transplantation. Chapter 12, Immunopathology, discusses the cellular and molecular basis of congenital and acquired immune deficiency diseases, the inappropriate responses of T cells and B cells in hypersensitivity diseases, and the relationships between specific major histocompatibility genes and specific diseases. Chapter 13, Cancer Biology and Immunology, describes cancer cells, our current knowledge of the mechanisms by which they arise, and the immune-related aspects of cancer, including future immunological approaches to cancer prevention, diagnosis, and therapy.

Using the Book

Each chapter in *Immunology* is comprised of four sections: Concepts, Selected Bibliographies, Problems, and Answers. The *Concepts* are text sections; they present the most important general principles of each subject first, followed by more detailed information in subparagraphs.

The *Selected Bibliographies* offer short "where to begin" sections that cite readable introductory materials, followed by references to longer reviews and specific journal articles. We have included seminal articles from the classical literature as well as many up-to-date references.

The *Problems* sections, we believe, contain much of the teaching value of the book. They provide from 4 to 21 problems each, and the problems are arranged in order of increasing difficulty. New concepts and techniques are presented in the introductions to the problems. Because many problems have been drawn from the contemporary literature, the reader is exposed to data analysis in many areas of modern immunology. All information required to work these problems is contained in the book.

The *Answers* sections provide readers with detailed feedback on their efforts to obtain solutions, often by describing the analytical process originally used to interpret data in the literature.

Audience

We have written *Immunology* with several audiences in mind: undergraduate, graduate, and medical students taking a first course in immunology; students of biological disciplines related to immunology, such as microbiology, cell biology, or molecular biology; and scientists and health professionals wishing a text suitable for self-instruction with which to review modern immunology. The organization of the text allows its use at several levels, from a quick scan of the Concepts and their opening statements as a review of principles in contemporary immunology, to detailed study of all the text and accompanying problems as a comprehensive introduction to the subject.

The immune system is complex, and immunologists have employed a complex terminology to describe it. We have taken pains to minimize the considerable problem that this terminology can pose for the nonimmunologist by defining all terms clearly when they are introduced and by avoiding jargon and unnecessary abbreviations.

For all readers, we feel that the emphasis on problem solving is a particularly valuable feature of the book. To gain an active working knowledge of immunology, we have found it essential for students to confront actual experimental data and solve concrete problems in addition to reading, listening to lectures, and learning factual material. Consequently, we have included both simple and challenging problems, with detailed answers, in each chapter of the book. Students in the immunology courses we have taught often report that they have learned more from solving these problems than from any other aspect of the course.

Acknowledgments

Many people have contributed to the creation of this second edition. Foremost among these are the immunology students and teaching assistants at Stanford and Caltech who helped refine the lectures and problem sets that form the basis of this book. Teaching assistants who made the major contributions to the effort are Eric Pillemer, Howard Gershenfeld, John Monaco, Carol Nottenburg, Tony Infante, Dave Maloney, and Geoff Kansas at Stanford, and Bev Sher, Henry Sun, and Tim Hunkapiller at Caltech. We are indebted to Jonathan Fuhrman, Mitchell Kronenberg, and Roger Perlmutter for writing many of the problems, to Henry Sun and Lance Fong for collating the index, and to Ellen Rothenberg and Carol Sibley for criticizing portions of the text. We are also indebted to Alfred Dorfman, Gerald Edelman, Sylvia Friedberg, George Gutman, Elias Lazarides, Arthur Olsen, Jan Orenstein, Robert Rouse, Willem van Ewijk, and Roger Warnke for making photomicrographs available.

Useful criticisms of the first edition were provided by a number of immunology instructors who used the book in their courses; in particular we are grateful for the reviews submitted by Rodney Dietert, Richard Karp, Julia Levy, and Susan Pierce. Most of the writing of this text took place in Aspen, Colorado, at the Given Institute of Pathology, and we are grateful to Don King and Joan Leatherbury, who were our gracious hosts. Barbara Norris and Georgeann Waggeman in Aspen transformed our crude drawings into finished artwork. Bernita Larsh, Connie Katz, Susan Mangrum, and Stephanie Canada at Caltech and Janice Mason at Stanford contributed expert secretarial assistance and somehow managed to organize reams of manuscript to the finished chapters demanded by our publisher. Jane Gillen and Mary Forkner provided invaluable editorial help. Finally, we appreciate the support and understanding of our families during the writing of this book.

Leroy E. Hood
Irving L. Weissman
William B. Wood
John H. Wilson

Brief Contents

Detailed Contents

Chapter 5

Molecular Recognition at Cell Surfaces   131

Concepts

Chapter 8

The Immune Response 282

Concepts

Chapter 9

Immune Effector Mechanisms and the Complement System 334

Concepts

Chapter 10

Tolerance and the Regulation of Immunity   366

Concepts

Chapter 11

Tissue Transplantation   402

Concepts

Chapter 12

Immunopathology   436

Concepts

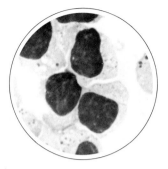

CHAPTER 1

The Immune System

Chapter Outline

Vertebrates possess a surveillance mechanism, called the *immune system*, that protects them from disease-causing (pathogenic) microorganisms such as bacteria and viruses, from parasites, and from cancer cells. The immune system specifically recognizes and selectively eliminates foreign invaders by a process known as the immune response. The immune response has three major characteristics: (1) it responds *adaptively* to foreign invaders, (2) it exhibits exquisite *specificity*, and (3) it displays a long-term *memory* of earlier contacts with specific

1

foreign pathogens. Immunology, the study of the immune system, has contributed significantly to modern medicine in areas such as blood transfusion, vaccination, organ transplantation, and the treatment of allergy, autoimmune disease, and cancer. Immunology also has made vital contributions to cell biology by advancing our understanding of differentiation, cell-cell cooperation, and the triggering of proliferation and differentiation by cell-surface receptors. This chapter presents an overview of the immune system and its response to foreign invaders.

Concepts

1-1   All organisms have nonadaptive defense systems against pathogens

Nonadaptive systems for organismic defense protect against infection in a fixed way. Elements of this system include external skin, internal defensive cells, and circulating proteins (Figure 1-1). Collectively, these elements must serve as the first line of defense against foreign invaders because the immune system, being adaptive, takes time to respond to a pathogen.

The skin is composed of highly keratinized epithelial cells that provide a passive barrier to penetration by pathogens. Defensive cells include both *phagocytes,* which bind, eat (*phago-*), and digest the great majority of invading organisms, and *natural killer cells,* which recognize and rapidly eliminate several kinds of parasitized cells and cancer cells. Phagocytes can be made more efficient in their recognition of foreign invaders by combining with products of the humoral immune response (Concept 1-2). Circulating or humoral factors in the nonadaptive defense system include proteins such as lysozyme, C-reactive protein, and properdin that bind to bacterial surfaces and initiate elimination reactions. Some of these humoral proteins are always present, whereas others are rapidly inducible.

1-2   Two systems of immunity protect vertebrates

Cellular and humoral immunity

Immune protection in vertebrates is provided by a dual system that maintains two basic defenses against foreign invaders. Both systems are adaptive and respond specifically to most foreign substances, although one response generally is favored. The *cellular immune response*

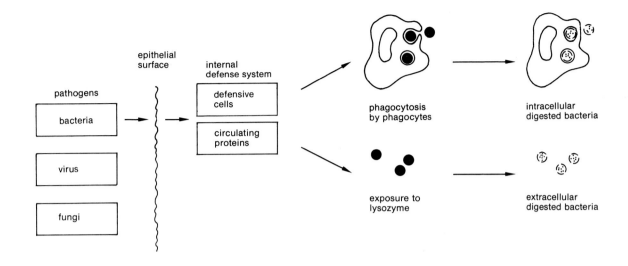

Figure 1-1

Nonadaptive systems of organismic defense against pathogens. The epithelial barrier and two specific defensive reactions against bacteria are illustrated.

is particularly effective against fungi, parasites, intracellular viral infections, cancer cells, and foreign tissue. The *humoral immune response* defends primarily against the extracellular phases of bacterial and viral infections.

Cellular immunity is provided by certain cells of the lymphoid system. Humoral immunity is provided by the proteins called *antibodies* that circulate through two body fluids: the serum, which is the fluid component of blood that remains after cells and fibrinogen have been removed by clotting and centrifugation, and the lymph, which is the fluid that bathes all tissue spaces. Thus the two systems of immunity are distinct but provide overlapping protection.

The cells of the immune system

The duality of the immune system results from two populations of morphologically indistinguishable lymphoid cells, called *lymphocytes.* One class of lymphocytes, the *T cells,* includes cells that mediate the cellular immune response. When the organism is invaded by a foreign substance that can alter the normal surface characteristics of host cells, some of the T cells that recognize it are activated and initiate reactions that include binding to and eliminating the altered cells (Figure 1-2). The other class of lymphocytes, the *B cells,* is responsible for the humoral immune response. Individual B cells, when activated by recognition of a foreign invader, differentiate to plasma cells that secrete antibodies. The antibodies bind specifically to the foreign sub-

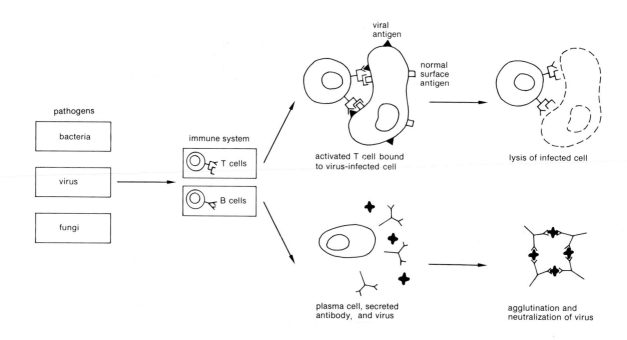

Figure 1-2

Differentiation, interaction, and elimination events that may occur upon stimulating T and B cells of the immune system.

stance and initiate a variety of elimination responses (Figure 1-2). Each lymphocyte in these two populations is poised to recognize and respond to one or a few closely related foreign substances. During a response, these cells first must proliferate and differentiate before they or their products are capable of eliminating foreign invaders.

In addition to lymphocytes, several other kinds of *accessory cells* are essential to the immune system (Figure 1-3). Their functions include accumulation of foreign substances in the body for presentation to lymphocytes, scavenging of foreign invaders attacked by the immune system, and mediation of physiological changes that accompany the immune response.

Phylogenetic occurrence of immunity

The dual system of T-cell and B-cell immunity appears to be restricted to vertebrates. Specific cellular and humoral immune responses are found in bony fishes and even in the lowest vertebrates. The extent to which cellular and humoral immunity occur in invertebrates is still unclear, although efficient cellular scavenging mechanisms, transplant rejection, and potent inducible antibacterial substances have been demonstrated in several subvertebrate species.

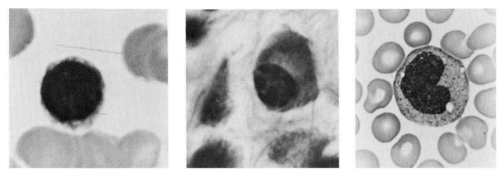

(a)　　　　　　　(b)　　　　　　　(c)

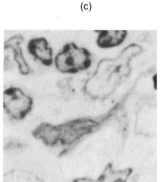

(d)　　　　　　　(e)　　　　　　　(f)

Figure 1-3

Cells associated with the vertebrate immune response: (a) blood lymphocyte (B or T), (b) plasma cells, (c) blood monocyte, (d) basophile, (e) polymorphonuclear leukocytes, (f) dendritic reticular cells, (g) large granular lymphocyte (natural killer cell). [Photomicrographs (a)–(e) courtesy of R. Rouse; (f) courtesy of G. Levine; (g) courtesy of J. Ortaldo.]

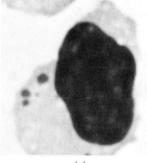

(g)

1-3　The immune system recognizes foreign substances by their molecular features

Antigen recognition by antibodies

The essence of the immune system is its capacity to recognize surface features of macromolecules that are not normal constituents of the organism. The components of the organism that carry out this specific recognition include the protein molecules called *antibodies*; the foreign

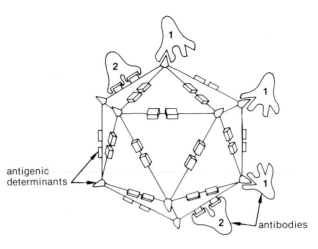

Figure 1-4

A virus interacting with antibodies specific for two types of antigen determinants.

entities that they recognize are termed *antigens.* That portion of the antigen to which an antibody binds is called an *antigenic determinant* (Figure 1-4). Antibodies recognize and bind antigens by molecular complementarity, which permits multiple noncovalent interactions of the same types that confer specificity on enzyme-substrate binding. An antigen complementary to a specific antibody is called a *cognate antigen.*

Immunogens and immunity

An antigen that elicits a response from the immune system is referred to as an *immunogen.* Macromolecules such as foreign proteins, nucleic acids, and carbohydrates are usually effective immunogens; molecules with molecular weights of less than 5000 are usually not. However, many small nonimmunogenic molecules, termed *haptens,* can stimulate an immune response if covalently attached to a large *carrier* molecule. For example, the 2,4-dinitrophenyl group is not immunogenic unless attached to a carrier protein such as serum albumin (Figure 1-5).

Animals that have an appropriate number of activated specific T cells or an appropriate concentration of specific antibody in their blood are *immune* to the cognate antigens.

Immunoglobulin molecules

Antibodies form the class of proteins called *immunoglobulins.* The basic unit of immunoglobulin structure is a complex of four polypeptides, two identical "light" (low molecular weight) chains and two identical "heavy" (high molecular weight) chains, linked together by disulfide bonds (Figure 1-6).

The amino-terminal (N-terminal) portions of the light and heavy chains differ substantially in amino acid sequence between individual species of antibody. These *variable* regions of the light and heavy chains combine to form the *antigen-binding sites* of an antibody mole-

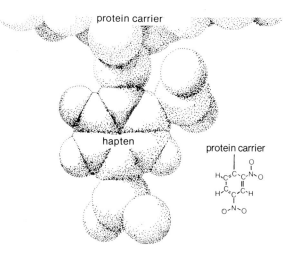

Figure 1-5

Three-dimensional representation of a simple hapten, the dinitrophenyl group, attached to a hypothetical protein carrier. The structural formula of the dinitrophenyl group is shown at right. [Adapted from G. Edelman, *Sci. Am.* **223,** 34(1970). Copyright © 1970 by Scientific American, Inc. All rights reserved.]

Figure 1-6

A two-dimensional representation of the antibody molecule. The heavy and light chains are joined by disulfide bridges. The N-terminal (NH_3^+) and C-terminal (COO^-) ends and the variable (V) and constant (C) regions of each chain are oriented as shown. The envelope around the immunoglobulin molecule approximates its three-dimensional shape.

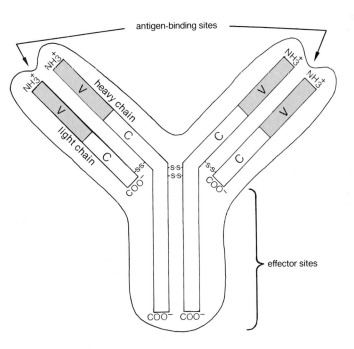

cule, as shown in Figure 1-6. The *valence* of an antibody is the number of identical antigen-binding sites per molecule, which is two for the basic unit. The *affinity* of an antibody combining site is a measure of the strength of its binding to an antigenic determinant. The term *avidity* is used to describe the net strength of interaction of a *multivalent* antibody with a *multideterminant* antigen.

The carboxyl-terminal (C-terminal) portions of the light and heavy chains, termed the *constant* regions, are identical or nearly identical for antibodies of the same class. The constant regions of circulating antibodies are responsible for the variety of characteristic *effector functions* that are involved in the elimination of foreign antigens. Immunoglobulins in mammalian serum can be divided into five classes on the basis of amino acid sequence differences in the constant regions of their heavy chains. These classes, designated IgM, IgG, IgA, IgD, and IgE, correspond to antibodies with different effector functions. One example of the diverse effector functions specified by heavy-chain constant regions is the differential transport of antibodies across tissues (Figure 1-7). IgA molecules (but not IgG molecules) may be transported across the intestinal lining into the lumen, whereas IgG molecules (but not IgA molecules) may be transported across the placenta to a fetus. The structures and molecular functions of antibody molecules are discussed in more detail in Chapter 2.

Antigen-binding sites

The antigen-binding sites of individual antibodies are unique combinations of light-chain and heavy-chain variable regions, and consequently these binding sites exhibit unique protein structures. If a specific antibody from one animal is injected as an immunogen into a suitable second animal, the injected antibody will elicit production of host antibodies. Some of these antibodies will be specific for the unique determinants of the variable regions of the injected antibody. Such antigenic determinants are known collectively as the *idiotype* of the injected antibody. Every species of antibody will exhibit unique idiotypic determinants, some of which are determined by its antigen-binding site and some of which are determined by structural features outside the binding site.

1-4 Each lymphocyte is predetermined to express a homogeneous set of membrane-bound receptors with a single specificity for antigen

The molecular nature of receptors

The cell surfaces of lymphocytes carry membrane-bound antibodies or antibodylike molecules that function as antigen receptors. The receptors of B cells are antibodies that are present on the membrane in a quantity of about 10^5 molecules per cell. The receptors of T cells appear to have similar properties, but their molecular nature is less well known. Each lymphocyte carries only one kind of specific receptor, and therefore it will respond to only a few closely related antigenic determinants. Binding of an antigen to a receptor initiates a humoral or a cellular immune response, depending upon whether a B-cell or a T-cell receptor is stimulated.

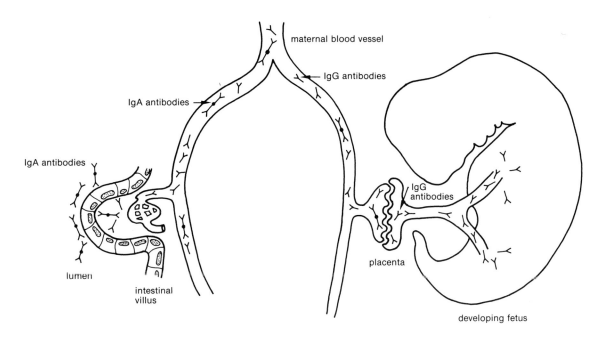

Figure 1-7 Two examples of different sites of concentration and effector functions for antibodies of different heavy-chain class. Circulating IgA molecules (>—●—<), which are a dimer of the basic antibody structural unit, are transported selectively to the intestinal lumen where they combine with food and bacterial antigens, whereas IgG molecules (Y) are transported selectively across the placenta to protect the developing fetus.

Diversity of receptor specificities

The lymphocyte population of a mammal consists of about 10^6 to 10^8 clones of cells with different receptor specificities. The number of cells in each clone is thought to range from 1 up to 10^6. In general more than one clone of lymphocytes will respond to a typical antigen because antigens usually display many determinants and because a given determinant can be recognized by more than one kind of antibody receptor. The total population of lymphocytes, which in a human may be as many as 10^{12} lymphocytes, collectively possesses the capacity to respond to a nearly infinite variety of antigens.

Clonal selection, proliferation, and differentiation

Lymphocytes that bind an antigen may be triggered to proliferate to form large clones of progeny lymphocytes that display surface receptors of the same specificity as the parent cell. Antigenic stimulation of preexisting clones of lymphocytes is known as *clonal selection* (Figure 1-8). It was originally proposed in the 1950s by Jerne, Burnet, Lederberg, and Talmage to account for the prominent characteristics of the humoral immune response and is now amply supported by experimental evidence.

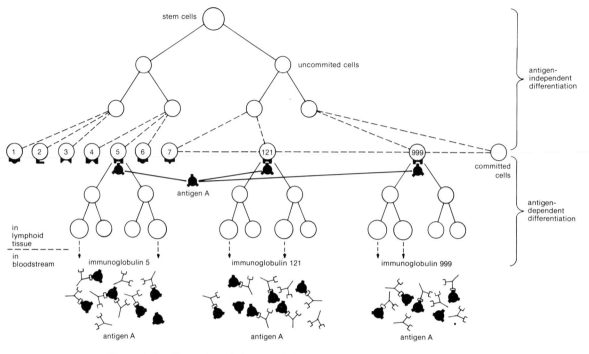

Figure 1-8 Formation of clones and their selection by antigen. Stem cells differentiate in an antigen-independent manner that ultimately commits each of 10^6 to 10^8 clones to the synthesis of one species of antibody (numbers). These antibodies are displayed as receptors on the cell surfaces. A particular antigen (A) usually interacts with several clones to initiate an antigen-dependent stage of differentiation, which leads to proliferation of clones of memory cells and clones of plasma cells that synthesize specific antibody molecules. [Adapted from G. Edelman, *Sci. Am.* **223,** 34(1970). Copyright © 1970 by Scientific American, Inc. All rights reserved.]

In the process of proliferation, some progeny lymphocytes differentiate into *effector cells* that carry out the immune response. The effector cells of B lymphocytes are *plasma cells* (Figure 1-3b), which secrete antibodies of the same antigen-recognition specificity as their cell-surface receptors (Figure 1-9). The T-lymphocyte population produces several types of effector cells with different functions (Figure 1-10). One of these types is the *cytotoxic* or *killer T cell* (T_C cell), which eliminates foreign cells directly. Other types of effector T cells are responsible for delayed hypersensitivity (T_D cells), for helping B-cell differentiation and proliferation (T_H cells), for amplifying killer T-cell differentiation and proliferation (T_A cells), and for suppressing immune responses (T_S cells). *T-cell recognition and action are mediated by cell-cell interactions.* The several known classes of effector T cells are programmed by cell-surface receptors to recognize other cells of the

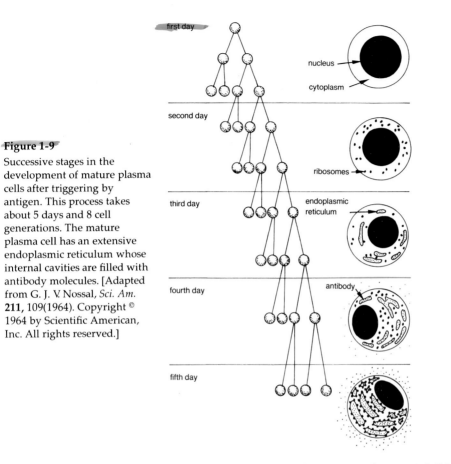

Figure 1-9
Successive stages in the development of mature plasma cells after triggering by antigen. This process takes about 5 days and 8 cell generations. The mature plasma cell has an extensive endoplasmic reticulum whose internal cavities are filled with antibody molecules. [Adapted from G. J. V. Nossal, *Sci. Am.* **211**, 109(1964). Copyright © 1964 by Scientific American, Inc. All rights reserved.]

immune system in order to stimulate or inhibit them (Figure 1-10). The functions and characteristics of the various classes of effector B and T cells are discussed in more detail in Chapters 8, 9, and 10.

Immunologic memory

Clonal selection underlies the phenomenon of *immunologic memory.* When a vertebrate first encounters an antigen, its so-called *primary immune response* generally exhibits the kinetics shown in Figure 1-11. However, if the animal encounters the same antigen after an interval of a few days or at any later time during its life, its specific response is both more rapid and of greater magnitude. The initial encounter causes specific B-cell and T-cell clones to proliferate and differentiate. The progeny lymphocytes include not only effector cells but also large clones of *memory cells,* which retain the capacity to produce both effector and memory cells upon subsequent stimulation by the original antigen. Effector cells live for only a few days, but memory cells have lifetimes of decades. Thus when an antigen is encountered a second time, its cognate memory cells quickly produce the large numbers of effector cells that account for the characteristically rapid and massive *secondary immune response.* In the humoral immune response, the ma-

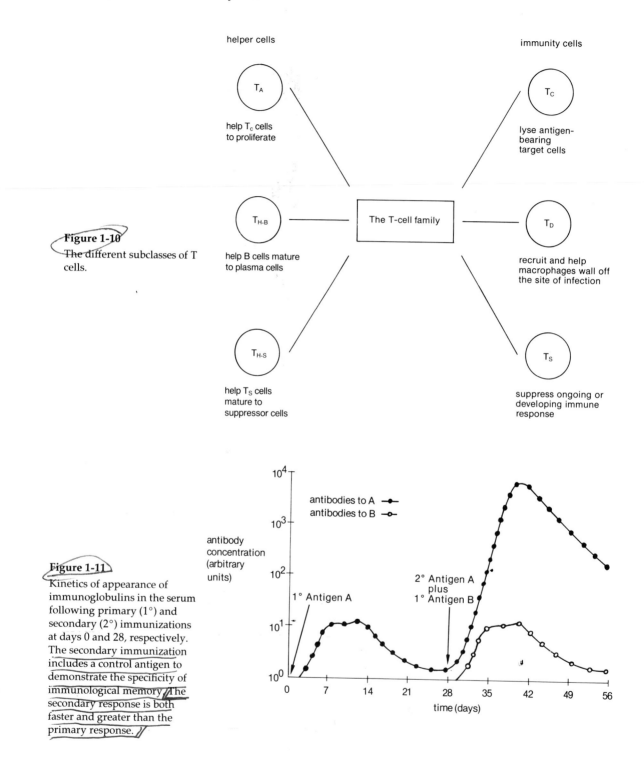

Figure 1-10
The different subclasses of T cells.

Figure 1-11
Kinetics of appearance of immunoglobulins in the serum following primary (1°) and secondary (2°) immunizations at days 0 and 28, respectively. The secondary immunization includes a control antigen to demonstrate the specificity of immunological memory. The secondary response is both faster and greater than the primary response.

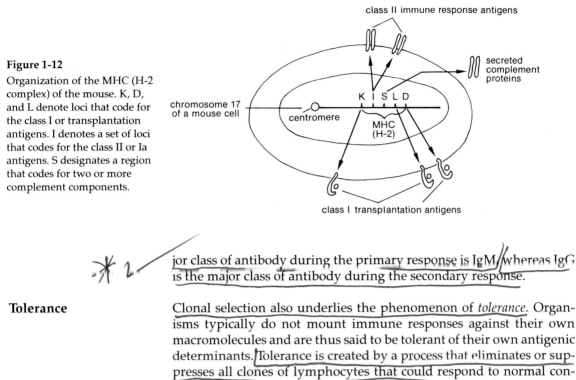

Figure 1-12
Organization of the MHC (H-2 complex) of the mouse. K, D, and L denote loci that code for the class I or transplantation antigens. I denotes a set of loci that codes for the class II or Ia antigens. S designates a region that codes for two or more complement components.

jor class of antibody during the primary response is IgM, whereas IgG is the major class of antibody during the secondary response.

Tolerance

Clonal selection also underlies the phenomenon of *tolerance*. Organisms typically do not mount immune responses against their own macromolecules and are thus said to be tolerant of their own antigenic determinants. Tolerance is created by a process that eliminates or suppresses all clones of lymphocytes that could respond to normal constituents of the organism.

1-5 Gene products of the major histocompatibility complex play a fundamental role in immune responses

The *major histocompatibility complex* (MHC) is a discrete chromosomal region encoding a variety of cell-surface proteins that mediate immune cell-cell interactions and trigger rejection of foreign tissue transplants (Figure 1-12). A subset of the transplantation antigens, called the class I MHC antigens, is present on virtually all cells of a vertebrate organism and appears to play an important role in T-cell surveillance for virally infected cells and cancer cells. Another subset of MHC-encoded proteins, called the class II or Ia (*immune response associated*) antigens, appears to regulate a number of the cellular interactions involved in immune responses. The MHC also encodes several components of the *complement* pathway, which is an effector mechanism activated by the humoral immune response (Concept 9-2).

These various MHC functions have been found in all vertebrates examined, but only some MHC-like functions have been found in advanced invertebrates. Thus the emergence of the vertebrate immune system is correlated evolutionarily with that of the MHC. This coincidental appearance is consistent with the fundamental role of the MHC in the differentiation, regulation, and expression of the immune response.

Selected Bibliography

Ada, G. L., and Byrt, P., "Specific inactivation of antigen-reactive cells with ¹²⁵I-labelled antigen," *Nature* **222**, 1291(1969).

Burnet, F. M., "A modification of Jerne's theory of antibody production using the concept of clonal selection," *Austral. J. Sci.* **20**, 67(1957).

Dutton, R. W., and Mishell, R. I., "Cellular events in the immune response. The *in vitro* response of normal spleen cells to erythrocyte antigens," *Cold Spring Harbor Symp. Quant. Biol.* **32**, 407(1967).

Edelman, G. M., "The structure and function of antibodies," *Sci. Am.* **223**, 34(1970).

Gowans, J. L., McGregor, D. D., Cowen, D. M., and Ford, C. E., "Initiation of immune responses by small lymphocytes," *Nature* **196**, 651(1962).

Jerne, N. K., "The immune system," *Sci. Am.* **229**, 52(1973).

Miller, J. F. A. P., "Immunological function of the thymus," *The Lancet* (September 30), 748(1961).

Problems

1-1   Indicate whether each of the following statements is true or false. Explain the error in each statement you consider to be false.
   (a)   An antibody molecule has one type of antigen-binding site.
   (b)   A large antigen can generally combine with many different antibody molecules.
   (c)   Antigens combine with specific antibodies and stimulate the production of these antibodies.
   (d)   A hapten can stimulate antibody production but cannot combine with antibody molecules.
   (e)   In a secondary immune response, IgM is the major class of antibody synthesized.
   (f)   Immunologic memory can last 20 years or more.
   (g)   The B-cell receptor molecule has not yet been identified conclusively.
   (h)   Plasma cells are the major effector cells of the B-cell response; several classes of small lymphocytes are the effector cells of the T-cell response.

1-2   (a)   When haptens are attached to a larger _____ molecule, they become immunogenic.
   (b)   _____ are the terminal effector cells of B-cell differentiation.
   (c)   T cells mediate _____ immunity.
   (d)   The clonal selection theory contends that lymphocytes commit themselves to the synthesis of one type of antibody molecule prior to exposure to _____ , but that _____ triggers the final stage of differentiation.
   (e)   _____ immunity is protective against extracellular bacterial infections.
   (f)   The presence of specific immunoglobulin response to antigen in the animal kingdom is thought to be limited to _____ .

1-3   For each of the following conditions, indicate whether a humoral or a cellular immune response is more effective or relevant.

(a) *Diphtheria* toxin
(b) Measles virus
(c) Heart transplant
(d) Streptococcal infection
(e) Salmonella infection of the GI tract
(f) Candidiasis caused by the fungus *Candida albicans*
(g) Fetal bacterial infection
(h) Poison oak hypersensitivity

1-4 The apparent range of different specificities in the immune system is enormous. The average concentration of serum antibody is about 15 mg/mL. Assume a molecular weight of 160,000 daltons for the antibody molecule, and assume that the average human has 5 L of serum.

(a) How many antibody molecules are present in each milliliter of serum? In the average human?

(b) Assume that there are 1,000,000 different types of antibody molecules and that each is represented equally in the population. How many molecules of each type are present in 1 mL of serum?

Answers

1-1 (a) True
(b) True
(c) True
(d) False. A hapten cannot stimulate antibody production by itself, but it can combine with a specific antibody.
(e) False. IgG is the major class of antibody synthesized in a secondary response.
(f) True
(g) False. The B-cell receptors for antigens are antibody molecules.
(h) True

1-2 (a) carrier
(b) Plasma cells
(c) cellular
(d) antigen; antigen
(e) Humoral
(f) vertebrates

1-3 (a) Humoral
(b) Cellular
(c) Cellular
(d) Humoral
(e) Humoral
(f) Cellular
(g) Humoral
(h) Cellular

1-4 (a) The number of antibody molecules in 1 mL of serum is $(15 \times 10^{-3} \text{ g/mL})/(16 \times 10^4 \text{ g/mole}) \times (6 \times 10^{23} \text{ molecules})/\text{mole} \cong 6 \times 10^{16}$ antibody molecules/mL. In an average human, the total number of antibody molecules is 6×10^{16} molecules/mL $\times 5 \times 10^3$ mL $= 3 \times 10^{20}$ antibody molecules.

(b) There are $6 \times 10^{16}/10^6 = 6 \times 10^{10}$ molecules of each type of antibody in 1 mL of serum.

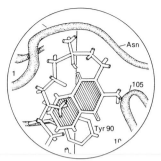

CHAPTER 2

Antibodies

Chapter Outline

The antibody molecule has evolved to perform two distinct functions—antigen recognition and antigen elimination. Antibody molecules can interact with a virtually unlimited number of antigens, yet antibodies destroy or eliminate antigens by a small number of effector mechanisms. The antibody molecule has evolved discrete globular domains to carry out these two functions. One of these domains binds antigen, and the others mediate effector functions. Thus the functional duality of the antibody molecule is reflected in its three-dimensional structure. This chapter considers antibody structure and its relation to antibody functions.

Concepts

2-1   Homogeneous antibodies can be obtained from myeloma or hybridoma tumor cells

Myeloma proteins from plasma cell tumors

The serum of a normal vertebrate contains a large variety of proteins (Figure 2-1). The γ-globulin fraction of these proteins includes five classes of immunoglobulins designated IgA, IgD, IgE, IgG, and IgM, which differ in the structures of their heavy-chain constant regions. The immunoglobulins are the organism's circulating antibody population. The basic structures and gross chemical properties of immunoglobulins are very similar, but their combining specificities vary widely, reflecting the spectrum of antigens that the individual has encountered during its lifetime.

The immunoglobulins are so similar and yet normally so heterogeneous that isolation of an individual molecular species for detailed chemical study is difficult. One possible source of homogeneous immunoglobulins results from an abnormal condition, a cancer of antibody-producing cells called *multiple myeloma*. In an individual afflicted with this disease, neoplastic transformation generally occurs in a single plasma cell or its immediate precursor, so that the resulting tumor secretes a homogeneous immunoglobulin (myeloma protein). This protein can comprise 95% of the serum immunoglobulin, and therefore it is easy to isolate in pure form. The myeloma protein from any afflicted individual is generally different from the myeloma proteins of all other individuals. Myeloma tumors have been observed in many mammalian species, including human, rat, mouse, horse, and dog.

Myeloma proteins are indistinguishable from normal immunoglobulins by all available criteria. All the types of polypeptide chains and genetic markers seen in normal immunoglobulins have been found in myeloma proteins. Extensive amino acid sequences are identical in normal and myeloma immunoglobulins. Some myeloma proteins bind known antigenic determinants. For example, about 5% of

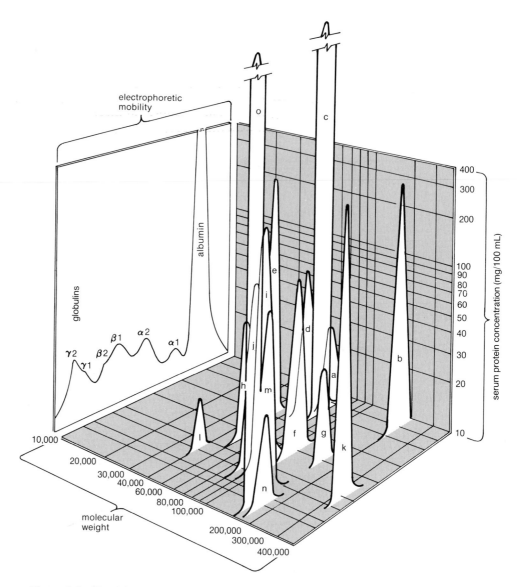

Figure 2-1 Some human serum proteins characterized by molecular weights, electrophoretic mobilities at pH 8.6, and concentrations in the blood serum. For purposes of comparison, the mobilities and concentrations of the globulins (α, β, γ) and albumin are shown at the rear. Proteins are identified by the following letters: a, prealbumin; b, α_1 lipoprotein; c, albumin; d, α_1 acid glycoprotein; e, α_1 antitrypsin; f, haptoglobulin; g, ceruloplasmin; h, α_2 HS glycoprotein; i, transferrin; j, hemopexin; k, fibrinogen; ℓ, β_2 glycoprotein; m, IgA; n, IgG.

the myeloma proteins from a particular inbred strain of mice react with cell-surface determinants of enteric bacteria such as phosphorylcholine and simple sugars. Presumably these myeloma tumors developed from lymphocytes that proliferated in response to specific antigens on intestinal bacteria. Some of these myeloma proteins have variable regions that are identical to those on antibodies induced by immunization with the appropriate hapten. This observation suggests that myeloma proteins are normal antibody molecules.

The utility of myeloma proteins for study of immunoglobulin structure was enhanced by the discovery that myeloma tumors can be induced artificially in two laboratory strains of mice (BALB/c and NZB) by injection of mineral oil into the peritoneal cavity (Figure 2-2). Because these mice are highly inbred, the immunoglobulin genes of all individuals from each strain are similar if not identical. Induced tumors can be transplanted from one mouse to many other individuals of the same strain to increase the production of a particular myeloma globulin. Myeloma tumors can be frozen without loss of viability, and banks of thousands of mouse tumors are now maintained. Study of myeloma proteins has provided a detailed picture of the structure of antibodies.

Monoclonal antibodies from hybridoma tumors

Another source of homogeneous antibodies is tumors or cultures of so-called *hybridoma cells*, which are produced artificially by cell fusion. Cells in tissue culture can fuse spontaneously at a low frequency, which can be greatly increased by adding fusion-promoting agents like polyethylene glycol. The immediate fusion products are *heterokaryons*, which are cells with two or more nonidentical nuclei. If the nuclei subsequently fuse to form a single nucleus, as they often do, the resulting cells can give rise to stable *hybrids* that multiply normally and express both parental genomes. To generate hybridoma cells, normal antibody-producing lymphocytes from the spleen of a recently immunized mouse or rat are fused to a myeloma cell line with two special properties (Figure 2-3). First, the myeloma cell line is deficient in the enzyme hypoxanthine-guanine phosphoribosyl transferase (HGPRT), which catalyzes reactions of the bases hypoxanthine and guanine with 5-phosphoribosyl-1-pyrophosphate to form the nucleotides inosine-5′-P (IMP) and guanosine-5′-P (GMP), respectively. The hybrid cells can be selected over either parental cell by culturing in a medium containing hypoxanthine, aminopterin, and thymidine (HAT medium). The myeloma cells, which lack HGPRT, cannot survive because the *de novo* synthesis of GMP is blocked by the folate antagonist aminopterin, and the normal lymphocytes grow very slowly in HAT medium. By contrast, hybrid cells, in which a functional HGPRT gene is supplied by the lymphocyte genome, grow rapidly and form large colonies readily distinguishable from those of

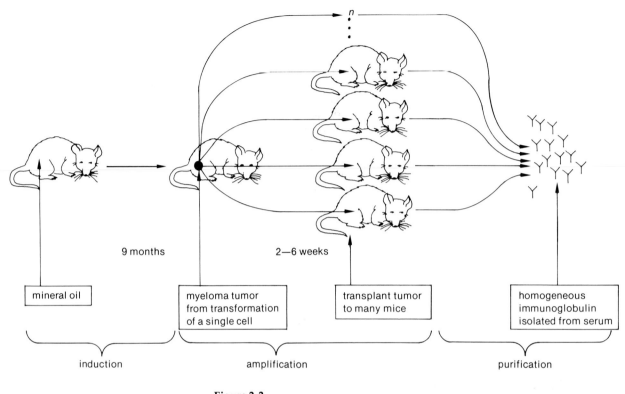

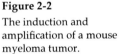

Figure 2-2
The induction and
amplification of a mouse
myeloma tumor.

the slowly growing lymphocytes. Second, the myeloma cell line does
not synthesize its own immunoglobulin. Hence the hybrid cell synthesizes only the antibody produced by the lymphocyte parent.
Clones of hybrid cells that produce a desired antibody can be identified by a suitable assay procedure and grown into larger cultures. The
homogeneous immunoglobulin produced by such a cloned hybrid is
termed a *hybridoma antibody* or *monoclonal antibody.*

Hybridomas are permanent cell lines with the potential for unlimited proliferative capacity. They can be injected into appropriate
mice and carried as solid tumors which, like myeloma tumors, secrete
large quantities of homogeneous antibody. The hybridoma technique
makes it possible to obtain virtually unlimited quantities of homogeneous antibody with specificity for any desired antigen.

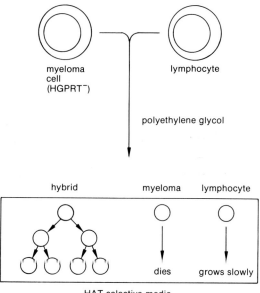

Figure 2-3
The cell-fusion technique for
generating hybridoma cell
lines.

2-2 Immunoglobulin molecules are composed of two kinds of polypeptides

Structure of IgG molecules

Immunoglobulin molecules of the most common class, IgG, are made up of two identical polypeptides of molecular weight 23,000 called light chains and two identical polypeptides of molecular weight 53,000 called heavy chains (Figure 2-4). Each light chain is linked to a heavy chain by noncovalent associations and also by one covalent disulfide bridge. In the IgG molecule, the two light-chain–heavy-chain pairs are linked together by disulfide bridges between the heavy chains. As shown in Figure 2-4, the molecule can be repre-

Figure 2-4

A schematic drawing of the human immunoglobulin molecule, showing its principal structural features. V and C indicate variable and constant regions, respectively, of the heavy (H) and light (L) chains, as explained in the text. Shaded segments indicate V regions; the remainder of each chain is C region. –S–S– symbols represent the 12 intrachain and 4 interchain disulfide bridges. Dark portions of the two heavy chains indicate the hinge region. CHO represents carbohydrate groups attached to the heavy chains.

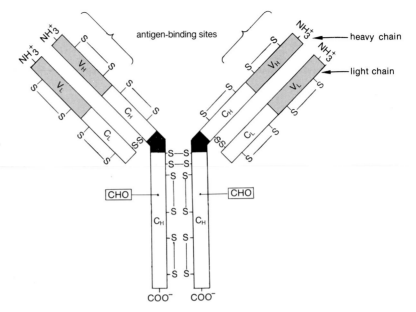

sented schematically in the form of a Y, with the amino (N) termini of the four chains at the top and the carboxyl (C) termini of the two heavy chains at the bottom. The portion of the molecule that includes the disulfide linkages between heavy chains where the three arms of the Y come together is called the *hinge region*. The arms of the Y are flexible. Twelve intrachain disulfide bridges are spaced periodically, two in each light chain and four in each heavy chain. Carbohydrate groups are attached through the side chains of asparagine residues in the two heavy chains at the positions shown in Figure 2-4. Thus immunoglobulins are glycoproteins.

Structures of IgA, IgD, IgE, and IgM molecules

A dimer of light-chain–heavy-chain pairs, (L–H)$_2$, is the basic structural subunit of all classes of immunoglobulin molecules. The structures of individual classes and subclasses differ in the positions and number of the disulfide bridges between heavy chains and in the number of (L–H)$_2$ subunits in the molecule (Figure 2-5). IgD and IgE molecules, like IgG, are composed of one (L–H)$_2$ subunit. The IgA molecule may have one, two, or three (L–H)$_2$ subunits. The serum IgM molecule has five (L–H)$_2$ subunits; that is, it is equivalent to an aggregate of five IgG-like molecules. The membrane-bound form of the IgM molecule has one (L–H)$_2$ subunit. In the polymeric forms of IgA and in IgM, the (L–H)$_2$ subunits are held together by disulfide bridges to a polypeptide called the J or joining chain. The heavy chains of the various classes of immunoglobulins differ in amino acid sequence and correspondingly in function (Concept 2-6).

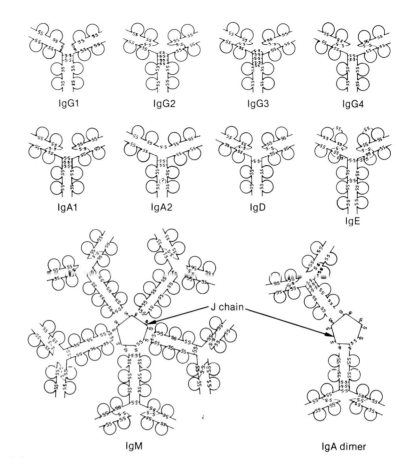

Figure 2-5
Subunit structures of various human immunoglobulins. –S–S– indicates a disulfide bridge. The question mark indicates that the interchain disulfide bridge structure is unknown. IgG1, IgG2, IgG3, and IgG4 are subclasses of IgG. IgA1 is the monomeric subclass of the IgA class. The J chain joins the higher polymeric forms of IgA as well as the five subunits of the IgM molecule. [Adapted from J. Gally in *The Antigens*, M. Sela (Ed.), Academic Press, New York, 1973, p. 209.]

2-3 The light- and heavy-chain subunits of immunoglobulin molecules are differentiated into variable and constant regions

Variable and constant regions

When the amino acid sequences of several myeloma light chains were first compared, a striking pattern emerged (Figure 2-6). In the N-terminal half of the polypeptide, the sequences were found to vary greatly from one light chain to another. By contrast, in the C-terminal half of the polypeptide the sequences of all the molecules were identical. These two segments of the molecule were named the variable (V_L) and constant (C_L) regions of the light chain, respectively. The V_L region begins at the N terminus and is approximately 110 amino acid residues in length. The C_L region makes up the remainder of the chain, and it is also about 110 residues in length.

Figure 2-6

A schematic representation of the variable and constant regions for light and heavy chains from ten IgG molecules. NH_3^+ indicates the N terminus and COO^- the C terminus. X, O, Δ, and □ indicate amino-acid-sequence differences. Lines without these symbols indicate sequence identity among the proteins compared. The lengths of the V and C regions are indicated by residue number, beginning with residue 1 at the N terminus.

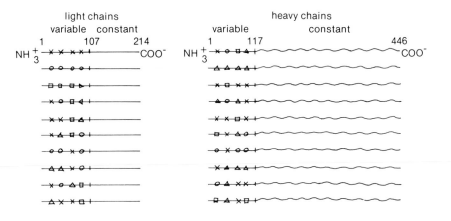

Heavy-chain sequences exhibit a similar pattern. A variable (V_H) region begins at the N terminus and is approximately the same length as the V_L region of the light chain, about 110 residues. The heavy-chain constant (C_H) region for the IgG molecule is about three times this length or about 330 residues.

Implications for antibody diversity

Because the N-terminal portions of each L–H pair comprise the antigen-binding sites in an immunoglobulin molecule (Figure 2-4), the sequence heterogeneity of the V_L and V_H regions accounts for the great diversity of antigenic specificities among antibody molecules. The C_H regions make up the portion of the immunoglobulin molecule that carries out effector functions, which are common to all antibodies of a given class (see Concept 2-6). Each immunoglobulin molecule has at least two identical antigen-binding sites. This bivalence permits antibodies to form cross-linked aggregates with antigens that carry two or more antigenic determinants. The flexibility of the arms of the antibody molecule allows it to bind antigenic determinants that are separated by various distances.

2-4 The antigen-binding site, formed by the light- and heavy-chain variable regions, can exhibit a broad range of specificities

Variability among active sites

X-ray crystallographic studies of several myeloma immunoglobulins that bind different haptens have shown that the active site is a crevice between the V_L and V_H regions (Figure 2-7) and that the dimensions of the crevice can vary significantly. The size and shape of the active

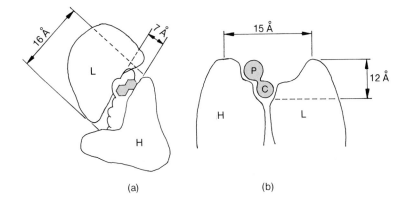

(a)   (b)

Figure 2-7 (a) A schematic top view of the shallow cleft between the heavy- and light-chain variable regions of the human myeloma protein NEW, which specifically binds the hapten, vitamin K$_1$OH (shaded). The dimensions of the binding site are 1.6 nm × 0.7 nm × 0.6 nm. [Redrawn from F. Richards et al., *The Immune System: Genes, Receptors, Signals*, E. Sercarz, A. Williamson, and C. Fox (Eds.), Academic Press, New York, 1975, p. 53.] (b) A schematic side view of the interaction of the variable regions of mouse myeloma protein MOPC603 with its specific hapten, phosphorylcholine (shaded). The dimensions of the binding site are 2.0 nm × 1.5 nm × 1.2 nm. [Redrawn from E. Padlan et al., *The Immune System: Genes, Receptors, Signals*, E. Sercarz, A. Williamson, and C. Fox (Eds.), Academic Press, New York, 1975, p. 7.]

site vary due to differences in the spatial relationship of the V_L and V_H regions and due to amino acid sequence variation in the V_L and V_H regions. Antibody specificity results from the molecular complementarity between determinant groups on the antigen molecule and amino acid residues in the active site.

Antigen binding by antibodies resembles substrate binding by enzymes in several ways. Both involve multiple, weak noncovalent associations, including ionic bonds, hydrogen bonds, van der Waals bonds, and hydrophobic interactions, which combine to give strong binding. Both antibodies and enzymes exhibit dissociation constants that range from 10^{-4} to 10^{-10} M, corresponding to standard free energy changes of binding of −6 to −15 kcal/mole. The binding sites of both antibodies and enzymes are predominantly nonpolar niches. In addition, both exhibit significant cross-reactivity with structurally related ligands.

Role of the hypervariable regions

The walls of the antigen-binding site are composed of *hypervariable* (hv) segments of the V_L and V_H regions (Figure 2-8). These regions of extensive diversity were initially defined by comparing immunoglob-

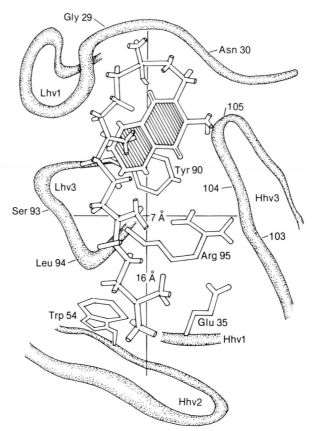

Figure 2-8

A schematic drawing of the hapten, vitamin K_1OH bound to a human IgG molecule. Lhv1, Lhv3, Hhv1, Hhv2, and Hhv3 designate the approximate locations of the hypervariable regions of the light and heavy chains, respectively. The quinone group (two fused six-membered rings) of the hapten is bound at the top in a shallow crevice (1.6 nm $\times$ 0.7 nm $\times$ 0.6 nm); the phytyl tail folds over the quinone and extends along most of the length of the binding site. [From I. M. Amzel et al., *Proc. Natl. Acad. Sci. USA* **71**, 1427(1974).]

ulin chains from a given class after alignment for sequence homology. Such a comparison is shown in Figure 2-9, using the common one-letter abbreviations for amino acid residues. These abbreviations, and the alternative three-letter amino acid designations, are defined in Table 2-1, which also lists the codons in messenger RNA (mRNA) that correspond to each amino acid. The diversity in hypervariable segments includes sequence insertions and deletions as well as amino acid substitutions. Three hypervariable segments are present in V_L regions, and three in V_H regions (Figure 2-10). Although hypervariable regions were initially identified by analysis of myeloma proteins, they have been confirmed by analysis of normal, homogeneous antibody molecules that can be produced by special immunization and cell-fusion procedures (Concept 2-1).

Two lines of evidence indicate that hypervariable regions comprise the antigen-binding sites of most antibody molecules. First, the X-ray analyses of two myeloma proteins that bind simple haptens (Figures 2-7 and 2-8) show that five of the six hypervariable regions constitute the walls of the antigen-binding crevice. Moreover, the three-dimensional structures of the V_L and V_H regions from all myeloma proteins analyzed so far, in species as diverse as mouse and

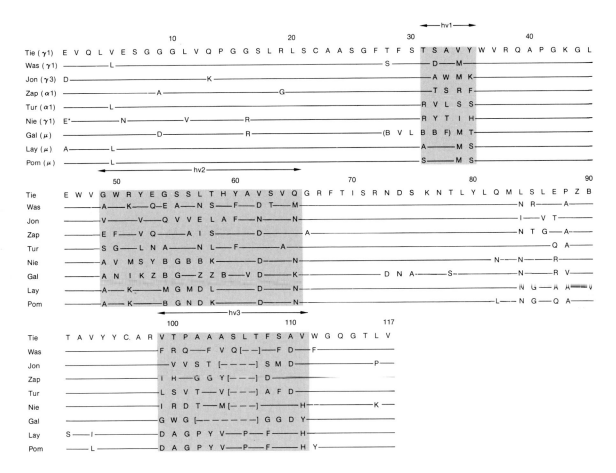

Figure 2-9

The V$_H$ sequences of nine human heavy chains. Unbroken lines signify identity with protein Tie. Dashes in brackets represent deletions of residues present in protein Tie. Sequence variations tend to cluster in the hypervariable segments (shaded). E* denotes pyrolidine carboxylic acid. A fourth hypervariable segment, residues 84–88, is located away from the antigen-binding site and has no known function. [From J. D. Capra and J. M. Kehoe, *Proc. Natl. Acad. Sci. USA* **71**, 4032(1974).]

man, are remarkably similar except for differences in the hypervariable segments. The second line of evidence comes from studies using antigens, which were constructed to include a chemical group that could link covalently to the antibody molecule at or near the antigen-binding site. Such antigens are known as *affinity labels*. A wide variety of affinity labels have been reacted with specific antibodies and found to attach only to residues in the hypervariable regions and not to other residues of the light or heavy chains.

Significance of combinatorial association

The antigen-binding sites of antibodies differ from the substrate-binding sites of most enzymes in one important way: two chains, rather than one, fold to make the antigen-binding site. Thus extensive

Table 2-1 Amino Acid Abbreviations and Codons[a]

Amino Acid	Three-Letter Abbreviation	Single-Letter Abbreviation	mRNA Codon
Alanine	Ala	A	GCX
Arginine	Arg	R	CGX, AGZ
Asparagine	Asn	N	AAY
Aspartic acid	Asp	D	GAY
Either Asp or Asn	Asx	B	—
Cysteine	Cys	C	UGY
Glutamic acid	Glu	E	GAZ
Glutamine	Gln	Q	CAZ
Either Glu or Gln	Glx	Z	—
Glycine	Gly	G	GGX
Histidine	His	H	CAY
Isoleucine	Ile	I	AUY, AUA
Leucine	Leu	L	CUX, UUZ
Lysine	Lys	K	AAZ
Methionine	Met	M	AUG
Phenylalanine	Phe	F	UUY
Proline	Pro	P	CCX
Serine	Ser	S	UCX, AGY
Threonine	Thr	T	ACX
Tryptophan	Trp	W	UGG
Tyrosine	Tyr	Y	UAY
Valine	Val	V	GUX

[a]In the mRNA codon sequences, A, C, G, and U represent the four common nucleotides; X represents any one of the four nucleotides; Y represents either pyrimidine nucleotide; and Z represents either purine nucleotide.

Figure 2-10

A linear map of hypervariable segments in the variable regions of light and heavy chains. Residue numbers indicate the approximate end points of these segments and the position of the central disulfide bridges. † indicates a hypervariable segment that is sometimes a part of the antigen-binding crevice.

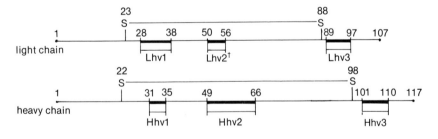

binding-site diversity can be generated by the *combinatorial association of light chains and heavy chains during antibody synthesis* (Figure 2-11). For example, if any light chain can associate with any heavy chain to produce a functional antibody, then 1000 different light chains and 1000 different heavy chains could combine in pairs to produce $10^3 \times 10^3 = 10^6$ different antibody molecules. The combina-

combinatorial association
of light and heavy chains

Figure 2-11
The generation of antigen-binding site diversity by combinatorial association of three different light chains and three different heavy chains. The total number of different binding sites that can be generated from p light chains and q heavy chains is $p \times q$.

light chains $p=3$

————— 1
————— 2
————— 3

heavy chains $q=3$

~~~~~ 1
~~~~~ 2
~~~~~ 3

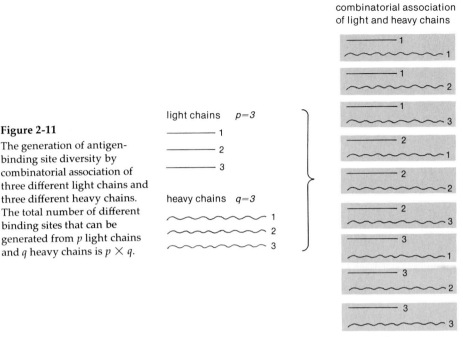

$p \times q = 9$

torial diversity increases as the product of the number of different light and heavy chains available.

Although it is not known whether every (L–H)$_2$ combination produces a functional antibody, it is likely that most of them do. Two independent observations support combinatorial association as an important mechanism for increasing antibody diversity. First, several hybrid cells that were derived from different antibody-producing parental cells have been shown to synthesize both parental and hybrid immunoglobulin molecules that include most of the possible L–H combinations (Figure 2-12). Second, the contact residues between associated V_L and V_H segments, which have been identified by X-ray analyses, are highly conserved in the antibody molecules analyzed so far. Thus most V_L and V_H regions appear capable of associating normally in an antibody-producing cell.

Multispecificity

The diversity of antigen-binding capability is increased still further by a biologically significant phenomenon called *multispecificity,* which is the ability of a single antibody molecule to combine with a spectrum of different antigens. Although a single antibody molecule has a unique three-dimensional structure, it can combine with the inducing antigenic determinant, determinants with similar structures (cross-reacting antigens), and perhaps even determinants with quite disparate structures. A stable antigen–antibody complex will result

Figure 2-12

The fusion of two myeloma tumor cells to yield a hybrid cell that produces both parental and hybrid immunoglobulin molecules. ■ and ∿ represent variable regions characteristic of the immunoglobulins produced by the two parental cell types. In addition to the four species of antibody shown here, there are six more possible species with two nonidentical binding sites.

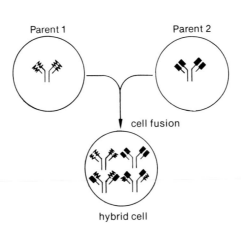

Figure 2-13

A schematic representation of multispecificity in a single antibody molecule.

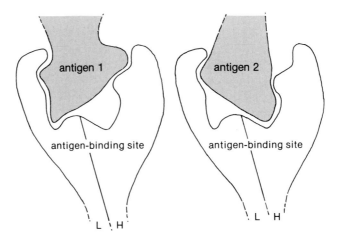

whenever there is a sufficient number of short-range interactions, regardless of the total fit. Within the antigen-combining site, a lack of fit in one region can be compensated for by increased binding elsewhere. Disparate antigens may fit into the antigen-binding crevice in different ways (Figure 2-13). Each species of antibody has a different spectrum of determinants with which it can combine.

Although individual antibodies are multispecific, the collection of antibodies induced in response to a particular antigen behaves in a highly specific manner, normally reacting only with the inducing antigen and very closely related structures. This apparent paradox can be explained as follows. Many different molecular species of antibody are normally induced in an immune response, and each will react with a different spectrum of antigens. Thus every antibody molecule will react with the inducing antigen, but each kind of antibody molecule will differ in the spectrum of disparate antigens it can bind. If each molecular species of antibody is present at the 1% level, the

Table 2-2 Hypothetical Specificity Profiles of Individual Antibody
Species Raised Against an Immunogen, Hapten A[a]

	Antibody Species					
	1	2	3	4	5	n
Specificities	A	A	A	A	A	A
	A′	A′	A′		A′	A′
	A″		A″	A″		A″
	B	C	F	J		T
	E		G	W	H	L
	Q	M	R	X	P	Y
	V	S	N	K	Z	U
	•	•	•	•	•	•
	•	•	•	•	•	•
	•	•	•	•	•	•
	•	•	•	•	•	•

[a]Letters represent antigenic determinants that are recognized by the various antibody
species. A′ and A″ represent determinants that are closely related in structure to
Hapten A. The recognition specificities for disparate determinants generally are not
common to different antibody species.

disparate reactions will be below the limits of detection for most routine immunologic assays (Table 2-2).

2-5 Homology units in immunoglobulins correspond to molecular domains with different functions

Homology units within light and heavy chains

On the basis of primary structure comparisons, light and heavy chains can be divided into two groups of *homology units* of similar amino acid sequence (Figure 2-14). Each of these units is about 110 residues in length and has a centrally placed disulfide bridge. One group consists of the V_L and V_H regions. In the IgG molecule, the other group consists of the C_L region and three subsegments of the C_H region, designated C_H1, C_H2, and C_H3.

The sequences of the two V-region homology units are similar, as are those of the four C-region homology units (Figure 2-15). Although the V- and C-region units have no apparent sequence homology to one another, some relationship is suggested by the observations that both homology units are roughly the same length and both have a centrally located intrachain disulfide bridge that spans about 60 residues. Direct support for homology is provided by X-ray crystallo-

Figure 2-14

A diagrammatic representation of the homology units and domains of the IgG molecule. Pairs of homology units fold together to form four globular domains termed V, C_H1, C_H2, and C_H3, as indicated by boxes in the figure. Limited proteolytic attack at the hinge region (shaded segment of heavy chains) cleaves the molecule into Fab and Fc fragments.

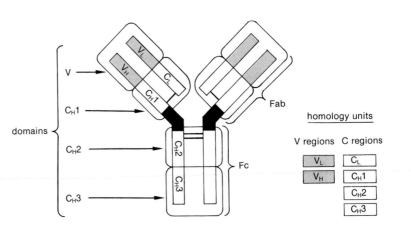

```
                                          110                                          120
Eu C_L    (Residues 109-214)   Thr Val Ala Ala Pro Ser Val Phe Ile Phe Pro Pro Ser
Eu C_H1   (Residues 119-220)   Ser Thr Lys Gly Pro Ser Val Phe  —  —  Pro Leu Ala
Eu C_H2   (Residues 234-341)   Leu Leu Gly Gly Pro Ser Val Phe Leu Phe Pro Pro Lys
Eu C_H3   (Residues 342-446)   Gln Pro Arg Glu Pro Gln Val Tyr Thr Leu Pro Pro Ser

                                                    130
Asp Glu Gln  —   —  Leu Lys Ser Gly Thr Ala Ser Val Val Cys Leu Leu Asn Asn Phe
Pro Ser Ser Lys Ser Thr Ser Gly Gly Thr Ala Ala Leu Gly Cys Leu Val Lys Asp Tyr
Pro Lys Asp Thr Leu Met Ile Ser Arg Thr Pro Glu Val Thr Cys Val Val Val Asp Val
Arg Glu Glu  —   —  Met Thr Lys Asn Gln Val Ser Leu Thr Cys Leu Val Lys Gly Phe

    140                                        150
Tyr Pro Arg Glu Ala Lys Val  —   —  Gln Trp Lys Val Asp Asn Ala Leu Gln Ser Gly
Phe Pro Glu Pro Val Thr Val  —   —  Ser Trp Asn Ser  —  Gly Ala Leu Thr Ser Gly
Ser His Glu Asp Pro Gln Val Lys Phe Asn Trp Tyr Val Asp Gly  —  Val Gln Val His
Tyr Pro Ser Asp Ile Ala Val  —   —  Glu Trp Glu Ser Asn Asp  —  Gly Glu Pro Glu

    160                                        170
Asn Ser Gln Glu Ser Val Thr Glu Gln Asp Ser Lys Asp Ser Thr Tyr Ser Leu Ser Ser
 —  Val His Thr Phe Pro Ala Val Leu Gln Ser  —  Ser Gly Leu Tyr Ser Leu Ser Ser
Asn Ala Lys Thr Lys Pro Arg Glu Gln Gln Tyr  —  Asp Ser Thr Tyr Arg Val Val Ser
Asn Tyr Lys Thr Thr Pro Pro Val Leu Asp Ser  —  Asp Gly Ser Phe Phe Leu Tyr Ser

    180                                        190
Thr Leu Thr Leu Ser Lys Ala Asp Tyr Glu Lys His Lys Val Tyr Ala Cys Glu Val Thr
Val Val Thr Val Pro Ser Ser Ser Leu Gly Thr Gln  —  Thr Tyr Ile Cys Asn Val Asn
Val Leu Thr Val Leu His Gln Asn Trp Leu Asp Gly Lys Glu Tyr Lys Cys Lys Val Ser
Lys Leu Thr Val Asp Lys Ser Arg Trp Gln Glu Gly Asn Val Phe Ser Cys Ser Val Met

    200                                        210
His Gln Gly Leu Ser Ser Pro Val Thr  —  Lys Ser Phe  —   —  Asn Arg Gly Glu Cys
His Lys Pro Ser Asn Thr Lys Val  —  Asp Lys Arg Val  —   —  Glu Pro Lys Ser Cys
Asn Lys Ala Leu Pro Ala Pro Ile  —  Glu Lys Thr Ile Ser Lys Ala Lys Gly
His Glu Ala Leu His Asn His Tyr Thr Gln Lys Ser Leu Ser Leu Ser Pro Gly
```

Figure 2-15 Amino-acid-sequence homologies of the four constant-region homology units of the human myeloma protein Eu. Deletions indicated by dashes have been introduced to maximize the homology. Identical residues are lightly shaded; dark shadings indicate alternative identities at a given position. [From G. M. Edelman et al., *Proc. Natl. Acad. Sci. USA* **63**, 78(1969).]

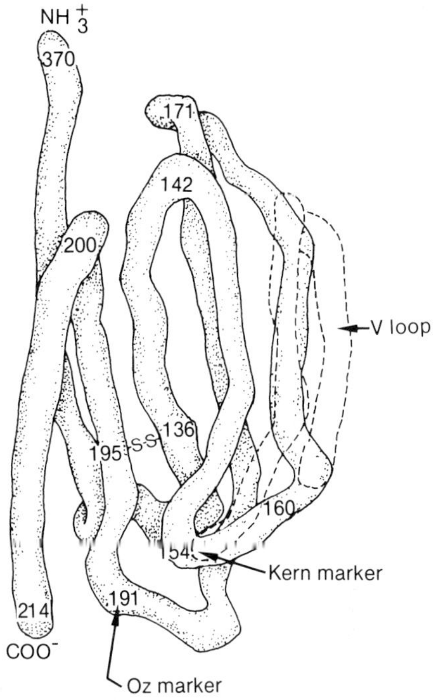

Figure 2-16 A diagrammatic representation of the basic immunoglobulin fold present in mammalian immunoglobulin molecules. Solid lines show the folding of the polypeptide chain in the constant regions C_L and C_H1. Dotted lines indicate the additional loop of polypeptide characteristic of the V_L and V_H regions. NH_3^+ and COO^- correspond to the N and C termini of these subunits, respectively. Numbers refer to positions at which residue substitutions are found in the C_L region. [From R. J. Poljak et al., *Proc. Natl. Acad. Sci. USA* **70,** 3305(1973).]

graphic studies on immunoglobulins of different classes from different animal species. These studies, which are at about 3-Å resolution, show that the V_L, V_H, C_L, and C_H1 regions are strikingly similar in their three-dimensional conformation. These homology units exhibit the characteristic *immunoglobulin fold* (Figure 2-16). The V regions differ from the C regions only by the presence of an extra polypeptide loop and by structural variation in the antigen-binding crevice. The three-dimensional structures of these homology units must have been highly conserved throughout vertebrate evolution because the genes that code for the C_H regions of different immunoglobulin classes (e.g., IgG and IgA) probably diverged from one another hundreds of millions of years ago.

Homologous polypeptides presumably reflect genes that diverged from a common ancestor at some past time. Accordingly, these homology relationships strongly suggest that present-day light-chain and heavy-chain genes evolved by duplication and divergence from a single primordial gene that coded for a polypeptide of about 110 residues (see Concept 4-8).

Globular domains of the immunoglobulin molecule

X-ray analysis shows that the immunoglobulin molecule is differentiated into discrete, compact, globular *domains* connected by short segments of more extended polypeptide chain (Figure 2-17). Each domain consists of a pair of corresponding homology units that are

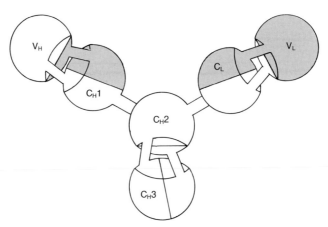

Figure 2-17
The domains of the human IgG
molecule as determined by
X-ray analysis at 6 Å. Shaded
regions indicate that portion of
each domain contributed by
light chains. [Reproduced by F.
J. Poljak et al., *Nature* **235,**
137(1972, Figure 3).]

tightly associated. The V_L and V_H homology units form the V domain; the C_L and C_H1 units form the C_H1 domain; two C_H2 units form the C_H2 domain; and two C_H3 units form the C_H3 domain (Figure 2-14). Thus the basic $(L–H)_2$ immunoglobulin unit is composed of six globular domains: two V, two C_H1, one C_H2, and one C_H3.

Proteolytic digestion under suboptimal conditions can cause limited cleavage of native immunoglobulin molecules between these globular domains. Presumably the compactly folded domains are protected from proteolysis, whereas the regions of more extended polypeptide structure between homology units are accessible. Early experiments with cleavage showed that the IgG molecule can be broken into three fragments by cleavage of the hinge region of the heavy chain (Figure 2-14). Two of these fragments, designated Fab (for antigen-binding fragment), are identical. Each consists of one V and one C_H1 domain so that each carries one antigen-binding site (Figure 2-18). The third fragment, which turns out to be readily crystallizable and is consequently designated the Fc fragment, consists of the C_H2 and C_H3 domains. Such fragmentation by mild proteolysis has allowed subsequent isolation of the combinations of globular domains listed in Table 2-3. These fragments have proven to be very useful in elucidating structure–function relationships in antibody molecules.

Functional roles of the different domains

The antigen-binding functions and effector functions of immunoglobulins are carried out by different domains of the molecule. The V domains are responsible for antigen binding, whereas the C domains carry out the various effector functions (Concept 2-6 and Chapter 9). These functions include the stimulation of B cells to undergo proliferation and differentiation; activation of the complement system; opsonization; transfer of IgG from mother to fetus across the placental barrier; transfer of immunoglobulin into milk, sweat, tears, saliva, and gastrointestinal secretions; and fixation of certain classes of antibodies to mast cells. Some of these functions are triggered by antigen–antibody combination (B-cell stimulation, mast-cell degranulation,

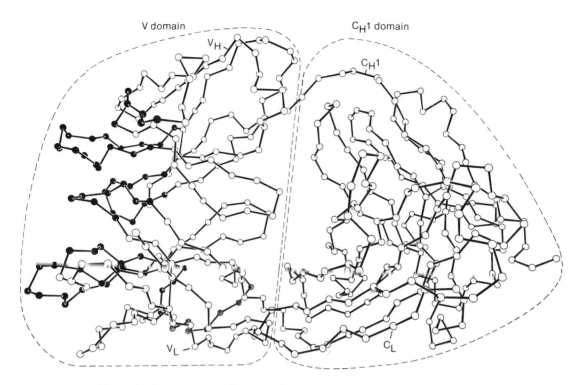

Figure 2-18 A drawing of the α-carbon backbone of the Fab fragment of the mouse myeloma protein MOPC603. The hypervariable regions associated with the antigen-binding site are indicated by black circles. A fourth hypervariable region, not associated with the antigen-binding site, is indicated by shaded circles. [From D. R. Davies et al., *Contemp. Top. Mol. Immunol.* **4,** 127(1976).]

Table 2-3 Domains Obtained from Immunoglobulin Molecules by Mild Proteolytic Digestion

Domain	Name of Fragment
V–C_H1[a]	Fab
C_H2–C_H3	Fc
$(V$–$C_H1)_2$	$(Fab')_2$
V–C_H1–C_H2	Fabc
C_H1	—
C_H3	Fc'
V	Fv
V_1[b]	—
C_1[b]	—

[a]The N-terminal half of the heavy chain, designated the Fd piece, can be isolated from the Fab fragment.
[b]Produced from proteolytic digestion of light chain.

and complement fixation), whereas others are not (placental transfer, epithelial transfer, and mast-cell fixation). It is likely, although unproven, that each of the C domains contains the active site for at least one effector function. There is some evidence that the C_H2 domain of the IgG molecule plays a role in complement activation. The C_H3 domain will bind to lymphocyte and certain macrophage membranes. Accordingly, the V domain must communicate with the C_H2 and C_H3 domains to trigger appropriate effector functions. Presumably this communication involves conformational changes that occur throughout the antibody molecule when an antigen is bound by the V domain. However, these conformational changes probably require binding of antigen to more than one V domain. Binding of univalent haptens does not activate complement or trigger B-cell activation. Apparently these effector functions are initiated by cross-linking the arms of a single antibody or by cross-linking two or more antibody molecules to each other.

2-6 The five classes of immunoglobulin molecules differ in the structures and functions of their heavy-chain constant regions

Heavy- and light-chain classes and structural differences

The five immunoglobulin classes are distinguished structurally by differences in their heavy-chain constant regions. Comparisons of C_H-region amino acid sequences show that there are five major heavy-chain classes, designated α, γ, δ, ϵ, and μ. These heavy-chain classes define the corresponding immunoglobulin classes IgA, IgG, IgD, IgE, and IgM, respectively (Table 2-4). The C_H amino acid sequences of these classes are homologous, but they differ by more than 60% of their residues. Some classes can be divided into subclasses, defined by C_H regions that are distinct but more similar in amino acid sequence; for example, in humans the γ class can be divided into $\gamma1$, $\gamma2$, $\gamma3$, and $\gamma4$ subclasses. The genes that code for heavy chains are known collectively as the *heavy-chain (H) gene family.*

In addition there are two major types of light chains based on comparisons of C-region amino acid sequence. These two types, designated κ and λ, differ by about 60% in their C_L amino acid sequences (Table 2-5). Like some heavy-chain classes, the λ-type light chains may be further divided into subtypes defined by distinct but very similar C_L sequences. Immunoglobulin light chains from various mammals can be assigned readily to the κ and λ types, based on sequence homology. The genes that code for these light-chain types comprise the κ gene family and the λ gene family, respectively.

Table 2-4 Subunit Structures of the Five Immunoglobulin Classes in Humans

Class	Heavy Chain	Subclasses	Light Chain	Molecular Formula
IgG	γ	$\gamma1, \gamma2$ $\gamma3, \gamma4$	κ or λ	$(\gamma_2\kappa_2)$ $(\gamma_2\lambda_2)$
IgA	α	$\alpha1, \alpha2$	κ or λ	$(\alpha_2\kappa_2)_n{}^a$ $(\alpha_2\lambda_2)_n{}^a$
IgM	μ	none	κ or λ	$(\mu_2\kappa_2)_5$ $(\mu_2\lambda_2)_5$
IgD	δ	none	κ or λ	$(\delta_2\kappa_2)$ $(\delta_2\lambda_2)$
IgE	ϵ	none	κ or λ	$(\epsilon_2\kappa_2)$ $(\epsilon_2\lambda_2)$

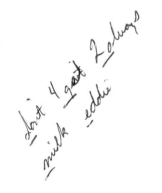

[a]n may equal 1, 2, or 3.

Table 2-5 The Amino-Acid-Difference Matrix for Various Mammalian C Regions[a]

	Human C_κ	Mouse C_κ	Rat C_κ	Human C_λ
Human C_κ				
Mouse C_κ	41			
Rat C_κ	38	28		
Human C_λ	60	65	61	
Mouse $C_{\lambda 1}$	56	68	61	39

[a]Numbers indicate the percentages of amino acid differences between the two chains compared. Differences between λ and κ chains (shaded rectangles), even from the same species, are more pronounced than λ–λ or κ–κ differences (unshaded rectangles).

Immunoglobulin classes are defined by their constituent heavy-chain subunits only (Table 2-4). The class of an immunoglobulin molecule is independent of the type of light-chain subunits that it contains. A single immunoglobulin molecule always has identical light and identical heavy chains. However, immunoglobulin molecules of a given class may contain either κ or λ light chains. The subunit compositions of the five immunoglobulin classes are listed in Table 2-4.

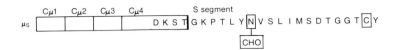

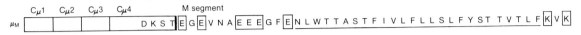

Figure 2-19   Carboxy-terminal amino acid sequences of μ_s and μ_m chains. The four C_H domains for the μ_s and μ_m chains are identical in amino acid sequence. The 20-residue tail following the C_H4 domain has no homology with the immunoglobulin domains, and it includes the cysteine (boxed) which links μ_s chains to the J chain in secreted IgM and the asparagine site of carbohydrate attachment (boxed CHO). The 41-residue M segment has no homology with the immunoglobulin domains or the μ_s C-terminal segment, and it includes the long hydrophobic sequence (underlined). Charged residues are boxed.

Expression of light and heavy chains in B cells

In general, a given B-cell clone produces only one type of light chain, κ or λ, and one of the five classes of heavy chain. At certain stages in their differentiation, however, B cells may simultaneously produce two classes of heavy chains and thus two classes of immunoglobulins. These stages may reflect switching of a clone from production of one heavy-chain class to another in the course of maturation. By contrast, no clone has ever been observed to produce more than a single type of light chain, as if the choice between expression of κ or λ gene families were made irreversibly very early in B-cell differentiation. A fully mature plasma cell invariably produces only a single class of heavy chain and a single type of light chain.

Secreted and membrane-bound forms of antibodies

Antibodies of several classes are produced in two structurally different forms, one secreted and the other membrane bound. Secreted IgM, for example, is pentameric (Figure 2-5) and must be sufficiently hydrophilic to circulate as a soluble serum molecule. By contrast, the membrane-bound IgM, which serves as the surface receptor that triggers B-cell differentiation, is monomeric and must be sufficiently hydrophobic to remain anchored in the cell membrane. The heavy chains of the membrane-bound (μ_m) and secreted (μ_s) forms each have four C_H domains, but they differ in the structures of their C-terminal tails (Figure 2-19).

The differences in aggregation state and cellular location of the secreted and membrane-bound forms of IgM are explained nicely by their distinctive C-terminal sequences. The difference in aggregation arises because the μ_s tail has a penultimate cysteine residue that can bridge to other μ_s chains or to the J chain to form the pentameric secreted IgM molecule. The μ_m tail lacks cysteine and, accordingly, is capable of forming only monomeric IgM molecules. The differences in cellular location arise because the μ_s tail, which is a hydrophilic 20-residue segment, allows the μ_s chain to pass completely through the membrane during its synthesis, whereas the μ_m tail, which is a hydrophobic 41-residue segment, interrupts the transfer of the μ_m chain across the membrane and anchors it in the membrane. The μ_m tail has an uncharged stretch of 26 amino acid residues that are hydrophobic and would be predicted to form an α helix. About 24 residues of α helix are required to span the plasma membrane. Moreover, this presumed transmembrane belt is flanked by a cluster of acidic residues on the external side and a cluster of basic residues on the cytoplasmic side, which serve to anchor the transmembrane belt in the lipid bilayer. In these respects, the transmembrane belt resembles the corresponding region of glycophorin, a well-known transmembrane protein of the red blood cell.

Other classes of heavy chains also employ hydrophilic and hydrophobic C-terminal tails for their secreted and membrane-bound forms, respectively. The mechanism by which one plasma cell can generate these alternative forms of the same heavy chain is discussed in Concept 4-4.

Correspondence of structural and functional class differences

The structural differences among the five classes of immunoglobulins correspond to functional differences in their sites of production and action, their relative levels of production in primary and secondary immune responses, and their roles as physiological effectors. For example, IgG is prevalent in both blood and tissue fluids, whereas IgM is confined to the blood and IgA is found primarily on epithelial surfaces. Chapter 9 discusses the various effector mechanisms that are mediated by the five different classes of immunoglobulins.

Selected Bibliography

General

Kabat, E. A., *Structural Concepts in Immunology and Immunochemistry*, Holt, Rinehart & Winston, New York, 1976.

Nisonoff, A., Hopper, J. R., and Spring, S. B., *The Antibody Molecule*, Academic Press, 1975.

Homogeneous antibodies

Kohler, G., and Milstein, C., "Continuous cultures of fused cells secreting antibody of pre-defined specificity," *Nature* **256,** 495(1975).

Krause, R. M., "The search for antibodies with molecular uniformity," *Adv. Immunol.* **12,** 1(1970).

Milstein, C., "Monoclonal antibodies," *Sci. Am.* **243,** 66(1980).

Potter, M., "Immunoglobulin-producing tumors and myeloma proteins of mice," *Physiol. Rev.* **62,** 631(1972).

Three-dimensional structures

Amzel, L., Poljak, R., Saul, F., Varga, J., and Richards, F., "The three-dimensional structure of a combining region-ligand complex of immunoglobulin NEW at 3.5 Å resolution," *Proc. Natl. Acad. Sci. USA* **71,** 1427(1974).

Davies, D. R., Padlan, E. A., and Segal, D. M., "Three-dimensional structure of immunoglobulins," *Annu. Rev. Biochem.* **44,** 639(1975).

Variable regions

Gearhart, P., Johnson, N., Douglas, R., and Hood, L., "IgG antibodies to phosphorylcholine exhibit more diversity than their IgM counterparts," *Nature* **291,** 29(1981).

Hilschmann, N., and Craig, L. C., "Amino acid sequence studies with Bence-Jones proteins," *Proc. Natl. Acad. Sci. USA* **53,** 1403(1965).

Kaartinen, M., Griffiths, G. M., Hamlyn, P. H., Markham, A. F., Karjalanen, K., Pelkonen, J. L. T., Makela, O., and Milstein, C., "Anti-oxazalone hybridomas and the structure of the oxazalone idiotype," *J. Immunol.* **130,** 937(1983).

Antibody specificity

Capra, J. D., and Edmundson, A. B., "The antibody combining site," *Sci. Am.* **236,** 50(1977).

Richards, F., Konigsberg, W., Rosenstein, R., and Varga, J., "On the specificity of antibodies," *Science* **189,** 130(1975).

Hypervariable regions

Wu, T. T., and Kabat, E. A., "An analysis of the se-quences of the variable regions of Bence-Jones proteins and myeloma light chains and their implications for antibody complementation," *J. Exp. Med.* **132,** 211 (1970).

Additional concepts and techniques presented in the problems

1. Urinary light chains (Bence-Jones) proteins. Problem 2-3.

2. Enzymatic cleavage of antibodies. Problem 2-4.

Problems

2-1   Indicate whether each of the following statements is true or false. Explain the error in each statement you consider to be false.
(a)   The hinge region joins light and heavy chains in the immunoglobulin molecule.
(b)   One immunoglobulin molecule can have light chains with two different V-region sequences.
(c)   The V_H region is twice the length of the V_L region.
(d)   Homology units of immunoglobulin polypeptides are encoded by nucleotide sequences of about 330 nucleotide pairs in length.
(e)   The immunoglobulin active site is composed primarily of the light chain.
(f)   The V and C regions of the light chain have very similar tertiary structures.
(g) V_λ regions are sometimes associated with C_κ regions.
(h)   IgG1 and IgG2 molecules are distinguished by differences in their light-chain sequences.
(i)   A single antigen generally evokes the synthesis of a single molecular species of antibody.
(j)   Myeloma proteins from different humans are always identical in sequence.
(k)   The presence of homology units in immunoglobulins suggests that genes for light and heavy chains evolved from a common precursor gene.

2-2   Supply the missing word or words in each of the following statements.
(a)   The diversity of antigen-binding sites is presumably reflected in the amino-acid-sequence diversity of the subunit _____ regions.
(b)   _____ are homogeneous immunoglobulins derived from organisms with plasma cell tumors.
(c)   The finding of _____ suggests that immunoglobulins evolved by a series of gene duplications.
(d)   The IgG antibody molecule folds into six discrete _____ .
(e)   The _____ regions fold to form the walls of the antigen-binding crevice.
(f)   The _____ functions of immunoglobulins from different classes are different, whereas the _____ function may be the same.
(g)   The two types of light chains are _____ and _____ .

2-3   A myeloma patient excretes large quantities of a protein in his urine. The kidney generally permits only those molecules smaller than 45,000 daltons to pass from the

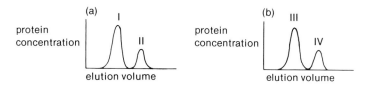

Figure 2-20 Gel filtration patterns of goat IgG after cleavage by (a) reduction and alkylation and (b) mild pepsin digestion (Problem 2-4). The fragments have the following molecular weights: I, 53,000; II, 23,000; III, ~ 100,000; and IV, ~ 50,000.

blood to the urine. Assuming that no proteolysis occurs in the blood or kidney, what could this protein be?

2-4   Goat antibodies of the IgG class are induced with bovine serum albumin (BSA). These antibody molecules have a molecular weight of about 160,000, and they can be fragmented into smaller pieces by chemical and enzymatic procedures. The patterns given in Figure 2-20 are obtained from gel filtration after the indicated chemical or enzymatic modification. Peak III can precipitate BSA from solution, whereas Peaks I, II, and IV do not combine with this antigen. Peak IV can fix complement (an effector function) under appropriate conditions, whereas none of the others can do so.

(a) Sketch a model of the goat IgG molecule based on the information given, and indicate the cleavage sites that would give patterns (a) and (b) in the figure.

(b) Suggest an explanation for the type of cleavage that occurs with mild pepsin digestion.

(c) Where are the antigen-binding and effector functions located on this immuno-globulin molecule? Are both light and heavy chains necessary for each of these functions?

(d) Papain digestion of the goat antibody gives two types of fragments that are about 50,000 daltons in molecular weight. Draw a model to explain this cleavage. The fragment with antigen-binding capacity can no longer precipitate BSA although it does associate with BSA. Explain.

2-5   As a physician in a large medical center you have access to large numbers of myeloma patients. You decide to investigate their myeloma proteins, which can be obtained easily in nearly pure form from their urine. You prepare antisera in rabbits against three of these light chains (A, B, C) and then analyze each of these antisera on Ouchterlony plates against a set of eight other myeloma proteins, with the results shown in Figure 2-21 (see Concept 3-1).

(a) Explain these results, based on your knowledge of human light chains. What experiments could you do to test your explanation?

(b) Suggest an explanation for the spur formation seen opposite Well 2 in Figure 2-21. What structural feature(s) of the light chain may correspond to this spur?

2-6   Myeloma tumors can be induced experimentally by injection of BALB/c mice with mineral oil. Various antigens have been added to the mineral oil in attempts to produce myeloma immunoglobulins with specific antibody activity, but all attempts have failed. However, a few myeloma immunoglobulins with apparently specific antibody activity have been found by screening large numbers of myeloma proteins against many different antigens. For example, one myeloma immunoglobulin with an affinity constant of 10^7 moles/liter for the dinitrophenyl group (Dnp) has been found. This affinity is similar to that exhibited by biologically induced antibody.

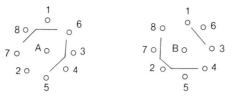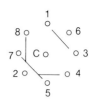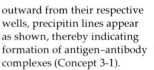

Figure 2-21   Analysis of three antisera to myeloma proteins on Ouchterlony plates (Problem 2-5). One of the three antisera, A, B, or C, is placed in the central well of each plate, and the peripheral wells are filled with solutions of the eight myeloma proteins. As the antigens and antibodies diffuse outward from their respective wells, precipitin lines appear as shown, thereby indicating formation of antigen–antibody complexes (Concept 3-1).

sequence			position		
	1	5	10	15	20
1	V K C A V V R S T A G M P S T A A A I L
2	V K C A L V R S T A G M P S T A A A I L
3	L R C A I V R T S A A F Y S A T S A V L
4	A D C A M V R G N A G M P S G G G A L L
5	V K C A V L R S T A G M P S T A A A I V
6	V P P P V I K S T G A F P S G V G V L S
7	V K C A L V R S T G G M P S T A A A I L
8	L R C G I V R T S A A F Y S A T S A V L
9	V K C A L L R S T A G M P S T A A A I L
10	V P P P V I K S T G A F P S G V A V L S

Figure 2-22

Homologous C_H sequences from imaginary gopher myeloma proteins (Problem 2-8).

(a) What functional and structural criteria must this myeloma protein fulfill to be considered a bona fide antibody?

(b) Suppose that this immunoglobulin satisfies all of the criteria for antibody. Then it is discovered that, in addition, it has a high affinity constant (5×10^5 moles/liter) for menadione (vitamin K), a compound with little apparent steric similarity to Dnp. Offer three explanations for this paradoxical binding of apparently different antigenic determinants.

(c) How could you test the possibilities that you suggest in part (b)?

2-7 You are given two preparations of antibody against hen ovalbumen, each raised under similar immunization conditions in a different guinea pig. The specificities and binding constants of these preparations appear identical, yet one preparation fixes complement after combination with antigen and the second does not. Explain how antibodies with identical antigen-binding properties can have distinct effector functions.

2-8 The imaginary homologous C_H sequences shown in Figure 2-22 might have been obtained from gopher myeloma proteins. By inspection, group these C_H sequences into classes by relatedness of sequence.

2-9 Assume that any light chain can combine with any heavy chain to generate antibody molecules with a spectrum of different combining sites. How many different antibody molecules could be assembled in an animal that could synthesize 10 different light and 10 different heavy chains? How many different antibodies could be assembled in an animal that could synthesize 100 of each chain? A thousand of each chain?

species															position								24
κ1	T	V	A	C	P	S	V	F	C	F	P	P	D	I	L	C	T	Q	S	P	C	S	L A
κ2	T	V	A	C	P	S	V	F	C	F	P	P	V	I	Q	C	T	Q	S	P	C	S	L A
λ1	T	L	A	C	T	S	I	F	C	Y	P	T	Q	S	A	C	T	Q	P	P	C	[]	L T
λ2	T	L	A	C	T	S	I	F	C	Y	P	T	N	S	S	C	T	Q	T	P	C	[]	L T
λ3	T	L	A	C	T	S	I	F	C	Y	P	T	Q	S	T	C	T	Q	P	P	C	[]	V T

Position 34 region:

γ1: T V A C S T V Y C F P P T V A C S T V Y C F P T T V A C T T V Y C F
γ2: T V A C S T V Y C F P P T V A C S T V Y C F P T T V A C T T V Y C F
γ3: T V A C S T V Y C F P P T V A C S T V Y C F P T T V A C T T V Y C F
μ1: T V G C S S V Y C F P P T V G C S S L Y C F P P T V G C S S V Y C F

Position 35 — 48 — 60:

γ1: P P E V Q C L E S G C G L S
γ2: P P A V Q C L Q T G C G L S
γ3: P P E I Q C L E S A C G V S
μ1: P P T V G C S S V Y C F P P E V Q C L E S G C G L S

Figure 2-23
Amino acid sequences of Pigmodian immunoglobulin molecules. Bars indicate disulfide bridges (Problem 2-10).

2-10 In the world of Pigmodia everything is small, creatures as well as molecules. Suppose, as a visiting expert biochemist, you are asked to examine and comment on the evolution of the representative Pigmodian antibody polypeptide chains in Figure 2-23.
(a) Can you distinguish V and C regions? How long are they?
(b) Are internal homologies evident in the light or heavy chains? If so, how long are they and how many homology units are present in each chain?
(c) Do the V and C regions appear evolutionarily related? How?

Answers

2-1 (a) False. The hinge region joins the N- and C-terminal halves of the heavy chain.
(b) False. The light chains of a single antibody molecule always are identical, as are the heavy chains.
(c) False. The V_L and V_H regions are approximately the same size.
(d) True
(e) False. Both chains contribute to the active site.
(f) True
(g) False. The V regions of one immunoglobulin family are never associated with the C regions of another family.
(h) False. The C_H regions distinguish the classes and subclasses of antibodies.
(i) False. The immune response to a single antigen usually consists of a heterogeneous array of different antibody molecules.
(j) False. Identical myeloma proteins from different humans have never been observed.
(k) True
2-2 (a) variable
(b) Myeloma proteins
(c) homology units
(d) domains

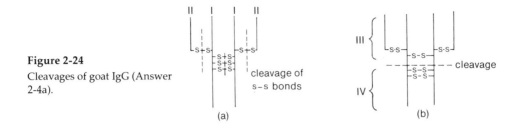

Figure 2-24

Cleavages of goat IgG (Answer 2-4a).

(e) hypervariable

(f) effector, antigen-binding

(g) λ and κ

2-3   This protein probably is a light chain. Some myeloma patients synthesize an excess of light chain along with the myeloma immunoglobulin. Other myeloma patients synthesize just a light chain. The 23,000-dalton light chain can pass through the kidney and is excreted in the urine. Urinary light chains from myeloma patients are called *Bence–Jones proteins,* after their discoverer. Early structural studies were carried out on Bence–Jones proteins because they were easily obtained and readily purified of minor urinary protein contaminants.

2-4   (a) Pattern (a), Figure 2-24; pattern (b), Figure 2-24.

(b) Pepsin cannot generally cleave regions of polypeptide chains with a compact structure (the Fab and Fc fragments), but it can cleave unstructured or randomly oriented regions such as the hinge region.

(c) Fragment III (Fab) binds antigen. It is composed of the two light chains and the N-terminal halves of the heavy chains. Fragment IV (Fc) carries effector functions and is composed of the C-terminal halves of the heavy chains. Thus both light and heavy chains are required for antigen binding, but heavy chains alone can carry out some effector functions.

(d) The sites of papain cleavage are shown in Figure 2-25a. To precipitate an antigen, antibody must be bivalent so an antigen–antibody lattice can form (Figure 2-25b). Papain digestion produces univalent Fab fragments that can bind to antigen; however, they cannot form the lattice necessary for precipitation (Figure 2-25c).

2-5   (a) The results show two antigenically distinct types of light chains: Proteins 1, 3, 4, and 8 react with Antiserum A, and Proteins 2, 5, 6, and 7 react with Antisera B and C. These classes correspond to the λ and κ types of light chains. To confirm this explanation you could carry out amino-acid-sequence analysis on each of the eight proteins to determine their types. This kind of serologic analysis first suggested that there are two types of light chains in humans.

(b) Myeloma Protein 2 has antigenic determinants that are not present in Proteins 5 and 7 but that must have been present in the protein used to prepare Antiserum C. There are two possible explanations for this observation. These determinants could be features of the V_L region of Protein 2 not present in Proteins 5 and 7 (i.e., idiotypic determinants). Alternatively, Antiserum C may be detecting a different type of C_L region in Protein 2. All humans have at least five different types of C_L regions: four C_λ subtypes and the C_κ type.

2-6   (a) Fab fragments (which carry the antigen-binding sites on true antibodies), prepared from the immunoglobulin, must be shown to bind the Dnp group.

Figure 2-25

(Answer 2-4d.) (a) Sites of papain cleavage of goat IgG. (b) Lattice formed by association of bivalent antibodies (Ab) with antigen molecules (Ag). (c) Association of monovalent antibody fragments with antigen.

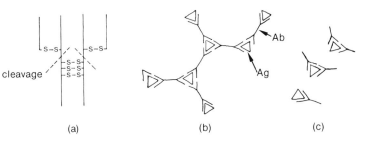

(a)   (b)   (c)

The Dnp group must be shown to bind in the active-site cleft. The hydrophobic Dnp group may associate nonspecifically with other hydrophobic clefts, which have nothing to do with the active site.

The stoichiometry of binding should be one mole of Dnp bound per mole of Fab, and the valence of the intact immunoglobulin should correspond to that of one of the known immunoglobulin classes. For example, IgG antibodies have a valence of 2 and IgM antibodies a valence of 10.

Upon binding to the antigen, the myeloma immunoglobulin should carry out the effector functions triggered by antigen binding to normal antibodies of the same immunoglobulin class. For example, complement fixation should occur with IgG1 molecules.

Normally the synthesis of antibodies is specifically induced by corresponding antigens. No one understands the nature of the induction process in myelomatosis. It would be interesting to make a specific antiserum (anti-idiotype) for the V regions of the myeloma protein and to determine whether similar molecules are induced in a normal immune response to the Dnp group.

(b) Dnp and menadione could share some unrecognized common structural features that permit binding to occur at the same antigen-binding site.

If menadione and Dnp have distinct antigenic determinants, there could be two distinct Fab binding sites, one for each antigen. Conversely, both antigens could bind to the same site in different orientations. The antigen-binding site could have two or more distinct subsites.

Menadione could bind nonspecifically to a region of the antibody molecule other than the active site.

(c) You could locate the binding site for menadione.

You could carry out a competition experiment to determine whether Dnp can bind in the presence of excess menadione. If the sites are the same or if they hinder one another sterically, competition will occur. If the sites are independent, no competition will occur.

You could make a structural analysis of the two antigen–antibody complexes by X-ray crystallography.

2-7 Some immunoglobulin classes can fix complement, whereas others cannot. Therefore, similar ovalbumen-specific V_H regions must be attached to different C_H regions in the two antibody preparations. This phenomenon, in general, allows the same antigen-binding site to be associated with many different types of effector functions. Thus antibody molecules allow a given antigen to trigger several different kinds of physiological responses.

2-8 There are four distinct classes. They are I: 1, 2, 5, 7, 9; II: 3, 8; III: 4; IV: 6, 10.

2-9 With random association, the number of different antibodies that could be assembled is $p \times q$, in which p = number of light chains and q = number of heavy chains.

Therefore, with 10 light and 10 heavy chains, $10^2 = 100$ antibodies could be formed; with 100 of each chain, $100^2 = 10^4$; and with 1000 of each chain, $1000^2 = 10^6$.

2-10   (a)   The V regions for each family are the C-terminal 12 residues. The C regions for light chains are 12 residues, whereas those for heavy chains are 36 (γ) and 48 (μ) residues.

(b)   The light chains are composed of two homology units, each 12 residues in length, with symmetrically placed disulfide bridges. The heavy chains have 4 (γ) or 5 (μ) similar homology units. The μ chain in man also appears to have 5 homology units.

(c)   The V regions and the C regions share at least two features: (1) they can be broken down into homology units 12 residues in length, and (2) these homology units have symmetrically disposed disulfide bridges that span four residues. The V regions are related to one another by sequence homology, as are the C-region homology units.

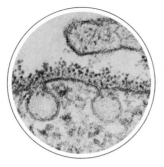

CHAPTER 3

Detection and Application of Antigen–Antibody Reactions

Chapter Outline

The exquisite specificity of antibody molecules has led to their widespread use for the immunoassay of biologically and medically relevant molecules. Moreover, two recently developed techniques—production of monoclonal antibodies from hybridomas and fluorescence-activated cell sorting—have made possible striking advances in the fundamental and clinical uses of antigen–antibody reactions. This chapter considers the currently important techniques for immunoassay and immunodiagnosis.

Concepts

3-1 Antigen–antibody reactions can be measured by the formation of insoluble complexes

The precipitin reaction

Precipitation of antigen–antibody complexes from solution (the *precipitin reaction*) can be used to estimate the amount of antigen or antibody in a test sample. Multivalent antigens may interact with multivalent antibodies to form large insoluble lattices (Figure 3-1a) or small soluble complexes (Figure 3-1b,c). When large antigen–antibody complexes precipitate out of solution, the amounts of antigen and antibody precipitated can be measured.

Complexes precipitate most completely at roughly equal concentrations of antigen and antibody. Excess antibody allows single antigen molecules to be coated by several antibodies and thus prevents lattice formation (Figure 3-1b). Excess antigen saturates all binding sites with different antigen molecules, again preventing lattice formation (Figure 3-1c). In the precipitin assay, a fixed quantity of antiserum is reacted with increasing concentrations of antigen, and the amounts of antibody or antigen in the precipitate are measured chemically by various assays for protein or carbohydrate, radiochemically if either reactant is labeled with a radioisotope, or biologically if the antigen exhibits, for example, a toxic or enzymatic activity that can be measured in the soluble fraction before and after precipitation.

Figure 3-2 shows a typical *precipitin curve* that might be obtained with standard solutions of antigen and antibody. In the example shown, 0.1-mL samples of antiserum against hemoglobin are added to increasing amounts of pure hemoglobin in a series of tubes (Figure 3-2a). These mixtures are incubated, and the resulting precipitates are collected by centrifugation and assayed. The supernatant fractions are assayed for the presence of residual antibody and antigen (Figure 3-2b). The amounts of precipitates are then plotted against the amounts of antigen added (Figure 3-2c). The tube in which neither antigen nor antibody is found in the supernatant fraction defines the *equivalence point* of the precipitin curve. This point generally does not

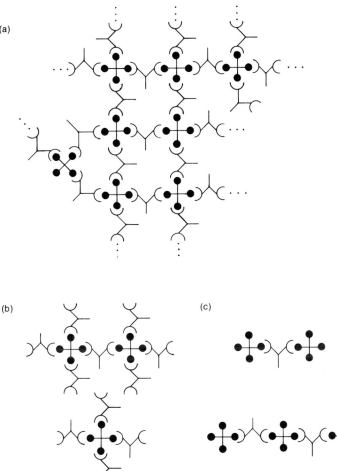

Figure 3-1

Complexes of antibody with antigen. Antigenic determinants are represented as solid circles and the antibody-binding sites that recognize them as open semicircles. (a) Lattice formation near the equivalence point. (b) Soluble complexes in the presence of excess antibody. (c) Soluble complexes in the presence of excess antigen. [Adapted from I. Roitt, *Essential Immunology*, 2nd ed., Blackwell, London, 1974, p. 6.]

correspond to the point of maximum precipitation, which usually occurs at a slight excess of antigen.

Once such a standard curve is prepared, precipitin assays can be used to estimate amounts of the antigen in test samples of unknown concentration. Using the standard antiserum in this example, equivalence is reached when the test sample added contains 40 μg of hemoglobin. Similar assays may be used to compare other serum samples to the standard antiserum; if dilutions of a test serum are added to tubes that each contain 40 μg of hemoglobin, the equivalence point will define the dilution of test serum in which the antibody concentration is the same as in the standard serum.

Ouchterlony double diffusion

Antigen–antibody precipitates can also be observed conveniently by allowing one reactant to diffuse into a gelatinous medium, such as

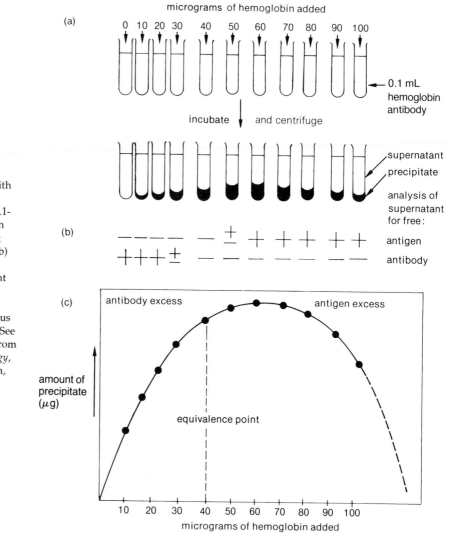

Figure 3-2

A precipitin curve for the reaction of hemoglobin with hemoglobin-specific antiserum. (a) Mixing of 0.1-mL aliquots of hemoglobin antiserum with increasing amounts of hemoglobin. (b) Separation of immune precipitate and supernatant fluid by centrifugation. (c) Precipitin curve plotted as amount of precipitate versus amount of antigen added. See text for details. [Adapted from I. Roitt, *Essential Immunology*, 2nd ed., Blackwell, London, 1974, p. 5.]

agar, that contains the other reactant. In the widely used *Ouchterlony double-diffusion* technique, antigen and antibody samples are placed in small wells cut into an agar slab. The antigen and antibody molecules diffuse out of their respective wells into the agar at a rate inversely proportional to their molecular weights if the molecules have no affinity for the agar itself. If an antigen reacts with an antibody, then a line of precipitation (*precipitin line*) will form where the two reactants diffuse together.

A diagram of such a test is shown in Figure 3-3. The antibody is a rabbit antibody against the κ light chain of mouse immunoglobins. The κ light chain is a common element of the three immunoglobulin

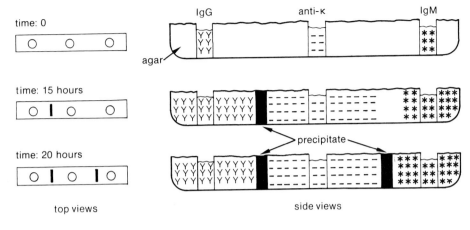

Figure 3-3 Ouchterlony double diffusion in an agar slab. The center well contains antibody against mouse κ chains. The outer wells contain IgM and IgG as antigens, both of which have κ chains that will complex with the antibody. See text for details.

classes IgG, IgA, and IgM (Concept 2-6). IgG and IgM, with molecular weights of 160,000 and 900,000, respectively, are used as test antigens in the experiment. The IgG and the anti-κ antibodies diffuse toward one another at equal rates and form a precipitate near the point at which the antibody and IgG fronts meet. The anti-κ front continues to diffuse and forms a second precipitate when it meets the more slowly diffusing IgM.

If serial dilutions of an antigen—for example, IgG—are tested against anti-κ antibody in this system, the distance between the antigen well and the precipitin line will decrease with decreasing antigen concentration. Because the diffusion gradient of anti-κ is constant, the location of the precipitin line will be determined by the diffusion gradient of the antigen, which will depend on its concentration in the well. Accordingly, this assay can be used to compare antigen concentrations in different samples.

The Ouchterlony technique can be used to determine whether two antigens are different or identical, or whether they share some but not all antigenic determinants. Three such experiments are shown in Figure 3-4.

In Experiment (a), anti-κ antibody forms a single continuous precipitin line against the test antigens IgG and IgM, thereby showing that the two antigen samples cannot be distinguished by this antiserum. This result is called a *reaction of identity*.

In Experiment (b), the antibody well contains a mixture of antibodies against IgG heavy chains (anti-γ) and IgM heavy chains (anti-μ). Because anti-μ precipitates IgM but not IgG, the antibodies migrate through the IgG precipitin line and precipitate IgM on the

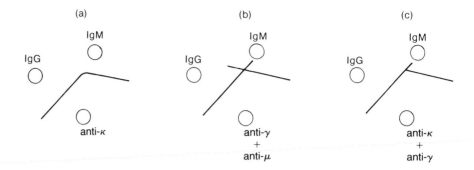

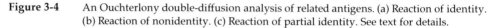

Figure 3-4 An Ouchterlony double-diffusion analysis of related antigens. (a) Reaction of identity. (b) Reaction of nonidentity. (c) Reaction of partial identity. See text for details.

other side. The reverse is true for the anti-γ antibodies, which precipitate IgG but not IgM. The resulting pattern of crossed precipitin lines indicates that the antibodies recognize at least one unique determinant on each of the two antigens. This result is termed a *reaction of nonidentity*.

In Experiment (c), the antibody well contains a mixture of anti-κ and anti-γ antibodies. The anti-κ precipitates both IgG and IgM, forming a continuous precipitin line. The anti-γ, however, migrates through the IgM zone to precipitate IgG behind it, thereby forming a spur. This result indicates that the antibody recognizes determinants in the left antigen well that are not present in the right well. This result is termed a *reaction of partial identity*.

Immunoelectrophoresis

The related technique of *immunoelectrophoresis* provides improved resolution for complex samples by combining electrophoresis of antigens in one dimension with subsequent double diffusion of antibodies and separated antigens in a second dimension. The experimental system is diagrammed in Figure 3-5. In this example, the mixture of antigens to be analyzed is whole serum.

Separation of serum components by gel electrophoresis alone is shown in Figure 3-5a. A serum sample is placed in the well near one end of a suitably buffered gel slab, and an electric current is applied across the gel. The various serum components migrate through the gel at rates proportional to their charge/mass ratios. Four major classes of proteins are resolved as distinct components: albumins migrate most rapidly, followed by α, β, and γ globulins. The amount of protein at each point in the gel can be determined by staining and measurement of light absorption (Figure 3-5b). All immunoglobulins are found in the γ- or β-globulin fractions.

An immunoelectrophoresis experiment is illustrated in Figure 3-5c. Four samples of serum are placed in wells near the left side of a

Figure 3-5
Immunoelectrophoresis in an agar slab. (a) Electrophoresis of a sample of whole serum. The sample is placed in a hole in an agarose gel, to which is applied an electric field. The relative migration of the various proteins is illustrated. (b) A quantitative assessment of the amount of protein that migrates across the gel. Four categories of proteins are noted; albumin, α globulins, β globulins, and γ globulins. Most antibodies are γ globulins. (c) Immuno-diffusion. Following electrophoresis, antibodies to serum protein are placed in the horizontal slots, and the antibodies and separated serum proteins diffuse toward each other to form precipitin lines. Antibodies directed against whole serum, which were placed in the center slot, form a large number of precipitin lines with various serum components. Antiserum specific for κ light chains, which was placed in the top slot, reveals only γ globulins that contain κ light chains. Notice that only a single line is formed, demonstrating complete binding of κ-specific antibodies by the first immunoglobulin it meets. Antiserum specific for μ heavy chains, which was placed in the bottom slot, detects γ globulins that contain γ chains. (d) A simplified anti-whole serum pattern, showing the relative positions of IgG, IgM, and IgA.

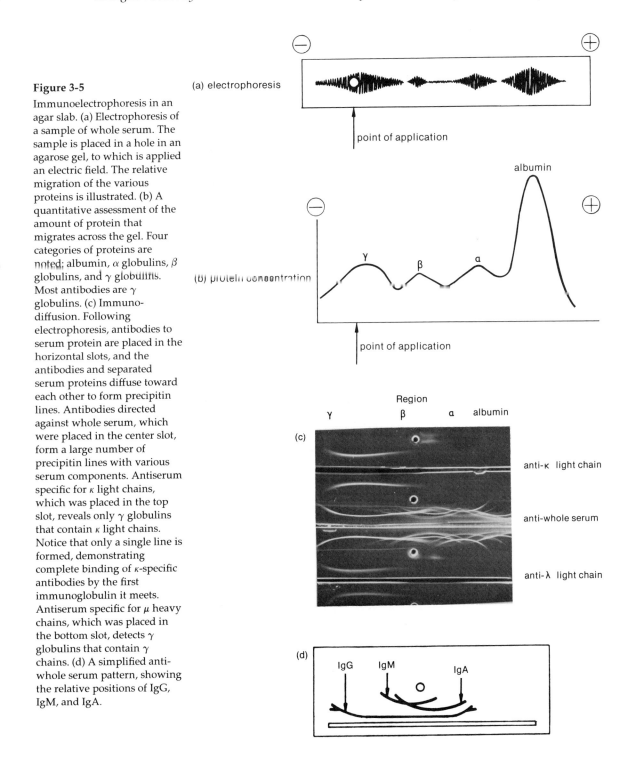

large gel slab and are subjected to electrophoresis in parallel. Slots are then cut into the gel parallel to the direction of electrophoresis and filled with various test antibody preparations. The antibodies and the separated antigenic components diffuse toward each other through the gel and form precipitin lines that indicate which of the antigenic serum components are reactive with the various antibodies. An idealized drawing of the precipitin lines that would be obtained with IgM, IgG, and IgA as antigens with antibody against whole serum is shown in Figure 3-5d. The spurs on the IgG precipitin line are due to the different subclasses of IgG antibody. The analysis of such patterns is considered further in Problem 3-6.

3-2 Antigen–antibody complexes can be detected by direct labeling of either component or by indirect methods

Assays with labeled antigen

Many analytical techniques involving antibodies require detection or quantitation of antibody–antigen complexes under conditions where a precipitate either will not form or will be present in amounts too small to be seen directly. One approach to detecting such complexes is to label the antigen, usually radioactively, react it with antibody, precipitate both free and complexed antibody under conditions that will not precipitate free antigen, and then measure the bound radioactive antigen in the precipitate.

The *Farr assay* employs 50% ammonium sulfate, which precipitates most immunoglobulins, but not haptens and many proteins. Figure 3-6a shows the results of a typical Farr assay with antiserum against the hapten *digoxin*, a drug that is commonly used to regulate the heart action of cardiac disease patients. For convenience, the hapten is labeled radioactively. Tests with a constant amount of the hapten in increasing dilutions of antiserum define the antibody concentration sufficient to precipitate 50% of the hapten under these conditions. Once such a standard curve is available, it can be used to compare the digoxin-specific antibody titer of other serum samples relative to that of the standard.

Precipitation can also be carried out with an immunoglobulin-specific antibody from another species (*heterologous anti-immunoglobulin*), often referred to as a secondary antibody. For example, if the specific antibody used for antigen–antibody complex formation is from a rabbit, it can be precipitated by a goat antibody specific for rabbit immunoglobulin, added at a concentration that gives maximum precipitation.

The preceding techniques can also be used to measure competitive binding for *quantitative radioimmunoassay* of a known antigen in the presence of many other components. An example is the clinically important method used to monitor serum levels of digoxin. Monitor-

Figure 3-6

(a) Measurement of antibody–hapten complex formation using the Farr assay. A standard amount of labeled digoxin (Dg^*) is added to each of a series of twofold dilutions of digoxin-specific antiserum. After several hours, free antibody and antibody–hapten complex are precipitated by bringing the solution to 50% saturation with ammonium sulfate. The percentage of radioactivity in the precipitate is then plotted against serum dilution. (b) A competitive radioimmunoassay using the Farr technique. The serum dilution that gives approximately 70% precipitation in (a) is added to a series of tubes that contain the standard amount of labeled digoxin and varying concentrations (0.4 to 6 ng/mL) of unlabeled digoxin. A standard curve is prepared by plotting the ratio of bound to free labeled digoxin against nanograms of unlabeled digoxin added. This standard curve can then be used to determine the concentration of unlabeled digoxin in samples of patient's serum. Current radioimmunoassays for digoxin use dextran-coated charcoal particles, which will bind free but not antibody-bound digoxin.

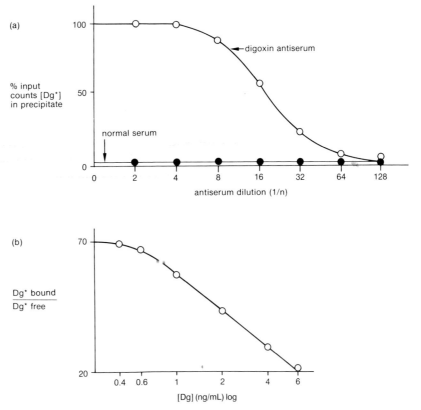

ing is crucial because the drug is highly toxic at levels not far above the therapeutic serum concentration. For the assay, radiolabeled digoxin is incubated with sufficient digoxin-specific antibody to precipitate 70–90% of the radioactivity in the Farr assay. A standard curve is then prepared by adding known amounts of unlabeled digoxin to the incubation mixture and measuring the decrease of radioactivity in the precipitate due to competition between labeled and unlabeled antigen for the antibody-binding sites (Figure 3-6b). Samples of serum from patients receiving digoxin can then be added to the assay mixture, and their digoxin content can be estimated from the observed decrease in bound radioactivity using the standard curve.

Research applications of antibodies often require identification or characterization of cognate antigens in complex mixtures, such as cell extracts. Immunoprecipitation with immunoglobulin-specific heterologous antibody allows separation of these antigens from other components of the mixture. If all components of the mixture are radioactively labeled, then the labeled precipitated antigens can be characterized by various microanalytical techniques, such as electrophoresis on calibrated polyacrylamide gels in the presence of the detergent sodium dodecyl sulfate (SDS) to estimate molecular weights.

Immunoprecipitation is used not only analytically, but also as a highly specific preparative technique. Antibody specific for one component in a complex mixture can be used to precipitate the component either directly, using ammonium sulfate, or indirectly, using an appropriate heterologous anti-immunoglobulin. The purified component can then be eluted from the precipitate, often by treatment with a competing hapten, a protein denaturant, or a buffer of low pH.

Assays with labeled antibody

In situations where a single, pure antibody species is available, such as a myeloma immunoglobulin or a monoclonal antibody, labeling of the antibody provides a convenient means for detecting or quantitating separated antigen–antibody complexes.

The antibody can be radioactively labeled either by culturing the cells that produce it in the presence of radioactive amino acids or by a nondestructive chemical reaction of the antibody with a radioactive ligand, such as ^{125}I, which adds to tyrosine side chains.

A radioactive antibody can be used to quantitate antigen–antibody complexes only if the procedure allows separation of complexes from free antibody. One method commonly referred to as *Western blotting* accomplishes this separation by immobilizing the antigen on a filter. This method also allows identification of a cognate protein antigen in a complex mixture of proteins. The components of the mixture are first denatured and electrophoretically separated on a thin polyacrylamide slab gel in the presence of SDS. The proteins are electrophoretically transferred from the gel to a nitrocellulose sheet, which is then incubated with antibody. Alternatively, the gel is dried onto a filter paper sheet and incubated with antibody directly. After being washed to remove free antibody, the gel or replica is dried, and the protein bands that reacted with antibody are made visible by autoradiography (Figure 3-7a). This method detects only antigenic determinants that are common to both the denatured and native forms of the proteins, such as covalently attached carbohydrate groups or determinants that are destroyed by denaturation but renature during the incubation with antibody.

As an alternative to radioactive labeling, antibodies can often be coupled to active enzymes that catalyze conversion of a soluble specific reagent to an insoluble product, which can be used to detect the presence of the antibody. For example, if a peroxidase-coupled antibody were used in a gel-replica experiment such as the one described in the preceding paragraph, the antigenic components that reacted to form antigen–antibody complexes could be made visible by treating the replica with hydrogen peroxide and a reagent, such as 3-diaminobenzidine, which forms an insoluble black precipitate in the vicinity of antibody-bound peroxidase (Figure 3-7b).

As another alternative, antibody can be labeled with a fluorescent ligand and either detected by exposure to light of an appropriate excitatory wavelength or quantitatively assayed in a fluorimeter. Fluores-

Figure 3-7

Immobilized antigens after electrophoretic separation. In this experiment thymus cells expressing allelic forms of the cell-surface glycoprotein, Thy-1, were lysed in a detergent (1% NP40) buffer, and the solubilized proteins were denatured in 1% sodium dodecyl sulfate at 100° before electrophoresis through polyacrylamide gels. Following electrophoresis the proteins were electrophoretically transferred from the gels to a sheet of nitrocellulose. Unoccupied regions of the nitrocellulose were then saturated with a protein-rich blocking reagent, and longitudinal strips of the nitrocellulose were cut out for incubation with antibodies and a radioactive marker for bound antibodies, [125]I Staphyloccus Cowan strain protein A. The bound ^{125}I protein A was revealed by autoradiography on sensitive X-ray film. The

two prototype mouse strains are listed as A (AKR/J=Thy-1.1) and C (C57BL/6J=Thy-1.2). Rabbit antibodies 86, 88, and 90 were raised by immunization with synthetic polypeptide antigens. Antibody 86 is directed against a 20 amino acid stretch shared by both Thy-1.1 and Thy-1.2 strains. Antibody 88 was raised against a 19 amino acid stretch containing a single amino acid difference from the immunogen used to raise antibody 90; antibody 88 binds to the peptide representing Thy-1.2 molecules, while antibody 90 binds to the Thy-1.1 synthetic peptide. Antibody 88 shows nearly absolute preference for Thy-1.2 cellular glycoproteins, while antibody 90 shows a significant preference for Thy-1.1 glycoproteins. [From Alexander, H., Johnson, D.A., Rosen, J., Jerabek, L., Green, N., Weissman, I. L., and Lerner, R. A. "Mimicking the

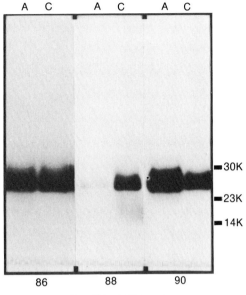

antipeptide antiserum

Alloantigenicity of Proteins with Chemically Synthesized Peptides Differing in Single Amino Acids." *Nature* **306**, 697, (1983).]

cent antibodies are especially useful for visualization of particular antigens in cells by microscopy. Preparation and use of these antibodies are described under Concept 3-5.

Indirect assay methods In the frequently encountered situations where labeling of neither the antigen nor the antibody is convenient, antigen–antibody complexes can often be detected using indirect methods that exploit a secondary antibody. These methods require separation of complexes from free primary antibody by one of the techniques described previously. The secondary antibody, a labeled immunoglobulin-specific heterologous antibody that will bind to the primary antibody, is then added, allowed to react, and again treated to separate complexes from unbound antibody. To allow detection and quantitation, the secondary antibody can be labeled as described previously by isotopes, coupled enzymes, or fluorescent ligands.

An even less direct but sometimes more convenient variation that takes advantage of antibody bivalence is the *enzyme–antienzyme method*. The most commonly used version, peroxidase–antiperoxidase, exploits the finding that antibodies to horseradish peroxidase will bind the enzyme tightly without inactivating it. As an example of this method, a mixture of components containing an antigen to be detected might be separated by gel electrophoresis, replicated onto nitrocellulose, treated with a rabbit primary antibody, and then washed free of unreacted antibody (Figure 3-8a). The bound antibody then would be detected first by incubating with excess secondary rabbit-specific goat antibody followed by washing (Figure 3-8b); second, by incubating with peroxidase-specific rabbit antibody, which complexes with free antigen-binding sites of the secondary antibody (Figure 3-8c); third, by incubating with peroxidase, which complexes to the bound peroxidase-specific antibody (Figure 3-8d); and finally, by incubating with a soluble peroxide reagent that forms a visible precipitate in the region of the bound enzyme (Figure 3-8e). This method is convenient because it does not require preparation of chemically modified antibodies.

3-3   The interaction between antigens and antibodies can be described algebraically

Measurement of antigen–antibody affinity

The affinity of antibody-binding sites for cognate monovalent antigens varies widely. Binding can be described by Equation 3-1:

$$\text{Ag} + \text{Ab} \underset{k_2}{\overset{k_1}{\rightleftharpoons}} \text{Ag} - \text{Ab} \tag{3-1}$$

in which Ag, Ab, and Ag–Ab represent unbound antigenic determinants, antibody-binding sites, and bound antigenic determinants, respectively, and k_1 and k_2 are rate constants for the association and dissociation reactions, respectively. The antigen–antibody *affinity* in such a reaction can be measured as the ratio of complexed to free reactants at equilibrium. The affinity constant K is defined by Equation 3-2:

$$K = \frac{[\text{Ag–Ab}]}{[\text{Ag}][\text{Ab}]} \tag{3-2}$$

K also is equal to k_1/k_2. Because K is an *association* constant, its value will be high for high-affinity complexes and low for low-affinity complexes. Typical K values vary from 10^5 to 10^{11} liters/mole.

Like any equilibrium constant, K is related to the standard free energy change of the binding reaction by Equation 3-3:

$$\Delta G'_0 = -RT \ln K \tag{3-3}$$

in which $\Delta G'_0$ is the standard free energy change in kilocalories per mole at pH 7, R is the gas constant (0.00198 kcal/mole/degree), and T is the absolute temperature.

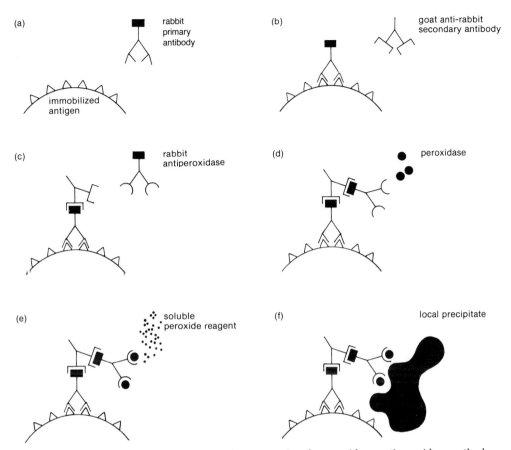

Figure 3-8   Detection of an immobilized antigen using the peroxidase–antiperoxidase method.

The affinity of an antibody-binding site for a monovalent hapten can be measured by *equilibrium dialysis* (Figure 3-9). A concentrated solution of antibody in a dialysis sac, which is permeable to hapten but not to antibodies, is placed in a known volume of buffer that contains hapten at a concentration in the range of $1/K$. At equilibrium, the concentrations of bound plus free hapten inside the sac [I] and free hapten outside the sac [O] will depend on the concentration and average affinity of the antibodies inside the sac.

Using equilibrium dialysis, one can determine both the average association constant K and the antibody valence n from the relationship described by Equation 3-4:

$$\frac{r}{c} = Kn - Kr \tag{3-4}$$

in which r is the ratio of moles of hapten bound per mole of antibody and c is the concentration of unbound hapten ($=$[O]). The moles of

Figure 3-9

Equilibrium dialysis. A concentrated solution of antibodies against a hapten (•) is placed in a sac of dialysis tubing, which is permeable to the hapten but not to the antibodies, and the sac is suspended in a known volume of hapten solution. When the system reaches equilibrium, the concentration of free hapten will be the same throughout, but the sac will contain bound hapten as well. The difference in total hapten concentration inside and outside the sac can be measured and used to calculate the average affinity of the antibodies for the hapten. See text for details.

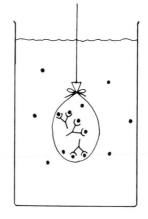

hapten bound are determined by subtracting [O] from [I]. Since Kn is a constant, a plot of r/c versus r for different hapten concentrations will approximate a straight line with slope $-K$, so that the association constant K can be determined as the negative of the slope and the antibody valence as the r intercept at infinite hapten concentration.

Avidity of multivalent antigen–antibody binding

Binding of antibody to a typical multivalent antigen is not as easily defined as binding to a monovalent hapten. Because several different affinities may be involved, the term *avidity* is used to designate the strength of multivalent antigen binding. The kinetics of such binding are complex because binding of one antigenic determinant affects the rates of binding of others on the same molecule. The net avidity of an antibody–multivalent antigen interaction is a complex function of the valences of both reactants and the affinities of the various determinants involved.

3-4 Binding of antibodies to cell-surface antigens can be detected by cell agglutination or complement-mediated lysis

Cell agglutination assays

Cells can be agglutinated by cross-linking with antibodies. Cell agglutination is the basis for several widely used assays. An agglutination assay is commonly used for the typing of human blood. Human red blood cells may carry the cell-surface antigens A and B, which define the well-known blood groups, AB, A, B, and O (Concept 5-3). If, for example, antibody specific for group A antigens is reacted with red cells that carry group A antigens, the resulting agglutination visibly alters the normal settling pattern of the cells in a test tube or in a well of a test tray (Figure 3-10). If the cells do not carry group A antigens,

Figure 3-10

The red-cell agglutination assay for typing of human blood groups. (a) At the microscopic level, divalent anti-A antibodies cross-link red cells that carry A antigen to form a lattice of agglutinated cells. (b) Agglutination affects the settling pattern of cells in a test tube or in the well of a test tray. Antibodies, like many proteins, adhere strongly to certain plastic and glass surfaces. The combination of surface-bound antibodies reacting with overlying red blood cells and the intercellular lattice shown in (a) prevents the free settling of the red cells to the bottom of the well. The property of antibody or antigen adherence to the surface of plastic or glass assay wells can be used for various solid phase immunoassays. (c) This effect can be exploited to type blood cells for A antigen using a tray test with several dilutions of anti-A serum.

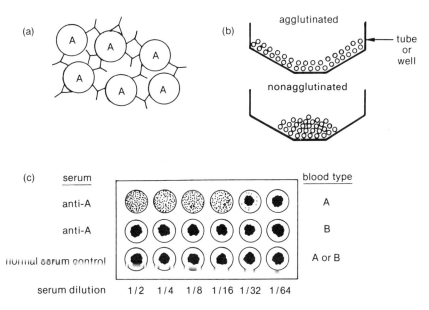

then no agglutination is observed. Type A and type B blood cells are identified as being agglutinated only by A-specific and B-specific antibodies, respectively. Type AB cells are agglutinated by both specific antibodies, and type O cells by neither. Thus all four blood types can be identified by these simple tests. Knowledge of blood types allows transfusions to be made only with serologically compatible blood, thereby avoiding induction of agglutinating antibodies in the recipient.

The cell-agglutination technique can be used to assay antibodies specific for antigens that either are normally present on a cell surface or can be coupled artificially to a cell surface. Coupling can be accomplished by treating red cells to promote electrostatic binding of proteins to their surfaces or by chemically cross-linking antigens to red cells. Appropriate dilutions of the unknown antibody sample are incubated with the antigen-bearing test cells, and the antibody concentration (titer) is determined by comparing the resulting agglutination responses to those obtained with a standard antibody sample of known titer.

The sensitivity of the agglutination reaction with antibody can be increased markedly by incubation with an immunoglobulin-specific heterologous antibody. This technique, known as the *Coombs test*, is particularly useful when agglutination by the first antibody is inefficient; nonagglutinated cells that have bound the first antibody will be agglutinated by the second (Figure 3-11).

Competitive inhibition of cell-agglutination reactions can be used to assay free antigens identical to those on the surface of a target cell. For example, if an agglutination reaction is set up with an amount of

Figure 3-11

Use of an immunoglobulin-specific heterologous antibody to agglutinate cells complexed with a nonagglutinating antibody. Some antibodies that bind to the cell surface are ineffective in promoting agglutination (Step 1). If secondary antibodies directed against the primary antibodies are then added, agglutination occurs (Step 2). This technique, called the *Coombs test*, is often used in clinical laboratories to detect cell-surface antigens.

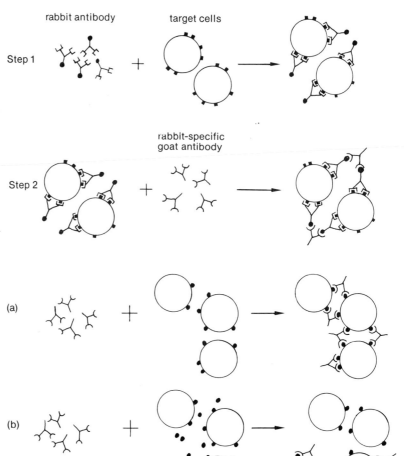

Figure 3-12

Competitive inhibition between cell-bound and free antigens. (a) Cells are agglutinated by antibodies against a cell-bound antigen. (b) Cells are not agglutinated when competing free antigen is present.

Figure 3-13

Complement-mediated cell lysis as an assay for antibody binding to cell-surface antigens. Target cells are preincubated with limiting amounts of antibody (Step 1) and then treated with complement (Step 2), which lyses only cells to which antibody has bound.

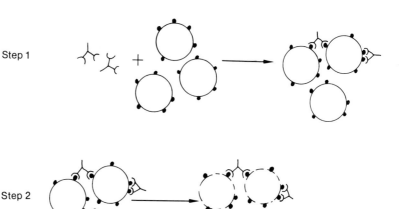

antibody just sufficient to agglutinate visibly, then minute amounts of competing free antigen in test samples can be detected by preincubating with the antibody and testing for inhibition of agglutination (Figure 3-12).

Assays using complement-mediated cell lysis

Cells that carry antibodies bound to cell-surface antigens may be lysed by complement. Complement refers to the set of serum proteins that are activated in a cascade of proteolytic reactions when the first component, C1q, binds to antigen–antibody complexes involving IgM and some IgG subclasses. When a complement-activating antibody binds to a cell-surface antigen, the terminal steps of the complement reaction lead to the lysis of the cell by interrupting the integrity of the cell membrane (Concept 9-2). Because several steps in the sequence are specific proteolytic cleavages, complement is consumed in the reaction. The ability of the terminal steps in the complement sequence to lyse target cells is the basis for a number of widely used assays for antigen–antibody reactions. Guinea pig serum is a commonly used source of complement.

Complement-mediated lysis of target cells, usually red blood cells, can be measured in a variety of ways. Lysis can be followed directly by decrease in optical density of a cell suspension, or by release of cell components, such as hemoglobin, enzymes, or a previously introduced isotope such as ^{51}Cr. Alternatively, loss of membrane integrity can be followed by failure to exclude vital dyes such as trypan blue or eosin, or by failure to concentrate compounds such as fluorescein diacetate that are converted to fluorescent derivatives (fluorescein in this example) by intracellular enzymes.

Complement-mediated lysis can be used as an assay for antibodies specific for antigens on the surface of target cells. As in the agglutination assays, these antigens may be either intrinsic membrane components or coupled artificially to target cells. In the assay, a sample to be tested for antibody is incubated with antigen-bearing target cells; complement then is added, and cell lysis or membrane disruption is measured (Figure 3-13, Step 1). If antibody is limiting, the degree of lysis will be a function of the sample's antibody concentration, which can be determined by comparison with a previously prepared standard curve that relates degree of lysis to a known antibody concentration.

The foregoing procedure can detect only antibodies of the complement-activating classes of immunoglobulins: IgM and some IgG subclasses. Nonactivating antibodies can be detected by including an additional step. Following incubation with the test antibody sample and before the addition of complement, the cells are incubated further with an immunoglobulin-specific heterologous antibody of a complement-activating class. Cell-bound test antibodies will in turn bind the heterologous antibody to produce complexes that will trigger complement-mediated cell lysis (Figure 3-13, Step 2).

Figure 3-14

The Jerne plaque assay for antibody-producing cells. In the example shown, spleen cells from a mouse immunized with Dnp coupled to a carrier protein are mixed with melted agar and enough red blood cells bearing coupled Dnp groups to give a continuous lawn of cells when poured onto an agar plate. (a) Dnp-specific plasma cells among the spleen cells continue to produce Dnp-specific antibodies, which bind to surrounding red blood cells. (b) When complement is added, these cells lyse to form a plaque, which indicates the presence of a plasma cell making Dnp-specific antibodies. (c) A photomicrograph of two plaques. The assay provides a convenient method for quantitating antigen-specific plasma cells produced in an immune response.

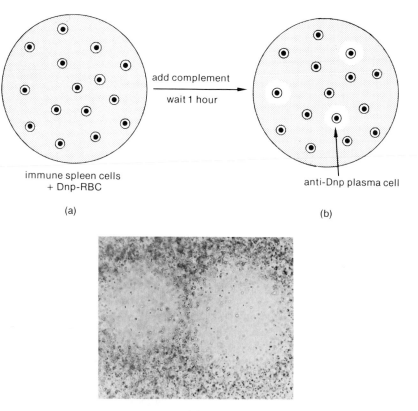

immune spleen cells
+ Dnp-RBC

(a)

add complement

wait 1 hour

anti-Dnp plasma cell

(b)

(c)

Complement-mediated lysis also can be used as an assay for lymphoid cells that produce antibodies specific to a cell-surface antigen (the *Jerne plaque assay*). An excess of red blood cells bearing the target antigen is mixed with a suspension of the lymphoid cells to be assayed, plated as a monolayer on a suitable surface, and incubated to allow plasma cells to release their immunoglobulins (Figure 3-14). The monolayer then is overlaid with complement, which creates a zone of red-cell lysis (a plaque) around any plasma cell that has secreted specific antibody (Figure 3-14b,c). The number of antibody-producing cells in the suspension will thus be indicated by the number of plaques observed in the monolayer. Cells producing antibodies that do not activate complement can also be assayed by treating the monolayer of red cells and lymphoid cells with an appropriate immunoglobulin-specific heterologous antibody prior to addition of complement. Specificity of the assay may be validated by demonstrating that preincubation of the lymphoid cell suspension with a free form of the target antigen prevents subsequent plaque formation. In addition, estimates of relative antigen–antibody avidity may be obtained by adding varying amounts of a competing soluble antigen to the test dish.

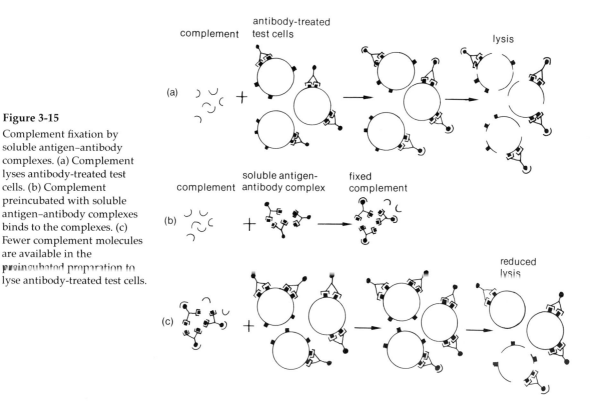

Figure 3-15

Complement fixation by soluble antigen–antibody complexes. (a) Complement lyses antibody-treated test cells. (b) Complement preincubated with soluble antigen–antibody complexes binds to the complexes. (c) Fewer complement molecules are available in the preincubated preparation to lyse antibody-treated test cells.

Any complex of a soluble antigen with a complement-activating antibody can be assayed by the technique of *complement fixation*. This assay is based on the principle that complement that has been activated (fixed) by soluble antigen–antibody complexes will be unavailable for subsequent complement-mediated cell lysis. A limiting amount of complement, known to cause lysis of a certain number of red blood cells treated with red blood cell-specific antibody, is incubated with the test antigen and a sample of the antibody preparation to be assayed. The mixture is then added to a suspension of antibody-treated red blood cells, and its capacity to cause lysis is assayed. Given appropriate controls to show that the test antigen alone does not affect complement activity, reduced red-blood-cell lysis indicates the presence of antibody specific for the test antigen in the sample assayed (Figure 3-15). The titer of this antibody can be determined quantitatively by comparison with an appropriate standard curve prepared using specific antibody of known titer.

An important clinical procedure is the assay of complement levels in human serum by determining the ability of serum samples to mediate lysis of red blood cells treated with specific antibodies. A sudden drop in serum complement activity usually indicates complement activation *in vivo*, presumably as the result of antigen–antibody reactions. In patients with some immunological diseases, a fall in complement activity usually heralds an immunologic crisis.

3-5   Cellular antigens can be detected directly by microscopy using specific labeled antibodies

All the methods described in Concept 3-2 for detecting immobilized antigens can be used in conjunction with microscopy to determine the presence of endogenous antigens in cell and tissue preparations. These methods—using specific antibodies labeled with fluorescent ligands, radioisotopes, covalently attached enzymes, or electron-opaque markers—provide powerful techniques both for determining the locations of antigenic structural components in basic research on cell and tissue ultrastructure and for identifying characteristic disease-related antigens in clinical diagnosis.

Fluorescent compounds (fluorochromes), such as fluorescein and rhodamine, can be coupled chemically to antibodies without affecting antigen binding. When illuminated with light of an appropriate wavelength, the antibody-bound fluorochrome absorbs light energy, attains an excited state, and then returns to its ground state by emitting light at a characteristic longer wavelength. Fluorescein is excited at 490 nm and emits at 517 nm to give a yellow-green fluorescence. Rhodamine is excited at 515 nm and emits at 546 nm to give a red fluorescence. A fluorescence microscope equipped with the appropriate excitatory light source and filters allows visualization of fluorochrome-labeled antibodies bound specifically to cells and tissues (Figure 3-16a). The presence of two different antigens can be monitored simultaneously using two specific antibodies labeled with fluorochromes that fluoresce at different wavelengths. Additional fluorochromes with distinctive absorption-emission spectra allow an even greater sampling of multiple antigens in a single specimen.

Antibodies also can be labeled radioisotopically without destroying their abilities to bind antigen. A common technique is chemical or enzyme-catalyzed iodination of tyrosine side chains on the antibody molecule, using either of two radioactive isotopes of iodine, ^{125}I or ^{131}I. Both these isotopes are γ emitters whose presence can be detected in a gamma counter. Both isotopes also emit short-range ionizing particles (Auger electrons and β particles, respectively), which can be detected photographically by *autoradiography* (also known as radioautography), taking advantage of the capacity of the emitted ionizing radiation to expose a photographic emulsion locally. If antigen-bearing cells are exposed to a specific labeled antibody and then washed to remove unbound molecules, gamma counting allows precise quantitation of the amount of antibody taken up by the cell population. Autoradiography provides additional information. If the treated cells

Figure 3-16
The direct visualization of antibody–antigen complexes. (a) Immunofluorescence identification of T lymphocytes in a lymph-node B-cell region [photograph by G. Gutman]. (b) Autoradiography of a lymphocyte with ^{125}I-bound antibody [photograph by G. Edelman].

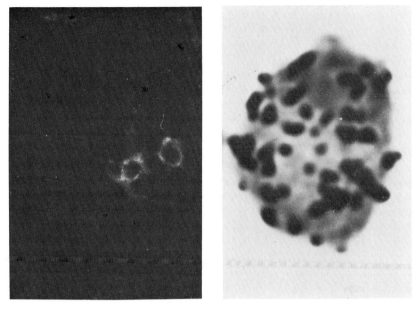

(a)   (b)

are spread on a suitable surface, covered with a photographic emulsion, and stored in the dark to allow exposure to the emitted ionizing radiation, then silver grains will appear on the developed film as an "autograph" that indicates the locations of bound antibodies. In this manner the distribution and number of antibody molecules bound to individual cells in the population can be determined (Figure 3-16b). The same technique can be used to determine the locations of specific antigenic structures in a tissue.

Enzymes that catalyze the formation of a microscopically visible product can be coupled to antibodies using bifunctional cross-linking reagents without destroying the activity of the enzyme or the antibody. For example, horseradish peroxidase coupled to a specific antibody and bound to a specific cell or tissue site will convert added hydrogen peroxide to oxygen-free radicals. These radicals can in turn react with a chromogenic precursor, such as 3,3′-diaminobenzidine or 4-chloro-1-naphthol, added with the peroxide to form an insoluble colored precipitate (Figure 3-17).

Antibodies can be made visible in the electron microscope by coupling to electron-dense or morphologically distinguishable particles. Antibodies coupled to ferritin, an iron storage protein from the spleen that consists of a protein shell with a ferric hydroxide core, are seen in the electron microscope as small dense spots (Figure 3-18). Antibodies can also be linked to hemocyanin, a large oxygen-carrying protein complex from crustacean hemolymph, to latex microspheres,

Figure 3-17
Horseradish peroxidase-coupled antibody to human secretory component reveals the subcellular locations of molecules of secretory component to be the perinuclear space (PNS), the plasma membrane, and the rough endoplasmic reticulum (RER) of human small intestinal epithelial cells (N, nucleus; BM, basement membrane). [Courtesy of W. R. Brown, Y. Isobe, and P. Nakane.]

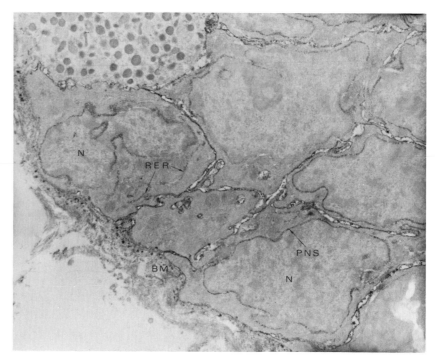

to small viruses, or to colloidal gold particles—all of which can be recognized by their characteristic appearance in electron micrographs.

Each of the four preceding techniques can be extended by indirect methods, which allow detection of unlabeled antibodies bound to a specific antigen by subsequent reaction with a labeled immunoglobulin-specific heterologous antibody (Figure 3-19a). Another modification called the *sandwich method* can be used to detect specific antibodies on the surfaces of plasma cells by incubating them, first with a cognate multivalent antigen and then with labeled soluble antibody specific for the same antigen (Figure 3-19b).

3-6   Monoclonal antibodies are powerful reagents for identification and isolation of interesting antigens

Monoclonal antibodies, synthesized by hybridoma cells produced as described in Concept 2-1, offer several advantages over heterogeneous serum antibodies raised by conventional immunization. Because hybridomas are immortal cell lines, unlimited quantities of homogeneous antibody of a defined isotype can be prepared. Appropriate

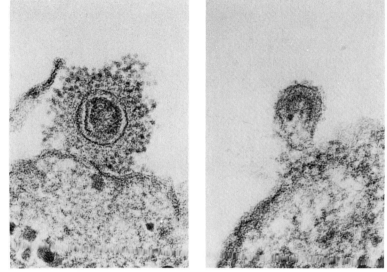

(a)   (b)

Figure 3-18

Ferritin-coupled antibody to mouse leukemia virus antigens used to demonstrate that: (a) a mouse virus carries these antigens; (b) a cat virus does not; (c) these antigens may be expressed on regions of a cell membrane. [From L. Oshiro, J. A. Levy, J. L. Riggs, and E. H. Lennette, *J. Gen. Virol.* **35**, 317(1977), © 1977 by Cambridge University Press.]

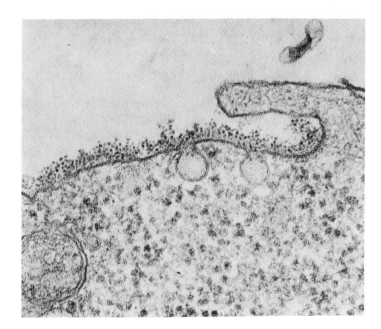

(c)

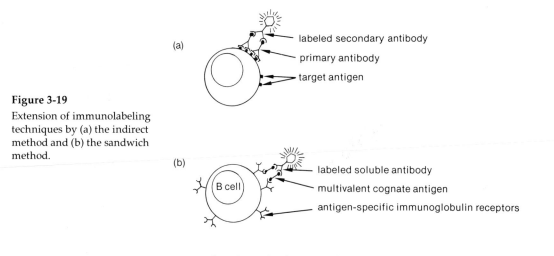

Figure 3-19

Extension of immunolabeling techniques by (a) the indirect method and (b) the sandwich method.

monoclonal antibodies can thus become standard reagents worldwide for specific diagnostic or therapeutic purposes. A mixture of antigens can be used for immunization in the preparation of hybridomas as long as a selective procedure can be devised for isolating clones of hybrid cells that synthesize a desired antibody (Figure 3-20). Therefore, the hybridoma technique is well suited for analysis of complex sets of antigens such as those found on the cell surface. Immunization with the entire set generates a set of hybridomas, each of which when cloned yields a single homogeneous antibody.

Because monoclonal antibodies consist of a single molecular species, their specificity can be far more precisely defined than that of a conventional antiserum. However, because of the phenomenon of multispecificity discussed in Concept 2-4, monoclonal antibodies are *not* monospecific. A monoclonal antibody isolated as reacting with a particular antigen may also react with quite disparate antigens that also bind to it with sufficient affinity. Therefore, caution must be exercised in interpreting evidence for presence of a particular antigen based only on reaction with a single cognate monoclonal antibody.

3-7 The fluorescence-activated cell sorter permits large numbers of cells to be separated on the basis of differences in cell-surface antigens

The fluorescence-activated cell sorter is a recently developed analytical and preparative instrument that can rapidly sort a subset of cells carrying a particular surface antigen from a mixed cell population. Prior to sorting, the cell suspension is reacted with a fluorescein-tagged antibody specific for the cell type of interest (Figure 3-21). The

(a) production of hybridomas

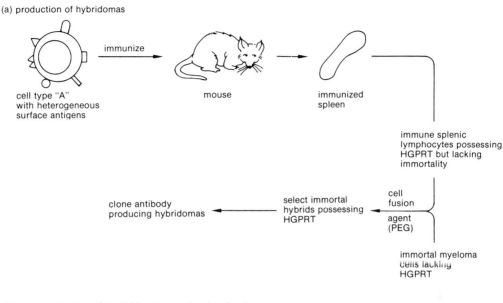

(b) assay for cell-specific hybridoma monoclonal antibodies

Figure 3-20 Production (a) and assay (b) of monoclonal antibodies specific for one of the many cell-surface antigens present on the cells used for immunization.

cells then pass single file through a small orifice that breaks the liquid stream into microdrops, each of which contains no more than one cell. The drops fall through a detector that uses a laser beam to determine by light scattering whether a cell is present in each drop and, if so, whether it carries fluorescent antibody. When used analytically, the cell sorter counts the fraction of reactive cells in the population (Figure 3-22). In the preparative mode, an electrical charge is applied selectively to the fluorescence-positive drops, which then are deflected by an electrical field into a separate receptacle. By this method,

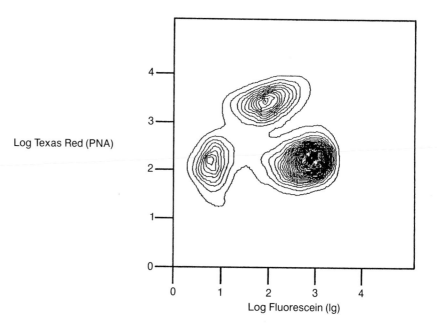

Log Texas Red (PNA)

Log Fluorescein (Ig)

Figure 3-21 Detection of fluorescein-antibody-tagged cells in a fluorescence-activated cell sorter. In this case, cells from lymphoid organs are assayed for their cell-surface expression of surface-accessible galactose residues with the lectin PNA labeled with the new fluorochrome Texas Red, and simultaneously for their expression of surface immunoglobulin with fluoresceinated antibody to mouse immunoglobulin. The cells in the lower left are small T lymphocytes which are PNA^{lo} and surface Ig^{lo}. The cells on top are germinal center B cells which are PNA^{hi} and surface Ig^{mid}. The cells in the lower right are small B cells which are PNA^{lo} and surface Ig^{hi}. The use of a logarithmic scale readout sharpens the distinctions between otherwise overlapping groups of cells. The number of concentric lines, and thus the intensity of each cell grouping, is related to the number of cells in that fluorochrome-determined category. [Provided by G. Kraal, R. Hardy, E. Butcher, and I. Weissman.]

rare subclasses of cells can be isolated as a homogeneous population in quantities suitable for biochemical analysis.

The cell sorter is proving valuable in a variety of applications, both in clinical and fundamental research. For example, it has allowed separation of B cells and T cells into many different subclasses. It has also been used to select rare mutants in a B-cell population. Clinically, it has been used to quantitate specific antigens on leukemic cells in human patients as an aid to distinguishing among different forms of leukemia.

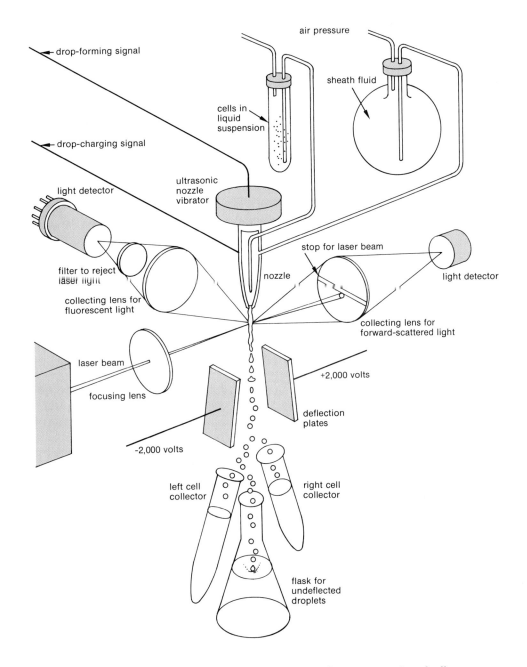

Figure 3-22 Sorting of fluorescein-antibody-tagged cells in a fluorescence-activated cell sorter. [From Leonard A. Herzenberg, Richard G. Sweet, and Leonore A. Herzenberg, "Fluorescence-Activated Cell Sorting," *Sci. Am.* **234,** 112, (1976). Copyright © 1973 by Scientific American, Inc. All rights reserved.]

Selected Bibliography

General

Farr, R. S., "A quantitative immunochemical measure of the primary interaction between I*BSA and antibody," *J. Infect. Dis.* **103**, 239(1958). The classic description of precipitation methods using radiolabel to estimate amounts of antibody and average antibody affinities.

Kabat, E. A., and Mayer, M. M., *Experimental Immunochemistry*, Charles C. Thomas, Springfield, Illinois, 1961. The classic text on antigen–antibody reactions.

Karush, F., "Immunologic specificity and molecular structure," *Adv. Immunol.* **2**, 1(1962).

Landsteiner, K., *The Specificity of Serologic Reactions*, Harvard University Press, Cambridge, Massachusetts, 1945.

Nisonoff, A., and Pressman, D., "Heterogeneity and average combining constants of antibodies from individual rabbits," *J. Immunol.* **80**, 412(1958).

Yalow, R. S., "Radioimmunoassay: a probe for the fine structure of biologic systems," *Science* **200**, 1236(1978).

Immunofluorescence and FACS

Beutner, E. H., "Defined immunofluorescent staining," *Ann. N. Y. Acad. Sci.* **177**, 1(1971). Proceedings of a symposium on the use of immunofluorescent techniques.

Coons, A. H., Creech, H. J., and Jones, R. H., "Immunological properties of an antibody containing a fluorescent group," *Proc. Soc. Exp. Biol. Med.* **47**, 200(1941). An early description of the use of immunofluorescence.

Herzenberg, L. A., Sweet, R. G., and Herzenberg, L. A., "Fluorescence-activated cell sorting," *Sci. Am.* **234**, 108(1976).

Radbruch, A., Liesegang, B., and Rajewsky, K., "Isolation of variants of mouse myeloma ×63 that express changed immunoglobulin class," *Proc. Natl. Acad. Sci. USA* **77**, 2909(1980). Application of immunofluorescence to a challenging immunologic problem.

Schroder, J., Nikinmaa, B., Kavathas, P., and Herzenberg, L. A., "Fluorescence-activated cell sorting of mouse-human hybrid cells aids in locating the gene for the Leu 7(HNK-1) antigen to human chromosome 11," *Proc. Natl. Acad. Sci. USA* **80**, 3421(1983). Using FACS to approach problems in molecular genetics.

Additional concepts and techniques presented in the problems

1. Antibody-antigen precipitation. Problem 3-3.
2. Rocket electrophoresis. Problem 3-4.

Problems

3-1 Indicate whether each of the following statements is true or false. Explain the error in each statement you consider to be false.
(a) Complete immunoprecipitation of an antigen is most nearly achieved by adding antibody in large excess.
(b) The Ouchterlony technique can be used to determine whether two antigens share some but not all determinants.
(c) An antigen that fails to precipitate with a primary rabbit immunoglobulin preparation can often be precipitated by adding secondary antibody produced in the secondary immune response of the animal to the same antigen.
(d) Techniques that identify protein antigens after blotting from denaturing gels following electrophoresis can detect only antigenic determinants that are not irreversibly denatured.

(e) Antigen–antibody affinity is commonly expressed as the dissociation constant of the antigen–antibody complex.

(f) In an equilibrium dialysis experiment to measure affinity of a hapten for a cognate antibody in a dialysis sac, the concentrations of free hapten inside and outside the sac at equilibrium will be equal.

(g) Complement fixation assays depend on consumption of complement during an antigen–antibody reaction.

(h) Monoclonal antibodies are useful reagents because of their unique specificity and uniform affinity for single antigenic determinants.

(i) To produce a monoclonal antibody, immunization must be carried out with a single defined antigen species.

3-2 Supply the missing word or words in each of the following statements.

(a) The _____ reaction can be used to estimate the amount of either antigen or antibody in a test sample.

(b) In the Ouchterlony test, crossed precipitin lines between two adjacent antigen wells indicates a reaction of _____ with antibodies from the antibody well.

(c) The _____ assay takes advantage of the fact that concentrated ammonium sulfate will precipitate most free and complexed antibodies but not free haptens.

(d) Heterologous anti-immunoglobulins are used in many immunochemical procedures as _____ antibodies.

(e) The _____ method for detecting antigens has the advantage that neither the antigen nor the antibodies used need to be chemically modified or radioactively labeled.

(f) The term _____ is used to describe the strength of binding of multivalent antibodies and antigens where several different affinities may be involved.

(g) Any complex of a soluble antigen with a complement-activating antibody can be assayed by the technique of _____ .

(h) Radioactively labeled, fixed antigens or antibodies can be detected by exposure to a photographic emulsion using the technique known as _____ .

(i) _____ coupled to a specific antibody and bound to a specific cell or tissue site will convert added _____ to oxygen-free radicals, which in turn can react with a chromogenic precursor to give an insoluble colored precipitate visible by microscopy.

(j) The fluorescence-activated cell sorter achieves preparative cell separations by selectively applying _____ to microdrops containing fluorescence-positive cells.

3-3 Proteins, although highly immunogenic, also are highly complex and difficult to purify without modern chromatographic techniques. Pioneering immunologists, who needed well-defined antigens to study the nature of antigen–antibody interactions, turned to hapten-carrier conjugates that elicit antibody specific for determinants on both the carrier and the hapten. By attaching the same hapten to several noncrossreactive carriers, one can study the interaction of antibodies with determinants of known conformation.

In one experiment, glucose and galactose were used as haptens. Derivatives of each were coupled to horse globulin or egg albumin. Rabbits were immunized with the glucoglobulin conjugate. The resulting antiserum was tested for its ability to precipitate various conjugates, as given in Table 3-1. In this semi-quantitative assay, the results are recorded as either $-$, $+$, $++$, $+++$, or $++++$ ($-$ indicating no reaction, $+++$ indicating the greatest antigen–antibody precipitate). Although inexact, this system is surprisingly reproducible in the hands of a careful immunologist,

Table 3-1   Precipitin Reactions of Anti-Glucoglobulin Antiserum (Problem 3-3)

Concentration of Antibodies	Hapten–Carrier Antigen		
	Glucoglobulin (Horse)	Gluco + Albumin (Egg)	Galacto + Albumin (Egg)
1:1,000	+ + ±	+ +	−
1:5,000	+ + + +	+ + + +	−
1:10,000	+ + + +	+ + + +	−
1:20,000	+ + + ±	+ + +	−
1:40,000	+ + +	+	−
1:50,000	+	±	−
1:100,000	±	−	−

[From O. Avery and W. Goebel, *J. Exp. Med.* **50**, 531(1930). © 1930 by the Rockefeller University Press.]

Figure 3-23

Rocket electrophoresis (Problem 3-4). Antigen migrates electrophoretically into a gel that contains antibody. The distance from the starting well to the front of the rocket-shaped arc is a function of antigen concentration. [Adapted from I. Roitt, *Essential Immunology*, 2nd ed., Blackwell, London, 1974, p. 105.]

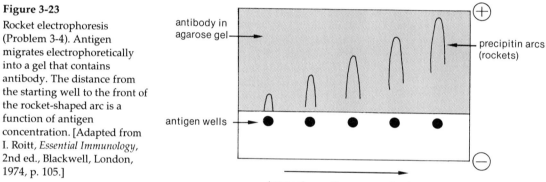

antibody in agarose gel · precipitin arcs (rockets) · antigen wells · increasing antigen concentration

and the difference between + + and + + + + reactions is significant.

(a) How do glucose and galactose differ in their chemical structures? What, then, does Table 3-1 show about the specificity of the antibodies?

(b) If free glucose is added to the rabbit antiserum, no precipitate forms. How can you determine experimentally whether the glucose binds to the antibodies? Why is there no precipitate when glucose is added?

(c) Assume that a specific site on the antibody molecule combines with a specific complementary determinant on the antigen. What are the limits on the number of combining sites per antibody molecule, or determinants per antigen, if a precipitation reaction is to occur?

(d) In Table 3-1, the amount of precipitate increases with increasing antibody concentration, but it suddenly decreases significantly when the 1:1000 dilution of antibody is tested. Can you suggest an explanation for a decrease in the total precipitate when the concentration of antibody is high?

(e) Assume that you are working in an isolated community hospital. On one phone the clinical chemistry lab informs you that it can no longer make chemical analyses of blood sugar, while on the other phone the emergency room assistant tells you that three diabetics found at home in coma are about to arrive. You must determine whether the diabetics are in coma because of too much insulin (low

Figure 3-24

The precipitin pattern in an Ouchterlony test (Problem 3-5). BSA, bovine serum albumin; BGG, bovine gamma globulin; HSA, human serum albumin; Dnp-BSA, Dnp-BGG, and Dnp-HSA designate the same proteins carrying covalently linked haptenic dinitrophenyl groups. The center well contains anti-Dnp-BSA.

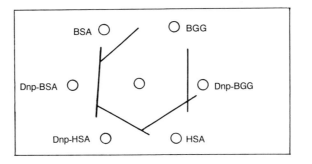

Figure 3-25

The precipitin pattern in an Ouchterlony test (Problem 3-6).

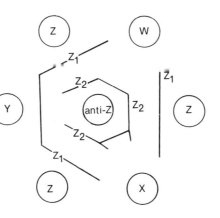

blood glucose) or too little insulin (high blood glucose and acids). You have available only glucose and the reagents defined in Table 3-1. What can you do?

(f) How could you proceed if you had radiolabeled glucose?

3-4 Figure 3-23 illustrates a technique known as *rocket electrophoresis*, in which antigen migrates under the influence of an electric field into a gel that contains antibody. Explain why the positions of precipitin lines vary with antigen concentration as shown in the figure.

3-5 Suppose that an animal is immunized with bovine serum albumin to which 2,4-dinitrophenol has been conjugated (Dnp-BSA). Immune serum is obtained and placed in the center well of an Ouchterlony plate, with antigens in the outer wells as shown in Figure 3-24. Explain the precipitin pattern obtained.

3-6 Suppose that as a physician you carry out the following experiments. You isolate a substance, called Z, from the plasma of a patient with a particular disease. You prepare an antiserum to Z (anti-Z) by injecting the substance repeatedly into a rabbit. You isolate similar substances—call them W, X, and Y—from three other patients suspected of having a disease similar to that of the patient from whom Z was prepared. You prepare an Ouchterlony plate and place the anti-Z antibody in the center well. You arrange antigen preparations W, X, Y, and Z in the antigen wells, as shown in Figure 3-25.

(a) What is the minimum number of antigens present in Z?

(b) How similar are these antigens? Compare preparations W, X, and Y to preparation Z in detail.

(c) Do you conclude that your patients have similar diseases?

3-7   A serum sample is taken from an individual who has just recovered from an unknown disease. This serum neither agglutinates nor precipitates a suspension of bacteria thought to cause the disease or a suspension of membrane fragments from these bacteria. When passively immunized with a transfusion of this serum, patients suffering from this disease recover much more rapidly than those who receive no treatment.
  (a) How can you show that immunoglobulins, and not some other serum proteins, are responsible for the therapeutic effect of the serum?
  (b) How can you determine whether the immunoglobulins in the serum bind to the bacteria thought to cause the disease?

Answers

3-1 (a) False. Precipitation is most complete when antigen and antibody concentrations are roughly equal.
    (b) True
    (c) False. Secondary antibody refers to a heterologous anti-immunoglobulin—that is, an immunoglobulin-specific antibody from another species.
    (d) True
    (e) False. The affinity constant for antigen–antibody complex formation is expressed as an association constant.
    (f) True
    (g) True
    (h) False. Due to the possibility of multispecificity, monoclonal antibodies often are not monospecific.
    (i) False. Immunization can be carried out with a complex mixture of antigens; hybridization and cloning of individual lymphocytes provide hybridomas that each produce a monoclonal antibody directed against one (or more) determinant in the immunizing mixture.

3-2 (a) precipitin
    (b) nonidentity
    (c) Farr
    (d) secondary
    (e) enzyme–antienzyme
    (f) avidity
    (g) complement fixation
    (h) autoradiography
    (i) Peroxidase; hydrogen peroxide (H_2O_2)
    (j) charge

3-3 (a) Glucose and galactose are epimers—that is, stereoisomers that differ only in the orientation of the OH group on Carbon 4. The total lack of cross–reactivity illustrates the exquisite specificity of the immune response.
    (b) You can show that radiolabeled glucose migrates with the antibody molecules through Sephadex columns or acrylamide gels, whereas radiolabeled galactose, the nonspecific hapten, does not. Essentially, each glucose molecule is a single antigenic determinant that can bind to a single antigen-binding site. Therefore, in the presence of glucose, no cross-linking can occur to form macromolecular aggregates or precipitates.
    (c) Both the antibodies and antigens must be at least bivalent for cross–linking and precipitation to occur. Even then, precipitation will not necessarily occur. There

are certain so-called nonprecipitating antibodies, which, for unknown reasons, will not precipitate under any conditions. The IgM molecule has ten antigen-binding sites; IgA has two, four, or six antigen-binding sites; all other immunoglobulins have two antigen-binding sites per molecule. There is no upper limit on the number of sites per antigenic molecule.

(d) In a large excess of antigen, a high proportion of antigen molecules will have only one antibody molecule bound to them. Soluble antigen–antibody complexes are formed (Ag–Ab–Ag), rather than macromolecular aggregates. Consequently the total amount of precipitate decreases.

(e) With the reagents in Table 3-1, you can set up a hapten-competition assay to measure free glucose concentrations, as follows. Using glucoglobulin at 1:20,000, find the highest dilution of antiserum that gives precipitation. Then add measured concentrations of glucose to tubes containing these concentrations of antigen and antiserum, and determine the concentrations of free glucose that reduce precipitation to $+++$, $++$, $+$, and $-$. You now have a standard set of measurements that you can compare with assays of patient serum and urine as sources of free glucose. You hope that the patients will still be alive by the time you get the results.

(f) If you had radiolabeled glucose (and a counter for detecting it), you could determine glucose concentrations with a Farr assay, which is more rapid and more sensitive than the method in part (e). You would first determine the concentration of antiserum that will coprecipitate 70% of added labeled glucose in the presence of 50% ammonium sulfate, and then you would proceed with competition assays using standards and unknowns as in part (e).

3-4 Precipitin lines will become visible only in a region of antigen–antibody equivalence. As each antigen sample electrophoretically migrates into the gel, it forms a gradient of decreasing antigen concentration from the sample well to the migrating front. The concentration near the front decreases as the front moves away from the well and the gradient becomes longer. Precipitin lines form at the point where the concentration at the front reaches the zone of equivalence. Because the antibody concentration is constant, this point will increase in distance from the well as antigen concentration in the well is increased. Ahead of the "rocket," antibody is in excess; in its trail, antigen is in excess.

3-5 The antiserum contains antibodies directed against the antigenic determinants on the native BSA and against the Dnp hapten. The anti-Dnp antibodies react with the Dnp hapten on the Dnp-BGG, Dnp-BSA, and Dnp-HSA. Because some of the antigenic determinants on BSA also are present on HSA, some of the anti-BSA antibodies can cross-react with HSA. The result is a line of partial identity. The Dnp-BSA spur indicates precipitation of Dnp-BSA molecules by antibodies specific for BSA unique determinants. None of the antibodies that could react with HSA fail to react with BSA, so there is only one spur. Similarly, reactions of partial identity are seen in comparing BSA and HSA with Dnp-BSA and Dnp-HSA, respectively. None of the anti-BSA antibodies cross-react with BGG; therefore, there is no precipitin line with this antigen. Both HSA and Dnp-BGG are precipitated, but by different antibodies, so there are overlapping spurs and no line of identity.

3-6 (a) Substance Z contains at least two separate antigenic components, as indicated by the presence of two precipitin lines, which can be called Z_1 and Z_2.

(b) W contains a component that appears antigenically identical to component Z_2; that is, W shows a reaction of identity with Z_2.

X contains a component that shares at least one antigenic determinant with component Z_2, but Z_2 contains at least one antigenic determinant that is nonidentical to those of X. The evidence for partial identity of X and Z_2 is the merging of the X line with the Z_2 line, but the Z_2 line has a spur that overlaps the X line.

Y contains a component that appears antigenically identical to component Z_1; that is, Y shows a reaction of identity with Z_1.

(c) Your information does not permit you to draw any conclusions. All you know is that the substances from the diseased patients have at least one similar antigen. Analysis of a similar control preparation from a healthy individual may indicate whether these substances are related to the disease process.

3-7 (a) To show that immunoglobulins are responsible, you could treat the immune serum with a heterologous anti-immunoglobulin—for example, rabbit anti-human-immunoglobulin—and demonstrate that the serum loses its protective effect as the immunoglobulins are removed. Alternatively, you could purify the immunoglobulin fraction (by ammonium sulfate precipitation, chromatography, starch gel electrophoresis, etc.) and show that the isolated immunoglobulin fraction gives as good or better protection than the whole serum.

(b) To demonstrate that the antibody binds to the bacteria, you could show that treatment of the serum with bacteria will absorb out the protective agent. One such experimental approach would be to attach bacteria to an insoluble matrix and pass the protective serum over a column of this material, called an *immunoabsorbent column*. If the antibodies bind to the bacteria, they should be removed, and the absorbed serum eluted from the column should have lost its protective power.

Another approach would be to use an appropriate heterologous anti-immunoglobulin labeled with a fluorescent dye (e.g., fluorescein). Bacteria would be incubated in the immune serum, washed, and then incubated with the fluorescent-labeled heterologous antibody. If the bacteria are stained specifically by the fluorescent antibody, then human immunoglobulins must be bound to the surface of the cells. The appropriate control to demonstrate specific binding is to incubate the bacteria first in a nonimmune human serum, and then to wash and add the fluorescent antibody. If the bacteria are stained under these conditions, then either the fluorescent antibodies or human immunoglobulins are being absorbed onto the bacteria in some nonspecific manner that would invalidate your results.

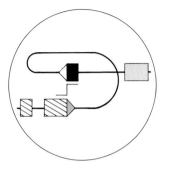

CHAPTER 4

Expression of Antibody Genes

Chapter Outline

Vertebrate immune systems are capable of synthesizing perhaps 10^8 different antibody molecules, which can collectively recognize a virtually unlimited number of antigens. How this vast antibody diversity might be generated has been a principal focus of immunological research. In 1965 Dreyer and Bennett predicted that antibody polypeptides would be encoded by two separate genes that were brought together during the differentiation of B cells. This remarkably prescient suggestion was the first speculation that eukaryotic genes might be "split" and might have to be rearranged for expression. Recent studies using serological, genetic, protein, and recombinant DNA techniques have verified and extended this hypothesis by providing a rather detailed picture of the organization and expression of antibody genes. Rearrangements of antibody genes are a key element in the generation of antibody diversity; moreover, they are associated with certain developmental changes in B-cell differentiation and provide useful insights into the molecular biology of development in a complex eukaryotic system. This chapter considers the organization, rearrangement, and expression of antibody genes.

Concepts

4-1 A precise developmental program generates B-cell clones that express antibody molecules with a single type of antigen-binding site

Antibody-producing cells in the adult differentiate continually along a pathway that has been partially defined by the chemical and serological analyses of expressed immunoglobulins (Figure 4-1). In the first stage, which is not dependent on the presence of antigen, stem cells from the bone marrow give rise to pre-B cells with cytoplasmic μ heavy chains. Later, these cells synthesize either κ or λ light chains and anchor the resulting monomeric IgM molecules in their membranes to serve as receptor molecules to trigger subsequent stages of differentiation and proliferation in response to cognate antigens. Cells at this stage are called virgin B_μ cells. (B cells and their derivatives are usually designated by a subscript that corresponds to the heavy chain of the expressed antibody.) As a population, these cells produce IgM molecules with all the antigen-binding specificities in the organism's repertoire. However, each cell synthesizes IgM molecules with a single type of antigen-binding site. In a process that is not yet well understood, those cells with binding specificities for self-antigens are eliminated or suppressed so that the organism normally does not mount an immune response against itself (see Chapter 10).

Virgin B_μ cells differentiate into mature $B_{\mu+\delta}$ cells, which express on their surface both IgM and IgD molecules with identical V domains and hence identical binding specificities. It is not yet known

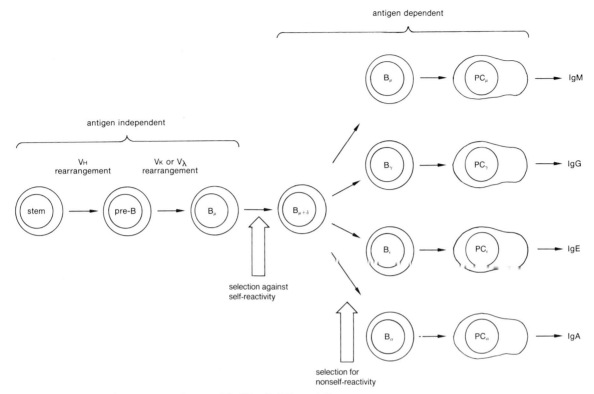

Figure 4-1   One model of B-cell differentiation.

whether this step is dependent on the presence of cognate antigen, but all subsequent steps certainly are. In response to bound antigen, mature $B_{\mu+\delta}$ cells differentiate into large dividing *blast cells* that express simultaneously both membrane-bound and secreted immunoglobulins with the same V domain. The activated B cells or their progeny then go through alternative terminal differentiation pathways to produce short-lived *plasma cells*, which each secrete only one type of antibody molecule, and long-lived *memory cells* for future protection. An activated B cell can give rise to plasma cells that produce antibody of any class or subclass. The process whereby a single B cell or its progeny shifts from the synthesis of one class of immunoglobulin to a second is called *class switching*.

One striking feature of B-cell differentiation is that each B cell may display on its membrane or secrete antibodies with a single type of V domain. For a given B-cell clone, although the antibody class may change during development, the characteristic V domain and the basic antigen-binding specificity remain the same. The light and heavy chains that comprise the V domain are synthesized from a single light-chain gene and a single heavy-chain gene. In an animal heterozygous for genetic markers on light and heavy chains, it can be clearly demonstrated that an individual B-cell clone expresses only one light-chain and one heavy-chain allele. This phenomenon is known as *allelic exclusion*. The maintenance of a single V domain and the other features of B-cell differentiation pose a series of fascinating questions concerning the regulation and expression of antibody genes.

4-2   Mammalian antibodies are encoded by three unlinked clusters of genes

Allotypes, isotypes, idiotypes

Genetic analysis of antibody genes has been carried out in mice, rabbits, and humans, using serologic reagents to follow the inheritance of distinctive antigenic markers on immunoglobulin molecules. These antigenic markers are of three types: allotypes, isotypes, and idiotypes. *Allotypes* are antigenic determinants that characterize the light or heavy chains from different forms of the same gene (alleles). Allotypes have been found on λ light chains in rabbits, on κ light chains in rabbits and humans, and on heavy chains in mice, rabbits, and humans (Table 4-1). Allotypic differences generally are localized

Table 4-1   Allotypes of Human, Mouse, and Rabbit[a]

Immunoglobulin Family	Alleles
	Human
κ	Inv(1), Inv(1,2), Inv(3)
λ	none identified
Heavy	
G1	Gm1, Gm(non-1); *Footnote b* Gm3, Gm17; *Footnote b* Gm2, 18, 20; *Footnote c*
G2	Gm23, Gm(non-23); *Footnote b*
G3	Gm21, Gm(non-21); *Footnote b* Gm5, Gm(non-5); *Footnote b* Gm11, Gm(non-11) Gm6, 10, 14, 15, 16, 24, 25; *Footnote c*
G4	Gm(4a) Gm(4b); *Footnote b*
A1	none identified
A2	Am(1), Am(−1); *Footnote b*
D	none identified
M	none identified
E	none identified

Immunoglobulin Family	Alleles
Mouse	
κ	none identified
λ	none identified
Heavy	
G1	$4^{a,c,d,e,f,g,h}$; 4^{b}; *Footnote d*
G2a	1^{a}, 1^{b}, 1^{c}, 1^{d}, 1^{e} 1^{f}, 1^{g}, 1^{h}
G2b	$3^{a,c,h}$, 3^{b}, 3^{d}, 3^{e}, 3^{f}, 3^{g}
G3	none identified
A	$2^{a,h}$, 2^{b}, $2^{c,g}$, $2^{d,e}$, 2^{f}
D	5^{a}, 5^{b}
M	6^{a}, 6^{b}
Rabbit	
κ	b4, b5, b6, b9
λ	c7, c21
Heavy	
V_H	a1, a2, a3; *Footnote e* x32, x— y33, y—
C_μ	n81, n82
C_α	f71, f72, f73; *Footnote f* g74, g75
C_γ	d11, d12; *Footnote f* e14, e15

[a]Adapted from R. Mage et al. in *The Antigens*, M. Sela (Ed.), Academic Press, New York and London, 1973, p. 300.

[b]Allelic pairs that are known or suspected to be caused by amino acid substitutions at homologous positions in the polypeptide chain (see Table 4-2).

[c]Allelic alternatives whose structural basis is unknown.

[d]The alleles for the various immunoglobulin classes are found on various inbred strains of mice. Many of the serological markers that define these alleles have been localized to their respective C_H regions. None have been localized to V_H regions.

[e]The a, x, and y serological markers are found on three different kinds of V_H regions. x— and y— indicate that an antiserum has not been raised to the allelic alternatives of x32 and y33, respectively.

[f]The f and g markers are located at two different positions in the C_α region. C_α regions exhibiting many combinations of the f and g markers have been found in various populations of rabbits. The d and e markers of γ chains also are located at two different positions, and γ chains with three of the four combinations of these markers have been identified.

Table 4-2   Amino Acid Substitutions That Correlate with Allotypes

Species	Immunoglobulin Family	Residue Position	Alternate Residues
Human	κ Inv (1), (1, 2), (3)	153, 191	V-A, V-L
	Heavy		
	GM (1)	355–358	RDEL[a]
	Gm(non-1)		REEM
	Gm(3)	214	R
	Gm(17)		K
	Gm(11)	296	F
	Gm(non-11)		Y
Rabbit	κ b4, b5, b6, b9	Multiple	Througout C_κ
	Heavy		
	a1, a2, a3	Multiple	Throughout V_H
	d11	225	M
	d12		T
	d14	309	T
	d15		A

[a]One-letter amino code is given in Table 2-1.

to the constant regions and, consequently, have been most useful for the genetic mapping of C genes (Table 4-2). Because allotypes result from allelic differences, they are inherited in a Mendelian fashion.

Isotypes are the antigenic determinants that distinguish the constant regions of the different heavy-chain classes and light-chain types. Because each isotype is encoded by a distinct gene that is present in every member of the species, all the isotypes characteristic of that species are found in the serum of every individual. Isotypes most likely arose by gene duplication and divergence during evolution. Isotypes that differ by a few amino acid changes, as do the four human C_λ regions (Figure 4-2), presumably arose more recently than those that differ more extensively, as do C_μ and C_γ.

Idiotypes are the antigenic determinants that distinguish one V domain from other V domains. These determinants are commonly located at or near the antigen-binding site because that is the region of the V domain where the hypervariable segments of the light and heavy chains fold together (Concept 2-4). However, idiotypic determinants can be located elsewhere on the V domain as well. Idiotypes have been most useful for mapping V genes.

The serologic reagents that are essential for identifying these antigenic markers have been obtained by appropriate immunizations. The subtle differences between allotypes or between idiotypes are

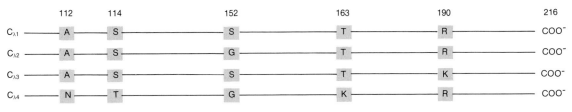

Figure 4-2 Amino-acid-sequence variations found in the C_λ regions of human immunoglobulins. Position 152 is designated the *Kern marker*. Position 190 is designated the *Oz marker*. For each of these variations, there is an antiserum that can detect one variant but not the other. Hence, for the Kern marker, glycine chains are designated + and serine chains −. Likewise, for the Oz marker, lysine chains are + and arginine chains −. Each of these four C_λ sequences is found in the serum of all humans. Thus this polymorphism represents isotypes coded by at least four C_λ genes present in every individual. [Adapted from J. Fett and H. Deutsch, *Immunochemistry* **12**, 643(1971).]

revealed best by immunization within the same species, a process known as *homologous* or *allogeneic immunization*. Because most of the immunoglobulin structure is shared between donor and host, the immune response is directed at the allotypic or idiotypic determinants. To generate antibodies that will react with the major antigenic differences between isotypes requires immunization of one animal species with the immunoglobulin chains of a second, a process known as *heterologous* or *xenogeneic immunization*. Cross-species hybridization is required because all members of the same species normally exhibit the same isotypes and thus will not mount an immune response against these determinants.

Three gene families shown by genetic analysis

Genetic analyses of allotypes, isotypes, and idiotypes have led to the conclusion that immunoglobulin polypeptides are coded by three unlinked clusters of autosomal genes. One cluster codes for heavy chains of all classes and subclasses, a second codes for κ light chains, and a third codes for λ light chains. These three gene clusters are called the H, κ, and λ gene families, respectively. Each of the three immunoglobulin gene families includes a cluster of V genes separated from one or more linked C genes. Although the precise number of V genes is still a matter of controversy (Concept 4-7), the number of functional C genes in various gene families has been determined by serological methods. For example, in mice the κ gene family appears to have a single C gene, whereas the λ gene family has four C genes, and the heavy-chain gene family has eight. The separation between the clusters of V and C genes within a family has been demonstrated, for example, in rabbits, which exhibit both V_H and C_H allotypes (Table 4-1). There it has been shown that germline recombination can give rise to new

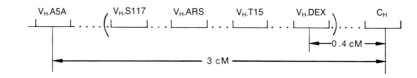

Figure 4-3   A genetic map of some V_H gene segment families on chromosome 12 of the mouse. V_H gene segments in a given family are generally greater than 85% homologous, whereas V gene segments from different families are generally less than 75% homologous. Many additional unidentified V_H gene segment families presumably exist. [Adapted from R. Riblet et al., *Eur. J. Immunol.* **5**, 778(1975).]

combinations of V_H and C_H genes. In addition, genetic analysis of idiotypes in mice has demonstrated more than twelve V_H markers that segregate in a Mendelian fashion and are closely linked to the C_H allotypic markers. Recombinational analysis of some of these idiotypes has permitted determination of their map order and estimation of the genetic map distance across this region (Figure 4-3). The results indicate that multiple V_H genes are linked to the C_H gene cluster in the DNA of mice.

Chromosomal locations of antibody genes

Somatic cell genetics has been used to elucidate the chromosomal location of immunoglobulin genes. Fusion of mouse B cells to human fibroblasts leads to formation of hybrid cells, whose chromosomes are randomly lost. By correlating the loss of a particular immunoglobulin gene with the loss of a particular mouse (or human) chromosome, one can determine the chromosomal locations of antibody gene families. In mice, the κ gene family is on chromosome 6, the λ gene family is on chromosome 16, and the H gene family is on chromosome 12. In humans, the κ gene family is on chromosome 2, the λ gene family is on chromosome 22, and the H gene family is on chromosome 14.

4-3   Recombinant DNA analyses have defined the arrangement of gene segments within the light-chain and heavy-chain families

Recombinant DNA techniques have permitted a direct analysis of the organization of the genes within the light- and heavy-chain families. In mice, the overall organization of these gene families as they exist in the germline before any developmental rearrangements have occurred is shown in Figure 4-4. Perhaps most striking is the segmental

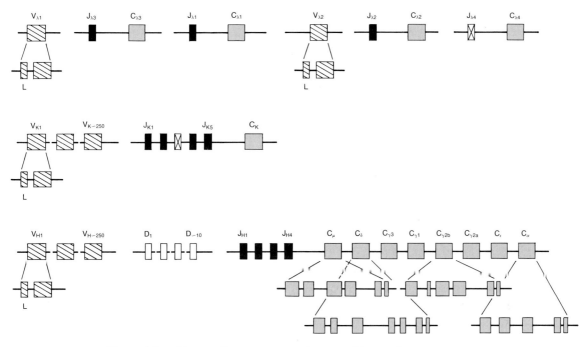

Figure 4-4 The germline arrangement in mice of the λ and κ light-chain gene families and the heavy-chain gene family. Boxed regions on the main line represent gene segments. The arrangement of exons (boxed) and introns in some gene segments is represented below the main line. Discontinuities in the main line represent nucleotide distances of undefined length. X denotes a pseudogene segment.

arrangement of coding information. Each light chain is encoded by 3 distinct gene segments, V, J, and C, and each heavy chain is encoded by 4 distinct gene segments, V, D, J, and C. The variable region of light chains is encoded by the V and J segments, whereas the variable region of heavy chains is encoded by the V, D, and J segments. The C gene segments encode the constant regions.

The V gene segments for both light and heavy chains are split into two coding segments as indicated in Figure 4-4. In eukaryotes, where many genes are split, the portions of a gene that become part of the mRNA are often referred to as *exons*, and the intervening stretches of DNA are called *introns*. During gene expression, exons in the primary RNA transcript of the gene are spliced together to form an mRNA as described in Concept 4-4. The first exon (L) of the V gene segment encodes the leader or signal sequence that directs the nascent protein products across the membrane of the rough endoplasmic reticulum (Concept 4-4). The second exon encodes the N-terminal 96 amino acids of the variable region. The J (joining) gene segments, which are separated from the V or D gene segments by an undefined length of

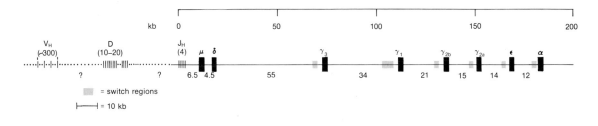

Figure 4-5 A diagram showing the organization of mouse C_H genes; kb denotes kilobases.

DNA, encode the last 10 or so amino acids of variable regions of light and heavy chains. The D (diversity) gene segments, which are separated from the V and J gene segments by an undefined length of DNA, encode from 1 to 15 amino acids in the variable region of the heavy chain between the V and J portions. The D gene segments are so named because they encode the most variable portion of the heavy-chain variable region.

The mouse λ light-chain gene family has only 2 V_λ gene segments and a pair of J_λ and C_λ gene segments that form two functionally independent units that are separated by an undefined physical distance. The $J_{\lambda 4}$ gene segment is nonfunctional. The human λ gene family contains 6 C_λ genes that are spread out over about 50 kb of DNA. Their functional organization with respect to V_λ and J_λ gene segments is not yet defined.

The mouse κ gene family, in contrast to λ, is organized into a single functional unit that contains 200–300 clustered V_κ gene segments, 5 clustered J_κ gene segments about 250 nucleotides apart, and 1 C_κ gene segment. Protein sequences of isolated κ light chains suggest that any V_κ gene segment can be joined to any one of the 4 functional J_κ gene segments, the middle J_κ gene segment being nonfunctional. The structure of this gene family in humans is quite similar to that of mice except that all 5 J_κ gene segments are functional.

Heavy-chain gene organization is similar to that for light-chain genes. In mice there are 200–300 V_H gene segments, 10–20 D gene segments, 4 J_H gene segments, and 8 C_H genes, whereas in humans there are 6 J_H gene segments and 10 C_H genes, the C_α and C_ϵ genes being duplicated. One C_ϵ gene is nonfunctional. The heavy-chain C_H genes, which encode the constant regions that define the various classes and subclasses of heavy chains, are distributed over approximately 200 kb of DNA (Figure 4-5). Unlike C_κ and C_λ genes, C_H genes are composed of multiple exons as illustrated for a few C_H genes in Figure 4-4. These exons correspond to structural domains in the antibody molecule. For example, each C_H gene has at its 3′ end 2 exons (labeled M) that together encode a hydrophobic C terminus that anchors membrane-bound antibodies to the membrane.

4-4 Antibody gene segments are joined together by DNA rearrangements during differentiation and RNA rearrangements during gene expression

Assembly of V genes

The differentiation of stem cells into B_μ cells requires two genetic rearrangements (Figure 4-1). The first DNA rearrangement, which assembles a functional heavy-chain gene, is associated with the differentiation of stem cells into pre-B cells. The second DNA rearrangement, which assembles a functional light chain, is associated with the differentiation of pre-B cells into B_μ cells. These genetic rearrangements occur by site-specific recombination between specific recognition sequences adjacent to V, D, and J segments (Concept 4-5). Because these rearrangements join V, D, and J segments in a random way, much antibody diversity is generated during the differentiation of B_μ cells (Concept 4-6).

Expression in B_μ cells

These rearranged genes are expressed in a manner common to all eukaryotic cells (Figure 4-6). RNA polymerase II copies the assembled gene into a nuclear transcript (nRNA), which is capped at the 5' end by a guanine nucleotide in a "backwards" 5'-5' triphosphate linkage and is tailed at the 3' end by a string of adenine nucleotides (poly A). Introns are removed from the nRNA, and exons are joined to create messenger RNAs (mRNAs) with contiguous coding sequences. These mRNAs are translated on the rough endoplasmic reticulum by virtue of the hydrophobic N-terminal leader segment, which initially attaches the ribosome-mRNA complex to the membrane and then leads the nascent chain across (Figure 4-7). Almost as soon as the leader sequence enters the lumen of the endoplasmic reticulum, it is removed by proteolytic digestion. Light chains pass all the way through the membrane into the lumen of the endoplasmic reticulum. In contrast, the heavy chains synthesized in virgin B_μ cells do not pass all the way through the membrane because of a hydrophobic C-terminal segment, encoded by two 3' exons, which stops transfer of the heavy chain and anchors it in the membrane. As a consequence, the assembled IgM molecules remain attached to the membrane with their antigen-binding sites exposed to the lumen of the endoplasmic reticulum (Figure 4-8).

IgM molecules in the endoplasmic reticulum are transported to the cell surface by cycles of vesicle formation and fusion that lead first to the Golgi apparatus and then to the plasma membrane (Figure 4-7). At all stages during transport, the antigen-binding sites face an external space within the cell and are never exposed to the cytoplasm. In the lumina of the endoplasmic reticulum and the Golgi apparatus, carbohydrate groups are attached in N-glycosidic linkage to specific

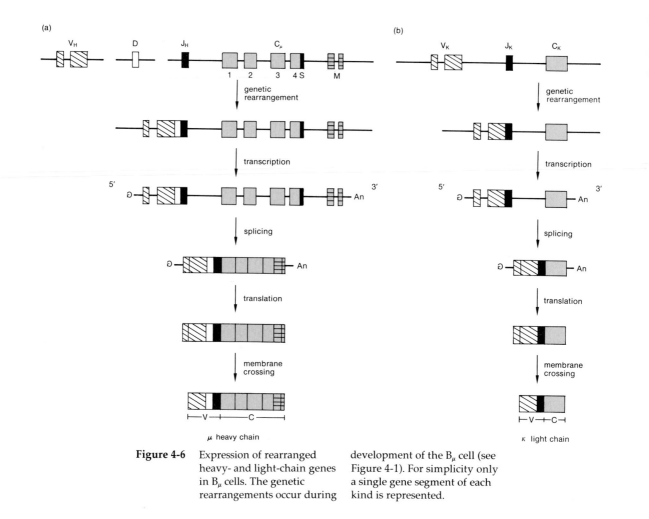

Figure 4-6 Expression of rearranged heavy- and light-chain genes in B_μ cells. The genetic rearrangements occur during development of the B_μ cell (see Figure 4-1). For simplicity only a single gene segment of each kind is represented.

amino acids in the antibody molecules as described in Concept 5-3. Interestingly, in pre-B cells, before a functional light chain has been made, the intracellular transport of heavy chains is blocked at an unknown stage so that they do not appear on the cell surface.

Differentiation from B_μ to $B_{\mu+\delta}$

Because the rearrangement of light- and heavy-chain variable segments is random, nearly the entire immune repertoire of antigen-binding sites is represented within the population of B_μ cells, with one binding site specificity displayed per cell. Thus many B_μ cells will display IgM molecules whose binding sites are complementary to self-antigens. Activation of these cells can have disastrous consequences for the organism as is illustrated by a number of autoimmune diseases (Concept 12-7). At this stage of differentiation, the immune system exerts a strong negative selection against cells with self-reactive anti-

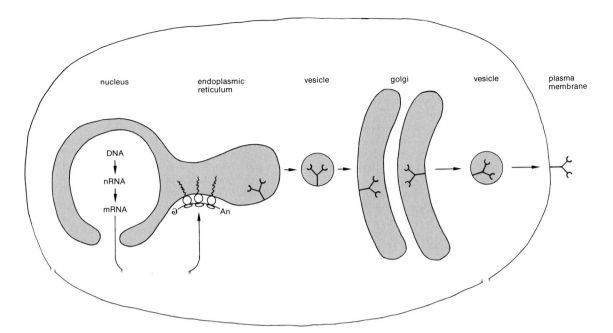

Figure 4-7 Pathway for expression of membrane-bound antibody. Shaded areas are topologically outside the cell. Thus the antigen-binding sites are never exposed to the cytoplasm of the cell.

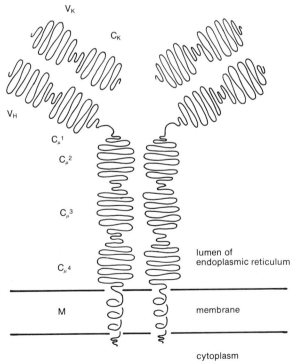

Figure 4-8

Schematic diagram of an IgM molecule anchored in the membrane. Note how the protein domains correspond to the exon structure of the gene (Figure 4-6).

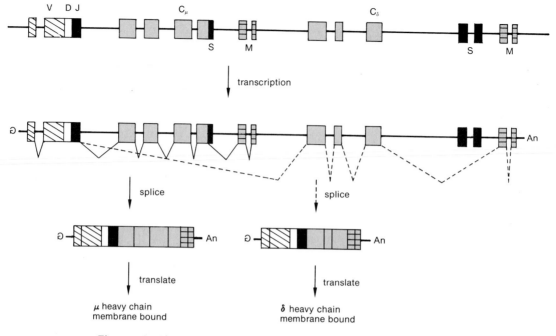

Figure 4-9   Alternative patterns of splicing to produce membrane-bound IgM and IgD. This diagram implies that both mRNAs can be spliced from a single transcript; however, the IgD may be produced preferentially from the long transcript illustrated here, whereas IgM is produced preferentially from a shorter transcript that ends just beyond the μM exon.

body. As a result, self-reactive B cells are eliminated or suppressed and the organism becomes tolerant of its own antigens (see Chapter 10).

B_μ cells that are not rendered unreactive eventually begin to synthesize membrane-bound IgD as well as IgM and thus become mature $B_{\lambda+\delta}$ cells (Figure 4-1). It is not known what triggers the differentiation of B_μ cells to $B_{\mu+\delta}$ cells or whether this step is dependent on stimulation by cognate antigen. Each $B_{\mu+\delta}$ cell displays only a single type of antigen-binding site, but that binding site is present on both kinds of membrane-bound antibodies. The simultaneous expression of μ and δ heavy chains with identical variable regions is accomplished by alternative patterns of RNA splicing (Figure 4-9). Differential splicing may be regulated indirectly by poly A addition as described next for membrane-bound and secreted forms of IgM antibody.

Clonal selection by antigen and further differentiation

The functional significance of membrane-bound IgM and IgD is unclear, but their simultaneous appearance on the surface of a B cell marks it as competent to trigger an immune response. $B_{\mu+\delta}$ cells that bind antigen are stimulated to differentiate further. One line of dif-

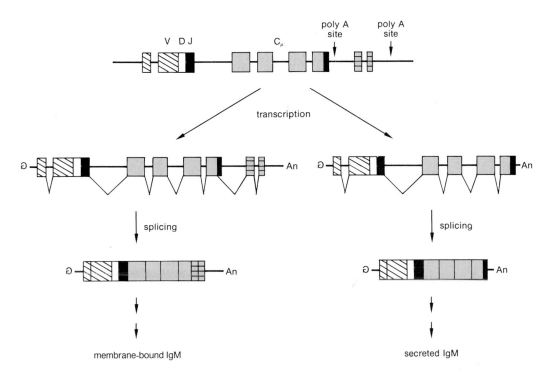

Figure 4-10   Alternative splicing of heavy chain transcripts to produce membrane-bound and secreted IgM. The splicing patterns are controlled by differential use of poly A addition sites: activation of the more 3′ site results in a membrane-bound antibody, whereas activation of the more 5′ site results in a secreted antibody.

ferentiation leads to plasma cells that secrete IgM, whereas a second line of differentiation leads to B cells that can secrete other classes of antibody with the same binding specificity. The detailed relationships among the activated B cells that arise in response to a particular antigen are not yet well defined.

The switch from membrane-bound IgM to secreted IgM is associated with plasma cell formation. Apparently, it is accomplished by alternative RNA splicing patterns, which in turn are regulated by developmentally controlled usage of two potential sequences (AAUAAA in RNA) for addition of poly A to nascent nuclear transcripts (Figure 4-10). In the C_μ gene segment, these two alternative poly A addition sites lie on either side of the pair of exons that encode the hydrophobic anchor sequence of 41 amino acids that holds IgM antibody in the membrane (Concept 2-6). Prior to antigen stimulation, the more distal poly A addition site is active so that the membrane exons are included in the initial transcript. Splicing of this nRNA replaces a short 3′ section of the $C_\mu 4$ exon with the pair of membrane exons, resulting in a membrane-bound antibody. After antigen stimulation, the more proximal poly A addition site is active so that the membrance exons are not included in the initial transcript. As a consequence, the $C_\mu 4$ exon remains intact and confers upon the antibody a hydrophilic C-terminal tail of 20 amino acids that allows the heavy chain to pass all the way through the membrane and the antibody to be secreted.

The differentiation of $B_{\mu+\delta}$ cells into B cells that express other classes of heavy chains is called *class switching*. It results from a second kind of DNA rearrangement that places the assembled V gene in front of different C_H genes as described in Concept 4-6. In individual B cells, the same light-chain gene and V_H gene are expressed throughout the process of class switching, thereby leading to expression of the same variable domain during the various stages of B-cell development. The other C_H genes, which are activated by class switching, also appear to employ alternative patterns of RNA splicing to generate their membrane and secreted forms. For example, 3 analyzed C_γ genes each have 2 membrane exons that encode hydrophobic membrane tails of 66 residues, the first 41 of which are homologous to the μ membrane anchor.

4-5   Variable genes are assembled by site-specific recombination at highly conserved recognition sequences

Rules for joining

The genetic rearrangements of heavy-chain and light-chain variable gene segments involve special recognition sequences at recombination sites that lie on the distal (3′) side of the V gene segments, the proximal and distal (5′ and 3′) sides of D gene segments, and the proximal (5′) side of J gene segments (Figure 4-11). These recognition sequences are of two types, in which a conserved palindromic heptamer is separated from a conserved nonamer by a nonconserved spacer sequence of either 12 or 23 base pairs. (A palindromic DNA sequence is one possessing an axis of twofold rotational symmetry so that the complementary strands are the same when read in the same direction; e.g., 5′–3′.) The distribution of these two types of sequences suggests a rule for recombination of gene segments: namely, that gene segments may be joined only if they are abutted by recognition sequences of opposite types. For example, V_κ gene segments are abutted by the 12 base pair recognition sequence, whereas J_κ gene segments are abutted by the 23 base pair recognition sequence (Figure 4-11). This rule also holds for rearrangements of heavy-chain gene segments, and it presumably ensures that a V_H gene may join to a J_H gene segment only through a D gene segment and never directly. The fundamental role these recognition sequences must play is underscored by their presence in all three gene families even though the families diverged from one another more than 500 million years ago.

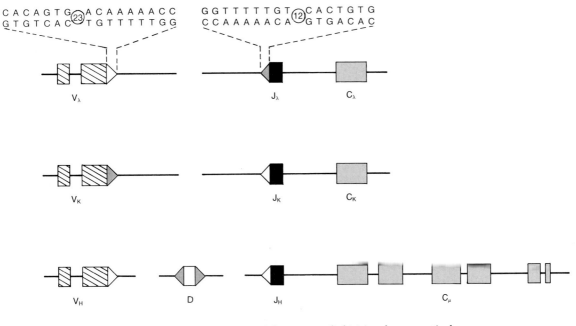

Figure 4-11   The arrangements of the two types of recognition sequences that are used in genetic rearrangements of variable genes. The recognition sequences containing 12 and 23 base pair spacers are represented by the dark and light triangles, respectively. The nucleotide sequences for oppositely oriented triangles are related by a 180° rotation. For simplicity only a single gene segment of each kind is represented.

Recognition sequences could mediate DNA rearrangements by providing homology for alignment by DNA pairing or by providing binding sites for recognition and alignment by proteins. Direct DNA pairing seems somewhat unlikely due to the rather small stretches of homology (7 and 9 nucleotides) and their separation by different lengths of spacer sequence. Thus it seems more likely that the sequences serve as binding sites for proteins that mediate the recombination process (Figure 4-12). It is striking that the lengths of the spacer sequences represent approximately one (12 base pairs) and two (23 base pairs) turns of the DNA helix. Perhaps the recognition proteins must see the conserved portions of the recognition sequences in identical orientations in the DNA helix. In any case, a one-turn spacer sequence must always interact with a two-turn spacer sequence. If the recognition sequences do act as binding sites for proteins that mediate the joining process, there remains the question of how two recognition sites, spatially separated by enormous distances on the chromosome, are brought into juxtaposition.

It is not yet clear whether the assembly of variable genes involves gene segments from the same duplex or from different duplexes. A recombination event within the same duplex could involve deletion

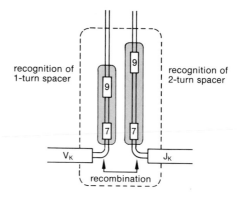

Figure 4-12

Two potential arrangements of recognition sequences for enzyme-mediated recombination of gene segments.

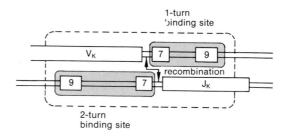

or inversion of a stretch of DNA, depending on the relative orientation of the gene segments, which is as yet undefined. If the gene segments all are oriented in the same direction as implied by the diagram in Figure 4-4, then recombination, for example between a V_κ gene segment and a J_κ gene segment, would cause the intervening sequences to be deleted from the chromosome (Figure 4-13a). If, on the other hand, the clusters of V_κ and J_κ gene segments are oriented in opposite directions, then a recombination between them would cause the intervening sequences to be inverted but not lost from the chromosome. As a consequence of the inversion, subsequent rearrangements involving these gene segments in the same cell or daughter cells could occur by inversion or deletion.

A recombination event between two different duplexes could involve duplexes in homologous chromosomes or, more likely, it could involve the duplexes that form the sister chromatids of one chromosome. Recombination between duplexes would result in no net loss of DNA sequences because those sequences deleted from one duplex would be duplicated in the other duplex (Figure 4-13b). It seems unlikely that recombination between duplexes could produce viable

(a) within a duplex

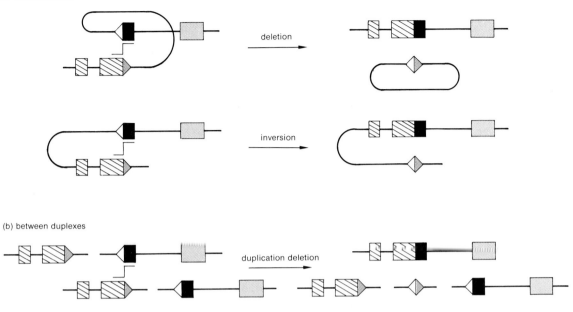

(b) between duplexes

Figure 4-13 Models for (a) intraduplex and (b) interduplex joining of gene segments. In each model an assembled variable gene is one product, but the reciprocal products differ. For simplicity only a single gene segment of each kind is represented.

progeny cells if clusters of gene segments were inverted relative to one another. A recombination between oppositely oriented gene segments would produce a dicentric chromosome and an acentric chromosome, neither of which could be segregated properly at mitosis.

Productive and nonproductive rearrangements

The genetic rearrangements that lead to V gene formation do not occur at a precise location relative to the recognition sequences. One consequence of the flexibility of joining is that several different nucleotide sequences can be generated at the junctions between gene segments as illustrated for the joining of V_κ and J_κ gene segments in Figure 4-14. The resulting differences in amino acid sequence make an important contribution to the generation of antibody diversity (Concept 4-7) because the region of polypeptide containing the amino acids forms a part of the antigen-binding site. The same joining flexibility is evident in assembled heavy chains as well (Figure 4-15). In addition, there are examples of assembled heavy-chain V genes that have extra nucleotides inserted at either the V–D or D–J junctions. The origin of these extra nucleotides is unknown, but one possibility is that they are added by an enzyme like deoxynucleotidyl terminal transferase, which adds nucleotides more or less randomly to the 3′ ends of DNA strands.

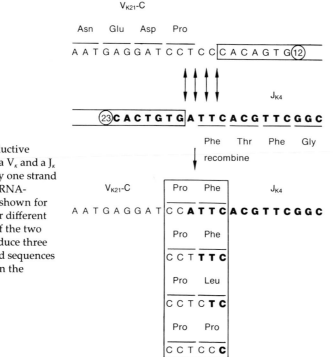

Figure 4-14

Four different productive rearrangements of a V_κ and a J_κ gene segment. Only one strand of the DNA (the mRNA-identical strand) is shown for simplicity. The four different in-phase joinings of the two gene segments produce three different amino acid sequences at the seam between the segments.

The rearrangements illustrated in Figures 4-14 and 4-15 all are termed *productive rearrangements* because the gene segments are joined in the correct reading frame so that they can be translated in phase with one another to produce a functional polypeptide. However, it is clear that gene segments can rearrange unproductively as well so that adjacent segments are joined in an incorrect reading frame or in such a way that a termination codon is generated downstream from the splice point. *Nonproductive* rearrangements may be expressed at the RNA level, but only rarely at the protein level. If joining were random in the local region around the recognition sequences, only one in three rearrangements would be expected to be productive.

The actual frequency of nonproductive rearrangements is unknown, but it is thought to be rather high based on analysis of chromosomes in functional B cells. For example, many myeloma cell lines have rearrangements of both chromosomes encoding heavy chains, one presumably rearranged productively and the other nonproductively. In addition, an analysis of a heterogeneous population of normal splenic B cells expressing immunoglobulins with κ light chains revealed that about 35% of the chromosomes encoding κ chains were unrearranged (germline), but only about 5% of the chromosomes encoding heavy chains were germline. Assuming that half of these chromosomes were rearranged productively, then 15% of κ-chain

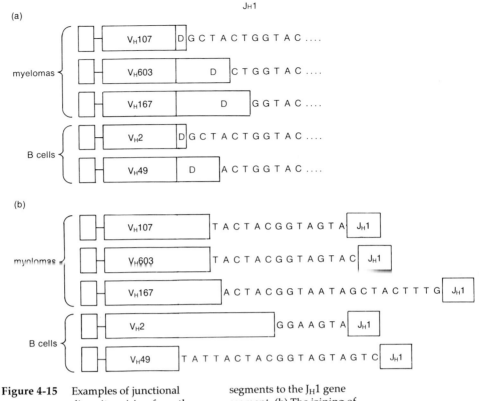

Figure 4-15 Examples of junctional diversity arising from the joining of J_H and D gene segments to form V_H genes. (a) The joining of D gene segments to the J_H1 gene segment. (b) The joining of homologous D gene segments to different V_H segments and the same J_H gene segment.

chromosomes and 45% of heavy-chain chromosomes were rearranged nonproductively. The higher frequency of nonproductively rearranged heavy-chain chromosomes might be expected because they require two rearrangements (V_H to D and D to J_H) as compared with one rearrangement for light-chain chromosomes.

Allelic exclusion

During development of B lymphocytes, antibody gene families are rearranged sequentially—first the heavy-chain family to produce pre-B cells and then a light-chain family to produce B_μ cells. Apparently the κ gene family is rearranged first and then, if no κ rearrangements were productive, the λ gene family is rearranged. This sequential order of expression of the light-chain gene families is suggested by observations on functional B cells where it is found that κ-expressing cells rarely have their λ chromosomes rearranged, whereas λ-expressing cells invariably have their κ chromosomes rearranged. The sequential rearrangement of antibody gene families during development suggests a carefully regulated process, although it is possible

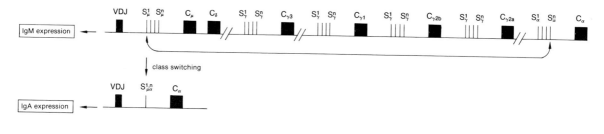

Figure 4-16   Class switching. S represents various switching regions. In this example, the C_μ gene is switched for the C_α gene.

that an apparent order could be achieved by a random joining process in which the probability of rearrangement in the H gene family is greater than in the κ gene family, which in turn is greater than in the λ gene family.

Regardless of how the developmental rearrangements of gene families are initiated, their termination must be regulated carefully because functional B cells never express more than one rearranged V_H gene and V_L gene. This phenomenon is known as *allelic exclusion.* The existence in B_μ cells of light- and heavy-chain gene families in their unrearranged germline configuration indicates that, after productive rearrangements have occurred, the enzymatic machinery responsible for genetic rearrangements must be turned off. The termination signals for heavy chains and light chains must be distinct because heavy-chain gene rearrangements are terminated before light-chain gene rearrangements are initiated. The termination signal for heavy-chain rearrangements is presumably linked to the appearance of heavy chains inserted into the endoplasmic reticulum, whereas the termination signal for light-chain rearrangements may be linked to the appearance of IgM molecules on the cell surface.

4-6   Class switching occurs by recombination between repetitive DNA sequence elements

Mechanism of class switching

Subsequent to antigenic exposure, $B_{\mu+\delta}$ cells differentiate and begin to synthesize other classes of antibodies that retain the same variable domain expressed by the parental B cell (Figure 4-16). Class switches occur by genetic recombination between switch (S) regions that lie from 2 to 3 kb in front of each C_H gene with the possible exception of the C_δ gene. These switch regions are rather large, but they are composed of multiple copies of short, repeated elements. For example, the S_α region is more than 1600 nucleotides long, but it is composed of at

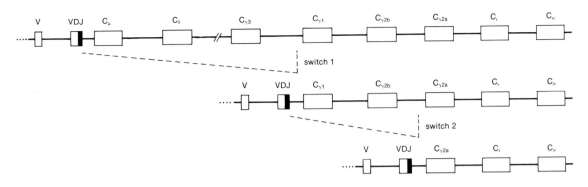

Figure 4-17   Two successive class switches.

least 15 repeated elements 80 nucleotides in length. These repetitive elements appear to be the active sites for switching because all the recombination events studied to date in the S_α region have occurred within one of the 80-nucleotide repeats. Other switch regions have similar structures: the four S_γ regions are composed of 49-nucleotide repetitive elements, which are distinct for each C_γ gene; the S_ϵ region is composed of 60-nucleotide repetitive elements; and the S_μ region is made up of two types of 5-nucleotide repeats, which, perhaps significantly, are scattered throughout some of the other switch regions.

In most characterized examples of class switching, an assembled V_H gene has been transferred from in front of the C_μ gene to one of the other C_H genes, with an accompanying deletion of the intervening DNA. These recombination events could occur within the same duplex or between two duplexes much as discussed for variable gene rearrangements (Concept 4-5). Presumably the actual recombination events are mediated either by direct DNA pairing between short homologies in the switch regions (for example, the 5-nucleotide long repeats) or, perhaps more likely, by a set of switching proteins that recognize and join distinct switch regions.

Occasionally two successive class switches have been observed. They have usually occurred between successively more distal C_H genes (Figure 4-17), as might be expected for an intraduplex deletion or a recombination between sister chromatids. However, more rarely the second switch has occurred from a more distal to a more proximal C_H gene, suggesting either a recombination between homologous chromosomes or a recombination within a heavy-chain gene cluster that already contained a duplicated segment as a result of a prior unequal sister chromatid exchange.

One particularly interesting series of observations, which may be relevant to the phenomenon of class switching, is that some B cells display combinations of antibody molecules other than IgM and IgD on their surface. For example, B cells have been observed to express

IgM and IgG, IgM and IgE, or IgM and IgA. These states could represent simply a transient stage in development before the newly synthesized antibody has replaced the original surface IgM. However, these observations have fostered the intriguing speculation that virtually any antibody molecule may be expressed in combination with IgM, perhaps by a set of events analogous to those that allow simultaneous expression of IgM and IgD (Concept 4-4). Thus class switches may first be "tested" at the level of RNA before a final commitment is made at the level of DNA. This hypothesis would seem to require extremely long nuclear RNA transcripts (over 200 kb in the case of IgM and IgA) or perhaps a novel method of transcription.

Somatic hypermutation accompanying class switching

The process of class switching may be correlated with a somatic hypermutation mechanism which can alter V genes after their assembly. The existence of somatic hypermutation has been demonstrated by the immune response of mice to the simple hapten phosphorylcholine. In mice the entire immune response to phosphorylcholine is derived from a single V_H gene segment, T15. However, out of 19 independently derived cell lines that make antibody directed against phosphorylcholine, only 10 V_H domains were found to be identical in amino acid sequence to that predicted by the nucleotide sequence of the germline T15 gene segment. The other 9 V_H domains differed by 1 to 8 amino acid substitutions (Figure 4-18). The differences were such that they could not have arisen by somatic recombination between the T15 gene segment and the 3 other most closely related V_H gene segments in the mouse genome. Thus a mutational mechanism must be responsible for some V-segment diversity.

Nucleotide sequence analysis of two variant V_H genes whose protein products differed by 8 (M167) and 3 (M603) amino acids differed from the germline T15 gene segment by 44 and 10 nucleotide changes, respectively (Figure 4-19). The mutational changes were localized to the rearranged V_H gene and the nearby flanking sequences. However, flanking sequences 5 kb on either side of the rearranged V_H gene, including the linked C_H gene, showed no mutations. Thus the somatic mutation mechanism seems to be capable of recognizing and introducing mutations selectively into the rearranged V_H gene.

The correlation with class switching derives from the observation that in this study all the variant V_H protein sequences were present in IgG and IgA molecules but not in IgM molecules (Figure 4-18). The process of somatic hypermutation appears to be associated only indirectly with class switching because, in immune responses where the predominant antibody class is IgM, somatic mutation can occur. For example, the number of mutations could simply be proportional to the number of cell divisions a particular B cell has undergone, and cells that have undergone more divisions are more likely to have experienced a class switch.

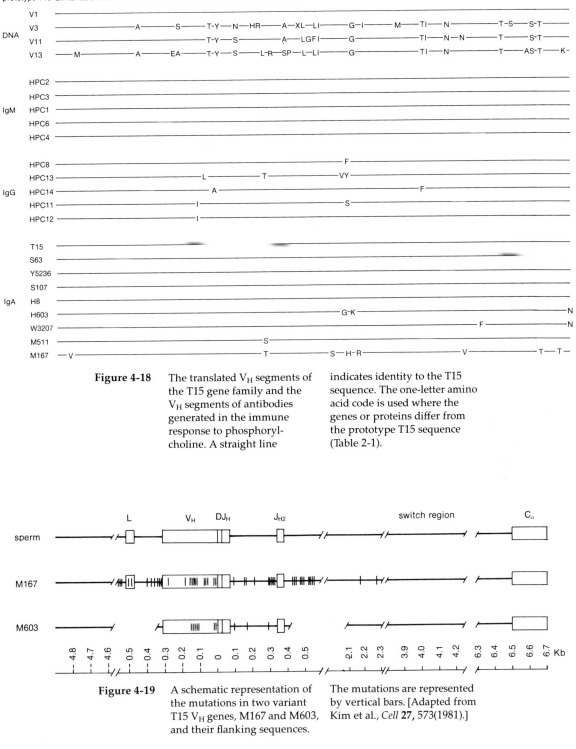

Figure 4-18   The translated V_H segments of the T15 gene family and the V_H segments of antibodies generated in the immune response to phosphorylcholine. A straight line indicates identity to the T15 sequence. The one-letter amino acid code is used where the genes or proteins differ from the prototype T15 sequence (Table 2-1).

Figure 4-19   A schematic representation of the mutations in two variant T15 V_H genes, M167 and M603, and their flanking sequences. The mutations are represented by vertical bars. [Adapted from Kim et al., *Cell* **27**, 573(1981).]

4-7 A variety of mechanisms contributes to antibody diversity

Historical perspective

The vertebrate immune system is capable of synthesizing at least 10^8 different antibody molecules, which can collectively recognize a virtually unlimited number of different antigens. How does an organism generate this vast antibody diversity? Many immunologists in the 1930s and 1940s favored the hypothesis that antigens could instruct the organism to make complementary antibodies by serving as templates around which antibody polypeptides might fold. However, the instructionist theories were ruled out in the early 1960s when it was shown that the three-dimensional structure of an antibody molecule is determined entirely by its amino acid sequence. Following this demonstration, attempts to explain antibody diversity became focused on the origin of amino-acid-sequence diversity among the V_L and the V_H regions.

In the late 1960s and early 1970s, two general theories were put forward to explain the observed amino-acid-sequence diversity of light-chain and heavy-chain variable regions. The *germline theory* postulated that most V genes were encoded separately in the germline of the organism. These genes were assumed to have arisen by gene duplication, mutation, and selection during vertebrate evolution. According to this theory, the diversity of V-region genes existed prior to the differentiation of each individual, and antibody synthesis required merely the activation of preexisting antibody genes in each lymphocyte. By contrast, the *somatic variation theory* postulated that V-region diversity developed from a relatively small number of germline genes, which diversified by mutational or recombinational processes during development of the immune system. According to this theory, V-region diversity was generated anew in each individual rather than passed from one generation to the next. Both the germline and the somatic theories assumed antigen-induced clonal expansion of lymphocytes that carried antigen-specific, cell-surface receptors. Therefore, both theories were compatible with induction of immune responses by clonal selection (Concept 1-4).

Calculation of diversity

Now that the structures and rearrangements of the antibody gene families are known, it is clear that elements of both theories are correct. There are *multiple germline gene segments*. Minimal estimates of the germline repertoire from the three antibody gene families in mice have come from combined protein and DNA analyses. In mice, the κ family has from 100 to 300 V_κ gene segments and 4 functional J_κ gene segments. The heavy-chain family has from 100 to 300 V_H gene segments, from 10 to 20 D gene segments, and 4 J_H gene segments. The λ family has 2 V_λ gene segments and 3 functional J_λ gene segments. Thus there is a substantial repertoire of germline diversity.

The gene segments within a family can be rearranged to create substantial diversity through *combinatorial joining*. Protein sequence data suggest that in the κ family any V_κ gene segment may be joined to any J_κ gene segment. The same is true in the heavy-chain family for the V_H, D, and J_H gene segments. Thus 250 V_κ gene segments could combine with 4 J_κ gene segments to produce 1000 V_κ genes. Likewise, 250 V_H, 10 D, and 4 J_H gene segments could combine to produce 10,000 V_H genes. (Because of its limited germline diversity, the λ gene family does not contribute significantly to antibody diversity in mice.) These calculations of diversity through combinatorial joining are minimum estimates because of the flexibility of joining at each junction between gene segments (Concept 4-5). This flexibility arises because of the variability in the precise points of joining and the possibilities for insertion of extra nucleotides at the junctions. If a conservative estimate of three different amino acids is used for each junction (see Figure 4-14), then the diversity associated with combinatorial joining rises to 3000 for V_κ genes and 90,000 for V_H genes.

These diversities of light and heavy chains are amplified still further by their *combinatorial association* to produce antibody molecules. Because any light chain seems able to combine with any heavy chain, the random association of 3,000 light chains with 90,000 heavy chains would generate 2.7×10^8 different antibody molecules. Thus a truly enormous diversity can be generated from a relatively few germline elements (518 in these calculations).

This baseline repertoire of antibody molecules can be expanded still further by *somatic hypermutation*, which seems to be activated by exposure to antigen (Concept 4-6). If somatic variants are produced in the presence of antigen, those variants with high affinity antigen-binding sites will be clonally expanded in preference to those with lower affinity binding sites. Thus the selective role of antigen in the presence of somatic mutation leads to a "fine tuning" of the immune response and to a virtually unlimited diversity of antibody molecules.

4-8 Antibody genes probably evolved from genes encoding membrane receptors

Plausible evolutionary sequence

One reason for thinking that antibody genes evolved from genes for membrane receptor proteins is that during development antibodies initially function as membrane receptors to trigger B-cell differentiation in response to antigen. The gene for this ancestral protein most likely contained three functional domains, each encoded by a separate exon: one (the L exon) encoding the leader or signal sequence to initiate transfer of the nascent peptide across the membrane of the endoplasmic reticulum; a second (the E exon) encoding the major external

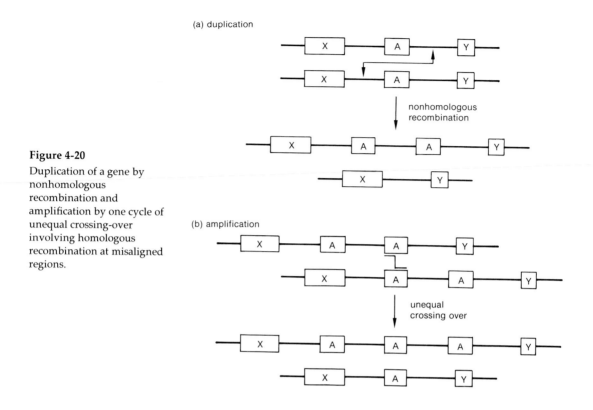

(a) duplication

nonhomologous
recombination

(b) amplification

unequal
crossing over

Figure 4-20

Duplication of a gene by nonhomologous recombination and amplification by one cycle of unequal crossing-over involving homologous recombination at misaligned regions.

domain of the protein responsible for receptor function; and a third (the M exon) encoding a membrane anchor to stop transfer of the protein across the membrane and to hold it in place. From this starting point, it is instructive to try to derive a plausible sequence of evolutionary events that can account for present-day antibody gene structure.

As described in Concept 2-5, the V and C domains of heavy and light chains are strikingly similar in tertiary structure, each possessing a typical immunoglobulin fold, and consequently they probably arose from a common ancestor. The evolution of antibody gene families presumably involved the duplication of gene segments and entire genes by recombination events that depended on minimal sequence homology, as well as the amplification of duplicated regions by cycles of unequal crossing over (Figure 4-20). Duplication of the entire gene presumably led to new genes for membrane receptor molecules. The genes encoding β_2–microglobulin, transplantation antigens, and Ia antigens all apparently evolved in this manner from an ancestral gene shared with antibodies as described in Chapter 6.

The first evolutionary event was presumably the duplication of the E exon to produce the primordial V and C exons, V' and C' (Figure 4-21). A second major evolutionary event was the creation of the J and D segments and the generation of the highly conserved recognition sequences used in their rearrangements. One attractive possibility is that these features

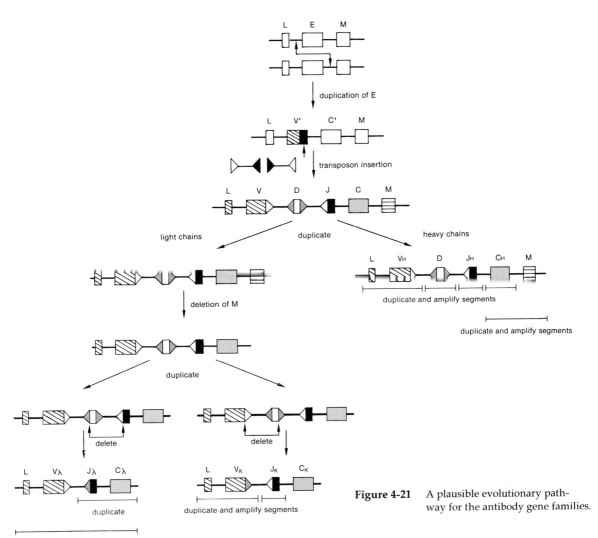

Figure 4-21   A plausible evolutionary pathway for the antibody gene families.

were created simultaneously by the insertion of a transposon near the distal end of the primordial V gene segment. Transposons are mobile genetic elements that have the capacity to move from place to place in a genome, and some transposons even encode enzymes that confer this mobility. Transposons generally have nucleotide sequence repeats at their ends, and they often show internal homologies of the type seen in the recognition structures for V gene formation. Thus a transposon could have inserted into the V′ gene to generate the primordial V, D, and J gene segments as well as the appropriate recognition sequences (Figure 4-21).

A duplication of this entire gene could have produced the ancestral genes for heavy and light chains. A second duplication of the ancestral light-chain gene, perhaps after deletion of the membrane exon, could have led to the primordial κ and λ genes. Within each primordial gene, specific portions of the original transposon would have had to be deleted and the remaining gene segments duplicated and amplified as suggested

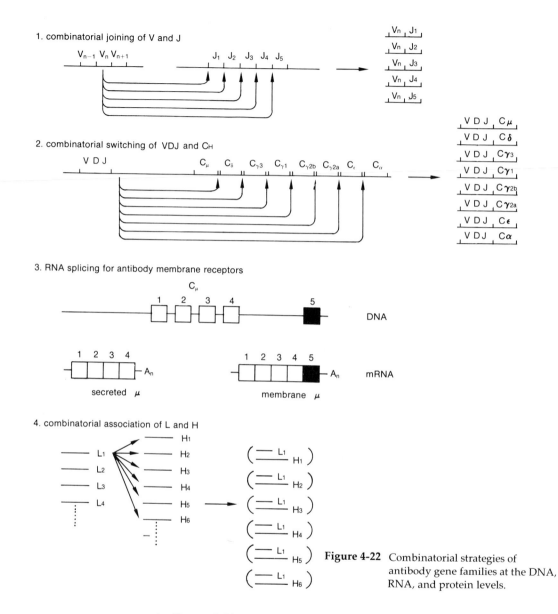

Figure 4-22 Combinatorial strategies of antibody gene families at the DNA, RNA, and protein levels.

in Figure 4-21 to generate the present-day κ and λ gene families. In the heavy-chain gene lineage, each of the gene segments would have had to be duplicated and amplified to generate the present-day heavy-chain gene family. In principle, exon duplication and exon shuffling or exchange provide a very rapid means for evolving new genes or gene families. This strategy has been used extremely efficiently in the evolution of antibody gene families.

Are there other split-gene families?

Antibody genes and polypeptides display a variety of combinatorial mechanisms for amplifying information (Figure 4-22). A key question is whether vertebrates have evolved these sophisticated mechanisms for

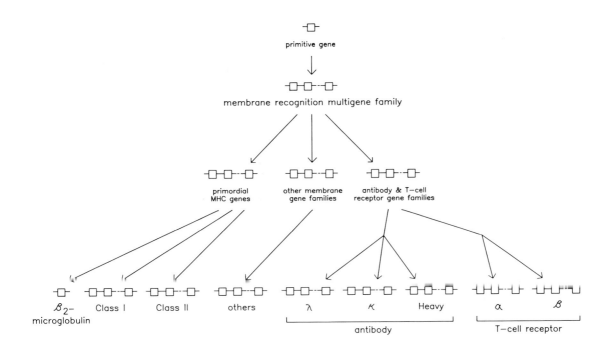

Figure 4-23   The supergene family encoding receptors of the immune system.

amplification of genetic information only in the antibody gene families. The first split-gene–multigene families with potential combinatorial strategies for information amplification may have arisen early in metazoan evolution in response to the requirement for more varied cell-surface receptor functions, such as cell-cell recognition, scavenging of debris, and hormonal triggering. Families of related genes probably evolved to carry out these diverse receptor functions, and antibody genes presumably developed as an offshoot of one of these families (Figure 4-23). If DNA rearrangement mechanisms can evolve by insertion of a transposon, then the duplication of gene segments, genes, and entire gene families could generate complex gene families that in time could encode diverse functions. Thus the multigene family becomes a unit of evolution in the sense that duplication of a part or all of it generates a new gene family, which in time can evolve new functions. This scheme ensures that the new gene family will have the potential to employ most, if not all, of the regulatory mechanisms (e.g., DNA rearrangement) of the ancestral gene family. If such evolutionary events occur, then the strategies of information amplification employed by the antibody gene system may well be employed by other complex eukaryotic systems, such as T-cell receptors, olfactory receptors, hormone receptors, tumor antigens, and molecules specifying neuronal interactions. Indeed, recently it has been demonstrated that the genes for T-cell receptors have V, D, J, and C gene segments and are homologous to their B-cell counterparts.

Selected Bibliography

General

Honjo, T., "Immunoglobulin genes," *Annu. Rev. Immunol.* **1**, 499(1983).

Leder, P., "The genetics of antibody diversity," *Sci. Am.* **246**, 102(1982).

Tonegawa, S., "Somatic generation of antibody diversity," *Nature* **302**, 575(1983).

Clonal expression of immunoglobulin

Gearhart, P. J., Hurwitz, J. L., and Cebra, J. J., "Successive switching of antibody isotopes expressed within the lines of a B-cell clone," *Proc. Natl. Acad. Sci. USA* **77**, 5424(1980).

Klinman, N., and Press, J., "The B-cell specificity repertoire: its relationship to definable subpopulations," *Transplant. Rev.* **24**, 41(1975).

Antibody genes

Blomberg, B., Traunecker, A., Eisen, H., and Tonegawa, S., "Organization of four mouse λ light-chain immunoglobulin genes," *Proc. Natl. Acad. Sci. USA* **78**, 3765 (1981).

Davis, M. M., Calame, K., Early, P. W., Livant, D. L., Joho, R., Weissman, I. L., and Hood, L., "An immunoglobulin heavy-chain gene is formed by two recombinational events," *Nature* **283**, 733(1980).

Early, P., Huang, H., Davis, M., Calame, K., and Hood, L., "An immunoglobulin heavy-chain variable region gene is generated from three segments of DNA: V_H, D, and J_H," *Cell* **19**, 981(1980).

Hood, L., Davis, M., Early, P., Calame, K., Kim, S., Crews, S., and Huang, H., "Two types of DNA rearrangements in immunoglobulin genes," *Cold Spring Harbor Symp. Quant. Biol.* **45**, 887(1981).

Hozumi, N., and Tonegawa, S., "Evidence for somatic rearrangement of immunoglobulin genes coding for variable and constant regions," *Proc. Natl. Acad. Sci. USA* **73**, 3628(1976).

Kurosawa, Y., and Tonegawa, S., "Organization, structure and assembly of immunoglobulin heavy-chain diversity DNA segments," *J. Exp. Med.* **155**, 201(1982).

Max, E. E., Seidman, J. G., and Leder, P., "Sequences of five potential recombination sites encoded close to an immunoglobulin κ constant region gene," *Proc. Natl. Acad. Sci. USA* **76**, 3450(1974).

Sakano, H., Maki, R., Kurosawa, Y., Roeder, W., and Tonegawa, S., "Two types of somatic recombination are necessary for the generation of complete immunoglobulin heavy-chain genes," *Nature* **286**, 676(1980).

Shimizu, T., Takahashi, N., Yamamaki-Kataoka, Y., Nishida, Y., Kataoka, T., and Honjo, T., "Ordering of mouse immunoglobulin heavy-chain genes by molecular cloning," *Nature* **289**, 149(1981).

Class Switching

Cory, S., Jackson, J., and Adams, J. M., "Deletions in the constant region locus can account for switches in immunoglobulin heavy-chain expression," *Nature* **285**, 450(1980).

Davis, M. M., Kim, S. K., and Hood, L., "DNA sequences mediating class switching in α immunoglobulins," *Science* **209**, 1360(1980).

Marcu, K. B., Lang, R. B., Stanton, W. L., and Harris, L. J., "A model for the molecular requirements of immunoglobulin heavy-chain class switching," *Nature* **298**, 87(1982).

Nikaido, T., Nakai, S., and Honjo, T., "The switch (S) region of the immunoglobulin C_μ gene is composed of simple tandem repetitive sequences," *Nature* **292**, 845(1981).

Rabbitts, J. H., Bently, D. L., and Milstein, C. P., "Human antibody genes: V gene variability and C_H gene switching strategies," *Immunol. Rev.* **59**, 69(1981).

Somatic mutation

Alt, F., and Baltimore, D., "Joining of immunoglobulin heavy-chain gene segments: implications from a chromosome with evidence of three D-J_H fusions," *Proc. Natl. Acad. Sci. USA* **79**, 4118(1982).

Crews, S., Griffin, J., Huang, H., Calame, K., and Hood, L., "A single V_H gene segment encodes the immune response to phosphorylcholine: somatic mutation is correlated with the class of antibody," *Cell* **25**, 59(1981).

Gearhart, P., and Bogenhagen, D., "Clusters of point mutations are found exclusively around rearranged antibody variable region genes," *Proc. Natl. Acad. Sci. USA* **80**, 3439(1983).

Gershenfeld, H., Tsukamoto, A., Weissman, I. L., and Joho, R., "Somatic diversification is required to generate the V_κ genes of MOPC511 and MOPC167 myeloma proteins," *Proc. Natl. Acad. Sci. USA* **78**, 7074(1981).

Kim, S., Davis, M. M., Sinn, E., Patten, P., and Hood, L. "Antibody diversity: somatic hypermutation of rearranged V_H genes," *Cell* **27**, 573(1981).

RNA splicing

Early, P., Rogers, J., Davis, M., Calame, K., Bond, M., Wall, R., and Hood, L., "Two mRNAs can be produced from a single immunoglobulin μ gene by alternative RNA processing pathways," *Cell* **20**, 313(1980).

Moore, K. W., Rogers, J., Hunkapiller, I., Early, P., Nottenburg, C., Weissman, I., Bazin, H., Wall, R., and Hood, L. E., "Expression of IgD may use both DNA rearrangement and RNA splicing mechanisms, " *Proc. Natl. Acad. Sci. USA* **78**, 1800(1981).

Rogers, J., Early, P., Carter, C., Calame, K., Bond, M., Hood, L., and Wall, R., "Two mRNAs with different 3' ends encode membrane-bound and secreted forms of immunoglobulin μ chain," *Cell* **20**, 303(1980).

Additional concepts and techniques introduced in the problems

1. Allotypes requiring multiple chains. Problem 4-10.
2. Genetic mapping with idiotypes. Problem 4-11.
3. Southern blot analysis. Problem 4-12.
4. Allelic exclusion. Problem 4-17.
5. T-cell idiotypes. Problem 4-18.
6. Northern blot analysis. Problem 4-19.
7. Expression of double antibody producers. Problem 4-20.

Problems

4-1   Indicate whether each of the following statements is true or false. Explain the error in each statement you consider to be false.

(a) Allotypes represent allelic alternatives of a single structural gene.

(b) Isotypes represent duplicated genes present in every individual.

(c) Idiotypes are antigenic determinants found only in the antigen-binding sites of antibodies.

(d) Pre-B cells contain cytoplasmic μ chains; they do not express light chains.

(e) Class switching arises when a B cell switches the type of light chain expressed.

(f) An individual germline light-chain gene has four distinct coding regions, whereas the somatically rearranged light-chain gene has three.

(g) The λ and κ gene families differ in that any functional J_κ gene segment may be expressed in association with the C_κ gene, whereas the J_λ gene segments may only be expressed with their paired C_λ gene.

(h) V_H gene formation requires a single DNA rearrangement.

(i) The IgM to IgG class switching requires a DNA rearrangement that joins the S_μ region directly to the 5' end of the C_α gene.

(j) The recognition sequences presumably mediating V gene formation are highly conserved in the light-chain gene families, but not in the heavy-chain gene family.

(k) A nonproductive V gene formation leads to a gene that cannot be expressed as an mRNA.

(l) Allelic exclusion is a phenomenon whereby each B cell expresses on its cell surface just one type of V domain.

(m) The S regions generally exhibit repeating sequences.

(n) The μ_m and μ_s mRNAs are derived from two distinct C_μ genes by alternative patterns of RNA splicing.

(o) IgM and IgD molecules with identical V domains may be expressed in the same B cell because the maternal and paternal H-chain chromosomes each rearrange the same V_H gene to the C_μ and C_δ genes, respectively.

(p) Antibody diversity arises from a variety of mechanisms including multiple germline V genes, combinatorial joining of the variable region gene segments, and somatic mutation.

(q) Junctional diversity may arise in each of the three hypervariable regions.

(r) Somatic mutation may occur in flanking as well as coding sequences of the rearranged V gene.

(s) The λ, κ, and H gene families probably arose from a common ancestor.

(t) Exon shuffling can lead to the creation of more complex C_H genes.

(u) Combinatorial strategies may be employed to generate C- as well as V-gene diversity.

(v) The T-cell receptor may be isolated by employing immunoglobulin gene probes.

4-2 Fill in the following blanks.

(a) Antibodies for allotypes are produced by _____ immunization.

(b) Antibodies for isotypes are produced by _____ immunization.

(c) B cells express as membrane or secreted immunoglobulin just one light-chain allele and one heavy-chain allele; this phenomenon is known as _____ .

(d) When a B cell shifts from the synthesis of IgM to IgA molecules, it is said to have undergone a _____ .

(e) The light-chain gene families are _____ and _____ .

(f) Unrearranged antibody genes are said to be in their _____ context.

(g) _____ brings the V_L and J_L gene segments into contiguous alignment.

(h) The V_H gene is composed of _____ , _____ , and _____ gene segments.

(i) Recognition sequences for V gene formation occur at the _____ end of V gene segments, the _____ and _____ ends of D gene segments, and the _____ end of J gene segments.

(j) The _____ model of V gene formation suggests that DNA is irreversibly lost.

(k) The _____ model of V gene formation predicts that after the DNA rearrangement, the resulting daughter cells will have different DNA sequences.

(l) A _____ rearrangement leads to a functional V gene.

(m) The _____ regions are joined in class switching.

(n) The μ_m and μ_s mRNAs differ only in their _____ ends.

(o) The C_μ gene contains _____ exons.

(p) The three general models to explain antibody diversity at the DNA level are _____ , _____ , and _____ .

(q) The _____ model suggests that any L chain may associate with any H chain.

(r) Somatic diversity arising by _____ may be associated in some cases with class switching.

(s) Two distinct types of gene duplication are called _____ and _____ .

(t) _____ suggests that the exons of the C genes may be rearranged during evolution to increase the potential rate of evolution for antibody genes.

(u) Combinatorial mechanisms for antibody diversification operate at the _____ , _____ , and _____ levels.

(v) The _____ receptor appears to share V idiotypes with its B-cell counterpart; however, it has proven impossible to isolate this molecule using immunoglobulin reagents and probes.

4-3 The combinatorial strategies offer enormous potential for the diversification of antibody genes and molecules. Assume the following: (1) any V gene segment may join to any J_L or D gene segment, (2) any D gene segment may join to any J_H gene segment, and (3) any L chain may associate with any H chain. Calculate the number of V_L and V_H genes and antibody molecules that may be generated by combinatorial strategies for the following:

(a) L: 10 V_L and 2 J_L
      H: 10 V_H, 2 D_H, and 2 J_H

(b) L: 100 V_L and 4 J_L
      H: 100 V_H, 20 D_H, and 4 J_H

(c) L: 1000 V_L and 4 J_L
      H: 1000 V_L, 20 D_H, and 4 J_H

4-4 (a) Diagram the DNA rearrangements necessary to create the mouse heavy-chain gene $V_3D_2J_3C_\epsilon$. Assume that the heavy-chain gene family has 5 V_H, 4 D, and 4 J_H gene segments. Depict the germline organization, the organization after V gene formation, and the organization after class switching. Show all genes and indicate sequences at recombination points.

(b) Depict the RNA splicing events necessary to generate an $\epsilon_{secreted}$ mRNA from the rearranged C_ϵ gene.

(c) Depict the RNA splicing events necessary to generate ϵ_m and ϵ_s mRNAs. Assume an M exon organization similar to that of the C_μ gene.

4-5 (a) To study the structure of mouse immunoglobulins, you set out to produce some specific antisera. Antiserum 1 (As1) is obtained by immunizing inbred strain-A mice with purified IgG Fc fragments from inbred strain-B mice. As2 is obtained by immunizing strain-B mice with purified IgG Fc from strain-A mice. Are As1 and As2 directed against an allotypic or idiotypic determinant(s)? On which homology region(s) of which chain(s) is the determinant(s) recognized by As1 and As2 located?

(b) As3 is obtained by immunizing A mice with purified κ chains from B mice. As4 is obtained by immunizing B mice with κ chains from A mice. Are As3 and As4 directed against an allotypic or idiotypic determinant(s)? On which homology region(s) of which chain(s) is the determinant(s) recognized by As3 and As4 located? Explain.

(c) Purified antigen X elicits a strong IgG response in A- and B-strain mice. The light-chain components of the anti-X antiserum are predominantly of the κ type. As5 is made by immunizing B mice with purified anti-X antibodies from strain A. As5 is then absorbed with strain-A normal serum immunoglobulins until it no longer reacts with them. However, the absorbed As5 still reacts with strain-A anti-X antibodies. What does the absorption step do? Is the absorbed As5 recognizing allotypic or idiotypic determinants? Explain.

(d) Strain-A and strain-B mice are crossed to produce (A $\times$ B)F_1 hybrids. Sera from (A $\times$ B)F_1 animals all react with As1, As2, As3, and As4. Does this contradict the principle of allelic exclusion? Why or why not?

(e) The F_1 hybrids are crossed to strain A to produce 24 (A $\times$ B)$F_1 \times$ B backcross progeny (BC 1–24). A serum sample is taken from each animal after immunizing with antigen X. Each sample is then tested for reactivity with As1, As2, As3, As4, and absorbed As5. (See results in Table 4-3.) If the reactivity against absorbed As5 is that shown in column (1), on which homology region(s) of which chain(s) is the determinant(s) recognized by As5 (absorbed) located? Explain.

(f) If the reactivity against absorbed As5 is that shown in column (2), on which

Table 4-3 Reactivities of Anti-X Sera from Backcross Mice with Various Allotype- and Idiotype-Specific Reagents (Problem 4-5)

Anti-X Serum	As1	As2	As3	As4	Absorbed As5	
A	−	+	−	+	+	
B	+	−	+	−	−	
(A × B)F$_1$	+	+	+	+	+	
					(1)	(2)
BC 1	+	+	+	−	+	−
2	+	+	+	−	+	−
3	+	−	+	−	−	−
4	+	+	+	+	−	+
5	+	−	+	+	−	−
6	+	+	+	−	+	−
7	+	−	+	+	−	−
8	+	+	+	−	+	−
9	+	−	+	−	−	−
10	+	−	+	−	−	−
11	+	+	+	+	+	+
12	+	+	+	+	+	+
13	+	−	+	+	−	−
14	+	−	+	−	−	−
15	+	+	+	−	+	−
16	+	−	+	+	−	−
17	+	+	+	−	+	−
18	+	−	+	+	−	−
19	+	+	+	−	+	−
20	+	+	+	+	+	+
21	+	−	+	+	−	−
22	+	+	+	+	+	+
23	+	−	+	−	−	−
24	+	−	+	+	−	−

homology region(s) of which chain(s) is the determinant(s) recognized by As5 (absorbed) located? Explain.

4-6 (a) The C$_{\lambda 1}$ and C$_{\lambda 3}$ regions of human λ chains are identical except for an arginine–lysine interchange at position 190 (Figure 4-2). Chemical analyses of the C$_\lambda$ regions from ten normal individuals reveal that each individual has λ chains of both the λ1 and λ3 types. Is it likely that this polymorphism is coded by alleles? Why? What is the probability of picking ten consecutive heterozygotes? (Assume that each variant represents 50% of the C$_\lambda$ genes in the human population.)

(b) Offer an alternative explanation for this C region polymorphism.

4-7 (a) Human heavy chains have C-region allotypes that can be recognized by serologic reagents or by sequence analysis. These allotypes represent variations within heavy-chain subclasses that are designated as G1^a or G1^b, G2^a or G2^b, G3^a or G3^b, G4^a or G4^b, and A1^a or A1^b. Most Caucasians have the G1^a, G2^a, G3^a, G4^a, and A1^a variants, whereas most Mongolians have the G1^b, G2^b, G3^b, G4^b, and A1^b variants. Caucasian–Mongolian mixed marriages yield F$_1$ offspring that pro-

Table 4-4 The Effect of Haptens and Other Small Molecules on the Reaction of $^{125}I-F(ab')_2$ Derived from D Antibodies of Rabbit 114 with Anti-D Serum (Problem 4-9)

	Final Molar Concentration of Competitor[a]		
Competitor	16×10^{-3}	5×10^{-4}	5×10^{-5}
	$^{125}I-F(ab')_2$ precipitated as % of control[b]		
p-(p'-Hydroxy)-phenylazobenzoate	32	39	61
Benzoate	95	101	108
p-Nitrobenzoate	72	72	86
m-Nitrobenzoate	85	90	112
o-Nitrobenzoate	98	106	98

[a]Refers to concentration prior to the addition of goat anti-rabbit Fc antiserum.
[b]Expressed as percentage of the quantity precipitated in the absence of competitor.
[From B. Brient and A. Nisonoff, *J. Exp. Med.* **132**, 951(1970). ©1970 by The Rockefeller University Press.]

duce both the a and b variants of each subclass. In a large-scale study, marriages between these F1 individuals and Caucasians (backcrosses) were found to yield offspring with the following phenotypes:

G1a and G1b, G2a and G2b, G3a and G3b, G4a and G4b, A1a and A1b; 337 offspring

G1a, G2a, G3a, G4a, A1a; 321 offspring

G1a and G2b, G2a, G3a and G3b, G4a, A1a and A1b; 1 offspring

What can you conclude about the genetic linkage of the heavy-chain genes that encode these allotypes?

(b) How can the last phenotype be explained? Can you derive a gene order on the chromosome from this phenotype?

4-8 The mammalian haploid genome consists of about 3.2×10^9 nucleotide pairs of DNA.

(a) How many V regions 107 residues in length could be encoded by this amount of DNA?

(b) What percent of the mammalian genome would be required to encode 1000 V_L and 1000 V_H genes?

4-9 Purified anti-p-azobenzoate antibodies (designated D) from donor rabbits will react with anti-idiotypic (anti-D) antisera. Suppose that you set out to determine which portions of the D antibody V regions combine with anti-D antisera. You purify D antibodies of the IgG class from a single donor rabbit. You prepare anti-D antiserum to these antibodies in allotypically matched recipient rabbits. You label $F(ab)_2$ fragments from these antibodies with ^{125}I and set up the following inhibition test. In a control experiment, you incubate $^{125}I-F(ab)_2$ fragments from D with anti-D serum, and you precipitate the resulting soluble complexes with goat anti-rabbit-Fc serum. You can determine the extent of the reaction by measuring the percent of the ^{125}I that is precipitated. This result establishes the fraction of the D antibodies that normally react with anti-D serum. You then repeat the experiment in the presence of various hapten inhibitors, with the results shown in Table 4-4. What are the implications of these data? Suggest two alternative interpretations.

4-10 An antigen Ms-1, discovered in a partially inbred rabbit colony, is inherited as an

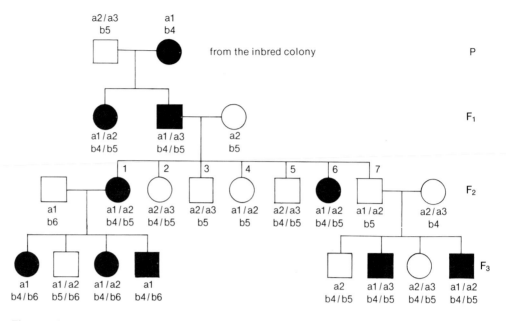

Figure 4-24 Family pedigree of a partially inbred rabbit and an outbred rabbit (Problem 4-10). Circles and squares represent females and males, respectively. Shaded symbols represent individuals that express the Ms-1 allotype. The markers a2, a3, and b5 are allotypes present in the outbred population. The designation a2/a3 indicates that an individual is heterozygous for allotypes a2 and a3; a2 indicates that the individual is homozygous for the a2 allotype.

allotypic variant of IgM molecules, but not of other immunoglobulin classes. All the rabbits of this colony have heavy chains of allotype a1 and 12 light chains of allotype b4 (Table 4-1). In matings between outbred rabbits and one of the partially inbred rabbits, the pedigree in Figure 4-24 was observed. With reference to this figure, answer the following questions.

(a) Does the Ms-1 specificity appear to be determined by the genes that code for the a1 V regions? Why?

(b) Propose a model for the observed pattern of inheritance. In particular, how can you account for the ability of two Ms-1-negative individuals (in the F_2 generation) to produce Ms-1-positive progeny?

(c) What regions in the IgM molecule might carry the Ms-1 specificity? How might you further localize the Ms-1 specificity?

4-11 (a) In mice, immunization with group A streptococcal carbohydrate elicits homogeneous antibodies of IgM and IgG classes. An idiotypic marker, designated A5A, has been defined for one clone of antibody-producing cells using an alloantiserum. This idiotype is variably expressed in mice of the A/J strain immunized with group A streptococci, but it is lacking in similarly immunized BALB/c mice. Interstrain matings were carried out with these two strains, and the results of immunization with respect to the concentration of A5A idiotype in immune sera for F_1, backcross, and parental mice are shown in Figure 4-25. Ig–1e

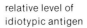

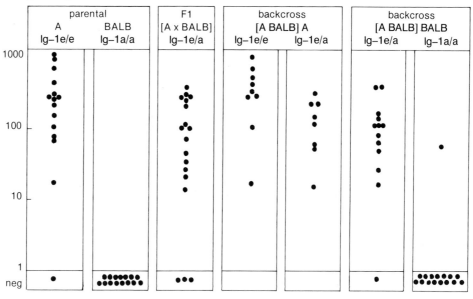

Figure 4-25 The expression of the A5A idiotype in the antibodies to group A streptococci from A/J(A) mice, F₁ hybrids, and backcross mice (Problem 4-11). Ig–1e and Ig–1a are two alleles of a C allotypic marker characteristic of the A/J and BALB/c strains, respectively. [Adapted from K. Eichmann and C. Berek, *Eur. J. Immunol.* **3**, 599(1973).]

Figure 4-26

A Southern blot analysis of the κ-producing myeloma DNAs and sperm DNA using a labeled cDNA probe including the four J$_k$ gene segments (Problem 4-12).

sperm	Myeloma 1	Myeloma 2
	—— 8 kb	—— 7 kb
—— 5 kb	—— 5 kb	
		—— 3 kb

and Ig–1a are two alleles of a C$_\gamma$ gene. What is the likely genetic basis for these results?

(b) Assume that 1 centimorgan is approximately equal to 1000 kb of mouse DNA, that the gene encoding the A5A heavy-chain variable region is at the far 5′ end of the V$_H$ gene family, and that V$_H$ genes are spaced about 20 kb apart in the germline. How many V$_H$ genes could be contained in the mouse genome?

4-12 The DNA from two myeloma tumors was examined by Southern blot analysis to investigate the mechanism of allelic exclusion (Figure 4-26). In this procedure, DNA is cleaved with a restriction enzyme (which cuts at specific nucleotide sequences) and electrophoresed on agarose to separate the DNA fragments by size. The size-separated DNA is then transferred to a nitrocellulose filter, denatured in place, and hybridized to a radiolabeled probe to identify the fragments containing sequences

Figure 4-27

Nucleotide sequences from V and J gene sequences (Problem 4-13).

```
V        10        20                                    50
TAC TAC TGT GCC AGA GACACAGTGAGGGAGCCTGCGACACAAACCTCTCTGCA

J        10        20        30        40        50
AGGTTTTTGTAAGGGGGGCGCAGTGATATGAATCACTGTGC TAC TGG TAC TTC GAT
```

complementary to the probe. The sizes of these fragments are generally indicated in kilobase pairs (kb). With reference to Figure 4-26, answer the following questions.

(a) How would you explain the results from the Southern blot analysis of sperm DNA?

(b) How would you explain the analysis of Myeloma 1 DNA? In view of these data, how would you explain allelic exclusion?

(c) How would you explain the analysis of Myeloma 2 DNA? How do these data alter your previous conclusion about allelic exclusion?

4-13 (a) Listed in Figure 4-27 are one sequence from the 3' end of a mouse V gene segment and one sequence from the 5' end of a mouse J gene segment. The codons representing the end of the V gene and the beginning of the J gene segments are spaced as triplets. Identify the V–J joining recognition sequences from the V and J gene segments. List the recognition sequences, the nucleotide numbers that the recognition sequences span, and the spacer lengths between the recognition sequences for the V and J gene segments.

(b) Given that these V and J gene segments belong to the same antibody gene family, from which family must they originate? Why?

(c) Write the protein sequence you would expect to result from V–J joining of the two segments shown in Figure 4-27 in the absence of junctional diversity.

4-14 Listed below are protein sequences from different variable regions which span the third hypervariable region and which derive from the V and J gene segments listed in Figure 4-27.

(a) TYR TYR CYS ALA ARG TYR TRP TYR PHE ASP

(b) TYR TYR CYS ALA ARG ASP TYR TRP TYR PHE ASP

(c) TYR TYR CYS GLY ARG TYR TRP TYR PHE ASP

(d) TYR TYR CYS ALA ARG ASP CYS TYR TRP TYR PHE ASP

(e) TYR TYR CYS ALA ARG GLY TYR TRP TYR PHE ASP

(f) TYR TYR CYS ALA SER TYR TRP TYR PHE ASP

(g) TYR TYR CYS ALA SER ASP TRP TYR PHE ASP

Which of these protein sequences derive from unmutated V and J gene segments?

4-15 Junctional diversity is an advantage of variable V–J joining. However, one consequence of this variability is that only a small percentage of rearrangements yield a V gene that preserves the reading frame. Calculate the probability of obtaining at least one in-frame rearranged heavy-chain gene and one in-frame rearranged light-chain gene in the same cell. Assume that the joining process is random so that rearrangement occurs with equal probability in all three reading frames. Also assume that all alleles rearrange but that each rearranges only once. Finally, assume that all V, D, and J gene segments have only one open reading frame.

4-16 (a) A mouse of strain X was crossed to a strain-Y mouse resulting in an $(X \times Y)F_1$ heterozygote. Antisera recognizing μ-chain allotypic determinants were used in a fluorescence-activated cell sorter (FACS) to isolate B lymphocytes from the $(X \times Y)F_1$ mouse expressing μ chains of the strain-X type. DNA was extracted from these B lymphocytes and analyzed by Southern blotting analysis. A partial restriction map of germline X and Y C_μ loci in relation to Bam HI and Eco RI cleavage sites is shown in Figure 4-28.

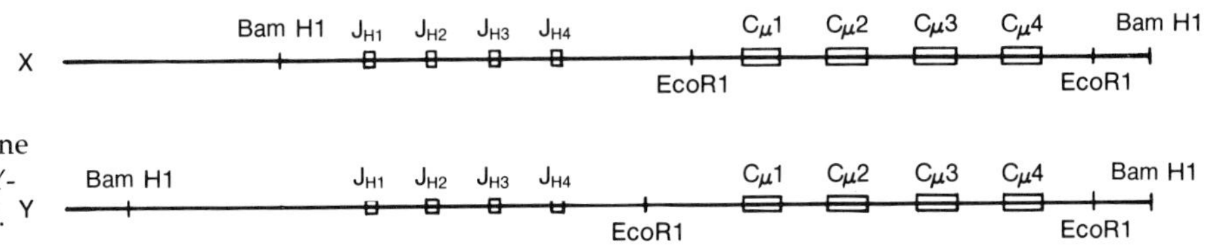

Figure 4-28

Restriction maps of germline C_μ loci from X-strain and Y-strain mice (Problem 4-16).

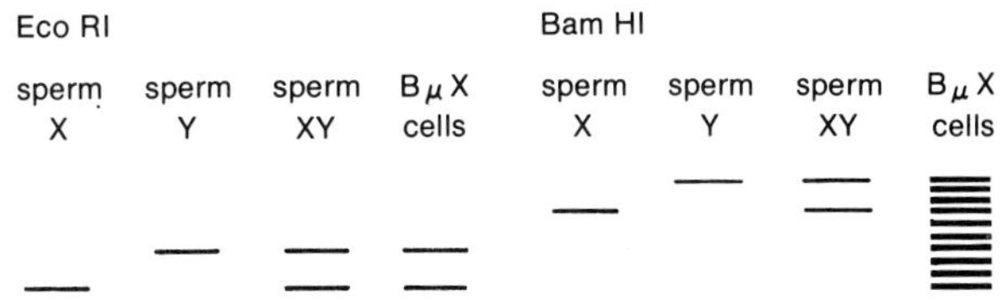

Figure 4-29

Southern blot analyses of X, Y, and $(X \times Y)F_1$ DNAs using a C_μ DNA probe (Problem 4-16).

What percentage of the B_μ cells from an $(X \times Y)F_1$ animal will express the C_μ X allotype? Why?

(b) Figure 4-29 shows the results of Southern blot analyses of germline X, Y, and $(X \times Y)F_1$ DNAs and DNA of B_μ X cells from the $(X \times Y)F_1$, using C_μ DNA as the probe. In the FACS-sorted B-cell population, what percentage of cells will have a rearranged C_μ X region? Why?

(c) In the FACS-sorted B-cell population, what percentage of the C_μ X genes will have a rearranged Eco RI restriction fragment? A rearranged Bam HI restriction fragment? Why?

(d) The right lane of the Bam HI Southern blot does not show any discrete bands; instead it shows a smear of hybridizing fragments. How do you interpret this result?

(e) There are two types of immunoglobulin gene rearrangements: V–D–J joining and C_H switching. In the FACS-sorted B-cell population, has the C_μ Y gene undergone a C_H switch rearrangement? How do you know?

(f) In the FACS-sorted B-cell population, has the C_μ Y gene undergone a V–D–J joining rearrangement? How do you know?

4-17 (a) One hypothesis for the mechanism of allelic exclusion proposes that only one heavy-chain, gene-containing chromosome (chromosome 12 in mice) will undergo rearrangement in any given B cell. To examine this process in more detail, Southern blots of DNA derived from several murine IgA-producing plasmacytomas in BALB/c mice were probed with a radiolabeled fragment of the murine C_α gene, and these results were compared with the pattern seen using DNA from sperm cells. The results of this experiment are shown in Figure 4-30. Are these results consistent with the "single-arrangement" theory of allelic exclusion? Why or why not?

(b) The 13 kb Eco RI fragment containing C_α sequence was cloned from plasmacytoma 1 and was found not to contain J_H, although the S_α switch region was present. A probe made from the unidentified DNA 5' to the S_α sequence hybridized with all of the 13 kb bands in the 7 plasmacytomas shown in Figure 4-30, as well as with a second band of 8 kb, which was present in all 7 plasmacytomas as well as the sperm DNA. Which bands in the Southern blot of Figure 4-30 represent the expressed heavy-chain encoding alleles?

Figure 4-30

Southern blot analysis of germline and plasmacytoma DNAs (Problem 4-17).

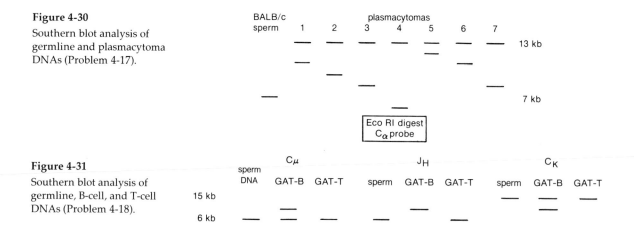

Figure 4-31

Southern blot analysis of germline, B-cell, and T-cell DNAs (Problem 4-18).

(c) Using a series of somatic cell hybrids between mouse and hamster cells containing various mouse chromosomes, it was possible to show that the 5′ probe described in part (b) was derived from chromosome 15. Describe the event that generated the 13 kb Eco RI C_α-containing fragment in the plasmacytomas. How could you determine if this event also occurred in normal B lymphocytes?

4-18 (a) Immune responses to most antigens involve the participation of both T lymphocytes and B lymphocytes. In one well-studied case, the production of antibodies against a synthetic polypeptide made up of glutamic acid, alanine, and tyrosine (GAT) is suppressed by T lymphocytes specific for the GAT antigen. Anti-idiotypic antibodies directed against GAT-specific antibodies have been shown to abrogate the suppressive effect of GAT-specific T lymphocytes. This experiment, like many other similar results obtained using other antigenic systems, suggests that T and B cells share the same idiotypic repertoire and hence may use the same receptors to recognize antigen. The following experiment was devised to test whether GAT-specific B cells and T cells use the same gene families to encode their antigen receptors.

DNA was extracted from GAT-specific T cells and GAT-specific B cells (both as hybridoma cell lines derived from the fusion of normal GAT-specific lymphocytes with malignant cells of either T- or B-cell origin) and subjected to Southern blot analysis using probes for C_μ, J_H, and C_κ. The results are shown in Figure 4-31. What can you conclude from these blots about the utilization of C_μ, J_H, and C_κ in T cells specific for GAT?

(b) Assuming that you had a probe for the V_H segment used in generating anti-GAT antibodies, how could you use this probe to determine if the same genetic element encodes part of the T-cell receptor for GAT?

4-19 A "Northern" blot is a technique used to examine the extent of transcription of particular genes and the size of the gene transcripts. In this procedure, mRNA molecules that carry poly(A) tails are isolated from total cellular RNA by adsorption to oligo(dT) cellulose and are subjected to electrophoresis in agarose under denaturing conditions. The mRNAs are thus separated by size and can be blotted directly onto nitrocellulose. Transcripts of interest are identified by hybridization of radiolabeled probes to the mRNA immobilized on the nitrocellulose filter.

Northern blots were performed using mRNA from three B-cell lymphomas, P1, P2, and P3. The probe in each case represented the C_H1 exon of the C_μ gene. RNA from a T-cell line was also examined. Figures 4-32a and b show the results of these experiments and describe the known characteristics of the lymphomas

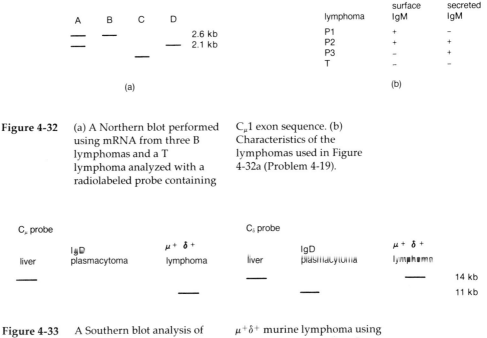

Figure 4-32 (a) A Northern blot performed using mRNA from three B lymphomas and a T lymphoma analyzed with a radiolabeled probe containing $C_\mu 1$ exon sequence. (b) Characteristics of the lymphomas used in Figure 4-32a (Problem 4-19).

Figure 4-33 A Southern blot analysis of Bam HI digested DNA from murine liver, a murine IgD-secreting plasmacytoma, and a $\mu^+\delta^+$ murine lymphoma using probes containing either C_μ or C_δ sequences (Problem 4-20).

used in these experiments. Match each lane of the Northern blot with the correct lymphoma described in Figure 4-32b. Knowing that C_μ is not rearranged in T cells, how would you interpret the results of the blot using the T-cell mRNA?

4-20 (a) The murine C_δ gene has been identified at a position 2 kb to the 3' side of the C_μ membrane exon in germline DNA. You are given an IgD-secreting plasmacytoma and a $\mu^+\delta^+$ lymphoma cell line, and you decide to examine the C_δ and C_μ genes in these cells using Southern blotting. Figure 4-33 shows the results obtained with Bam HI-digested DNA. What has happened to the C_δ gene in the plasmacytoma? What has happened to the C_μ gene in the plasmacytoma?

(b) How is the C_δ mRNA generated in the lymphoma cell line?

(c) In a similar experiment, IgE^+ B cells from immune mice were selected using the fluorescence-activated cell sorter, and DNA from these cells was examined by Southern blotting using a C_ϵ probe. No evidence of rearrangement of the C_ϵ gene was found. How large must the primary transcript from these IgE-secreting cells be?

(d) From the evidence in parts (a), (b), and (c), how is the synthesis of alternative immunoglobulin heavy-chain classes managed in B cells as compared with plasma cells?

4-21 There is some evidence that V–J and V–D–J joining can occur interchromosomally. In addition, the recognition sequences for rearrangement are similar in V and J gene segments. Would you expect rearrangement to occur between similar gene segments—for example, V gene segments to other V gene segments? Do you think that rearrangement can occur between families—for example, V_κ to J_λ? Assume that none of these potential translocation events is lethal.

Answers

4-1   (a) True

  (b) True

  (c) False. Idiotypic determinants may be within or outside the antigen-binding site.

  (d) True

  (e) False. Class switching occurs when a B cell switches from the expression of one heavy-chain class to the expression of a second.

  (f) True

  (g) True

  (h) False. V_H gene formation requires two DNA rearrangements—one joining V_H to D and a second joining D to J_H.

  (i) False. The IgM to IgA class switch requires a DNA rearrangement which joins the S_μ and S_α regions (see Figure 4-17).

  (j) False. The recognition sequences are highly conserved in all three gene families.

  (k) False. A nonproductive rearrangement leads to a V gene that cannot be expressed as a functional polypeptide; it is often expressed at the RNA level.

  (l) True

  (m) True

  (n) False. The μ_m and μ_s mRNAs are derived from a single C_μ gene by alternative patterns of RNA splicing.

  (o) False. The simultaneous expression of IgM and IgD molecules in a single B cell arises from a special RNA splicing mechanism.

  (p) True

  (q) False. Junctional diversity occurs as a result of flexible joining of the variable-region gene segments (V–J or V–D–J) and consequently only arises in the third hypervariable region.

  (r) True

  (s) True

  (t) True

  (u) True

  (v) False. B-cell immunoglobulin probes suggest that the corresponding B-cell genes are not necessarily expressed or rearranged in T cells.

4-2   (a) homologous

  (b) heterologous

  (c) allelic exclusion

  (d) class switch

  (e) λ and κ

  (f) germline

  (g) V gene formation

  (h) V_H, D, and J_H

  (i) 3′; 3′ and 5′; 5′

  (j) intramolecular deletion

  (k) interchromosomal sister chromatid exchange

  (l) productive

  (m) switch (S)

  (n) 3′

  (o) six

  (p) germline, combinatorial joining, and somatic mutation

  (q) combinatorial association

  (r) somatic hypermutation

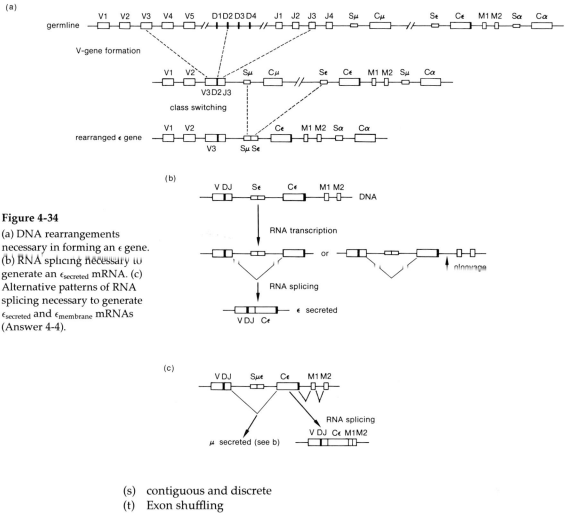

Figure 4-34

(a) DNA rearrangements necessary in forming an ε gene. (b) RNA splicing necessary to generate an ε$_{secreted}$ mRNA. (c) Alternative patterns of RNA splicing necessary to generate ε$_{secreted}$ and ε$_{membrane}$ mRNAs (Answer 4-4).

       (s)   contiguous and discrete
       (t)   Exon shuffling
       (u)   DNA, RNA, and protein
       (v)   T-cell

4-3   (a)   20 V_L
              40 V_H
              800 antibodies
       (b)   400 V_L
              8,000 V_H
              3,200,000 antibodies
       (c)   4,000 V_L
              80,000 V_H
              320,000,000 antibodies

4-4   (a)   See Figure 4-34.
       (b)   See Figure 4-34.
       (c)   See Figure 4-34.

4-5   (a)   As1 and As2 recognize allotypic determinants located on the C_H2 or C_H3 domains.
       (b)   As3 and As4 also recognize allotypic determinants, which may be located either

Figure 4-35

Recombination between genes for human C_H allotype (Answer 4-7).

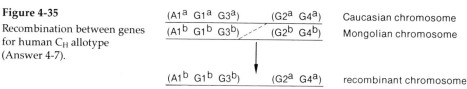

(A1^a G1^a G3^a) (G2^a G4^a)	Caucasian chromosome
(A1^b G1^b G3^b) (G2^b G4^b)	Mongolian chromosome
(A1^b G1^b G3^b) (G2^a G4^a)	recombinant chromosome

in the constant region domains or in the framework portion of the variable region. Unimmunized mice do not in general express enough of any particular variable region to permit the elicitation of anti-idiotypic antibodies using total light chains as an immunogen.

(c) The absorption step removes anti-allotype antibodies from As5 and hence leaves an antiserum with specificity for idiotypic determinants on anti-X antibodies.

(d) There is no contradiction here. Allelic exclusion applies only to individual cells, not to the organism as a whole.

(e) According to these results, the determinants recognized by As5 segregate with the heavy-chain marker defined by As2. Thus the As5 determinants are present on the γ chain and, since this is an idiotypic marker, on the V_H domain of the γ chain.

(f) According to these results, reactivity requires both heavy- and light-chain determinants. Thus the idiotypic marker is composed of components from both V_H and V_κ. Note that BC4 is a recombinant animal.

4-6 (a) It is unlikely that these variants are allelic forms of the same structural gene. If each variant represents 50% of the C_λ genes in the human population, then the probability of picking ten consecutive heterozygotes is $(1/2)^{10}$ or $1/1024$. If the variants were present in unequal frequencies in the population, then the probability of selecting ten consecutive heterozygotes would be even lower.

(b) This polymorphism may be coded by duplicate germline genes that have diverged by one base substitution.

4-7 (a) These genes must be closely linked because each group of polymorphisms segregates as a unit.

(b) The last individual must carry one Caucasian chromosome and a recombinant chromosome that arose in the F_1 parent, as shown in Figure 4-35. The phenotype of this individual suggests that the genes in parentheses are grouped together although a precise order cannot be determined.

4-8 (a) Specification of a V region 107 residues in length requires a gene of at least 321 nucleotide pairs. The maximum number of such genes that could be encoded by the mammalian haploid genome is

$$\frac{3.2 \times 10^9}{3.2 \times 10^2} = 10^7 \text{ V genes}$$

(b) If the entire haploid genome represents 10^7 V gene equivalents, then the percent of haploid DNA required for 1000 V_L and 1000 V_H genes is

$$\frac{2 \times 10^3}{10^7 \times 100\%} = 0.02\%$$

For random association of V_L and V_H regions, this percentage of the genome could provide the information for 10^6 different antibody molecules.

4-9 Haptens related structurally to the immunizing antigen compete with the anti-D antibody for binding to the D antibodies. This result might be explained in either of the following two ways:

1. The region of the combining site of the D antibody may include a major fraction of its idiotypic antigenic determinants. If so, the presence of hapten could sterically inhibit the reaction with anti-D antibody.

2. Combination of the hapten with the active site of the D antibody may cause a conformational change that alters idiotypic determinants, which need not be confined to the region of the active site.

X-ray structural studies indicate no variable-domain conformational changes upon reaction of an antibody with a hapten. Accordingly, most immunologists favor the first explanation.

4-10 (a) The Ms-1 allotype does not appear to be coded by a1 V genes because several a1 individuals in the pedigree are Ms-1-negative; for example, individuals 4 and 7 in the F_2 generation.

(b) Ms-1 must be a variant of the μ constant region because the Ms-1 allotype is observed only on IgM molecules. However, expression of the Ms-1 allotype occurs only in individuals that produce the b4 light-chain allotype as well. Individuals that carry only the Ms-1 C_μ gene or the b4 C_κ gene alone do not exhibit the Ms-1 allotype. The two mated Ms-1-negative individuals in the F2 generation each contribute one of the genes necessary to produce Ms-1-positive progeny. Close linkage between the V_H and C_H (including C_μ) genes accounts for the observation that a1 and Ms-1 always segregate together in these experiments.

(c) The $C_\mu 1$ and C_κ regions are the only constant-region homology units that interact with one another in the IgM molecule. Therefore, the Ms-1 specificity probably is produced by the interaction of these two homology units. This supposition could be verified by testing Fab and Fc fragments of the IgM molecule for the Ms-1 specificity and, if possible, by isolating and testing the $C_\mu 1$ domain alone.

4-11 (a) The A5A marker segregates in a Mendelian fashion with dominant or codominant expression. These results suggest that the A5A marker identifies a V_H gene that is linked to the C_H alleles.

(b) Of the 25 backcross mice that are either Ig–1 e/e or Ig–1 a/a, one apparent crossover event was observed. This event implies a recombination frequency of 4%, equivalent to 4000 kb of DNA between the A5A and C_H markers. This amount represents enough DNA to encode about 200 V_H genes if the average spacing between genes is 20 kb.

4-12 (a) The germline restriction fragment including the J_κ gene segments is 5 kb in length.

(b) Plasma cells are diploid and contain two copies (maternal and paternal) of the κ-chain chromosome. One chromosome has productively rearranged to generate an 8-kb DNA fragment containing the rearranged V_κ gene. The second chromosome is in the germline configuration. Allelic exclusion might arise when only one κ-chain chromosome rearranges productively. Perhaps there is a mechanism which permits only one DNA rearrangement in each B cell for the κ gene family.

(c) Both chromosomes appear to have rearranged to give different sized fragments carrying V_κ sequences. Such observations lead to the view that if the first κ-chain chromosome rearrangement is unproductive, yielding a nonfunctional V_κ gene, then a second rearrangement can occur. If this rearrangement is productive, the resulting plasma cells will carry rearrangements in both κ-chain chromosomes.

4-13 (a) $\overset{18}{C}ACAGTG-11-ACACAAAC\overset{45}{C}$ is the V recognition region

$\overset{2}{G}GTTTTTGTA-22-CACTGT\overset{25}{G}$ is the J recognition region

(b) Because the V segment has an 11-base spacer and the J segment a 22-base spacer between the 7-mer and 9-mer recognition elements, these sequences must derive from the κ gene family.

(c) TYR TYR CYS ALA ARG TYR TRP TYR PHE ASP

4-14 Sequences (a), (b), (d), (e), and (f) reflect junctional diversity generated during V–J joining. Sequences (c) and (g) must result from somatic mutation events superimposed on the V–J joining process.

4-15 For the light chain there are four possible alleles: two κ and two λ. Any one rearrangement has a 1/3 probability of being in-frame and a 2/3 probability of being out-of-frame. The probability P_L of at least one in-frame light-chain allele is one minus the probability that all four will be out-of-frame.

$$P_L = 1 - (2/3)^4$$
$$= 0.8025$$

For the heavy chain there are two possible alleles and two rearrangements, V–D and D–J for each. Each rearrangement has a 1/3 probability of being in-frame; hence for each allele the probabilities for the combined rearrangement are 1/9 that it is in-frame and 8/9 that it is not. The probability P_H of at least one in-frame heavy-chain allele is

$$P_H = 1 - (8/9)^2$$
$$= 0.2099$$

The probability P_{LH} of at least one in-frame light-chain and one in-frame heavy-chain allele is

$$P_{LH} = P_L \times P_H$$
$$= 0.802 \times 0.210$$
$$= 0.168$$

4-16 (a) Due to allelic exclusion, 50% will express the C_μ X allotype and 50% will express the C_μ Y allotype.

(b) One hundred percent will have a rearranged C_μ X region because the cells were selected for expression of the C_μ X allotype.

(c) From the restriction map, none will have a rearranged Eco RI fragment; all will have a rearranged Bam HI fragment due to juxtaposition of V_H sequences with the J region.

(d) The smear represents heterogeneity in the various C_μ-containing Bam HI fragments as a result of the juxtaposition of different V_H sequences in different cells with the J_H–C_μ sequence.

(e) Because the C_μ Y Eco RI fragment is still intact, C_H switching has not occurred.

(f) V–D–J joining must have taken place because the C_μ Y gene Bam HI fragment is not intact.

4-17 (a) The results are not consistent with a single rearrangement theory because the germline C_α fragment is missing in the plasmacytomas.

(b) Because the 13-kb Eco RI fragment in plasmacytoma 1 does not contain J_H, it cannot encode the heavy chain. Also, because the sequence 5' to the S_α region in this clone is also present in the 13-kb Eco RI fragments from the other tumors, these fragments also probably do not encode the heavy chain. The variable sized bands on the Southern blot are consistent with different V–D–J joining events, and these fragments, therefore, represent the expressed heavy-chain encoding alleles.

(c) A translocation must have occurred in the plasmacytomas, which brought a portion of chromosome 15 into juxtaposition with the S_α region of chromosome 12. We could test for the presence of this translocation (if at high frequency) in normal B cells by Southern blot analysis of DNA from B cells isolated using the cell sorter, using the C_α and 5' probes.

4-18 (a) If C_μ, J_H, and C_κ are used, they are not rearranged and hence must be transcribed very differently in T cells than in B cells.

(b) Two methods could be used. First, you could look for rearrangement of the V_{GAT} using Southern blots; second, you could try to determine if mRNA transcripts of V_{GAT} are present in GAT-specific T cells (see question 4-19).

4-19 A = P2; B = P1; C = T cell; D = P3.

C_μ is apparently transcribed to some extent in T cells even though it is not rearranged. Note that the transcript is smaller than the normal $\mu_{secreted}$ transcript.

4-20 (a) The C_δ gene is rearranged in the plasmacytoma; therefore, a class switching event must have occurred at the DNA level. The C_μ gene has been deleted.

(b) Because no rearrangement has occurred in the lymphoma DNA, synthesis of both IgM and IgD must be accomplished through processing of the primary RNA transcript to yield different mRNAs.

(c) If true, this result implies that the primary transcripts in IgE-secreting B cells would be in excess of 200 kb.

(d) Class switching in B cells appears to result from RNA processing. Class switching in plasma cells involves a DNA rearrangement.

4-21 Within families, V segments probably could not join to each other because their spacers are the same size (thus the 1-turn–2-turn rule would be violated). V_κ would not rearrange to J_λ for the same reason. V_λ could potentially rearrange to D segments interchromosomally, as could V_κ rearrange to J_H. Such events have not been observed to date.

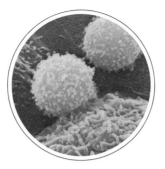

CHAPTER 5

Molecular Recognition at Cell Surfaces

Chapter Outline

131

In the vertebrate immune system, diverse immunologic functions are initiated by events at the lymphocyte cell surface. These functions include the transmission of positional information by cell-cell recognition, as in the homing of B cells and T cells to specific areas of lymphoid tissue, and the triggering of differentiation and proliferation by specific macromolecules, as in the response of B-cell and T-cell precursors to a circulating cognate antigen. Because new genes evolve from previously existing genes, the vertebrate immune system almost certainly had its origins in more primitive recognition systems. A variety of evidence indicates that such recognition systems operate in the development and physiological functioning of all metazoan organisms; moreover, they appear to be mediated by recognition elements embedded in cell-surface plasma membranes. This chapter considers the general structure and function of the plasma membrane and the characteristics of some simple metazoan cellular-recognition systems.

Concepts

5-1 Membranes are fundamental components of biological organization

Membrane functions

Membranes perform a variety of general functions in all cells and tissues. Most importantly, membranes separate cells from their environment and from one another, and they permit the specialization of cellular function that is characteristic of metazoa (Figure 5-1). In addition, membranes partition the interior of eukaryotic cells into areas of distinct specialization, such as the nucleus, the mitochondria, the endoplasmic reticulum, the Golgi apparatus, and a variety of smaller vesicles. Finally, plasma membrane and its associated cytoskeletal elements mediate cell movement. In the many types of eukaryotic cells that are capable of amoeboid movement, the plasma membrane is a dynamic structure that appears to be sending out pseudopodia in all directions, as if to explore its environment (Figure 5-2).

Cell membranes function as barriers because their lipid core, although relatively permeable to water and to small hydrophobic molecules, is relatively impermeable to macromolecules and polar molecules. The protein components of membranes mediate specific membrane functions. Membrane proteins mediate the transport of ions, metabolites, and macromolecules into and out of cells. Membrane pumps and gates allow active or passive transport, respectively, of certain ions and metabolites (Figure 5-1b). In nerve and muscle-cell membranes, the cooperative action of pumps and gates leads to propagation of action potentials along cells. Endocytosis and exocytosis

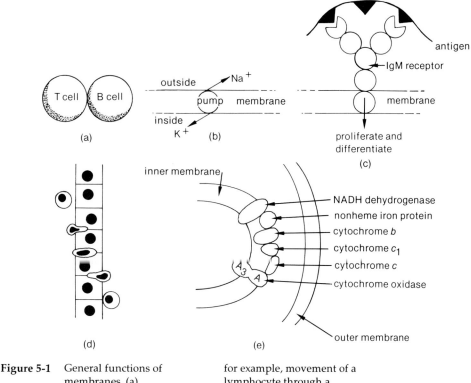

Figure 5-1 General functions of membranes. (a) Compartmentalization of cells to permit functional specialization. (b) Transfer of materials into and out of cells. (c) Transfer of signals from the environment into cells. (d) Mediation of cell movement; for example, movement of a lymphocyte through a postcapillary venule. (e) Organization of proteins; for example, organization of the electron transport enzymes in the inner mitochondrial membrane.

move macromolecules into or out of cellular compartments, respectively.

In addition, plasma membrane proteins mediate transfer of information from the exterior to the interior of cells. Most eukaryotic cells carry a variety of membrane-associated receptor molecules that are capable of transducing external stimuli into appropriate cellular responses. Cells within a tissue recognize and specifically adhere to one another via cell-surface structures. Certain cells, such as T cells, B cells, and macrophages, recognize one another and communicate differentiation signals at the cell surface (Figure 5-1a). Finally, small molecules or macromolecules can interact with cell-surface receptors to produce an appropriate cellular response, as in the stimulation of target cells by hormones, the triggering of lymphocyte differentiation by antigen (Figure 5-1c), and the initiation of action potentials at nerve synapses.

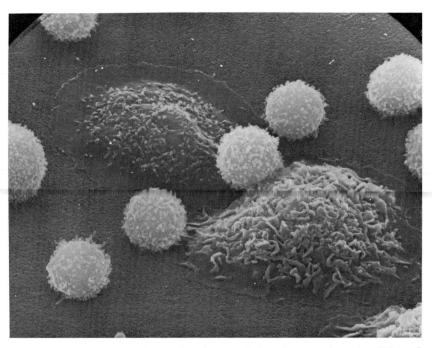

Figure 5-2 A scanning electron micrograph of several lymphocytes (round cells) and macrophages. [Courtesy of J. Orenstein and E. Shelton.]

Lipid components

Lipids are responsible for the sheetlike structure of membranes and for their general properties as hydrophobic barriers. Most membranes are 30–50% lipid by weight. Lipid molecules in membranes are amphipathic; that is, they have distinct polar and nonpolar regions. Such lipids can aggregate spontaneously in aqueous solution to form a bilayer with their nonpolar hydrocarbon "tails"—often represented by wavy lines—abutting in the interior, and their polar "heads"— usually represented by a circle—on either surface (Figure 5-3). Hydrophobic interactions of the tails, which remove them from the aqueous environment, are primarily responsible for the strong tendency toward bilayer formation.

The three major membrane lipids are *phospholipids, glycolipids,* and *cholesterol.* Phospholipids are derived from either of the two small molecules—glycerol or serine—to which are attached two fatty acids and a phosphorylated alcohol (Figure 5-4). The most common phospholipids, which are derived from glycerol, are called *phosphoglycerides.* The hydroxyl groups at C1 and C2 of glycerol are esterified to the carboxyl groups of two fatty acids (forming a diglyceride), and the C3 hydroxyl group is esterified through a phos-

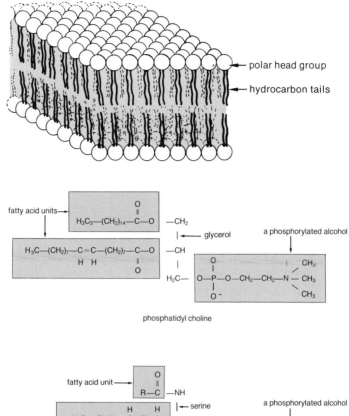

Figure 5-3

Diagram of a section of a bilayer membrane formed from phospholipid or glycolipid.

Figure 5-4

Two types of phospholipids (see text).

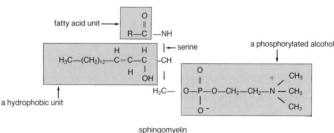

phate group to any one of several alcohols (Figure 5-5). For example, the phosphoglyceride with choline as the alcohol is phosphatidyl choline, a common membrane phospholipid. The only phospholipid not derived from glycerol is sphingomyelin, which is derived from serine. The amino group and α carbon of serine are attached to two fatty acids (forming a ceramide), and the serine hydroxyl is esterified through a phosphate group to choline (Figure 5-4). The fatty acid chains in phospholipids usually contain between 14 and 24 carbon atoms and may be saturated or unsaturated. Double bonds are nearly always in the *cis* configuration, which produces a kink in the fatty acid chain.

Glycolipids are derived from a ceramide by the attachment of one or more sugar units to the serine hydroxyl (Figure 5-6). Cholesterol, a steroid, is the biosynthetic precursor of bile acids and steroid hor-

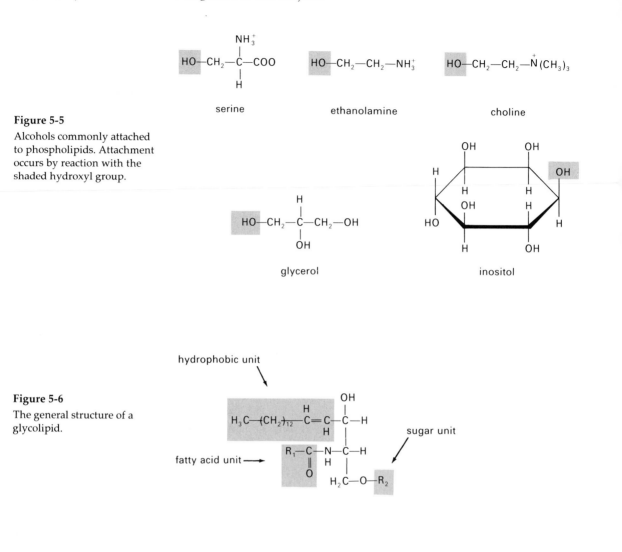

Figure 5-5
Alcohols commonly attached to phospholipids. Attachment occurs by reaction with the shaded hydroxyl group.

serine

ethanolamine

choline

glycerol

inositol

Figure 5-6
The general structure of a glycolipid.

hydrophobic unit

sugar unit

fatty acid unit

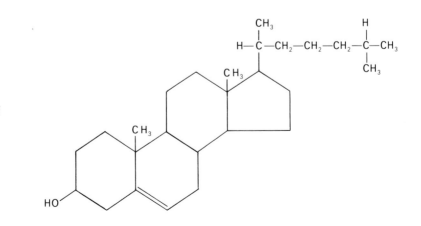

Figure 5-7
The structural formula of cholesterol.

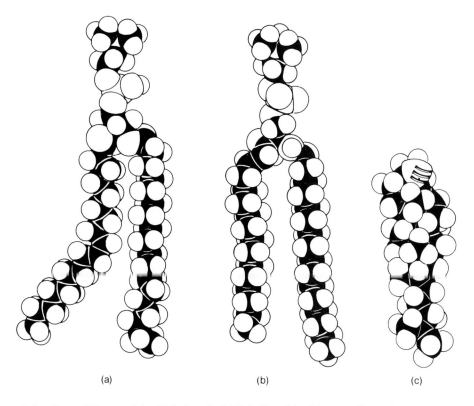

(a)   (b)   (c)

Figure 5-8   Space-filling models of (a) phosphatidyl choline, (b) sphingomyelin, and (c) cholesterol.

mones, as well as an important component of eukaryotic cell membranes (Figure 5-7). The polar head region of cholesterol is provided by its hydroxyl group. Membrane lipids are similar in three-dimensional configuration, which is roughly that of a cylinder (Figure 5-8).

Protein components   Membrane proteins are designated integral or peripheral depending on the nature of their association with the lipid bilayer. *Integral proteins* can generally be dissociated from the bilayer only by agents such as detergents and organic solvents that disrupt hydrophobic interactions. By contrast, *peripheral proteins* can be dissociated from the bilayer by mild techniques, such as changing the ionic concentration of the medium or adding a chelating agent such as ethylenediaminetetracetate (EDTA). Thus integral proteins presumably interact directly with the membrane lipids, whereas peripheral proteins are probably attached to the polar surfaces of the bilayer (Figure 5-9). It is difficult to define the set of peripheral proteins precisely because many of them may be attached so loosely that they are lost during membrane isolation.

Figure 5-9

Possible locations of peripheral and integral membrane proteins.

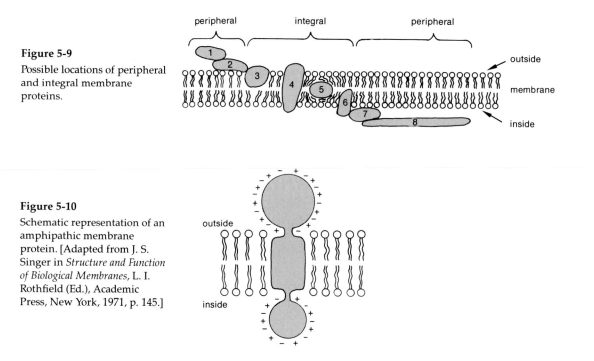

Figure 5-10

Schematic representation of an amphipathic membrane protein. [Adapted from J. S. Singer in *Structure and Function of Biological Membranes*, L. I. Rothfield (Ed.), Academic Press, New York, 1971, p. 145.]

Integral membrane proteins, like membrane lipids, have an amphipathic structure that permits them to associate simultaneously with hydrophobic membrane lipids and the hydrophilic external environment (Figure 5-10). In principle, an integral protein could be positioned in several different ways relative to the lipid bilayer; however, the most common arrangement appears to span the membrane (Figure 5-9, type 4). One of the first identified and best-studied transmembrane proteins is *glycophorin*, a red blood cell protein. Its polypeptide chain of 131 amino acid residues is divided into three distinct domains. The N-terminal portion of the molecule forms the external domain; the middle forms the hydrophobic membrane domain; and the C-terminal portion forms the internal domain (Figure 5-11). Thus the glycophorin molecule is linearly amphipathic. Although this arrangement is a common one, it is not the only arrangement for integral membrane proteins.

Different plasma membranes differ in the types and the amounts of proteins present, corresponding presumably to the distinct functions that various plasma membranes perform. For example, the red blood cell, the lymphocyte, and the kidney tubule cell plasma membranes have quite distinct membrane–protein compositions. The molecular weights of membrane proteins vary from approximately 10,000 to several hundred thousand. A few membrane proteins are present in high concentrations of 10–50% of total membrane protein, but most are present at concentrations of only a fraction of a percent.

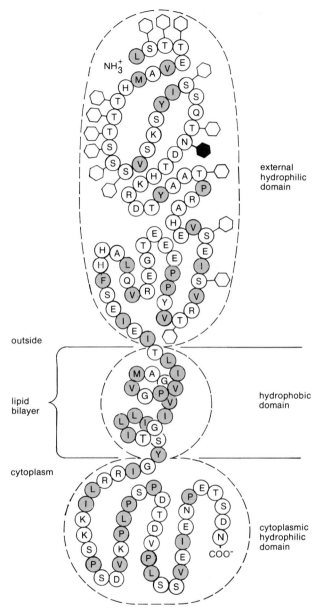

Figure 5-11

A diagrammatic representation of the three domains of glycophorin, an integral amphipathic membrane protein of the red blood cell. The single-letter designations for amino acid residues are as listed in Table 2-1. Hydrophobic residues are shaded to show their distribution more clearly. Hexagons connected to certain amino acids indicate attached carbohydrate groups.

The fluid mosaic structure of membranes

The general structure of the plasma membrane is a mosaic of proteins "floating" in a lipid bilayer (Figure 5-12). In a fluid membrane, both the lipid and protein components are capable of rapid rotational and translational diffusion in the plane of the membrane, but they undergo transverse diffusion (flipping) from one side of the membrane to the other much less rapidly. In artificial bilayers, the rate of lipid flipping is 10^9 times slower than the rate of translational diffusion.

Figure 5-12

The fluid-mosaic model of membrane structure. Black lipid molecules represent glycolipids; large white inclusions are protein molecules "floating in the bilayer, with their hydrophobic regions contacting lipid side chains and their hydrophilic regions exposed to the external medium." [Adapted from J. S. Singer in *Cell Membranes: Biochemistry, Cell Biology and Pathology*, G. Weissmann and R. Clairborne (Eds.), H. P. Publishing Co., Inc., New York, 1975, p. 35.]

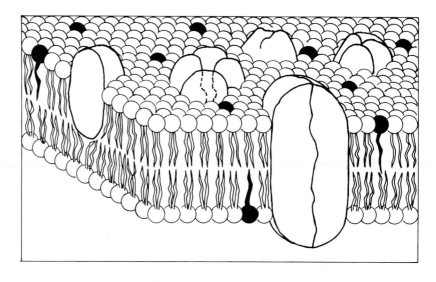

However, in biological membranes, lipid flipping is probably catalyzed by membrane proteins. By contrast, proteins in biological membranes probably flip extremely rarely, if at all, because of the high free energy of activation required to transport hydrophilic domains through the hydrophobic lipid bilayer.

The fluidity of membranes is determined by the packing of the nonpolar portions of the lipids in the membrane interior. Lipids with long saturated fatty acid chains decrease membrane fluidity because their straight hydrocarbon tails can form van der Waals bonds with one another along their full length (Figure 5-13a). Shorter chain fatty acids increase membrane fluidity because they interact less strongly than longer ones; each additional methylene group adds about 0.5 kcal/mole to the energy of interaction of adjacent chains (Figure 5-13c). Similarly, fatty acids with *cis* double bonds also increase membrane fluidity because they cause kinks that interfere with the packing of adjacent fatty acids (Figure 5-13b). Cholesterol tends to decrease the fluidity of natural membranes because it packs well with kinked fatty acid side chains.

Animals can apparently adjust the lipid composition of their membranes to maintain an optimal fluidity in response to the surrounding environmental temperatures. For example, Lapland reindeer have significantly more unsaturated fatty acids in the membranes of cells in their extremities than in membranes of their other body cells. Likewise, poikilothermic (cold blooded) animals increase the fraction of unsaturated fatty acids in their membranes at colder temperatures.

Membrane asymmetry

All cellular membranes are asymmetric in the sense that their inner (cytoplasmic) and outer (external) surfaces differ in all their major

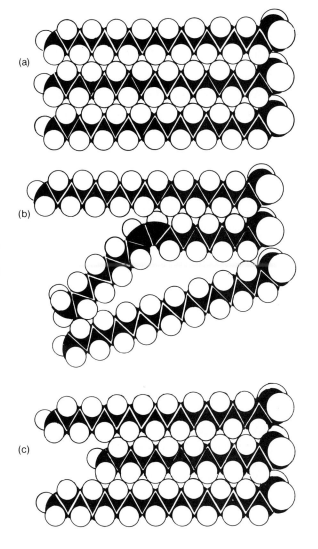

Figure 5-13

Space-filling models illustrating the packing of various fatty acid chains. (a) Three molecules of a saturated C_{18} fatty acid. (b) An unsaturated C_{18} fatty acid with a single double bond between two saturated C_{18} fatty acids. (c) Two molecules of a saturated C_{18} fatty acid separated by a C_{14} fatty acid.

components: proteins, phospholipids, and carbohydrates. Membrane proteins of like kind all are oriented in the same way relative to the two sides of the membrane. Therefore, the two surfaces of a membrane display different protein domains and different enzymatic activities. This asymmetry comes about because all membrane proteins are inserted in a defined orientation from the cytoplasmic side and do not flip thereafter.

Phospholipids are generally distributed unevenly between the surfaces of a membrane. For example, in the red blood cell membrane, choline phospholipids predominate in the external half of the lipid bilayer, whereas amino phospholipids predominate in the cytoplasmic half. If the flipping of lipids is catalyzed by proteins in natural membranes, then the uneven distribution of lipid species may reflect differences in the environment on the two sides of a membrane.

Glycolipids and glycoproteins, which do not flip from one side of the membrane to the other, are found only on external membrane surfaces because carbohydrates are added to lipids and proteins only in the lumen of the endoplasmic reticulum and Golgi apparatus (Concept 5-2). Upon transport of membrane material to the cell surface, the luminal surfaces of these intracellular compartments become the external surface of the cell.

5-2 Lipids and proteins are distributed to cellular membranes by flow processes involving membrane budding and fusion

Membrane biosynthesis and flow

Membrane components are in a constant state of turnover. The half-life of lipids in the membrane may be on the order of minutes, whereas the proteins have half-lives ranging from hours to days. The mechanisms of turnover and the factors that control the rates for various membrane components are poorly understood. However, the fact of turnover implies that membranes are renewed continually.

Although membrane biosynthesis is not clearly understood, most membrane components appear to be synthesized and inserted first into the endoplasmic reticulum. Lipid components are probably synthesized in the cytoplasmic leaflet of the bilayer and become distributed between the two leaflets by catalyzed flipping. Most of the transmembrane proteins that reach the plasma membrane are inserted into the membrane of the endoplasmic reticulum during synthesis by membrane-bound ribosomes. These proteins and others that are inserted into or through the membrane of the endoplasmic reticulum are sorted out to their final cellular location according to signals that are for the most part undefined. The mechanisms for protein sorting are a current focus of intensive research in cell biology.

Membrane material that is bound for the plasma membrane travels first to the Golgi apparatus and then to the plasma membrane via a series of vesicle formations and fusions. Small vesicles that are coated with the protein *clathrin* may mediate this membrane flow. Clathrin assembles into a protein basket on the cytoplasmic surface of vesicles to form *coated vesicles,* which appear to be important in the transport of material from the endoplasmic reticulum to the Golgi apparatus and from the Golgi apparatus to the plasma membrane, as well as being important in the reverse flow from plasma membrane to lysosomes during certain endocytotic events. Each vesicle formation and fusion occurs with conservation of asymmetry; that is, the cytoplasmic surface always remains in contact with the cytoplasm, and the luminal surface always faces the interior of an intracellular compartment until it finally fuses with the plasma membrane and becomes part of the external surface of the cell.

Membrane budding and fusion

Membrane budding and fusion are fundamental aspects of plasma membrane physiology (Figure 5-14). Besides playing a role in membrane flow, budding and fusion are also important in many normal processes that increase or decrease the number of membrane-bounded compartments in a cell or tissue: *exocytosis* and *endocytosis* involve vesicle fusion with and budding off from the plasma membrane, respectively (Figure 5-14a,b). Cell division requires one membrane-bounded compartment to bud into two (Figure 5-14c). Reproduction requires the fusion of sperm and egg membranes (Figure 5-14d). During embryonic development, somatic cells can fuse to form syncytial tissues, as in the fusion of myoblasts to form myotubules in muscle development and the fusion of osteoblasts in vertebrate bone development. Membrane fusion also is involved in the phagocytic response of macrophages to foreign antigen (Concept 9-2).

5-3   Oligosaccharide components of glycoproteins and glycolipids are added in the lumina of the endoplasmic reticulum and the Golgi apparatus

Sugar components and oligosaccharide diversity

The many different kinds of oligosaccharides found on glycoproteins are constructed from only nine components (Figure 5-15). Six are simple sugars; two, N-acetylglucosamine and N-acetylgalactosamine, are amino sugars that carry an acetyl group; and one, N-acetylneuraminic acid or sialic acid, carries a carboxyl group and provides most membranes with most of their negative charge.

In principle, these building blocks are capable of generating an enormous diversity of oligosaccharide sequences because each monomer possesses several hydroxyl groups that permit branching and a variety of potential linkages for each unit. However, oligosaccharides are constructed on specific substrates in stepwise fashion by a series of enzymatic reactions in which individual glycosyl transferases add carbohydrate monomers that have been activated by conversion to nucleotide derivatives (Figure 5-16). Because each transferase is specific for the sugar to be added and a particular acceptor sequence, each distinct kind of linkage requires a distinct glycosyl transferase. This practical requirement that a protein catalyze each step limits the actual diversity of oligosaccharides, which nevertheless is large.

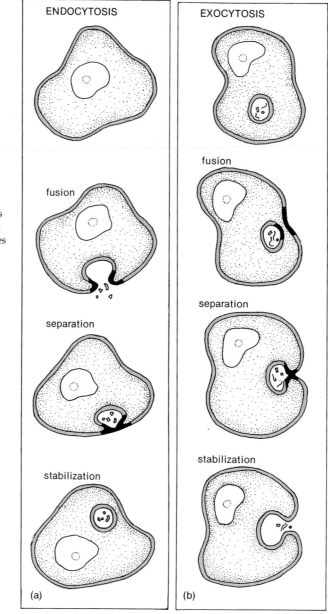

Figure 5-14
Membrane fusion in processes of normal cellular physiology. Shaded portions of membranes denote sites of membrane fusion. [Adapted from J. A. Lucy in *Cell Membranes: Biochemistry, Cell Biology and Pathology*, G. Weissmann and R. Clairborne (Eds.), H. P. Publishing Co., Inc., New York, 1975, p. 75.]

The sequence of saccharides on a particular protein in a cell is determined by the set of glycosyltransferases expressed by that cell. If compartmentalization of glycosylation does not occur within that cell, the same sequence of saccharides will be attached to each protein that has the appropriate recognition site for the first glycosyltransferase. However, each transferase is able to catalyze its reaction only when

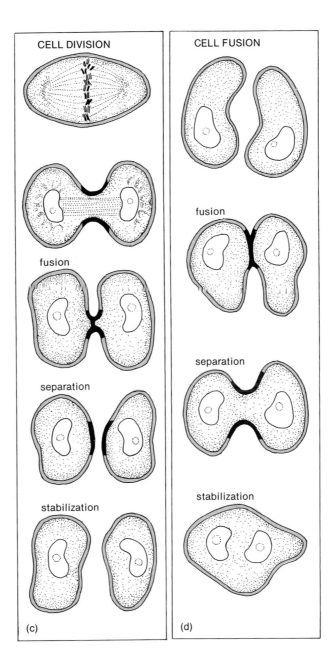

the preceding steps of synthesis have occurred and, under physiological conditions, there is variable completion and therefore a significant heterogeneity among oligosaccharide chains.

N-linked and O-linked oligosaccharides

Carbohydrates are attached to nearly all plasma membrane proteins during their transit through the endoplasmic reticulum and Golgi

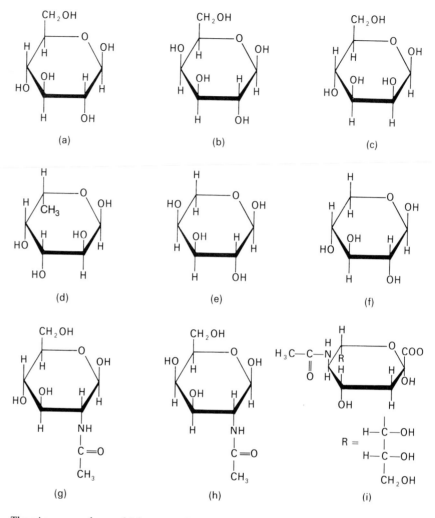

Figure 5-15 The nine sugars from which membrane oligosaccharides are constructed. (a) D-glucose (Glc); (b) D-galactose (Gal); (c) D-mannose (Man); (d) L-fucose (Fuc); (e) L-arabinose (Ara); (f) D-xylose (Xyl); (g) N-acetyl-D-glucosamine (GlcNAc); (h) N-acetyl-D-galactosamine (GalNAc); and (i) N-acetylneuraminic acid or sialic acid (NANA).

apparatus. Typically, one or a few oligosaccharide units are attached in N-glycosidic linkage to asparagine through N-acetylglucosamine (Figure 5-17a), or in O-glycosidic linkage to threonine or serine through N-acetylgalactosamine (Figure 5-17b), to serine through xylose, to hydroxylysine through galactose, or to hydroxyproline through arabinose.

In contrast to the highly diverse and less-well-studied O-linked oligosaccharides, there is an underlying pattern to N-linked oligosac-

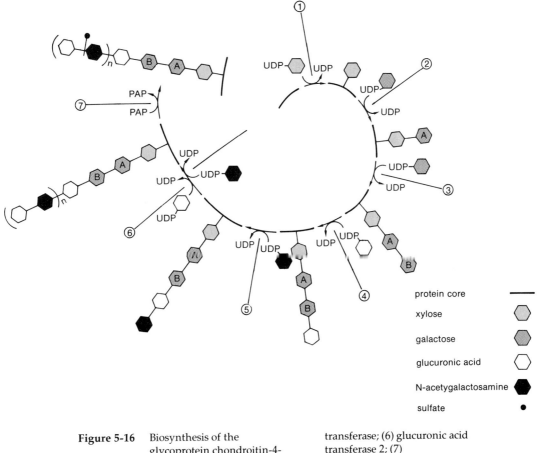

protein core ──────

xylose

galactose

glucuronic acid

N-acetygalactosamine

sulfate

Figure 5-16 Biosynthesis of the glycoprotein chondroitin-4-sulfate. The enzymes that catalyze the seven numbered steps are: (1) xylose transferase; (2) galactose transferase 1; (3) galactose transferase 2; (4) glucuronic acid transferase 1; (5) N-acetyl-D-galactosamine transferase; (6) glucuronic acid transferase 2; (7) sulfotransferase. UDP is uridine diphosphate. PAP designates the sulfate donor 3-phosphoadenosine 5'-phosphosulfate. [Courtesy of A. Dorfman.]

charide addition. Initially, a core oligosaccharide is constructed on the lipid carrier, dolichol phosphate, by the sequential action of specific transferases as just described (Figure 5-18a). This core oligosaccharide is then transferred as a unit to asparagine residues of Asn-X-Ser or Asn-X-Thr sequences in newly synthesized proteins as they enter the lumen of the endoplasmic reticulum. The terminal branches of the core structure are trimmed, partly in the endoplasmic reticulum and partly in the Golgi apparatus, and new carbohydrate monomers are added in the Golgi apparatus to produce the final N-linked oligosaccharide structure (Figure 5-18b).

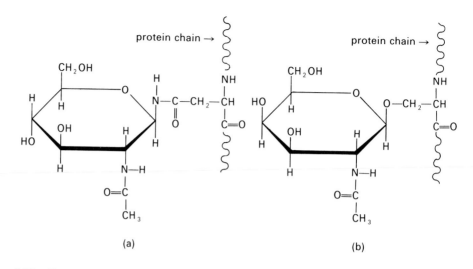

Figure 5-17   Two types of carbohydrate linkage to glycoproteins. (a) N-glycosidic linkage of N-acetylglucosamine to asparagine. (b) O-glycosidic linkage of N-acetylgalactosamine to serine.

Two experimentally useful antibiotics have been used to interfere with addition of N-linked oligosaccharides. *Tunicamycin*, which is a hydrophobic analog of UDP-N-acetylglucosamine, blocks addition of N-acetylglucosamine to dolichol phosphate at the first step in construction of the core oligosaccharide. *Bacitracin*, which blocks conversion of dolichol pyrophosphate to dolichol phosphate, interferes with the recycling of the lipid carrier after it has donated the core oligosaccharide to a protein.

Blood-group antigens   The human blood-group substances, also called the ABO and Lewis antigens, are cell-surface oligosaccharides whose genetics and chemistry are better understood than those of any other cell-surface carbohydrate system. These oligosaccharides are attached to glycolipids in the plasma membranes of red blood cells and other human cells. In addition, they may be attached to soluble glycoproteins that are found in secretions such as saliva, tears, and gastric juice. Large quantities of soluble glycoproteins that exhibit blood-group specificities can be obtained from certain individuals with ovarian cysts or tumors. These glycoproteins contain 85% by weight of carbohydrate in the form of multiple short oligosaccharides attached to a polypeptide backbone.

Five distinct blood-group specificities related to the ABO and Lewis systems can be detected by "natural" antibodies present in humans who lack the corresponding cell-surface antigens. These specificities are designated A, B, H(O), Le[a] (Lewis a), and Le[b] (Lewis b). Antibodies that react with four of these specificities can be inhibited by prior reaction with the corresponding monosaccharide (Table 5-1).

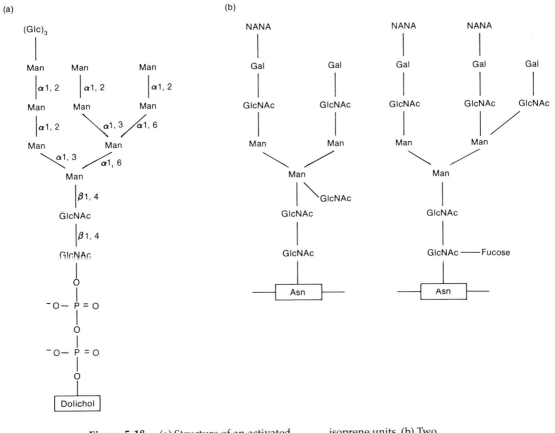

Figure 5-18   (a) Structure of an activated core oligosaccharide. Dolichol is a polyisoprenoid lipid alcohol containing about 20 isoprene units. (b) Two examples of Asn-linked oligosaccharides in mammalian glycoproteins.

Table 5-1   Monosaccharides That Inhibit Antibodies to Specific Blood-Group Substances

Blood-Group Specificity	Inhibiting Monosaccharide
A	N-Acetyl-D-galactosamine
B	D-Galactose
H	L-Fucose
Le[a]	N-Acetyl-D-glucosamine

Table 5-2 Relation Between Genotype, Red Blood Cell Antigens, and Serum Antibodies in the ABO Blood-Group System

Group (Phenotype)	Possible Genotypes	Antigens on Red Cells	Antibodies in Serum
A	AA AO	A	anti-B
B	BB BO	B	anti-A
AB	AB	AB	neither anti-A nor anti-B
O	OO	—	anti-A and anti-B

Figure 5-19

Two types of precursor oligosaccharides for the ABO and Lewis blood-group substances. Gal, D-galactose; GlcNAc, N-acetyl-D-glucosamine; GalNAc, N-acetyl-D-galactosamine.

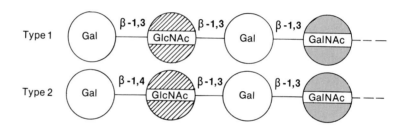

All natural antibodies to these blood-group antigens are IgM immunoglobulins. Because they are specific for relatively common saccharides, these antibodies are probably induced by environmental polysaccharide antigens, which would explain both their ubiquitous presence and their IgM nature (Concept 8-5). These natural antibodies are absent only from individuals with congenital or acquired agammaglobulinemia (Concept 12-4), and they are therefore useful in the diagnosis of these disorders. The relationships among ABO phenotypes, genotypes, and natural serum antibodies are given in Table 5-2.

Three genetically unlinked but functionally related gene systems—designated ABO, Hh, and Lewis—code for glycosyltransferases that determine the structure of blood-group oligosaccharides for the ABO and Lewis systems (Table 5-2). Each of these glycosyltransferases operates on two closely related oligosaccharides, which are the precursors to the blood-group substances (Figure 5-19). The synthetic pathways of the various blood-group oligosaccharides are given in Figure 5-20.

The multiple precursor oligosaccharides on a single polypeptide backbone are modified to differing extents by the transferases. For example, in an individual with A, B, H, and Le genes, the A, B, H, Le[b],

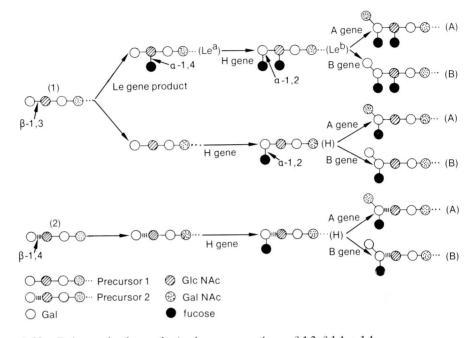

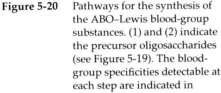

Figure 5-20 Pathways for the synthesis of the ABO–Lewis blood-group substances. (1) and (2) indicate the precursor oligosaccharides (see Figure 5-19). The blood-group specificities detectable at each step are indicated in parentheses. β-1,3, β-1,4, α-1,4, and α-1,2 indicate linkages between adjacent sugar residues. Gal, galactose; GlcNAc, N-acetyl-D-glucosamine; GalNAc, N-acetyl-D-galactosamine.

and even Le^a specificities can be detected on the same glycoprotein molecule. Because the glycosyltransferase systems are not very efficient, carbohydrate chains are completed to varying extents on the same glycoprotein backbone. Accordingly, some oligosaccharide chains are finished to the extent of expressing the Le^a specificity, others to the extent of expressing the H specificity, and so on (Figure 5-20). Thus the normal process of synthesis generates a family of closely related glycoproteins (or glycolipids). As indicated in Table 5-3, the transferase alleles O, h, and le represent a lack of the corresponding enzyme functions. Consequently, when these alleles are present in the homozygous state, oligosaccharide synthesis is blocked at specific sites of monosaccharide addition.

An additional gene, secretor (Se), plays a different role in determining the expression of blood-group specificities. The effects of this gene indicate that there are two distinct systems for the synthesis of blood-group substances. The *soluble* blood-group substances attached to glycoproteins and found in various body secretions are produced by the *secretory blood-group system*. The *insoluble* blood-group substances, attached to glycolipids and found on certain plasma mem-

Table 5-3 Gene Systems, Alleles, and Gene Products Responsible for the ABH and Lewis Specificities

Gene System	Alleles	Gene Product
ABO	A	N-Acetyl-D-galactosamine transferase
	B	D-Galactosyl transferase
	O	No functional gene product
Hh	H	L-Fucosyl transferase
	h	No functional gene product
Lewis	Le	L-Fucosyl transferase
	le	No functional gene product

branes such as those of the red blood cells, are produced by the *membrane blood-group system.* The secretor gene, in its homozygous (Se/Se) or heterozygous (Se/se) state, allows blood-group substances to be secreted in the soluble system. An individual homozygous for the recessive form of this gene (se/se) is termed a nonsecretor and has no A, B, or H specificities in his secretions although these specificities are expressed on his red blood cells. It appears that the se/se genotype leads to a lack of H gene activity in the secretory system.

The Le glycosyltransferase acts only in the secretory system. The resulting glycoproteins are adsorbed from the serum onto the red blood cell membrane to confer the Le specificity on these cells. Most of the structural studies just described have been carried out on glycoproteins obtained from various secretions. More recent studies on glycolipids from the red blood cell membrane suggest that the oligosaccharides responsible for the membrane ABO specificities are identical to those found in secretions.

The ABO–Lewis blood-group systems demonstrate that a relatively limited number of glycosyltransferases can generate a variety of different genetically controlled oligosaccharides. The function of the blood-group antigens is still unknown; individuals who are homozygous for the alleles O, h, le, and se do not appear to suffer ill effects from their lack of the corresponding enzymes. However, these antigens do exhibit the diversity and genetic regulation that are fundamental requirements for any cell-surface recognition system.

Lectins

Lectins are plant proteins or glycoproteins that bind to various sugars and sugar residues in oligosaccharides. The remarkable specificity of lectins has made them useful in studying the architecture of cell surfaces. Moreover, studies with cellular slime molds (Concept 5-7) suggest that lectinlike molecules may play a role in cell-cell recognition. Table 5-4 gives the specificities, sources, and molecular weights of some commonly used lectins.

Table 5-4   Properties of Some Commonly Used Lectins

Lectin	Source	Approximate Molecular Weight	Saccharide Specificity[a]
Abrin	*Abrus precatorius*	134,000	D-Gal
Concanavalin A (Con A)	*Canavalia einsformis* (Jack bean)	55,000	α-D-Man, α-D-Glc
DBA	*Dolichos biflorus*	135,000	α-D-GalNAc
Soybean agglutinin (SBA)	*Glycine max* (soybean)	110,000	D-GalNAc, D-Gal
Lentil lectins (LCA)	*Lens culinaris* (lentil)	42,000–60,000	α-D-Man, α-D-Glc
LP	*Limulus polyphemus*	400,000	sialic acid
Lima bean agglutinins	*Phaseolus limensis*	270,000	D-GlcNAc, D-Man
Phytohemagglutinin (PHA)	*Phaseolus vulgaris* (red kidney bean)	140,000	D-GlcNAc
Pokeweed mitogen (PWM)	*Phytolacca americana*	32,000	
RCA$_1$	*Ricinus communis* (castor bean)	60,000–120,000	β-D-Gal
RCA$_{11}$ ricin			D-Gal, D-GalNAc
Wheat germ agglutinin (WGA)	*Triticum vulgaris* (wheat germ)	23,000	(D-GlcNAc)$_2$, sialic acid

[a]See legend to Figure 5-15 for saccharide names. [Condensed from G.L. Nicolson, *Int. Rev. Cytol.* **39**, 89(1974).]

5-4 Membranes appear to be associated with a filamentous cellular cytoskeleton

Microtubules, microfilaments, intermediate filaments

Beneath the plasma membrane, higher eukaryotic cells have a *cytoskeleton* that consists of three types of filamentous structures: *microtubules, microfilaments,* and *intermediate filaments* (Figure 5-21). These elements of the cytoskeleton interact with the plasma membrane, various cytoplasmic organelles, and each other to carry out a variety of cellular functions.

Microtubules, which are about 25 nm in diameter, are hollow cylinders constructed from dimers of α and β *tubulin*. Microtubules effect shape changes in some cells by polymerization and depolymerization, and they may serve as static tracks along which other elements move through the cytoplasm. They are the main structural elements of the mitotic spindle and are responsible for the seg-

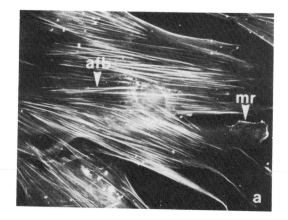

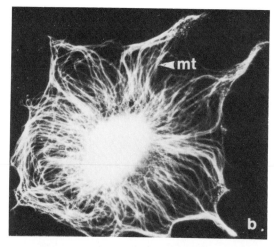

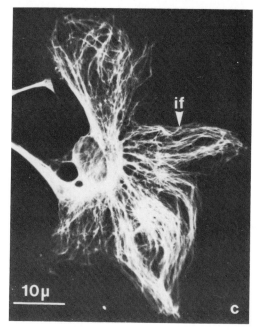

Figure 5-21

Distribution of cytoplasmic filaments in cultured cells as seen by indirect immunofluorescence. (a) A human skin fibroblast stained with anti-actin antibodies. The antibodies reveal the presence of actin in filament bundles (afb), known also as stress fibers, that frequently span the length of the cell. Actin is also seen to be present in a diffuse form in the main locomotory organ of these cells, the membrane ruffle (mr). (b) A human skin fibroblast stained with anti-tubulin antibodies. The antibodies show that microtubules (mt) emanate from the perinuclear region and extend out to the plasma membrane. (c) A chicken fibroblast stained with antibodies to the fibroblast-specific intermediate filament subunit known as vimentin. Intermediate filaments (if) extend throughout the cytoplasmic space upon the plasma membrane forming a dense network. This network is resistant to extraction by nonionic detergents and high salt buffers that solubilize the other two types of filaments. For this reason, the network is presumed to serve a cytoskeletal function connecting various cytoplasmic organelles. [From E. Lazarides, *Nature* **283**, 249 (1980).]

regation of chromosomes to the two daughter cells during mitosis. They are also the main structural and motive elements of the flagellae of sperm and of the cilia on a variety of cells, for example, in oviduct and tracheal epithelia. In cilia and flagellae, microtubules generate motion by sliding past one another in an ATP-requiring process mediated by a structural ATPase known as *dynein*.

Microfilaments, about 7.5 nm in diameter and composed of actin, are found as networks or bundles in a region called the *cell cortex*, just beneath the plasma membrane. Actin filaments have been implicated in a variety of cellular functions, including motility, endocytosis and exocytosis, membrane ruffling, and cytoplasmic streaming. They may also confer form or structural rigidity to the plasma membrane and may restrict the movement of integral membrane proteins. These diverse functions correlate with the state of the actin filament network, which is a dynamic structure that can range from a loose mesh to a highly structured gel. The dynamic properties of this network are mediated by proteins that regulate the rate of formation of individual filaments from actin monomers, the interaction of adjacent filaments to form bundles, and the interaction of filaments with the plasma membrane.

As is the case with muscle cells, most motile phenomena in nonmuscle cells are mediated by the generation of tension through the interaction of actin thin filaments with myosin thick filaments. The ability of myosin to interact with actin is regulated by the alternate phosphorylation (on-state) and dephosphorylation (off-state) of myosin. This cyclic process in turn is regulated by the level of Ca^{++} in the cell; high levels of Ca^{++} activate the phosphorylation of myosin, whereas lower levels activate dephosphorylation. This mechanism of regulating the activation of myosin is common to many nonmuscle cells as well as to smooth muscle cells, but it is distinctly different from the regulation of actin and myosin interaction in skeletal muscles.

Intermediate filaments, which are about 10 nm in diameter, are composed of a variety of protein subunits that are characteristic of the differentiated cell in which they are found. For example, epithelial cells contain 10-nm filaments composed of *keratins*, whereas neurons and glial cells contain 10-nm filaments composed of their own characteristic subunits. Muscle 10-nm filaments are composed of a protein known as *desmin*, whereas most other cell types—including lymphocytes, macrophages, and endothelial cells—contain a 10-nm filament protein known as *vimentin*. These filaments appear to link various parts of the plasma membrane with cytoplasmic organelles such as the nucleus and mitochondria. In muscle cells, desmin filaments may link myofilaments at their Z lines to each other or to the plasma membrane.

Cytoskeleton interaction with membranes

The cytoskeleton may interact with integral membrane proteins to alter their mobility. One well-studied example is the erythrocyte membrane. *Spectrin*, a protein composed of two polypeptides with approximate molecular weights of 240,000 and 220,000, is found on the inner surface of the plasma membrane in all adult mammalian and avian erythrocytes. There it forms, in association with actin and several other proteins, a network believed to be responsible for maintaining the shape of mature erythrocytes. Spectrin interacts with the plasma membrane through its association with *ankyrin*, a protein which in turn binds to a subset of the transmembrane anion channels (Figure 5-22). This interaction of spectrin with the transmembrane

Figure 5-22

A possible mode of interaction of spectrin (dark rods) with integral membrane proteins of the human red blood cell. [Adapted from J. S. Singer in *Cell Membranes: Biochemistry, Cell Biology and Pathology*, G. Weissmann and R. Clairborne (Eds.), H. P. Publishing Co., Inc., New York, 1975, p. 35.]

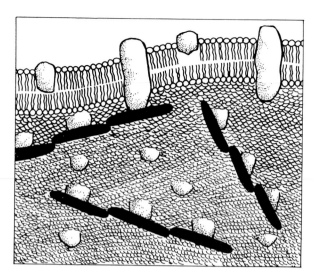

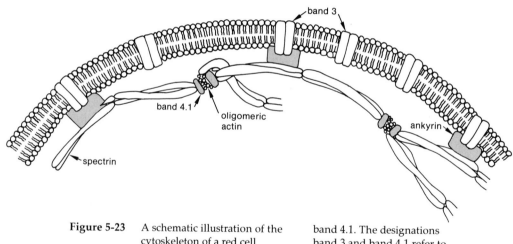

Figure 5-23   A schematic illustration of the cytoskeleton of a red cell membrane. Spectrin oligomers are linked to the cell membrane via ankyrin and band 3, a transmembrane ion channel. Spectrin oligomers are linked to one another through oligomeric actin and band 4.1. The designations band 3 and band 4.1 refer to the position these proteins occupy on a gel under standard electrophoretic conditions. [Adapted from B. Geigen, *Trends in Biochem. Sci.* **11**, 389 (1982).]

anion channel through ankyrin restricts the mobility of all these polypeptides in the plane of the membrane. Recent experiments have suggested that spectrin occurs in a variety of avian and mammalian nonerythroid cells, including neurons, muscle cells, lens cells, epithelial cells, and endothelial cells (Figure 5-23). Thus spectrin may mediate cytoskeleton–membrane interactions in a variety of diverse cell types.

Another well-studied example of restricting membrane protein mobility is the effect of the plant lectin *concanavalin A* on the capping and endocytosis of receptor immunoglobulins. Concanavalin A does not bind directly to receptor immunoglobulins, and yet its binding to the cell surface inhibits the capping and endocytosis of receptor immunoglobulins. The inhibition of capping is also achieved if concanavalin A is applied to only a small portion of the cell surface. This inhibition can be reversed by the addition of *colchicine,* a drug that depolymerizes microtubules. Although the molecular mechanisms involved in these effects are not known, it is apparent that concanavalin A can somehow restrict the mobility of the receptor immunoglobulins (perhaps of other integral membrane proteins as well) by attaching to a small fraction of its binding sites on a B cell. The finding that colchicine reverses this effect suggests that microtubules may be involved, although the drug effects of colchicine are complex.

5-5 Cell-surface receptor molecules share a number of general properties

Protein receptors

Responses to the many extracellular signals that coordinate metazoan growth and development begin at the cell surface. Hormones, drugs, neurotransmitters, and antigens are some examples of such extracellular signals. The cell-surface receptor molecules that recognize these signals must be highly specific because a given stimulus usually triggers only a highly selective cellular response. In addition, these molecules must be as diverse as the population of external signals to be received. This dual requirement for specificity and diversity argues strongly that cell-surface receptor molecules must be proteins.

Domain model for transduction

Receptor proteins must transduce information from the external environment into meaningful intracellular signals. To do so, these molecules must recognize a specific external stimulus, transduce the signal across the plasma membrane, and initiate a response inside the cell (Figure 5-24). Although only a few receptor proteins have been characterized at the molecular level, several reasonable assumptions can be made about their common properties. It seems likely that these receptors are integral proteins that span the membrane and that they have discrete domains for stimulus recognition, signal transduction, and response initiation. The specific interaction of the recognition domain with the external stimuli in the form of molecular ligands presumably involves the usual molecular complementarity typical of

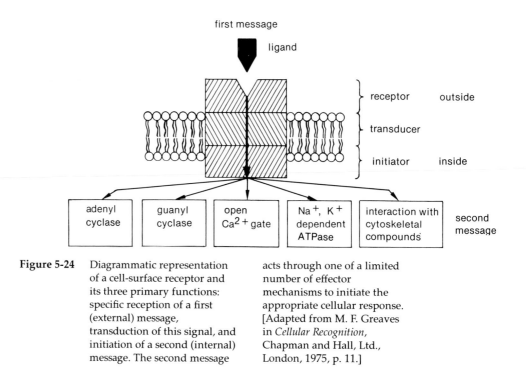

Figure 5-24 Diagrammatic representation of a cell-surface receptor and its three primary functions: specific reception of a first (external) message, transduction of this signal, and initiation of a second (internal) message. The second message acts through one of a limited number of effector mechanisms to initiate the appropriate cellular response. [Adapted from M. F. Greaves in *Cellular Recognition*, Chapman and Hall, Ltd., London, 1975, p. 11.]

enzyme–substrate and antigen–antibody interactions. Transduction of the external binding signal across the membrane probably involves conformational changes in the transducer domain, induced directly by ligand binding or indirectly through ligand-mediated aggregation of identical membrane receptors (Figure 5-25). The initiator functions of receptor proteins could act on any of a number of intracellular effector pathways. Several possibilities include direct interaction with the cytoskeletal system to initiate or terminate movement, opening or closing specific ion gates, activation or deactivation of specific ion pumps, and activation of nucleotide cyclases to produce the "second messengers," cyclic AMP or cyclic GMP, which in turn modulate the activities of soluble enzymatic or regulatory proteins.

Immunoglobulin receptors

Immunoglobulins are the most thoroughly characterized cell-surface receptors. The receptor immunoglobulin molecules associated with the plasma membrane of a given lymphocyte are identical to the specific antibodies secreted by the same cell or its clonal descendants, apart from the distinct membrane and secreted carboxyterminal tails (Concept 4-2). The number of receptor immunoglobulins on a lymphocyte has been estimated to be between 5×10^4 and 2×10^5 molecules. All the classes and subclasses of immunoglobulin molecules are capable of being expressed as membrane receptors (Concept 4-4). The general structure of immunoglobulin receptors is similar to

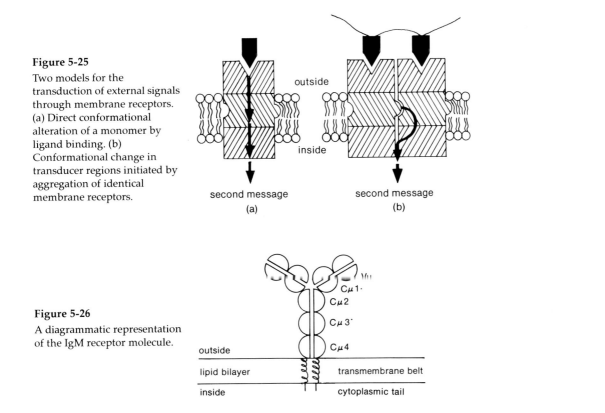

Figure 5-25

Two models for the transduction of external signals through membrane receptors. (a) Direct conformational alteration of a monomer by ligand binding. (b) Conformational change in transducer regions initiated by aggregation of identical membrane receptors.

Figure 5-26

A diagrammatic representation of the IgM receptor molecule.

that of the IgM receptor, which is the best characterized in that its complete amino acid sequence has been determined (Concept 4-4). The variable domain and the four distinct constant region domains all lie external to the membrane (Figure 5-26). A hydrophobic transmembrane belt spans the lipid bilayer, and the cytoplasmic domain consists of just two or three amino acid residues. Thus receptor immunoglobulins exhibit properties expected of cell-surface receptors in general. Given that immunoglobulins probably evolved from more general recognition systems, it is fruitful to explore organisms simpler than vertebrates for immunoglobulinlike receptor molecules and for recognition events analogous to antigen–antibody interactions.

5-6 Cell-cell recognition occurs through complementary molecular interactions

Cell-cell recognition

In all organisms that are multicellular or that go through a multicellular stage in their life cycle, positional information appears to be transmitted through cell-cell recognition via cell-surface receptors. The

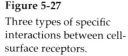

Figure 5-27

Three types of specific interactions between cell-surface receptors.

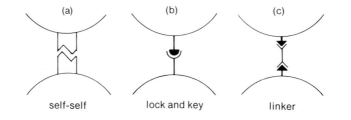

molecular basis for this recognition must be complementary interaction between cell-surface components. The possible recognition mechanisms can be classified conveniently into three types (Figure 5-27).

Self-self interaction may occur between identical receptor molecules on two different cells to form an intermolecular complex with twofold rotational symmetry (Figure 5-27a). A familiar example of such an interaction is the association of two $\alpha\beta$ dimeric subunits of hemoglobin to form the $\alpha_2\beta_2$ tetramer. Cell-cell recognition via self-self interaction requires only one gene product, which is expressed on the surface of all associating cells.

Complementary interaction may occur between a receptor protein on one cell and a different macromolecule on another (Figure 5-27b). Familiar examples of such complementary interactions include the association of the hemoglobin α chain with the β chain and the recognition of a macromolecular carbohydrate by an enzyme or a specific antibody molecule. Cell-cell recognition via complementary interaction requires a minimum of two different gene products. Both may be expressed on all cells, or each may be expressed on only one of two populations of cells that interact.

A special case of complementary interaction may involve identical or nonidentical surface-receptor molecules that recognize a *heterologous linker* molecule (Figure 5-27c). Such recognition also requires a minimum of two gene products but could involve three: one or two for the receptors and another one for the linker. *Fibronectins*, large asymmetric glycoproteins, are an example of linker proteins. They are multidomain molecules consisting of two similar or identical subunits of molecular weight 220,000 daltons (Figure 5-28a). Although flexible, fibronectins contain multiple domains that can bind with various cellular and extracellular components (Figure 5-28a). Fibronectins have been implicated in a wide variety of cellular properties, particularly those involving the interactions of cells with extracellular materials (Figure 5-28b). These properties include cell adhesion, morphology, oncogenic transformation, cytoskeletal organization, migration, differentiation, and phagocytosis.

Metazoan cell-surface interactions

Complex metazoa, which require many distinct sets of cell-cell recognition elements, must have multiple genes to code for these molecules. Conceivably, the genes for cell-surface receptors have evolved as

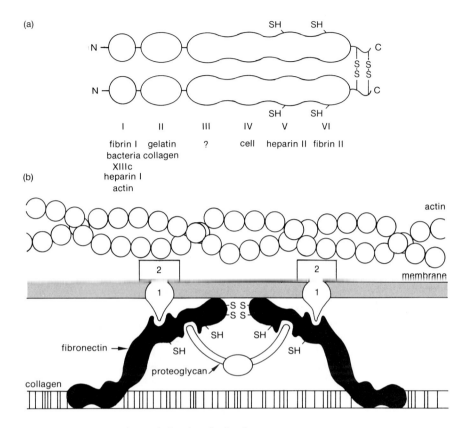

(a)

I	II	III	IV	V	VI
fibrin I	gelatin	?	cell	heparin II	fibrin II
bacteria	collagen				
	XIIIc				
	heparin I				
	actin				

(b)

actin

membrane

fibronectin →

proteoglycan

collagen

Figure 5-28 (a) A current working model for the modular structure of fibronectins. The molecules are composed of elongated subunits linked by disulfide bonds near the carboxyl terminus. Some regions are extremely sensitive to proteolysis and are depicted as extended chains (thin lines). Other regions are compact and globular and contain specific binding sites for other molecules. Two protease-resistant domains (I and II) are well defined and readily purified. The remainder of the molecule is less well analyzed, but it appears to contain regions that are relatively sensitive to proteolysis (constrictions) and other less sensitive regions that can be isolated by virtue of their binding affinities. The locations of the different binding sites on the molecule are indicated. (b) Hypothetical scheme showing fibronectin acting as a ligand, connecting the cell to the extracellular matrix. An elongated dimeric fibronectin molecule is depicted interacting through its N-terminal domains with collagen and through other binding sites with a heparin sulfate proteoglycan (PG) and with cells. One or more free sulfhydryl groups may also become involved in disulfide bonding. The nature of the cell-surface binding site is unknown; it is depicted here as an integral membrane protein (1), but it could be a protein, a glycolipid, or an assemblage of several molecules. The figure also shows one possible form of transmembrane interaction between fibronectin and actin microfilaments, involving a transmembrane "fibronectin receptor" and a molecule binding the microfilaments to the inner face of the membrane (2). Although the figure is consistent with known experimental data, the details are speculative. [Taken from R. O. Hynes and K. M. Yamada, *J. Cell Biol.* **95,** 369(1982).]

multigene families like those of the immunoglobulins, so that new recognition specificities or families of specificities can be generated readily. Whether or not such multigene families exist, all three of the recognition mechanisms require that genes or the portions that code for complementary recognition elements must *coevolve*, so that complementarity is maintained in the course of inevitable evolutionary changes. In view of this requirement for coevolution, recognition systems might be expected to evolve relatively slowly. Evidence in support of a slow evolutionary rate is the lack of species specificity among cells of a given tissue in vertebrate embryos. For example, if cells of embryonic liver and kidney tissue from two unrelated species are dissociated, mixed, and allowed to re-sort, the kidney cells from the two species will recognize each other as "self" and cohere, as will the liver cells.

5-7   Slime molds exhibit specific cellular interactions that are mediated by cell-surface molecules and their receptors

Life cycle

The life cycle of the cellular slime mold *Dictyostelium discoideum* begins with a vegetative phase in which unicellular amoebae consume bacteria and divide about every 3 hours. When the food supply is exhausted, the amoebae aggregate over the next 9–12 hours into a multicellular slug that is motile and phototactic. The 10^5 cells that make up the slug form stable intercellular contacts and then differentiate into prespore and prestalk cells. During the next 12 hours, the slug becomes sessile and the cells rearrange to form a stalk topped by a sporangium that contains stable spores (Figure 5-29). Because cells can be isolated in the vegetative state and at various stages during the development of the cohesive multicelled organism, slime molds are an excellent model system for studying the development of cellular cohesiveness.

Systems for cohesion

Cohesion in *Dictyostelium* appears to be mediated in four ways: through contact sites A and B, which are defined by specific antibodies; by the discoidin lectins; and by a 95,000-dalton membrane protein. The roles of these four systems in cohesion have been partially defined through the use of temperature-sensitive mutants and antibodies. Contact site A appears responsible for the initial aggregative cohesion. In the slug, cohesion appears to be mediated by the 95,000-dalton membrane protein. Contact site B probably binds bacteria prior to phagocytosis and may play a role in cell-to-substrate adhesion. The roles of the lectins in slime mold cohesion are uncertain.

The expression of these various types of cohesion is controlled developmentally. For example, there is a developmentally regulated shift from contact site A to the 95,000-dalton protein in going from the

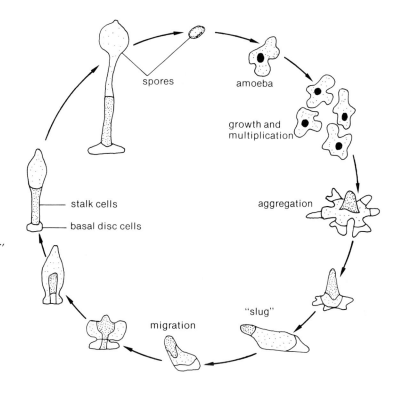

Figure 5-29
The life cycle of the cellular slime mold *Dictystelium discoideum*. [Adapted from James D. Watson, *Molecular Biology of the Gene*, 3rd ed., copyright © 1976 by J. D. Watson: W. A. Benjamin, Inc., Menlo Park, Calif., p. 508.]

stalk cells
basal disc cells

spores
amoeba
growth and multiplication
aggregation
"slug"
migration

early aggregate to the slug stage of development. In addition, several experiments suggest that the discoidin also appears in a developmentally regulated fashion. Indeed, there is also evidence for developmentally regulated high affinity cell-surface receptors for the discoidins. Vegetative cells are not significantly agglutinated by added discoidins but, as the cells differentiate, they become increasingly agglutinable. Thus both the lectins and their receptors appear to be developmentally controlled.

5-8 Metazoan development depends on specific cell-cell interactions

Cell-surface interactions in development

Metazoa are made up of many cells that specifically rearrange themselves and differentiate into distinct cell types during development. These differentiation events appear, at least in part, to be mediated by specific cell-surface molecules. In a few systems, the most general features of cell-cell interactions are becoming apparent.

The construction of tissues and organs in vertebrate embryos involves extensive cell migrations and rearrangements. Many organs, including the heart, gonad, adrenal medulla, and various components

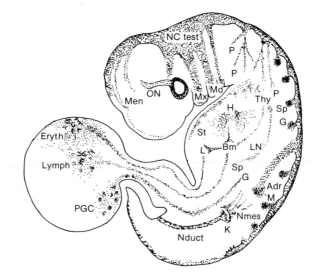

Figure 5-30

The migration pathways of various cells in the vertebrate embryo. [Courtesy of A. A. Moscona.]

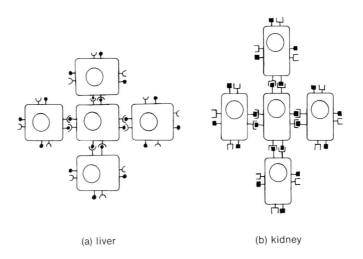

Figure 5-31

A diagram of tissue-specific, cell-surface recognition systems utilizing lock-and-key interactions.

(a) liver   (b) kidney

of the skeletal and nervous systems, arise in the embryo from cells that are distant from their final location (Figure 5-30). These cells migrate to predetermined sites and selectively aggregate with other cells to form tissue primordia.

One potential explanation for specific embryonic cell recognition is that each tissue has characteristic cell-surface *recognition molecules* that allow appropriate cells to aggregate into tissues and organs (Figure 5-31). The discriminating properties of these recognition molecules may increase as development progresses. For example, initially cells of the three embryonic layers—the ectoderm, mesoderm, and endoderm—may recognize cells of their own type specifically. Then

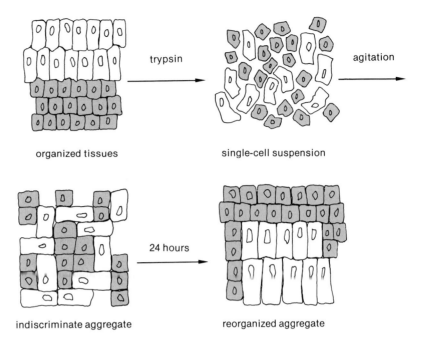

Figure 5-32

In vitro dissociation and reaggregation of an embryonic tissue with two layers of different cell types.

organized tissues

single-cell suspension

indiscriminate aggregate

reorganized aggregate

these embryonic layers further differentiate into the major tissue classes, and finally the cell types within tissues sort out.

Tissue-specific cell-surface antigens, termed *differentiation antigens*, have been demonstrated in several systems. Rabbit antisera raised against mouse embryonic neural retina tissue, after absorption with heterologous tissues, react with the surfaces of neural retinal cells but do not react with other cell types. Similar antisera have been prepared for myocardium, liver, and skeletal muscle. Regardless of the actual functions of the differentiation antigens, their existence is consistent with the hypothesis of cell-surface recognition systems.

In vitro cell aggregation experiments

The specific aggregation patterns of embryonic cells have been studied *in vitro* by examining associations among whole cells or by measuring the binding of radiolabeled plasma membrane vesicles, prepared from one type of embryonic cell, to whole cells. Both kinds of study indicate that there are *tissue-specific* and *cell type-specific* cell-surface recognition molecules. For example, when the embryonic neural retina, which is composed of three layers of discrete cell types, is dissociated into a single-cell suspension by trypsin treatment, it reassociates specifically (Figure 5-31). The cells go through two stages of reaggregation (Figure 5-32). Initially, cells send out microvilli that contact other cells of the various cell types (Figure 5-33). Over the next 24 hours, the cell types in these mixed aggregates sort out to reconstitute the initial retinal tissue pattern with similar cells associated in discrete layers. Almost all mammalian and avian embryonic tissues

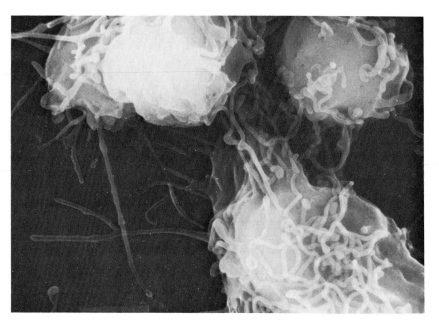

Figure 5-33 A small aggregate of retinal cells formed after 30 minutes of reaggregation. Note the microvilli interconnecting these cells. [From Y. Ben-Shaul and A. A. Moscona, *Exp. Cell Res.* **95,** 191(1975).]

sort out in a similar manner. The cell type-specific and tissue-specific recognition molecules implied by these studies have apparently been *highly conserved* during evolution because mixed suspension of neuronal retinal cells from chick and mouse reassociate to give the normal tissue pattern with the avian and mammalian cells intermingled.

These kinds of studies also suggest that recognition molecules in a particular cell type may change in a developmentally programmed manner. For example, chick plasma membrane vesicles from 7-, 8-, and 9-day-old optic tectum and neural retina show specificity for homologous cells of the same age. Seven-day membrane vesicles do not interact with 8- or 9-day-old cells, whereas 8- or 9-day membrane vesicles react only weakly with 7-day-old cells. Similarly, neural retinal cells isolated from 7-, 10-, and 14-day chicken embryos show a progressive decline in their ability to associate specifically. There is a corresponding loss in the fluidity of the cell membrane as these embryonic cells mature. These two changes may be related because cell–cell recognition appears to require clustering of receptors, which in turn requires mobility of receptors in the membrane. Thus cellular association could be regulated either by the expression of specific cell-interaction molecules or by altering the fluidity, and thus the potential distribution, of receptors in the cell membrane.

The specific aggregation patterns of embryonic cells appear to be governed in part by glycoproteins. One glycoprotein that specifically promotes the reaggregation of chicken neural retinal cells, but not other embryonic cells, has been isolated from the membranes of neural retinal cells and from the medium over monolayers of these cells grown in tissue culture. This 50,000-dalton glycoprotein binds to the surface of neural retinal cells but not to any other embryonic cells. In addition, antibodies to the glycoprotein bind only to neural retinal cells. A second 50,000-dalton glycoprotein, which was isolated from chicken cerebral cells, specifically promotes reaggregation of those cells. The similar sizes of these two glycoproteins raises the intriguing possibility that they may be related members of a family of specific cell-recognition molecules.

Selected Bibliography

Where to begin

Singer, S. J., "Architecture and topography of biologic membranes," in *Cell Membranes: Biochemistry, Cell Biology and Pathology,* G. Weissmann and R. Clairborne (Eds.), H. P. Publishing Co., Inc., New York, 1975, p. 35. A clear summary of the fluid mosaic model of membrane structure.

General

Capaldi, R. A., "Structure of intrinsic membrane proteins," *Trends in Biochem. Sci.* **7**, 292(1982).

de Mendoza, D., and Cronan, Jr., J. E., "Thermal regulation of membrane lipid fluidity in bacteria," *Trends in Biochem. Sci.* **8**, 49(1983).

Hartmut, M., "Crystallization of membrane proteins," *Trends in Biochem. Sci.* **8**, 56(1983).

Meyer, D. I., "The signal hypothesis—a working model," *Trends in Biochem. Sci.* **7**, 320(1982).

Porter, K. R., and Tucker, J. B., "The ground substance of the living cell," *Sci. Am.* **244**, 56(1981).

Rice-Evans, C. A., and Dunn, M. J., "Erythrocyte deformability and disease," *Trends in Biochem. Sci.* **7**, 282(1982).

Rothman, J. E., "The Golgi apparatus: two organelles in tandem," *Science* **213**, 1212(1981).

Ruoslahti, E., Pierschbacher, M., Hayman, E. G., and Engvall, E., "Fibronectin: a molecule with remarkable structural and functional diversity," *Trends in Biochem. Sci.* **7**, 188(1982).

Oligosaccharides

Sharon, N., "Carbohydrates," *Sci. Am.* **243**, 90(1980).

Watkins, W. M., "Blood-group substances," *Science* **152**, 172(1966). An old but well-written paper on the human ABO system.

Cytoskeleton

Cleveland, D. W., "Treadmilling of tubulin and actin," *Cell* **28**, 689(1982).

Craig, S. W., and Pollard, T. D., "Actin-binding proteins," *Trends in Biochem. Sci.* **7**, 88(1982).

Lazarides, E., "Intermediate filaments as mechanical integrators of cellular space," *Nature* **283**, 249(1980).

Receptors

Brown, M. S., Anderson, R. G. W., and Goldstein, J. L., "Recycling receptors: the round-trip itinerary of migrant membrane proteins," *Cell* **32**, 663(1983).

Kaplan, J., "Polypeptide-binding membrane receptors: analysis and classification," *Science* **212**, 14(1981).

Kühn, L. C., and Kraehenbuhl, J. P., "The sacrificial receptor—translocation of polymeric IgA across epithelia," *Trends in Biochem. Sci.* **7**, 299(1982).

Molecular recognition

Edelman, G. M., "Cell adhesion molecules," *Science* **219**, 450(1983).

Hood, L., Huang, H. V., and Dreyer, W. J., "The area-code hypothesis: the immune system provides clues to understanding the genetic and molecular basis of cell recognition during development," *J. Supramol. Struct.* **7**, 531(1977). Some ideas about cell-recognition molecules and how their genes are organized and expressed.

Additional concepts and techniques presented in the problems

1. Membrane fluidity. Problem 5-4.

2. Carbohydrate synthesis. Problem 5-5.

3. Blood group carbohydrates. Problems 5-6, 5-7, and 5-8.

4. Tissue aggregation. Problem 5-9.

Problems

5-1 Indicate whether each of the following statements is true or false. Explain the error in each statement you consider to be false.

(a) The plasma membrane is generally impermeable to polar molecules.

(b) Cholesterol has a molecular shape that is very different from the shapes of other membrane lipids.

(c) Glycoproteins form spontaneous bilayers in aqueous solution.

(d) The loose association of peripheral proteins with the plasma membrane makes it difficult to define precisely the outer and inner limits of the cell surface.

(e) Glycophorin is an integral membrane protein with linearly distributed hydrophilic and hydrophobic domains.

(f) Most membrane glycoproteins attach their oligosaccharide chains through serine, threonine, or asparagine residues.

(g) Lipids may flip-flop across the membrane almost as rapidly as they diffuse in a translational direction.

(h) Membranes with predominantly saturated fatty acids are more fluid than those with a higher degree of unsaturated fatty acids.

(i) Microfilaments appear to have direct connections with the plasma membrane and therefore may be involved in cellular movements.

(j) Slime molds have cell-surface recognition molecules with lectinlike properties.

(k) When dissociated liver and retinal cells from chick and mouse embryos are mixed together and gently agitated, the two species of liver cells specifically associate with one another but not with either species of retinal cells.

(l) Interaction of anti-Le^b antibodies and the Le^b human blood-group specificity can be inhibited by a monosaccharide.

(m) Clathrin is a protein that plays a role in the transport of material from the Golgi apparatus to the membrane.

5-2 Supply the missing word or words in each of the following statements.

(a) The three major kinds of membrane lipids are _____ , _____ , and _____ .

(b) _____ interactions are primarily responsible for the thermodynamic tendency of lipid bilayers to form in aqueous solutions.

(c) _____ molecules have distinct hydrophobic and hydrophilic regions.

(d) Membrane proteins can be divided into two categories: _____ and _____ .

(e) _____ confers a significant negative charge on most plasma membranes.

(f) The two types of carbohydrate linkages to glycoproteins are _____ and _____ .

(g) Oligosaccharide synthesis is not mediated by a template mechanism; instead, _____ are responsible for the enzymatic synthesis of these macromolecules.

(h) _____ are plant proteins or glycoproteins that exhibit specificities for monosaccharides.

(i) _____ are submembranous elements composed of actin that appear to be involved in various cell movements.

(j) A membrane receptor must carry out three distinct functions: _____ , _____ , and _____ .

(k) The _____ of the receptor immunoglobulin is attached to the lymphocyte membrane.

(l) The five distinct blood-group specificities of the Lewis and ABO systems are _____ , _____ , _____ , _____ , and _____ .

(m) The monosaccharide that determines the A blood-group specificity is _____ .

(n) Two general mechanisms of specific cellular association are _____ and _____ recognition.

(o) _____ is a protein found on the inner surface of the plasma membrane in adult mammalian erythrocytes and is believed to play a role in maintaining the shape of these cells.

(p) _____ are asymmetric linker proteins that play a role in the interactions between cells and extracellular materials.

5-3 (a) Consider Table 5-2 and then suggest a plausible scheme for human blood transfusions between individuals of different blood groups. Who is a universal donor? Who is a universal recipient? Explain.

(b) What other factors should be considered in blood transfusions apart from the ABO blood groups?

5-4 Which member of each of the following pairs of membrane components will make a membrane more fluid when it is present as part of the structure?

(a) (1) $CH_3(CH_2)_7CH = CH(CH_2)_7COO^-$ or (2) $CH_3(CH_2)_{16}COO^-$

(b) (1) $CH_3(CH_2)_{16}COO^-$ or (2) $CH_2(CH_2)_{14}COO^-$

(c) (1) $CH_5(CH_2)_{16}COO^-$ or (2) the compound shown in Figure 5-34

5-5 (a) Figure 5-35 shows a hypothetical polypeptide chain with two attached oligosaccharides. Assume that the carbohydrate residues are linked through the same hydroxyl groups in both oligosaccharides. How many glycosyl transferases would be necessary to synthesize these chains?

(b) To which amino acid would these oligosaccharides be linked?

5-6 Why must individuals who exhibit a strong Le^a specificity on their red blood cells be nonsecretors?

5-7 The carbohydrates shown in Figure 5-36 can be derived from alkaline or acid hydrolysis of various human blood-group substances. Each carbohydrate has the ability to inhibit the hemagglutination test for a specific blood-group specificity. Identify the specificity blocked by each carbohydrate.

5-8 (a) Six groups of individuals are distinguishable on the basis of the ABO and Lewis (Le^a or Le^b) red-cell phenotype and the A, B, H, Le^a, and Le^b activities present in secretions (see Figure 5-20). Table 5-5 presents results of serological tests on red blood cells (RBC) and secretions from these six groups. Predict the probable genotype for each group (H or h/h; Le or le/le; Se or se/se).

(b) Why is Le^b not expressed in group 2?

(c) Why is Le^b not expressed in group 5?

Figure 5-34

The structural formula of a membrane component (Problem 5-4).

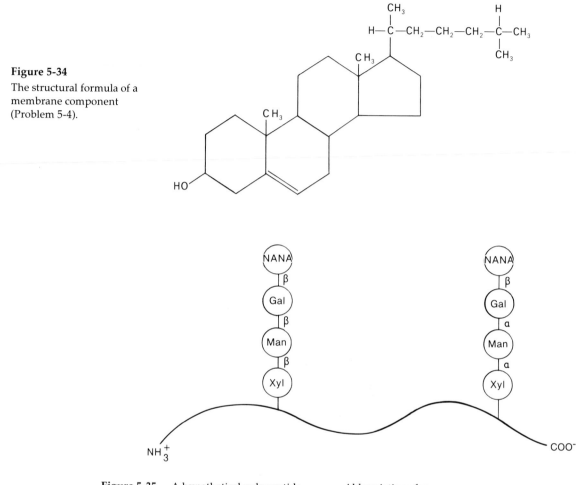

Figure 5-35   A hypothetical polypeptide chain with two oligosaccharides (Problem 5-5). α and β denote configurations of glycosidic linkages.

Abbreviations for monosaccharide residues are explained in the legend to Figure 5-15.

(d) What blood-group specificities cannot be present in the secretions of individuals with se/se genotype?

(e) Individuals of group 4 have in their secretions substances that are closely related chemically to the A, B, H, and Le^a substances. What may these substances be?

(f) Will the A and/or B genes be present in some individuals of groups 5 and 6? Why?

5-9 (a) Embryonic tissues can be dissociated by mild proteolysis or other treatments to yield suspensions of single cells that will reaggregate and eventually reproduce many of the features of the original tissue. When aggregates are prepared from cells derived from two different tissues, these cells will eventually segregate into two homotypic aggregates. Little is known about the molecules that mediate these

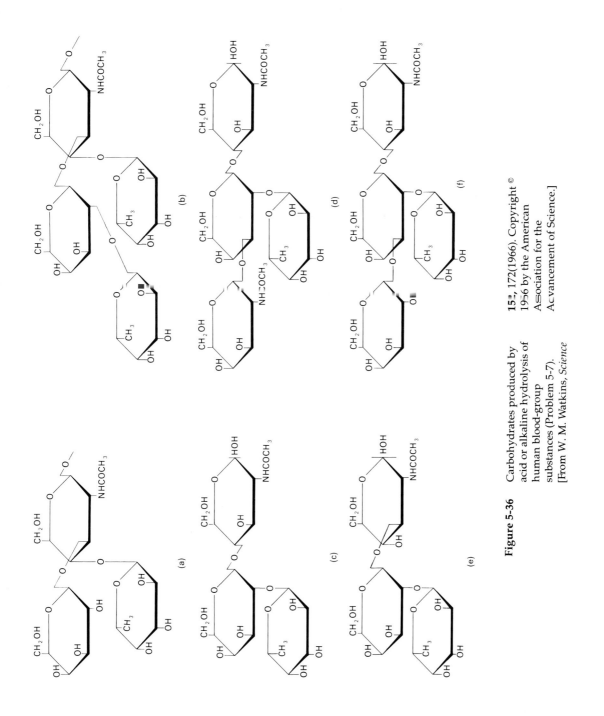

Figure 5-36 Carbohydrates produced by acid or alkaline hydrolysis of human blood-group substances (Problem 5-7). [From W. M. Watkins, *Science* **152**, 172(1966). Copyright © 1966 by the American Association for the Advancement of Science.]

Table 5-5 Red-Cell Phenotypes in Six Groups of Individuals[a] (Problem 5-8)

Group	Probable Genotype	Antigen Detectable on RBC			Specificities Detectable in Secretions		
		ABH	Le^a	Le	ABH	Le^a	Le
1	?	+++	−	++	+++	+	++
2	?	+++	+++	−	−	+++	−
3	?	+++	−	−	+++	−	−
4	?	+++	−	−	−	−	−
5	?	−	+++	−	−	+++	−
6	?	−	−	−	−	−	−

[a] +++, strong specific activity; +, weak specific activity; −, no activity; ABH +++ indicates A+H, B+H, or just H.

Figure 5-37

Effects of membrane preparations on retinal cell aggregations (Problem 5-9). 1.5 × 10⁵ neural retinal cells were incubated in 3 mL of medium with no additions ●; with cerebellar fraction B-1 (0.1 mg of protein) O; or with retinal fraction B-1 (0.1 mg of protein) ■. The percent remaining single cells is plotted as a function of time. [From R. Merrell and L. Glaser, *Proc. Natl. Acad. Sci. USA* **70,** 2794(1973).]

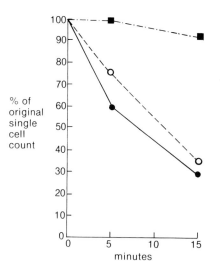

cell-cell interactions. Plasma membrane fractions have been prepared from neural retina and cerebellum to determine what effect, if any, they have on the formation of homotypic aggregates. Cell aggregation is measured by determining the fall in the single-cell count over the time period of the experiment. The effects of membrane fragments on the aggregation of retinal cells and cerebellar cells are shown in Figures 5-37 and 5-38, respectively. What effects do the plasma membrane preparations have on the aggregations of retinal and cerebellar cells?

(b) Figure 5-39 measures the binding of ³H-retinal plasma membranes to retinal and cerebellar cells. What is observed?

(c) What general conclusions can you draw from the results observed in Figures 5-37, 5-38, and 5-39?

Figure 5-38

Effects of plasma membrane preparations on cerebellar cell aggregation (Problem 5-9). Conditions are identical to those of Figure 5-37 except that cerebellar cells are used. ●, no addition; ■, 0.1 mg of retinal fraction B-1; O, 0.1 mg of cerebellar fraction B-1. [From R. Merrell and L. Glaser, *Proc. Natl. Acad. Sci. USA* **70**, 2794(1973).]

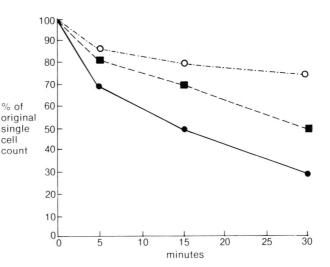

Figure 5-39

The binding of radioactive membranes to cells (Problem 5-9). 6×10^5 cells were incubated in 3 mL of medium with ^3H glucosamine-labeled retinal fraction B-1 (20 μg of protein, 15,000 dpm). At each time point, the aggregation was stopped by three-fold dilution; cells with attached membranes were collected by centrifugation. The pellet was washed, dissolved, and counted. ●, cerebellar cells; ▲ retinal cells. [From R. Merrell and L. Glaser, *Proc. Natl. Acad. Sci. USA* **70**, 2794(1973).]

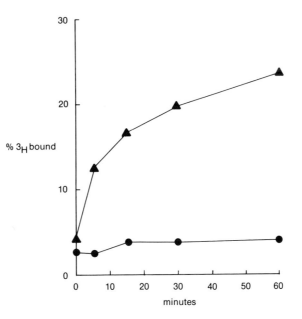

(d) What is the effect of trypsin on inhibition of aggregation (Figure 5-40)?

(e) Retinal membranes have also been isolated from 7-, 8-, and 9-day embryos and examined for their ability to inhibit the aggregation of 7-, 8-, and 9-day retinal cells (Figure 5-41a). Likewise tectal membranes have been isolated from 8- and 9-day embryos and examined for their ability to block the aggregation of 7-, 8-, and 9-day-old tectal cells (Figure 5-41b). What conclusions can you draw from the results?

Figure 5-40

The effect of trypsin on membrane activity (Problem 5-9). A suspension (0.1 mL) of 8-day retinal membranes (0.1 mg of protein) was incubated for 10 minutes at 37°C with trypsin. Soybean trypsin inhibitor was added and the membranes were assayed for their ability to inhibit aggregation of 8-day retinal cells. O, no addition; ▲, intact membranes (0.1 mg protein); ●, trypsin-treated membranes; △, membranes treated with a preincubated mixture of trypsin and trypsin inhibitor. [From D. I. Gottlieb et al., *Proc. Natl. Acad. Sci. USA* **71**, 1800(1974).]

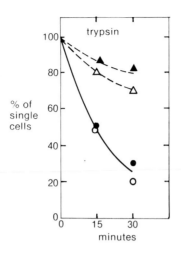

Answers

    5-1 (a) True
        (b) False. Cholesterol, phospholipids, and glycolipids all have a cylindrical shape (see Figure 5-8).
        (c) False. Few if any glycoproteins have the shape and solubility properties required for spontaneous bilayer formation.
        (d) True
        (e) True
        (f) True
        (g) False. The flip-flop of lipids across the membrane is about 10^9 times slower than translational diffusion.
        (h) False. Unsaturated fatty acids are "kinked" and therefore increase membrane fluidity.
        (i) True
        (j) True
        (k) True
        (l) False. The Le^b specificity is produced by the action of two gene products, H and Le, which add two sugar residues to the precursor oligosaccharide (see Figure 5-20). Consequently, Le^b-anti-Le^b interaction may be blocked by an appropriate disaccharide but not by a monosaccharide.
        (m) True
    5-2 (a) phospholipids, glycolipids, and cholesterol
        (b) Hydrophobic
        (c) Amphipathic

Figure 5-41

The effect of embryonal age on membrane specificity (Problem 5-9). All experiments were carried out with membranes prepared from whole neural retina, obtained from 7-, 8-, or 9-day-old embryos. The membranes were used to inhibit aggregation of either retinal or tectal cells of the ages indicated. [From D. I. Gottlieb et al., *Proc. Natl. Acad. Sci. USA* **71**, 1800(1974).]

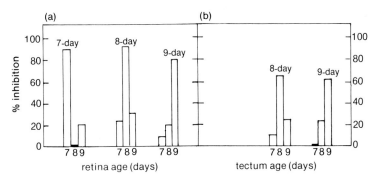

(d) integral and peripheral
(e) Sialic acid (or N-acetylneuraminic acid)
(f) N-glycosidic and O-glycosidic
(g) glycosyltransferases
(h) Lectins
(i) Microfilaments
(j) recognition, transduction, and initiation of effector mechanisms
(k) C-terminal domain (see Figure 5-26)
(l) A, B, O, Le^a, Le^b
(m) N-acetyl-D-galactosamine
(n) complementary and self-self
(o) Spectrin
(p) Fibronectins

5-3 (a) It is best to transfuse blood between individuals of identical ABO genotype. However, O individuals are universal donors because they have neither A nor B antigens; therefore, their cells will not be agglutinated by anti-A or anti-B antibodies when transfused into individuals with other ABO genotypes. AB individuals can accept red blood cells from any donor because they lack antibodies and the ability to make antibodies to the A and B antigens.

(b) A mismatch of other blood-group specificities can lead to a transfusion reaction (agglutination and lysis of the foreign cells). The presence of natural antibodies to these antigens can be checked simply by determining whether serum from the recipient agglutinates donor cells.

5-4 Components a(1), b(2), and c(2) will make a membrane more fluid. The compound shown in Figure 5-34 is cholesterol.

5-5 (a) Six glycosyl transferases would be necessary to synthesize the oligosaccharides shown in Figure 5-35. Separate transferases would be required for: (1), addition of the initial xylose residues of both oligosaccharides; (2) and (3), addition of the mannose residues in α and β linkage, respectively; (4) and (5), addition of the galactose residues in α and β linkage, respectively; and (6), addition of the N-acetylneuraminic acid (sialic acid) residues to both oligosaccharides.

(b) Xylose residues in oligosaccharides always are linked to glycoproteins through O-glycosidic bonds to the hydroxyl group of a serine residue (Figure 5-17).

5-6 Individuals who exhibit strong Le^a specificity must lack the fucose transferase coded by the H gene, which normally converts the Le^a specificity to the Le^b specificity (Figure 5-20). Lack of H-gene activity, in turn, indicates an se/se (nonsecretor) genotype.

5-7 Each carbohydrate will block agglutination of the blood-group substances whose structure it most closely resembles. See Figure 5-20 for the structures of the blood-group substances.

(a) Le^a
(b) Le^b
(c) H
(d) A
(e) H
(f) B

5-8 (a) Group 1 H*, Le, Se
                  2 H, Le, se/se
                  3 H, le/le, Se
                  4 H, le/le, se/se
                  5 h/h, Le, Se or se/se
                  6 h/h, le/le, Se or se/se

*H can be H/H or H/h; Le can be Le/Le or Le/le; Se can be Se/Se or Se/se.

(b) Le^b is not expressed in group 2 individuals because the se/se genotype blocks the activity of the H fucose transferase, which is necessary for the formation of the Le^b specificity.

(c) Le^b is not expressed in group 5 individuals because the H fucose transferase is not synthesized in individuals of h/h genotype.

(d) H, A, B, and Le^b.

(e) They appear to be the precursor oligosaccharides unmodified by any of the transferases (see Figures 5-19 and 5-20 and Table 5-3).

(f) The A and/or B genes are present in some of these individuals. They cannot be expressed because the H transferase is necessary to produce the precursor groups on which the A and B transferases act.

5-9 (a) The plasma membranes from neural retina almost totally inhibit retinal cell aggregation (Figure 5-37) and have a much smaller inhibitor effect on cerebellar cell aggregation (Figure 5-38). Cerebellar membranes inhibit the aggregation of cerebellar cells, but they have virtually no effect on the aggregation of retinal cells.

(b) The retinal plasma membranes bind significantly to retinal cells and only slightly to cerebellar cells.

(c) The specific site responsible for cellular recognition in embryonic cells can be retained in isolated plasma cell membranes. This recognition site appears to be highly specific for cell type. It binds rapidly to homotypic cells.

(d) Trypsin abolishes the inhibitory effects of plasma membranes on the aggregation of homotypic cells. The effect of the enzyme depends on its proteolytic activity because trypsin in the presence of a specific proteolytic inhibitor does not abolish membrane inhibition activity. Trypsin presumably exerts its effect by destroying cell-surface protein molecules.

(e) The surface specificity responsible for cell aggregation changes rapidly during development, either due to changes in cell types or due to changes in the surfaces of preexisting cells.

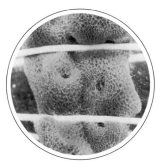

CHAPTER 6

Genes and Proteins of the Major Histocompatibility Complex

Chapter Outline

6-8 Exons of class II genes correlate well with the domains of the encoded proteins
Exons and domains
Homology of class I, class II, β_2-microglobulin, antibody, and Thy-1 genes

6-9 The class II genes constitute a small multigene family
Chromosomal arrangement of genes
Comparison of the genetic and physical maps

The major histocompatibility complex (MHC) is a chromosomal region that controls the immunological rejection of transplanted organs, such as kidneys or hearts. This finding, and the obvious need for medical science to understand and ameliorate its effects, has provided a major driving force for the development of the field of immunology. Experimental analysis of this system using the tools of immunogenetics has revealed the MHC to be complex and to play a role in virtually every aspect of the immune response. The major histocompatibility complex encodes three families of genes denoted class I, class II, and class III. The class I and class II genes encode cell-surface molecules that participate in recognition of nonself (antigens) by T cells, whereas the class III genes encode several components in the activation portion of the complement cascade. In the last few years, the techniques of recombinant DNA have permitted an unraveling of fundamental features of the genes and proteins of the MHC. The tools of molecular biology, when employed in conjunction with the well-developed assays of cellular immunology, provide a unique opportunity to dissect the functions of the multigene families involved in self-nonself recognition phenomena. This chapter considers the general problem of self-nonself recognition with emphasis on the genes and proteins of the major histocompatibility complex.

Concepts

6-1 Self-nonself recognition systems are found throughout metazoa

All metazoa appear to exhibit cell-surface recognition systems capable of discriminating between self and nonself. For example, the Hawaiian sponge, *Callyspongia diffusa*, a very primitive metazoan, has cells with a deep purple pigment that is lost upon cell death. When branches from two genetically identical *Callyspongia* are juxtaposed, rapid fusion of the branches occurs and a single individual sponge results (Figure 6-1). When branches from two genetically distinct *Callyspongia* are joined, fusion does not occur. Rather, a junctional region with dead cells is rapidly produced, as indicated by the attendant loss of purple pigment. More than 900 pairs of genetically disparate sponges have been grafted to one another and, in each case, the grafts were incompatible. Thus, the self-nonself recognition system in *Callyspongia* appears to exhibit three fundamental features in common

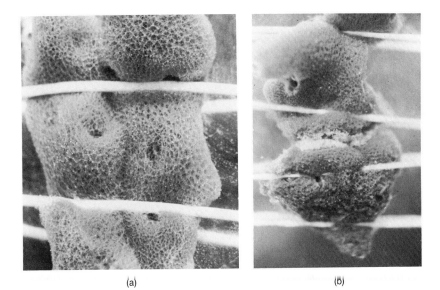

(a)　　　　　　　(b)

Figure 6-1
The grafting of genetically identical (a) and genetically disparate (b) sponges of the species *Callyspongia diffusa.* [Photos provided by William Hildemann.]

with mammalian recognition systems. (a) Self-nonself recognition appears to be mediated by cell-surface recognition molecules. (b) The identification of nonself activates effector mechanisms that lead to the death of adjacent cells. (c) The recognition system is highly polymorphic in that many different individuals within a given species appear to have distinct self-recognition markers.

Higher invertebrates such as the colonial ascidian, *Botryllus,* also exhibit self-nonself recognition systems with similar features. These systems may be of fundamental importance for invertebrates in preserving the integrity of individuals growing in densely populated environments (see book cover and legend, p. iv).

The self-nonself recognition systems of the major histocompatibility complex may have evolved from these primitive self-nonself recognition systems of invertebrates. The MHC carries out fundamental effector and regulatory roles in the vertebrate immune response. It will be interesting to determine to what extent the self-nonself recognition systems of vertebrates and invertebrates share structural and regulatory features.

6-2 Mice with special genetic features have provided a detailed genetic map of the major histocompatibility complex

Phenomenology of graft rejection

The major histocompatibility complex (*histo* = tissue) was initially defined by the graft rejection assay using inbred (genetically identical) strains of mice. Grafts between genetically identical or *syngeneic* indi-

Figure 6-2

Complexities of organization and expression of the H-2 complex. (a) The two H-2 chromosomes in an individual heterozygous for the H-2 complex. A, B, and C denote H-2 antigens. The superscripts ᵃ and ᵇ designate particular H-2 alleles. The constellation of alleles on a particular H-2 chromosome is termed a haplotype. (b) A cell expressing both alleles of the three H-2 genes.

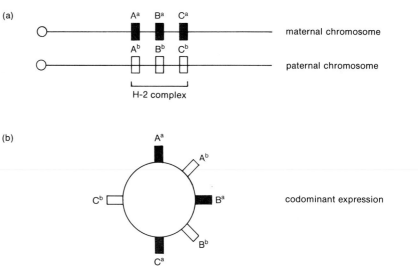

viduals are readily accepted, whereas grafts between genetically distinct or *allogeneic* individuals are rejected and ultimately destroyed. The graft rejection process is mediated by cell-surface structures termed histocompatibility (H) antigens, which are encoded by histocompatibility genes.

Three genetic factors have complicated attempts to study the histocompatibility proteins and genes. First, there appear to be 50–100 distinct histocompatibility loci in mice, with histocompatibility genes located on virtually every mouse chromosome (see Figure 11-3). However, one of these histocompatibility loci, which was initially denoted H-2, encodes cell-surface antigens leading to rapid graft rejection. The other histocompatibility genes encode antigens that lead to chronic or delayed tissue rejection. Accordingly, the H-2 locus was denoted the *major* histocompatibility locus, and the others were designated *minor* histocompatibility loci. The H-2 locus encodes the self-nonself recognition systems discussed throughout the remainder of this chapter. Very little information is available on the minor histocompatibility loci (see Chapter 11). Second, the H-2 locus actually contains multiple genes encoding histocompatibility antigens or self-nonself recognition structures (Figure 6-2). Thus the H-2 locus is actually a gene complex and, accordingly, has been denoted the H-2 complex. Finally, the most striking feature of graft rejection is the enormous polymorphism of the histocompatibility antigens of the H-2 complex. For example, virtually any randomly chosen pair of wild mice will rapidly reject mutual grafts. Randomly chosen mice are often heterozygous and have two allelic forms for most of the histocompatibility genes encoded by the H-2 complex (Figure 6-2). Because individual histocompatibility alleles on both chromosomes are expressed in all tissues (Figure 6-2), either or both histocompatibility antigens may mediate

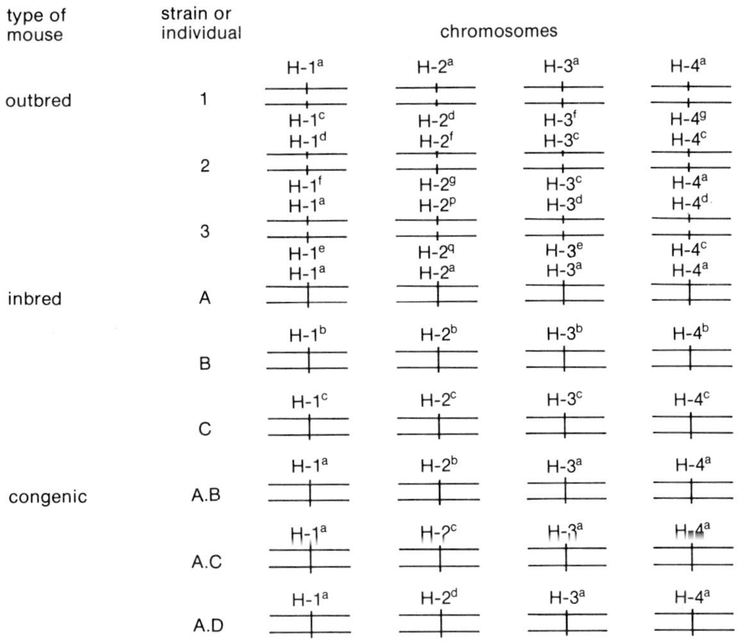

Figure 6-3

Schematic representations of histocompatibility loci in outbred, inbred, and congenic mice. The individual and strain designations are chosen arbitrarily. Four chromosomes are depicted. H-1 through H-4 denote four histocompatibility loci. Superscripts denote particular alleles.

type of mouse	strain or individual	chromosomes			
outbred	1	$H\text{-}1^a$ / $H\text{-}1^c$	$H\text{-}2^a$ / $H\text{-}2^d$	$H\text{-}3^a$ / $H\text{-}3^f$	$H\text{-}4^a$ / $H\text{-}4^g$
	2	$H\text{-}1^d$ / $H\text{-}1^f$	$H\text{-}2^f$ / $H\text{-}2^g$	$H\text{-}3^c$ / $H\text{-}3^c$	$H\text{-}4^c$ / $H\text{-}4^a$
	3	$H\text{-}1^a$ / $H\text{-}1^e$	$H\text{-}2^p$ / $H\text{-}2^q$	$H\text{-}3^d$ / $H\text{-}3^e$	$H\text{-}4^d$ / $H\text{-}4^c$
inbred	A	$H\text{-}1^a$	$H\text{-}2^a$	$H\text{-}3^a$	$H\text{-}4^a$
	B	$H\text{-}1^b$	$H\text{-}2^b$	$H\text{-}3^b$	$H\text{-}4^b$
	C	$H\text{-}1^c$	$H\text{-}2^c$	$H\text{-}3^c$	$H\text{-}4^c$
congenic	A.B	$H\text{-}1^a$	$H\text{-}2^b$	$H\text{-}3^a$	$H\text{-}4^a$
	A.C	$H\text{-}1^a$	$H\text{-}2^c$	$H\text{-}3^a$	$H\text{-}4^a$
	A.D	$H\text{-}1^a$	$H\text{-}2^d$	$H\text{-}3^a$	$H\text{-}4^a$

graft rejection. Thus the graft rejection phenomenon appears to be mediated by self-nonself recognition system(s) with each of the three fundamental characteristics identified in simpler metazoa—cell-surface recognition structures, cytotoxic effector mechanisms, and extensive polymorphism.

Genetic construction of special mouse strains

In order to study the individual histocompatibility genes and proteins of the MHC, it was necessary to deal with the problems of multiple histocompatibility loci, extensive H-2 polymorphism, heterozygosity of the H-2 genes, and multiplicity of genes within the H-2 complex. These problems were circumvented by constructing three special types of mouse strains—*inbred, congenic,* and *recombinant congenic.* Because of these special strains, the MHC of the mouse is better understood than the MHCs of any other vertebrate. Hence in this chapter the mouse MHC is considered almost exclusively.

Outbred or wild mice often display heterozygosity and extensive genetic polymorphism (Figure 6-3). Through 20 or more brother–sister matings, inbred strains of mice that are greater than 99% homozygous and generally express just a single form of each type of histocompatibility antigen (Figure 6-3) can be generated. Because these individual strains of inbred mice are homozygous for particular H-2 haplotypes (the collection of alleles on one chromosome), they eliminate the problem of heterozygosity of histocompatibility antigens. So-called congenic mice can be constructed from two distinct strains of mice (for example, A and B). Figure 6-4 illustrates the steps

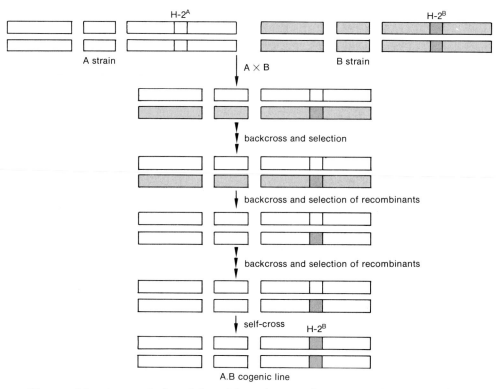

Figure 6-4   Diagram of the steps required to produce a congenic A.B strain of mice. Pairs of chromosomes for the inbred A and B strains are designated by open and dark rectangles, respectively. The MHC is designated by boundary lines on one chromosome. With an appropriate assay system (e.g., allograft rejection), the B-strain MHC from F_1 progeny can be followed through repeated backcrosses to the A strain. This backcrossing process leads to the loss of all B-strain chromosomes other than the one that carries the H-2 locus and the loss of B genes from the B chromosome that carries the H-2 locus by crossing over with the homologous A chromosome. These two processes are depicted as occurring successively although they actually occur simultaneously. After a large number of backcrosses, the B chromosome that carries the H-2 locus will have primarily A genes except in the H-2 complex of one chromosome. Two such F_1 animals can be crossed to produce a homozygous congenic strain.

by which the H-2 complex of strain B can be superimposed on the background genes of strain A. These congenic mice are denoted A.B, where the first letter denotes the background strain and the second the strain from which the H-2 complex was originally derived. In this manner, a series of different H-2 complexes can be superimposed on the same genetic background (e.g., A.B, A.C, A.D, A.E, etc.). Congenic mice permit one to study the effects of varying the H-2 complex on a background of identical genes (Table 6-1). Recombinant congenic mice are produced by mating two congenic strains that differ at the H-2 locus. Recombinant chromosomes are occasionally generated, and after appropriate breeding they give homozygous recombinant

Table 6-1 Congenic Inbred Strains: H-2 Haplotype, H-2 Donor Strain, Background Strain, and Inbred Strains with the Same H-2 Haplotype

Strain	H-2 Type	H-2 Donor	Background Strain	Inbred Strains with the Same H-2 Type
C57BL/10(B10)	b	C57BL/10(B10)	C57BL/10(B10)	129, C57BL/6 (B6), LP, A.BY, C3H.SW
B10.D2	d	DBA/2	B10	DBA/2, BALB/c
B10.A	a	A/WySn	B10	A/J
B10.M	f	Not inbred	B10	A.CA
B10.BR	k	C57BR	B10	C3H, CBA, AKR
B10.Q	q	DBA/1	B10	DBA/1, SWR
B10.RIII(71NS)	r	RIII	B10	RIII, LP.RIII
B10.S	s	A.SW	B10	A.SW, SJL
B10.PL	u	PL	B10	
A/WySn(A)	a	A/WySn	A/WySn(A)	A/J
A.BY	b	B10	A	C57BL/10, B6, 129, LP, C3H.SW
A.CA	f	Caracul	A	B10.M
A.SW	s	Swiss	A	B10.S, SJL

[Adapted from O. G. Bier et al., *Fundamentals of Immunology*, Springer-Verlag, New York (1981), p. 134.]

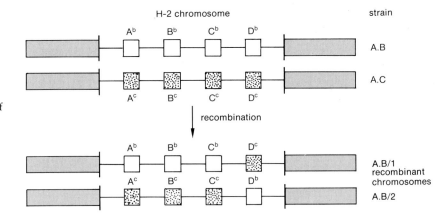

Figure 6-5

A model for the generation of recombinant congenic chromosomes.

congenic strains that differ from the parental strains by just one or a few histocompatibility genes (Figure 6-5, Table 6-2). These strains can be used to assess the effects of changing one or a few histocompatibility genes on a constant genetic background. Overall, more than 150 different inbred strains of mice are now available; approximately 75 strains that are congenic for the H-2 complex are available; and more than 275 recombinant congenic strains have been produced. In addition, about 100 strains with mutant histocompatibility antigens have been identified.

Table 6-2   H-2 Recombinant Strains and Their Origin

F₁-Hybrid Origin	H-2 Type	H-2 Complex Alleles K A_β A_α E_β J E_α S D								New H-2 Haplotype K A_β A_α E_β J E_ϵ S D								Strain	H-2 Type
$\frac{X^a}{Y}$	$\frac{k}{d}$	k	k	k	k	k	7	k	k	k	k	k	k	k|b	7	d	d	B10.A	a
		d	d	d	d	d	7	d	d										
$\frac{B10.A}{B10}$	$\frac{a}{b}$	k	k	k	k	k	7	d	d	b	b	b	b|	k	7	d	d	B10.A(5R)	i5
		b	b	b	b	b	0	b	b										
$\frac{B10.A}{B10}$	$\frac{a}{b}$	k	k	k	k	k	7	d	d	k	k	k|	b	b	0	b	b	B10.A(4R)	h4
		b	b	b	b	b	0	b	b										
$\frac{B10.A}{B10}$	$\frac{a}{b}$	k	k	k	k	k	7	d	d	k	k	k	k	k	7	d|	b	B10.A(2R)	h2
		b	b	b	b	b	0	b	b										
$\frac{B10.A}{T138}$	$\frac{a}{q}$	k	k	k	k	k	7	d	d	q|	k	k	k	k	7	d	d	B10.AQR	y1
		q	q	q	q	q	0	q	q										
$\frac{DBA/2}{C3H}$	$\frac{d}{k}$	d	d	d	d	d	7	d	d	k	k	k	k	k	7	k|	d	A.AL	a1
		k	k	k	k	k	7	k	k										
$\frac{A.AL}{A.SW}$	$\frac{a1}{s}$	s	k	k	k	k	7	k	d	s|	k	k	k	k	7	k	d	A.TL	t1
		s	s	s	s	s	0	s	s										
$\frac{A.AL}{A.SW}$	$\frac{a1}{s}$	k	k	k	k	k	7	k	d	s	s	s	s	s	0	s|	d	A.TH	t2
		s	s	s	s	s	0	s	s										
$\frac{A.TL}{B10.S}$	$\frac{t1}{s}$	s	k	k	k	k	7	k	d	s	s	s	s	s|	7	k	d	B10.HTT	t3
		s	s	s	s	s	0	s	s										
$\frac{B10.A}{B10.S}$	$\frac{a}{s}$	k	k	k	k	k	7	d	d	s	s	s	s	s	0	s|	d	B10.S(7R)	t2
		s	s	s	s	s	0	s	s										
$\frac{A.TL}{A.CA}$	$\frac{t1}{f}$	s	k	k	k	k	7	k	k	s	k	k	k	k	7	k|	f	A.TE	an1
		f	f	f	f	f	0	f	f										
$\frac{B10.AKR}{M}$	$\frac{k}{q}$	k	k	k	k	k	7	k	k	k	k	k	k	k	7	k|	q	B10.AKM	m
		q	q	q	q	q	0	q	q										
$\frac{DBA/2}{C3H}$	$\frac{d}{k}$	d	d	d	d	d	7	d	d	d	d	d	d	d	7	d|	k	C3H.OH	02
		k	k	k	k	k	7	k	k										
$\frac{DBA/2}{C3H}$	$\frac{d}{k}$	d	d	d	d	d	7	d	d	d	d	d	d	d	7|	k	k	C3H.OL	01
		k	k	k	k	k	7	k	k										

[a]The H-2 haplotype of B10.A was already existent before inbreeding; the parental strains of the F₁-hybrid are not known.
[b]Bar designates position of crossover. [Adapted from O. G. Bier et al., *Fundamentals of Immunology*, Springer-Verlag, New York (1981), p. 139.]

Genetic mapping of the H-2 complex

The availability of inbred, congenic, and recombinant congenic mice has permitted antisera and monoclonal antibodies to be raised against H-2 antigens. Because the antisera are raised in genetically distinct animals of the same species, they are denoted *alloantisera*. For example, cells may be injected from the hypothetical recombinant congenic strains A.B/1 or A.B/2 (Figure 6-5) into the parental A.B strain (Figure

6-6). In the immunization with A.B/c-1, alloantisera or monoclonal antibodies to D^c can be raised; in the immunization with A.B/c-2, anti-A^c, anti-B^c, and anti-C^c antibodies can be raised. These alloantisera or monoclonal antibodies are useful in two regards: (a) they can be used to detect H-2 antigens directly on cells (e.g., by radioimmunoassays or fluorescent assays) and (b) they can be used to isolate the radiolabeled histocompatibility antigen by indirect immunoprecipitation (see Problem 6-9).

Alloantisera and monoclonal antibodies have been used to map the genes of the MHC through the analysis of H-2 antigens on cells from recombinant congenic mice and their parent strains. Whenever two serological specificities characteristic of a parental strain are separated in the recombinant strain and are unaltered by the recombinational event, the specificities are assumed to be controlled by genes at two distinct loci; that is, the genes are not alleles (Figure 6-5, Table 6-2). Biological assays such as graft rejection can also be used in these kinds of genetic mapping studies. Immunogeneticists have used serological and biological assays of recombinant congenic strains to construct a detailed map of the MHC of the mouse (Figure 6-7). The MHC of the mouse is located on chromosome 17 about 7 centimorgans (cM) from the centromere. The MHC is divided into two major subcomplexes: (a) the classically defined H-2 complex and (b) the Tla complex (Figure 6-7). By recombination analysis, the H-2 complex is about 0.5 cM in length and the Tla complex is about 1 cM in length. Each of these complexes contains several regions that encode one or more homologous genes. The H-2 complex contains four regions—K, I, S, and D—whereas the Tla complex contains three regions—Qa-2,3, Tla, and Qa-1.

The MHC encodes three classes of genes—I, II, and III. The class I gene products include the transplantation antigens K, D, and L (L is encoded in the D region), which are responsible for the phenomenon of graft rejection initially used to define the MHC, and the hematolymphoid differentiation antigens Qa-1, Qa-2,3, and TL (encoded by the Tla gene). Transplantation antigens are found on virtually all nucleated somatic cells, and they provide the essential context of self in which foreign cell-surface antigens (e.g., those produced during viral infection) can be recognized by cytotoxic T cells which then destroy the antigen-bearing cells (see Chapter 8). The TL antigens are found on thymocytes at an early developmental stage and on certain leukemic cells, whereas the Qa-1 and Qa-2,3 antigens are found on many different types of lymphoid cells. The function of these molecules is completely unknown.

The class II genes—A_α, A_β, E_α, and E_β—are located in the I region. Class II molecules—which are found on macrophages, T cells, and B cells—provide self-recognition elements that allow these cells to interact in the presence of foreign antigen in specific combinations to produce antibody-secreting plasma cells, to stimulate proliferation of cytotoxic T cells, or to generate suppressor T cells (see Chapters 8 and

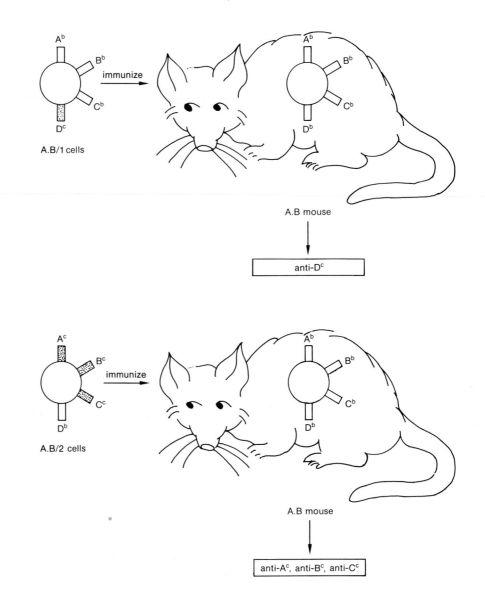

Figure 6-6 A hypothetical scheme for the production of alloantisera. Cells from two recombinant congenic mice are used to immunize one parental congenic line. This immunization takes advantage of the identical genetic backgrounds in congenic and parental mice and the partial differences in the H-2 complex from the recombinant congenic strain relative to either of the parental inbred strains.

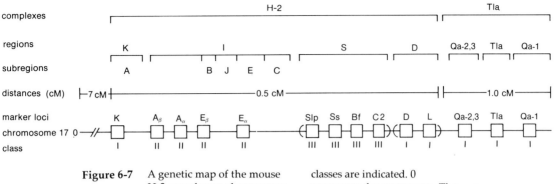

Figure 6-7 A genetic map of the mouse H-2 complex on chromosome 17. Map distances in centimorgans, marker loci, regions, subregions, and classes are indicated. 0 represents the centromere. The order of marker loci within parentheses is not known.

10). The class III genes—Ss, Slp, C2, and Bf—are located in the S region. These genes encode a subset of the serum proteins involved in the complement system, which is an important effector mechanism of the immune system (see Chapter 9). The Ss gene, which is expressed constitutively, and the Slp gene, which is induced by the steroid hormone testosterone, encode two different forms of the complement factor, C4.

6-3   The MHC has been highly conserved throughout vertebrate evolution

Vertebrate MHCs

An evolutionary tree of chordata, showing the presence or absence of the MHC, where known, is given in Figure 6-8. All vertebrates exhibit graft rejection. These rejections may be chronic or rapid. Chronic rejections exhibit a delayed onset of months and a prolonged rejection process that often takes several weeks. Rapid rejections have rapid onset of 1 to 3 weeks and a short rejection process, often of a few days. Rapid graft rejection is observed in some fish, some amphibia, birds, and mammals, and it correlates with the presence of an MHC. Therefore, rapid graft rejections probably indicate the presence of mammalianlike transplantation antigens with their attendant cytotoxic effector mechanisms for the destruction of foreign grafts. These same animals also give strong mixed lymphocyte reactions, a biological assay that probably indicates the presence of class II molecules (see Concept 11-2). Thus the vertebrate class I and class II molecules appear to have evolved together. In addition, the complement system is present in all vertebrates studied to date. Few data are available as to whether any of the complement components are encoded in the MHC. If the class I, II, and III genes have remained clustered in the MHC complex over the more than 600 million years of vertebrate

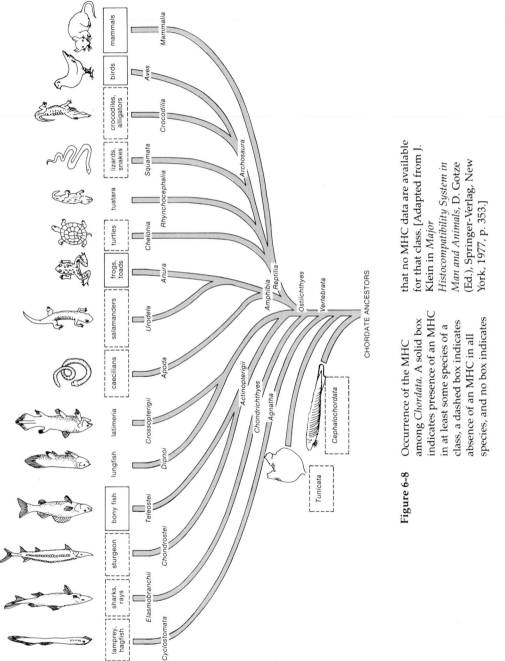

Figure 6-8   Occurrence of the MHC among *Chordata*. A solid box indicates presence of an MHC in at least some species of a class, a dashed box indicates absence of an MHC in all species, and no box indicates that no MHC data are available for that class. [Adapted from J. Klein in *Major Histocompatibility System in Man and Animals*, D. Gotze (Ed.), Springer-Verlag, New York, 1977, p. 353.]

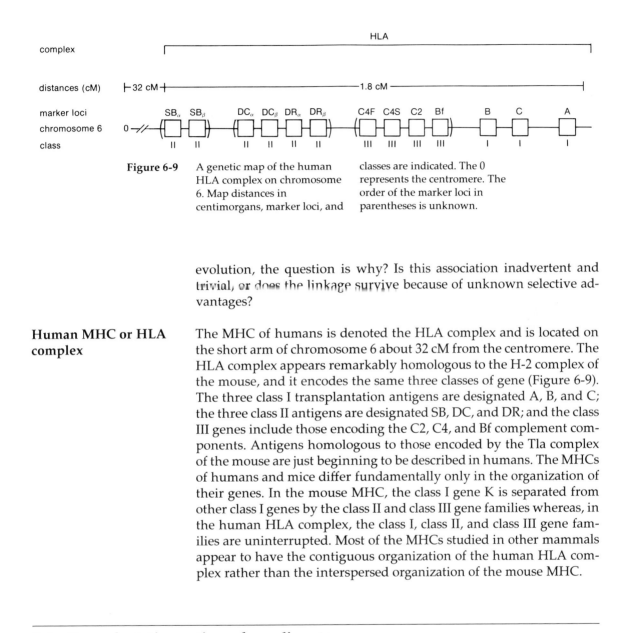

Figure 6-9   A genetic map of the human HLA complex on chromosome 6. Map distances in centimorgans, marker loci, and classes are indicated. The 0 represents the centromere. The order of the marker loci in parentheses is unknown.

evolution, the question is why? Is this association inadvertent and trivial, or does the linkage survive because of unknown selective advantages?

Human MHC or HLA complex

The MHC of humans is denoted the HLA complex and is located on the short arm of chromosome 6 about 32 cM from the centromere. The HLA complex appears remarkably homologous to the H-2 complex of the mouse, and it encodes the same three classes of gene (Figure 6-9). The three class I transplantation antigens are designated A, B, and C; the three class II antigens are designated SB, DC, and DR; and the class III genes include those encoding the C2, C4, and Bf complement components. Antigens homologous to those encoded by the Tla complex of the mouse are just beginning to be described in humans. The MHCs of humans and mice differ fundamentally only in the organization of their genes. In the mouse MHC, the class I gene K is separated from other class I genes by the class II and class III gene families whereas, in the human HLA complex, the class I, class II, and class III gene families are uninterrupted. Most of the MHCs studied in other mammals appear to have the contiguous organization of the human HLA complex rather than the interspersed organization of the mouse MHC.

6-4   Transplantation antigens have discrete domains and are associated with a small immunoglobulinlike polypeptide β_2-microglobulin

Domain structure

The class I gene products are integral membrane glycoproteins ranging in molecular weight from 40,000 to 45,000 (Figure 6-10). They are associated noncovalently with β_2-microglobulin, a peptide 96 amino

Figure 6-10

A model for the association of class I molecules with β_2-microglobulin. The three external domains and the cytoplasmic domain of the class I molecule are indicated by circles. β_2-microglobulin is about the same size as one of the external class I domains. Intrachain disulfide bridges are present in two of the class I domains and in β_2-microglobulin. Carbohydrate side chains are attached to the first two external domains. Charged amino acid residues lock the transmembrane domain into the lipid bilayer. The black boxes in the third external domain indicate residues 199 to 222 and 254 to 273, which surround the two cysteine residues involved in the disulfide bridge formation and show significant homology to immunoglobulin domains. [Adapted from Strominger et al., *Scand. J. Immunol.* **11**, 573–592 (1980).]

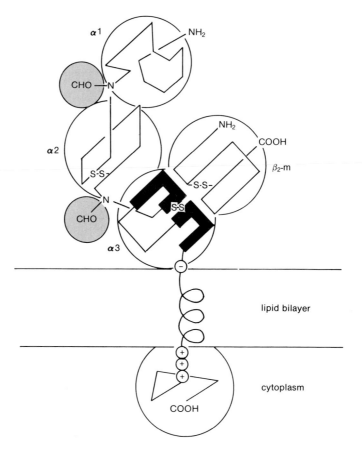

acid residues in length that exhibits significant homology to the C_H homology units of the antibody molecule (Concept 2-5). The class I polypeptide is often termed the heavy chain and the β_2-microglobulin the light chain. The transplantation antigens are divided into five distinct domains or regions (Figure 6-10). There are three external domains, each about 90 residues in length, denoted $\alpha 1$, $\alpha 2$, and $\alpha 3$. These domains are approximately the size of antibody homology units. Moreover, the $\alpha 2$ and $\alpha 3$ domains have centrally placed disulfide bridges that span about 60 amino acid residues, a second feature characteristic of antibody homology units. A fourth domain of about 40 residues spans the membrane and includes an uncharged, hydrophobic transmembrane segment, and a fifth domain about 30 residues in length is positioned in the cell cytoplasm.

The transplantation antigens probably fold with paired domains—$\alpha 1$ with $\alpha 2$ and $\alpha 3$ with β_2-microglobulin. This pairing is demonstrated most clearly for $\alpha 3$ and β_2-microglobulin, which have been shown to be physically associated. Their paired structure probably resembles the individual domains of antibody molecules because both $\alpha3$ and β_2-microglobulin are, by amino-acid-sequence analysis, homologous to the constant region homology units of immunoglobulins. Indeed, perhaps the constraints imposed by the interactions of the $\alpha3$ and β_2-microglobulin domains have preserved this distant ancestral relationship. In addition, a proteolytic fragment of a transplantation antigen—including the $\alpha1$, $\alpha2$, $\alpha3$, and β_2-microglobulin domains—has been crystallized and demonstrates by X-ray analysis a twofold axis of partial symmetry consistent with a paired domain structure. The intriguing homologies between the immunoglobulins and transplantation antigens raise the possibility that these gene families share a common evolutionary origin.

Polymorphism

The transplantation antigens of mice exhibit extensive genetic polymorphism and induce strong serological responses following allogeneic immunization. For this reason, transplantation antigens also are termed *serologically defined (SD) molecules.* Each transplantation antigen carries a number of determinants that are antigenic to most allogeneic hosts. These determinants, which can be defined by the alloantisera they elicit, fall into two categories, (a) *private* determinants that are unique to the immunizing haplotype and (b) *public* determinants that are shared by other haplotypes (Table 6-3). Allogeneic immunization studies in mice have defined 56 distinct alleles at the K locus and 45 alleles at the D locus. These analyses suggest that the worldwide population of mice may have more than 100 different alleles at each of these loci—a polymorphism more extensive than that of any other known gene system.

Both the transplantation antigens and hematolymphoid differentiation antigens were initially denoted class I molecules because of their common cell-surface location, similarity in size, and their distinctive association with β_2-microglobulin. However, the hematolymphoid antigens do not display the extensive polymorphism of the transplantation antigens, and they do not elicit strong humoral responses following allogeneic immunization.

6-5 Exons of class I genes correlate well with the domains of the encoded proteins

Exons and domains

A typical class I gene is composed of eight coding regions or exons separated by seven intervening DNA sequences or introns (Figure 6-11). There is a striking correlation between most of the exons and the protein domains of class I molecules. The first exon encodes the signal peptide that directs insertion of the protein into the endoplasmic reticulum during translation; exons 2 through 4 encode the $\alpha1$,

Table 6-3   K and D Antigenic Determinants of the Mouse[a]

H-2 Haplotype	K Determinants — Public																				K Determinants — Private	D Determinants — Public															D Determinants — Private
	1	3	5	7	8	11	25	27	28	29	34	35	36	37	38	39	42	45	46	47		1	3	5	6	13	27	28	29	35	36	41	42	43	44	49	
b	—	+	—	—	—	—	+	+	+	+	+	—	—	+	—	—	—	—	+	—	33	—	—	+	+	+	+	+	+	—	—	—	—	—	—	—	2?
d	—	+	—	—	—	+	+	+	+	+	—	—	—	+	—	—	—	—	+	+	31	—	+	+	+	+	+	+	+	+	+	+	+	+	+	+	4
f	—	—	—	+	+	+?	+?	+?	•	—	+	—	—	+	—	—	—	—	+	+	?	—	—	+	+	+	+?	−?−?	−?−?	—	—	—	—	—	+	—	9
j	+?	c	—	+	—	•	•	•	•	—	—	—	—	—	—	—	+	+?+?	—	—	15	•	•	•	+	+	+	+	+	—	—	—	—	—	—	—	2
k	+	+	+	+	—	—	—	—	—	—	+	—	+	+	—	+	+	+	—	—	23	+	+	+	+	+	+	+	+	+	+	+	+	+	+	+	32
p	+	+	+	+	—	—	—	—	+	+	—	—	—	+	—	—	+	•	—	—	16	+	+	—	+	+	+	—	c	—	c	—	—	—	+	+	?
q	+	+	+	—	+	—	—	—	—	—	+	—	+	—	—	—	—	—	+	—	17	—	+	+	+	+	+	+	+	+	+	+	+	+	+	+	30
r	+	+	+	+	+	—	—	—	—	—	—	—	—	—	+	—	+	+	—	+	•	+	—	+	+	+	+	+	—	—	—	—	—	+	+	—	18?
a	+	+	—	—	—	—	—	—	—	—	—	—	—	—	+	+	—	—	—	—	19	—	—	+	+	+	+	+	+	c	—	42	—	+	+	+	12
u	c	—	+?	+?	—	—	—	—	—	—	+	+	—	—	—	+	•	•	—	—	20	—	+	—	—	+?+?	+?+?	+	—	c	—	+	+	+	+	—	4
v	+	+	—	—	—	—	•	•	•	+	—	—	—	—	—	—	—	+?	—	—	21	—	—	•	•	−?+?	−?+?	•	—	—	—	—	—	—	—	+	30
z	—	+	—	—	—	—	+	+	+	—	—	—	—	—	—	—	—	+	—	+	•	—	—	+	+	•	•	•	—	—	—	—	—	—	•	•	•

[a](+) = presence of an antigen; (—) = absence of an antigen; (•) = unknown; (?) = presence or absence of antigen is uncertain; (c) = some antisera cross-react with the indicated H-2 haplotype.

[From J. Klein, *Biology of the Mouse Histocompatibility-2 Complex*, Springer-Verlag, New York, 1975, p. 126.]

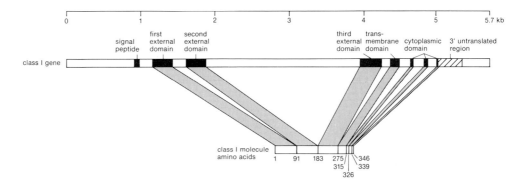

Figure 6-11 A comparison of the exons of a class I gene with the domains and regions of a class I polypeptide.

$\alpha 2$, and $\alpha 3$ external domains; exon 5 encodes the transmembrane domain; and exons 6 through 8 encode the cytoplasmic domain. This correlation between the exon structure of class I genes and the domain structure of the protein product is reminiscent of the similar correlation between antibody gene and protein structure (Figure 4-8), and it is consistent with a common ancestral origin for these two gene systems.

The overall homology between genes that map to the Qa-2,3 and Tla regions and genes encoding transplantation antigens (K, D, L) is 70–85%, and their exon–intron structures are identical. Thus the Qa-2,3 and Tla genes are as closely related to genes encoding the transplantation antigens as they are to one another. This homology firmly establishes the classification of Qa and Tla genes as class I genes.

Alternative patterns of RNA splicing

Three exons encode the cytoplasmic domain of a class I protein and, in this regard, they resemble the multiple 3' exons of the antibody C_H genes (Figure 4-10). Antibody heavy-chain genes are transcribed and differentially processed by RNA splicing at their 3' ends to generate the membrane and secreted forms of immunoglobulins. Several intriguing observations suggest that class I genes may also undergo alternative patterns of RNA splicing at their 3' ends. The C-terminal amino acid sequences derived from purified class I polypeptides and individual cDNA clones are heterogeneous in length and exhibit blocks of amino-acid-sequence differences (Figure 6-12a). Such differences would be expected if different exons encoded the C termini of these polypeptides. In addition, comparison of two mouse class I cDNA clones reveals a notable difference. Although the 3' ends of these two cDNA clones are homologous to one another, they differ by an insertion in one clone of 139 base pairs, which corresponds precisely to the seventh intron of a class I gene (Figure 6-12b). Thus it is attractive to suggest that the seventh intron was not spliced out of the mRNA represented by clone pH-2II, whereas it was removed from

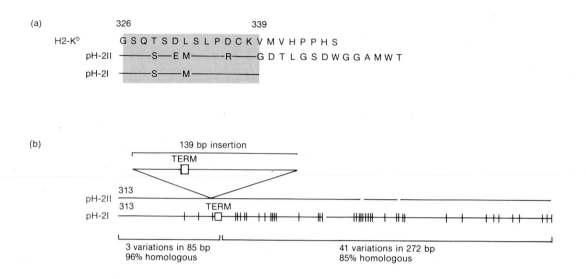

(a)

	326											339							
H2-Kᵇ	G	S Q T S D L S L P D C K	V M V H P P H S

pH-2II ——S——E M————R——G D T L G S D W G G A M W T

pH-2I ——S———M——

(b)

139 bp insertion
TERM

313
pH-2II ————————————————————————

313
pH-2I

3 variations in 85 bp
96% homologous

41 variations in 272 bp
85% homologous

Figure 6-12 Heterogeneity at the C termini of class I molecules. (a) Comparison of C-terminal sequences of the Kᵇ molecule and the translated class I cDNA clones, pH-2I and pH-2II. The shaded region from codon position 326 to 339 indicates the sequences encoded by the second cytoplasmic exon (exon 7). Only amino acid differences are indicated in this region. (b) Comparison of the DNA sequences at the 3′ ends of the cDNA clones, pH-2I and pH-2II. They are homologous except for a 139-bp insertion in clone pH-2II. The termination codons are boxed. Nucleotides in pH-2I that differ from pH-2II are indicated by vertical bars. [Adapted from M. Steinmetz et al., *Cell* **25**, 683(1981).]

Figure 6-13

A model for the generation of two different mRNAs from the same class I gene. The pH-2II-like mRNA would be generated by inclusion of intron 7 in the spliced product, whereas in pH-2I-like mRNAs this intron would be spliced out (see Figure 6-12). [Adapted from M. Steinmetz et al., *Cell* **24**, 125(1981).]

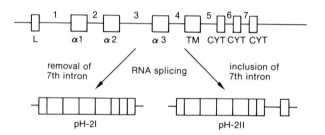

the mRNA represented by clone pH-2I (Figure 6-13). Alternative patterns of RNA splicing would lead to class I C-terminal sequences that differ in size and sequence. To be sure, it remains to be demonstrated that alternative forms of mRNAs can result from the transcription of the *same* class I gene. Nevertheless, the possibility of alternative patterns of RNA processing of class I gene transcripts leads to the intriguing speculation that heterogeneity in the cytoplasmic domains of class I molecules might be important for different effector functions through interactions with different components of the cytoplasm or cytoskeleton. Alternative patterns of RNA splicing may represent a general mechanism for generating alternative forms of proteins from the same gene.

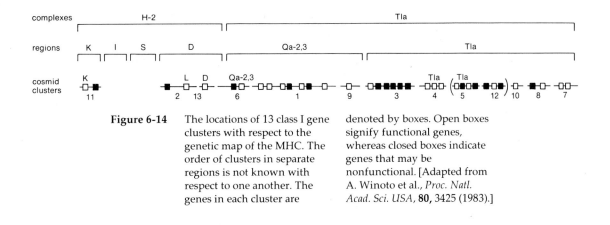

Figure 6-14 The locations of 13 class I gene clusters with respect to the genetic map of the MHC. The order of clusters in separate regions is not known with respect to one another. The genes in each cluster are denoted by boxes. Open boxes signify functional genes, whereas closed boxes indicate genes that may be nonfunctional. [Adapted from A. Winoto et al., *Proc. Natl. Acad. Sci. USA*, **80**, 3425 (1983).]

6-6 Class I genes form a multigene family

Chromosomal arrangement of genes

Thirty-six class I genes have been located within the MHC as illustrated in Figure 6-14. Although the map is not yet completely filled in, some principles are clear. Most of the class I genes (80%) are located within the Tla complex, making it much larger than expected from previous genetic analysis. Based on the demonstrated linkages, the contiguous members of the family appear to be oriented uniformly in the same direction. Similar arrangements are common in other gene families. The functional genes corresponding to the serologically defined K, D, L, Qa-2,3, and TL molecules have been identified; however, the Qa-1 gene has not yet been located. In the H-2 complex, only the K, D, and L genes are functional (open boxes in figure). By contrast, in the Tla complex there are many apparently functional genes, only three of which correspond to the previously identified genes. The functions of the other active genes in this region are completely unknown.

Activity has not been detected from many of the identified class I genes. Some of these apparently dead genes may actually function in a way that has not yet been assayed. Others are *pseudogenes,* which are nonallelic but recognizable relatives of known genes that have suffered inactivating mutations and appear functionally dead. Pseudogenes are a common feature of many gene families, for example, the α and β globin gene clusters. All class I genes identified so far map to the MHC, so that there are as yet no examples of so-called *processed pseudogenes,* which are nonfunctional gene relatives that lack introns and have been dispersed in the genome by an undefined mechanism, apparently involving an mRNA-like intermediate. Processed pseudogenes have been identified in other gene families, such as the antibody, globin, and tubulin gene families.

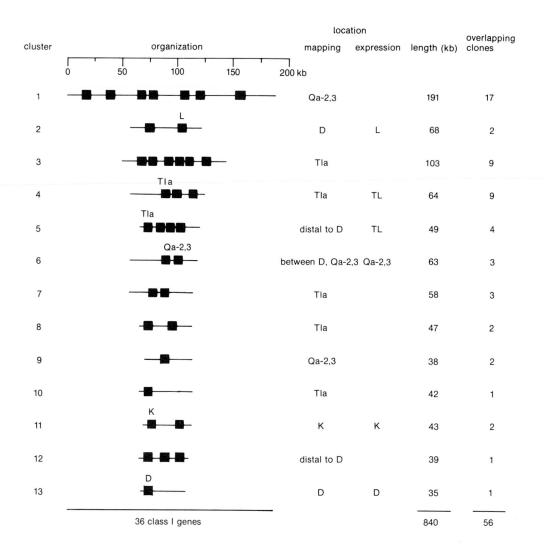

cluster	organization	location mapping	expression	length (kb)	overlapping clones
1		Qa-2,3		191	17
2	L	D	L	68	2
3		Tla		103	9
4	Tla	Tla	TL	64	9
5	Tla	distal to D	TL	49	4
6	Qa-2,3	between D, Qa-2,3	Qa-2,3	63	3
7		Tla		58	3
8		Tla		47	2
9		Qa-2,3		38	2
10		Tla		42	1
11	K	K	K	43	2
12		distal to D		39	1
13	D	D	D	35	1
	36 class I genes			840	56

Figure 6-15   Summary of the organization of 13 class I gene clusters of the MHC of the BALB/c mouse. Class I genes in the 13 clusters are indicated by black boxes. The numbers of overlapping cosmid clones in the cluster is also indicated. The lengths of the clusters are given in kilobase pairs (kb) together with the number of overlapping cosmid clones constituting a given cluster. The location of the 13 gene clusters was determined by restriction enzyme site polymorphism mapping (see text). The identification of certain expressed class I gene products was carried out by gene transfer to mouse L cells and serological analyses (see text). [Adapted from M. Steinmetz et al., *Cell* **28**, 489(1982).]

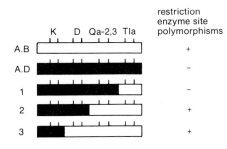

Figure 6-16   Genetic mapping by the correlation of serological and restriction enzyme polymorphisms in different recombinant congenic mice. The MHC is depicted for five congenic mice that are identical genetically except for the MHC. For the parental congenic mice A.B and A.D, the MHC from inbred mouse strains B and D, respectively, have been superimposed on an A-strain background. Recombinant congenic mice 1, 2, and 3 represent various recombinations between the two distinct parental MHCs. In the recombinant strains, crossing-over events have separated each of the four regions and thus permit a definitive assignment of these regions as distinct genes or clusters of genes. A restriction enzyme site polymorphism can be correlated with corresponding region. In the example given, the restriction enzyme site polymorphism correlates with the Qa region and indicates that this restriction enzyme site and the corresponding cosmid cluster map to that region. [Adapted from A. Winoto et al., *Proc. Natl. Acad. Sci. USA*, **80**, 3425 (1983).]

Genetic mapping

The arrangement of genes within the MHC was determined in several stages. Clusters of class I genes were identified in two steps. First, large 30- to 50-kilobase (kb) segments of chromosomal DNA from a BALB/c mouse were cloned into special (cosmid) vectors and the fragments containing class I genes were identified by hybridization to a previously cloned class I cDNA probe. Second, restriction maps of the fragments were generated and compared to determine which fragments overlapped. The 56 clones containing class I genes could be ordered into 13 gene clusters containing 36 distinct class I genes in a total of 840 kb of DNA (Figure 6-15).

The gene clusters were positioned relative to the genetic map of the MHC by exploiting sequence differences (polymorphisms) that exist between the parental strain from which the fragments were derived and related congenic strains. For each cluster, several congenic strains were screened until a restriction enzyme site polymorphism was identified. Appropriate recombinant congenic strains were then tested for the presence or absence of the polymorphism. The idealized experiment illustrated in Figure 6-16 shows the results for a restriction enzyme site polymorphism located in the Qa-2,3 region.

The restriction enzyme site polymorphisms themselves were identified in two steps. First, DNA segments that hybridize to only one or a few genomic restriction fragments were subcloned from each cluster to simplify the analysis. Then these probes were used to examine the DNAs of congenic mice for restriction enzyme site polymor-

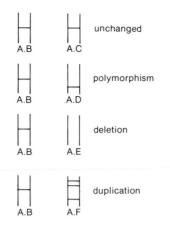

Figure 6-17   Hypothetical blot analyses of various congenic mouse DNAs with a single-copy DNA probe. The DNAs are cleaved with a restriction enzyme, electrophoresed on agarose gels to separate the fragments by size, transferred to a special nitrocellulose filter by blotting, hybridized against a radiolabeled probe, and then, after removal of the excess radiolabeled reagent, the fragments containing the complementary sequences are visualized by autoradiography. Various hybridization patterns can be identified by single-copy probes in different inbred strains. A.B, A.C, A.D, A.E, and A.F are congenic inbred strains with the same background genes but different MHC regions. Strains A.B and A.C have no detectable polymorphisms. In strain A.D, the fragment detected by blotting shows a size variation. In strain A.E, the probe sequence has been deleted, and, in strain A.F, a duplication of the sequence detected by the probe has occurred. [Adapted from A. Winoto et al., *Proc. Natl. Acad. Sci. USA*, **80,** 3425 (1983).]

phisms. Three types of polymorphism were observed, (a) a change in size of the restriction fragment (mutation), (b) a loss of the restriction fragment (deletion), or (c) an increase in number of restriction fragments (duplication) (Figure 6-17). Restriction enzyme site polymorphisms were detected with considerably greater frequency in the K and D regions than in the Qa-2,3 and Tla regions, which is in complete accordance with the extensive serological polymorphism of K and D molecules and the limited serological polymorphism of Qa-2,3 and TL molecules. Thus the extensive polymorphism evident in the K and D gene products and the limited polymorphism of the Qa-2,3 and Tla gene products are also reflected by similar degrees of polymorphism in the sequences flanking these genes.

To establish which genes were functional, each gene was transferred individually into mouse cells with a different haplotype. The genes, which were isolated from a BALB/c mouse (d haplotype), were transferred into thymidine kinase-negative mouse L cells (k haplotype) by cotransfer with a herpes virus thymidine kinase gene using the calcium phosphate transfer technique (Figure 6-18). Under appropriate selection conditions, only cells expressing the herpes vi-

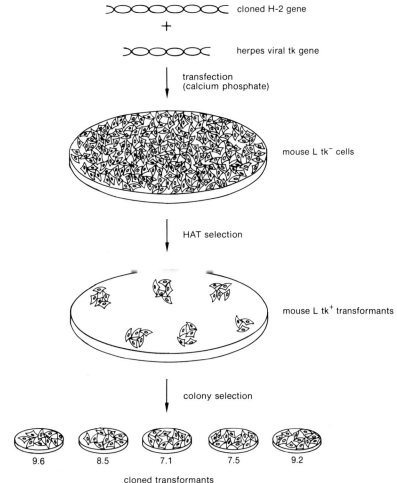

cloned H-2 gene

+

herpes viral tk gene

transfection
(calcium phosphate)

mouse L tk⁻ cells

HAT selection

mouse L tk⁺ transformants

colony selection

9.6   8.5   7.1   7.5   9.2

cloned transformants

Figure 6-18

A schematic diagram of the gene transfer technique. Cloned genes are transferred into mouse L cells lacking the thymidine kinase gene. The cloned class I gene and a herpes thymidine kinase gene are transferred under conditions such that about 1 in 10^5 mouse L cells incorporate both genes randomly into their chromosomes. Under appropriate selective conditions (HAT media), only those cells taking up the thymidine kinase gene can grow. About 90% of these cells have also taken up the class I gene. These cells are cloned and the class I cell-surface product identified by serological analyses.

rus thymidine kinase gene will grow. Only about 1 in 10^4 to 10^5 L cells expresses the viral thymidine kinase and grows under these conditions, but about 90% of these cells also express the newly introduced class I gene product on the cell surface. The gene products were assayed in two ways (Figure 6-19). The serologically defined molecules, K, D, L, Qa-2,3, and TL, were identified using specific monoclonal antibodies. The gene products that had not been defined serologically were detected indirectly by increased β_2-microglobulin on the surface of the transformed cells. In addition to identifying active genes, gene transfer should allow molecular biologists to begin to dissect the interactions among the transplantation antigens, T-cell receptors, and foreign antigens. *In vitro* exchange of exons between different class I

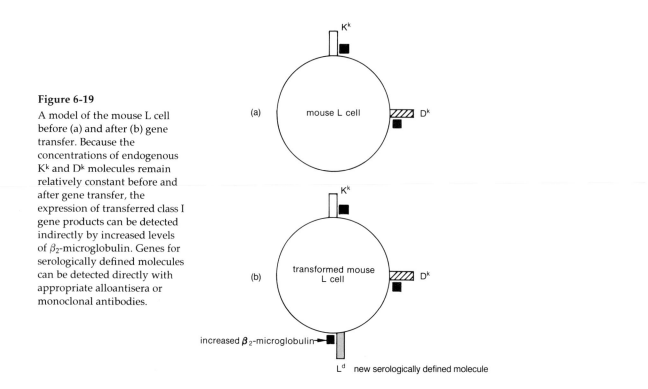

Figure 6-19

A model of the mouse L cell before (a) and after (b) gene transfer. Because the concentrations of endogenous K^k and D^k molecules remain relatively constant before and after gene transfer, the expression of transferred class I gene products can be detected indirectly by increased levels of β_2-microglobulin. Genes for serologically defined molecules can be detected directly with appropriate alloantisera or monoclonal antibodies.

genes and *in vitro* mutagenesis of specific sites within genes should provide insights into the nature of these complex interactions.

Genetic mechanisms for class I polymorphism

Amino-acid-sequence analyses on the N termini of transplantation antigens have established that the alleles of a particular gene generally differ by 5–10% of their sequence. These extensively differing alleles are denoted complex allotypes and stand in striking contrast to the alleles of most genes, such as the hemoglobins and haploglobins, which generally differ by only one or two residues. K and D alleles cannot be distinguished by virtue of their N-terminal sequences, and yet the transplantation antigens of the mouse exhibit species-specific residues that readily distinguish them from their human counterparts. Thus multiple class I genes appear to evolve in a coordinated or coincidental manner in each evolutionary line (Figure 6-20a).

The existence of complex allotypes, the lack of K-ness or D-ness, and the presence of species-associated residues suggest that several distinct genetic mechanisms are at work. Repeated *unequal crossing over* within a gene family can homogenize the gene family, and, in separate evolutionary lines, it could lead to species-associated characteristics (Figure 6-20b). Unequal crossing over has been demonstrated in some gene families, and the expansions and contractions (duplica-

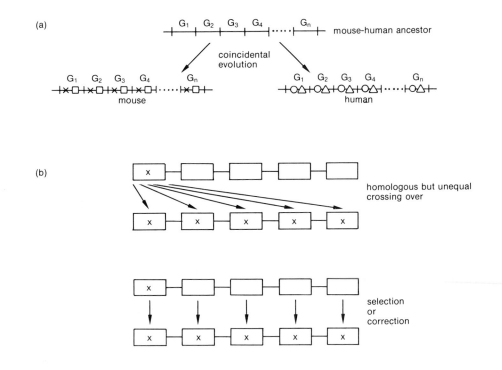

Figure 6-20 Coincidental evolution in a multigene family. (a) A diagrammatic representation of coincidental evolution during the divergence of the mouse and human evolutionary lines. X, □, O, and Δ represent coincidental changes in the respective evolutionary lines. (b) Two models for coincidental evolution.

tions and deletions) characteristic of unequal crossing over are evident in the duplication and deletion polymorphisms among mouse haplotypes. At the same time, nonallelic class I genes apparently exchange blocks of sequences, perhaps generating extensive differences among alleles and obscuring the distinctions between K and D alleles. Such nonallelic exchanges, which are commonly referred to as *gene corrections* or *gene conversions*, have been demonstrated in this gene family and in others. Indeed, one "function" of pseudogenes may be to serve as a reservoir of related sequence information. Preferred or directional transfers of information could also contribute significantly to the overall homogenization of the family (Figure 6-20b). The different degrees of polymorphism in the Tla and H-2 complexes suggest that *natural selection* may resist the rise of genetic rearrangements more severely in the Tla complex than in the H-2 complex. In principle, natural selection could also account for species-specific differences. Other as yet unknown genetic mechanisms may also contribute to class I polymorphisms.

6-7   Ia antigens are heterodimers with discrete domains

Class II subregions

The I region of the MHC contains the class II genes, and it has been divided by genetic analyses into five subregions denoted I-A, I-B, I-J, I-E, and I-C (Figure 6-7). The I-A and I-E subregions contain the genes for the class II molecules that have been well characterized by serological and biochemical methods. A third subregion, I-J, appears to encode polypeptides that are subunits of the suppressor factors secreted by suppressor T cells. These factors suppress various types of immune responses. Although the I-J polypeptides have been characterized in functional assays, their biochemical characterization is only beginning. The characterization of suppressor factors and their genes has been of vital interest because it may represent a unique opportunity to study one form of the T-cell receptor. The I-B and I-C subregions have been defined exclusively on the basis of their ability to modulate certain immune responses in mice, and some immunologists question whether these subregions exist.

Class II molecules

Two class II molecules, denoted I-A and I-E, are heterodimers composed of α and β chains. The α chains range in molecular weight from 30,000 to 33,000 daltons, and the β chains from 27,000 to 29,000. A third type of polypeptide termed the *invariant* (I_i) *chain,* which has a molecular weight of approximately 33,000, appears to be associated with the α and β polypeptides prior to their association and display on the cell surface. Because I_i polypeptides are not expressed on plasma membrane with Ia antigens, it has been suggested that the I_i chain plays an important role in the maturation of α and β chains or in their transport to the cell surface. The A_α, A_β, and E_β genes are contained within the I-A subregion, whereas the E_α gene is located within the I-E subregion (Figure 6-7).

The mouse I-A and I-E molecules are homologous to the human DC and DR molecules, respectively (Figure 6-9). The counterpart to the third human class II molecule, SB, has not been found in the mouse. Each class II polypeptide is composed of two external domains—$\alpha 1$ and $\alpha 2$ or $\beta 1$ and $\beta 2$—each about 90 amino acid residues in length, with a transmembrane domain of about 30 residues and a very short cytoplasmic domain of about 10–15 residues (Figure 6-21). Three of the four external domains ($\alpha 2$, $\beta 1$, and $\beta 2$) have centrally placed disulfide bridges.

The A_α, A_β, and E_β genes are highly polymorphic, whereas the E_α gene is not. If an animal is heterozygous for the A_α and A_β genes, then four different class II, I-A molecules can be displayed on its cell surface. The same is true of the I-E molecules, and this fact makes it possible to have as many as eight different Ia molecules in animals

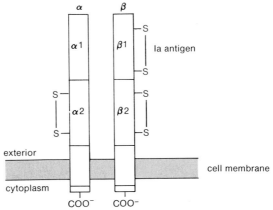

Figure 6-21

A model of the Ia molecule. The α and β chains are divided into two external domains (α1 and α2 or β1 and β2), a transmembrane domain, and a cytoplasmic domain. The cysteine residues that participate in disulfide bridge formation are indicated by S.

heterozygous at all four class II loci. Many inbred strains of mice fail to express I-E, molecules, although all express I-A molecules.

As described in Chapter 8, the heterodimeric structure of class II molecules allows molecular complementation of defects in immune response genes. For example, one inbred mouse strain may have a defective A_α gene required for an immune response to a particular antigen, whereas a second inbred mouse strain may have a defect in the A_β gene for the same immune response. The F_1 offspring from these two defective strains possess one functional A_α gene and one functional A_β gene, thus complementing one another to produce a functional I-A molecule that can restore immune responsiveness to an antigen to which the parental strains are blind.

6-8 Exons of class II genes correlate well with the domains of the encoded proteins

Exons and domains

The α and β genes each contain five exons (Figure 6-22). For both the α and β genes, the first exon encodes the leader peptide, and the second and third exons encode the α1 and α2 or β1 and β2 domains. For α genes, the fourth exon encodes the transmembrane domain, the short cytoplasmic domain, and a portion of the 3' untranslated region of the mRNA. The fifth exon encodes the remainder of the 3' untranslated region. In contrast, for β genes, the fourth exon encodes the transmembrane domain and a portion of the cytoplasmic domain, whereas the fifth exon encodes the remainder of the cytoplasmic domain and the 3' untranslated region. Once again there is a striking correlation between the exons and protein domains or regions (compare Figures 6-21 and 6-22).

Figure 6-22

Structure of the class II α and β genes. L indicates leader; $\alpha 1$, $\alpha 2$, $\beta 1$, and $\beta 2$, the external domains; TM, transmembrane; CYT, cytoplasmic; and 3'UT, 3' untranslated sequences. Slashes indicate that the distance of separation is unknown.

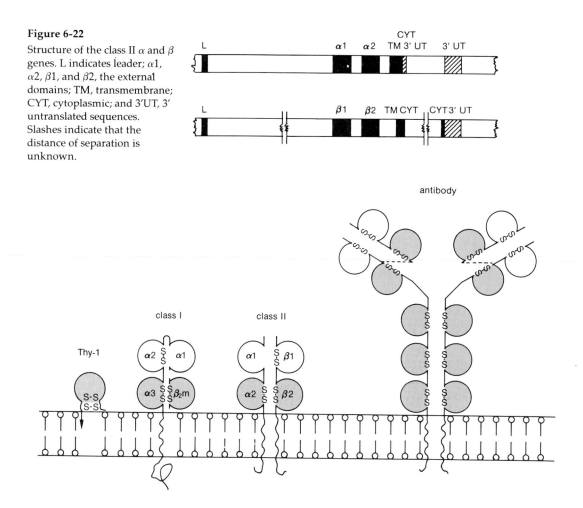

Figure 6-23 A schematic representation of the domain structures and membrane orientations of Thy-1, class I, class II, and antibody molecules. Thy-1 is a T-cell differentiation antigen. Shaded domains indicate sequence homologies that suggest a common evolutionary ancestry (see text). It is likely that the multidomain molecules fold to have interacting pairs of domains—$\alpha 1$ with $\alpha 2$ in class I, $\alpha 1$ with $\beta 1$ in class II, etc.

Homology of class I, class II, β_2-microglobulin, antibody, and Thy-1 genes

There are several similarities among class I, class II, β_2-microglobulin, and antibody genes (Figure 6-23). All these genes exhibit a precise correlation between exons and the protein domains they encode, and the sizes of the external domains and the central placement of the disulfide bridges are similar. During expression of all these genes, RNA splicing always occurs between the first and second base of the junctional codons. In addition, the DNA sequences of the class I $\alpha 3$ exons, the class II $\alpha 2$ and $\beta 2$ exons, and β_2-microglobulin are homologous to the exon sequences

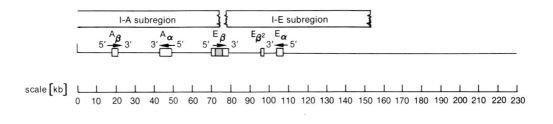

Figure 6-24   Physical map of the I region of the BALB/c mouse. Boxes indicate identified class II genes and give the maximum region that hybridizes to the probes used for identification. [Adapted from M. Steinmetz et al., *Nature* **300,** 35(1982).]

encoding antibody constant regions. Although the class I $\alpha 1$ and $\alpha 2$ exons and the class II $\alpha 1$ exons do not show significant sequence homology to one another or to antibody genes, their sizes are similar to those of the other class I, class II, and antibody exons. These observations suggest that class I, class II, and antibody genes share a common ancestor and that marked changes have occurred after divergence of the genes to fulfill different functions. The gene products also show homology to the T-cell differentiation antigen, Thy-1, at the protein level (Figure 6-23). Because of the sequence and structural relationships of these genes, it is attractive to speculate that all of them—class I, class II, β_2-microglobulin, immuno-globulin, and Thy-1—have descended from a common ancestor and are therefore members of a supergene family (see Figure 4-23).

6-9   The class II genes constitute a small multigene family

Chromosomal arrangement of genes

The chromosomal arrangement of class II genes was determined in the same way as that of the class I genes. Restriction enzyme site polymorphisms were identified between strains, and the appropriate recombinant congenic strains were screened to relate the genetic and physical maps (see Figure 6-16). The five identified class II genes are located within a 90-kb region near one end of a continuous 230-kb stretch of BALB/c chromosomal DNA (Figure 6-24). This chromosomal region must contain nearly the entire I region because it includes the serologically defined I-A and I-E region genes. The A_β and A_α genes are contained in the I-A region, and the E_α gene is contained in the I-E region, as expected, along with a new gene, $E_{\beta 2}$, which appears to be a pseudogene. Most curiously, the E_β gene seems to straddle the junction between the I-A and

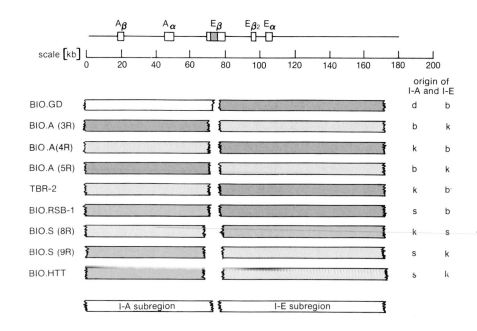

Figure 6-25 Physical maps for nine inbred mice exhibiting recombination points between the right boundary of the I-A subregion and the left boundary of the I-E subregion. All recombination events have occurred within a stretch of 8 kb or less of DNA. [Adapted from M. Steinmetz et al., *Nature* **300**, 35(1982).]

I-E regions. In addition, by cross-hybridization criteria, the class II gene family may have up to three more β-like members, at least some of which are located beyond the left end of the cloned I region.

The class II gene family differs from the class I gene family in several ways. This family is much smaller and the genes are not oriented in the same direction. However, it is similar to the class I gene family in that different genetic regions have characteristic degrees of polymorphism; I-A region genes are highly polymorphic, whereas the I-E region gene is not.

Comparison of the genetic and physical maps

The junction between the I-A and I-E regions, as derived from comparisons of nine recombinant haplotypes, apparently splits the E_β gene (Figure 6-25), leaving only about 2 kb of DNA to encode the I-B and I-J subregions. The discrepancy in the separation of the I-A and I-E subregions on the genetic and physical maps suggests that a recombination anomaly exists between these two subregions. The genetic map is based on the assumption that recombination events are distributed uniformly along the chromosome. Therefore, a bulge in the genetic map relative to the physical map indicates that recombination events occur more frequently than expected in the affected region, suggesting a recombination hotspot at the junction of the I-A and I-E subregions.

The junctional region of 2 kb seems remarkably small to encode a typical eukaryotic gene, let alone two, raising the distinct possibility that the I-B and I-J subregions are artifactual or have been incorrectly mapped. However, the serological evidence for the I-J subregion in particular seems convincing. Given the strange genetic properties of the junctional region and the genetic evidence for the existence of subregions at the junction, a close examination of all possibilities is warranted. Some of the ways in which the I-B, I-J, or both subregions could be accommodated within the junctional region include: (a) as distinct genes that overlap the E_β gene in the same or opposite orientation, (b) as distinct exons that are spliced into the transcript from the E_β gene, and (c) as noncoding stretches of DNA that represent binding sites for important regulatory molecules. These possibilities and others will be resolved only by further analysis.

Selected Bibliography

Where to begin

Cunningham, B. A., "The structure and function of histocompatibility antigens," *Sci. Am.* **237,** 96(1977).

Hood, L., Steinmetz, M., and Goodenow, R., "Genes of the major histocompatibility complex," *Cell* **28,** 685 (1982).

Matzinger, P., and Zamoyska, R., "A beginner's guide to major histocompatibility complex function," *Nature* **297,** 628(1982).

Robertson, M., "The evolutionary past of the major histocompatibility complex and the future of cellular immunology," *Nature* **297,** 629(1982).

Textbooks

Klein, J., *Biology of the Mouse Histocompatibility-2 Complex*, Springer-Verlag, New York, 1975. A well-written book that clearly introduces the general principles as well as the finer details of the mouse MHC.

Snell, G. D., Dausset, J., and Nathenson, S., *Histocompatibility*, Academic Press, New York, 1976. A book that covers every aspect of mammalian histocompatibility.

Invertebrate immunity

Burnet, F. M., "Self-recognition in colonial marine forms and flowering plants in relation to the evolution of immunity," *Nature* **232,** 230(1972).

Hildemann, W. H., Johnston, I. S., and Jokiel, P. L., "Immunocompetence in the lowest metazoan phylum: transplantation immunity in sponges," *Science* **204,** 420(1979).

Scofield, V. L., Schlumpberger, J. M., West, L. A., and Weissman, I. L., "Protochordate allorecognition is controlled by a MHC-like gene system," *Nature* **295,** 499(1982).

A series of papers that probe the ancient origins of the immune system.

Uses and construction of special mouse strains

Green, E. L., "Breeding Systems," in *Biology of the Laboratory Mouse*, E. L. Green, Ed., McGraw-Hill, New York, 11(1966). A concise description of the construction of inbred and congenic inbred strains of mice.

Klein, D., Sewarson, S., Figueroa, F., and Klein, J., "The minimal length of the differential segment in H-2 congenic lines," *Immunogenetics* **16**, 319(1982). A thorough attempt to analyze the length of the donor chromosome segment in a series of MHC congenic strains.

Snell, G. D., "Studies in Histocompatibility," *Science* **213**, 172(1981). A Nobel Prize lecture detailing some early experiments with congenic strains of mice.

Genetics of the MHC

Duncan, W. R., Wakeland, E. K., and Klein, J., "Histocompatibility-2 system in wild mice. VIII. Frequencies of H-2 and Ia antigens in wild mice from Texas," *Immunogenetics* **9**, 261(1979). Quantitative measurements of the polymorphism of MHC genes.

Klein, J., Juretic, A., Baxevanis, C. N., and Nagy, Z. A., "The traditional and a new version of the mouse H-2 complex," *Nature* **291**, 455(1981). A widely cited review that attempts to unify the genetic, cellular, and molecular studies on the MHC.

Melief, C., "Remodelling the H-2 map," *Immunol. Today* **4**, 57(1983). A good account of a scientific meeting on the MHC with particular emphasis on studies with spontaneous class I mutants.

A comparison of the major histocompatibility complex between different species

Götze, D., *The Major Histocompatibility System in Man and Animals*, Springer-Verlag, New York, 1977.

Klein, J., "The major histocompatibility complex of the mouse," *Science* **203**, 516(1979).

Thorsby, E., "Biological function of HLA," *Tissue Antigens* **11**, 321(1978).

Class I molecules and genes

Hood, L., Steinmetz, M., and Malissen, B., "Genes of the major histocompatibility complex of the mouse," *Annu. Rev. Immunol.* **1**, 529(1983).

Maloy, W. L., and Coligan, J. E., "Primacy structure of the H-2D^b alloantigen," *Immunogenetics* **16**, 11(1982). This paper contains a comparison of the class I DNA and protein sequences available in 1982.

Nathenson, S. G., Uehara, H., Ewenstein, B. M., Kindt, T. J., and Coligan, J. E., "Primary structural analysis of the transplantation antigens of the murine H-2 major histocompatibility complex," *Annu. Rev. Biochem.* **50**, 1025(1981).

Steinmetz, M., Moore, K. W., Frelinger, J. G., Sher, B. T., Shen, F. W., Boyse, E. A., and Hood, L., "A pseudogene homologous to mouse transplantation antigens: transplantation antigens are encoded by eight exons that correlate with protein domains," *Cell* **25**, 683(1981). This paper details the structure of a gene encoding a class I molecule.

Class II molecules and genes

Mathis, D. J., Benoist, C. O., Williams, V. E., II, Madge, R. K., and McDevitt, H. O., "The murine E$_\alpha$ immune response gene," *Cell* **32**, 745(1983).

Shackelford, D. A., Kaufman, J. F., Korman, A. J., and Strominger, J. L., "HLA-DR antigens: structure, separation of subpopulations, gene cloning and function," *Immunol. Rev.* **66**, 133(1982).

Steinmetz, M., Minard, K., Horvath, S., McNicholas, J., Ferlinger, J., Wake, C., Long, E., Mach, B., and Hood, L., "A molecular map of the immune response region from the major histocompatibility complex of the mouse," *Nature* **300**, 35(1982).

Additional concepts and techniques presented in the problems

1. Antigenic modulation. Problem 6-3.
2. Absorption analyses. Problems 6-4, 6-5, and 6-11.
3. Five laws of transplantation. Problem 6-6.
4. F$_1$ test. Problem 6-7.
5. Indirect immunoprecipitation. Problems 6-9 and 6-10.
6. Hemopoietic chimeras. Problem 6-12.
7. Restriction enzyme analyses. Problem 6-13.
8. Mutant transplantation antigens. Problem 6-14.
9. T-killer assays. Problems 6-16 and 6-21.
10. Southern blot analyses. Problem 6-17.
11. I-J polypeptide. Problem 6-18.
12. DNA-mediated gene transfer. Problems 6-19 and 6-20.

Problems

6-1 Indicate whether each of the following statements is true or false. Explain the error in each statement you consider to be false.

(a) The MHC has been found in all mammals studied to date.

(b) Two congenic strains that differ at the H-2 complex may also differ in genes closely linked to the H-2 complex.

(c) The H-2 complex has sufficient DNA to code for 10–20 genes 600 nucleotides in length.

(d) A single D gene product from the mouse may contain multiple public and private serological specificities.

(e) All vertebrates exhibit the ability to destroy allografts by an acute rejection process.

(f) The gene products of the K and D alleles of the mouse are examples of complex allotypes.

(g) Minor histocompatibility loci encode cell-surface antigens.

(h) The genes encoding minor histocompatibility antigens are present only on chromosome 17.

(i) Inbred mice generally exhibit greater than 99% homozygosity.

(j) The TL antigen is highly polymorphic.

(k) T_H cells recognize antigen in the context of class II molecules.

(l) The human HLA complex is organized differently from its mouse counterpart.

(m) The twofold axis of symmetry of the transplantation antigen suggests that it folds into paired external domains.

(n) The inbred BALB/c mouse appears to have approximately six class I genes.

(o) DNA-mediated gene transfer has been used to identify serologically defined class I genes.

(p) Novel class I gene products are not associated with β_2-microglobulin.

(q) Coincidental evolution indicates that multiple genes evolve in a parallel or co-ordinate fashion.

(r) The E_β gene lies in the I-E subregion.

(s) The invariant (I_i) chain is associated with class II polypeptides during their transport from the Golgi apparatus to the plasma membrane.

(t) The class II alleles are codominantly expressed.

(u) One class III gene lies 90 kb to the left of the E_α gene.

(v) The I-J polypeptide must be encoded between the I-A and the I-E subregions.

(w) Crossing over is randomly distributed throughout the class I region.

(x) The MHC contains sufficient DNA to encode additional multigene families beyond the three already described.

6-2 Supply the missing word or words in each of the following statements.

(a) The MHC of humans is designated _____ , and that of mice is designated _____ .

(b) _____ mice are genetically identical except for a single chromosomal region.

(c) A unique combination of alleles at loci within the MHC is termed a _____ .

(d) Regions and subregions of the H-2 complex are defined by _____ events among distinct genes.

(e) The class III regions of the MHC code for certain _____ components.

(f) Serological specificities shared by many class I molecules are said to be _____ specificities.

Table 6-4 An Absorption Analysis of Rabbit Anti-Mouse Red Blood Cell (RBC) Serum (Problem 6-4)

Mouse Test Cells	Rabbit Anti-Mouse RBC Serum				
			Absorbed with		
Source	Unabsorbed	RBC	Liver	Kidney	Brain
RBC	+a	—	+	+	+
Liver	+	—	—	—	—
Kidney	+	—	—	—	—
Brain	+	—	+	+	—

a+ indicates a positive reaction between the rabbit anti-mouse RBC serum and mouse red blood cells; — indicates a negative reaction.

(g) The I-J subregion appears to code for an antigen-specific T-cell _____ .

(h) The primary structures of the transplantation antigens of mice and humans are _____ to one another.

(i) _____ allotypes are those that differ by multiple amino acid residues.

(j) The three families of MHC genes are denoted _____ , _____ , and _____ .

(k) Both alleles of the K locus are expressed _____ on individual cells.

(l) The serologically defined class II genes are denoted _____ , _____ , _____ , and _____ .

(m) _____ and _____ are two duplicated forms of the C4 gene in the mouse.

(n) The two categories of class I gene products are _____ and _____ .

(o) Cytotoxic T cells recognize antigen in the context of a _____ molecule.

(p) The class I gene of the mouse has _____ exons; these exons generally correlate with the _____ structures of the class I molecule.

(q) Two techniques that have been used to locate class I genes within the MHC are mapping by _____ and _____ .

(r) Three mechanisms to explain coincidental evolution are _____ , _____ , and _____ .

(s) The class II molecule has _____ and _____ chains.

(t) The α and β class II genes contain _____ exons.

(u) Portions of class I, class II, and antibody genes are _____ .

(v) The BALB/c mouse appears to contain less than _____ class II genes.

6-3 A new alloantigen, S, is discovered on the spleen cells of the A inbred strain of rats, and it is missing on the corresponding cells of the B inbred strain. This alloantigen is expressed in (A $\times$ B)F$_1$ individuals and segregates in a classical Mendelian fashion. Two surprising observations are made. (a) Occasional leukemias that arise in the B strain express the S antigen. (b) Rats of the B strain can be immunized with lethally irradiated cells of an S$^+$ B-strain leukemia; these rats then produce anti-S antibodies that will kill S$^+$ B-strain leukemia cells *in vitro*. However, when such immunized rats are injected with S$^+$ B-strain leukemic cells, the rats are killed by the leukemia. Leukemic cells taken from these rats are S$^-$. However, the S$^+$ phenotype of these

Table 6-5 An Absorption Analysis of Anti-X Serum: Distribution of the Reaction (+ Versus −) of the Serum with Cells of Four Mice from Different Inbred Strains, 1–4 (Problem 6-5)

Test Cells from Each of Four Inbred Strains	Anti-X Serum				
	Unabsorbed	Absorbed with Test Cells of Strain:			
		1	2	3	4
1	+	−	+	−	+
2	+	+	−	−	+
3	+	+	+	−	+
4	+	−	−	−	−

cells reappears upon passage of the tumor through nonimmune hosts. What conclusions can you draw from these observations?

6-4   (a)   Suppose that you inject mouse red blood cells into a rabbit and then carry out the analysis shown in Table 6-4. What is the minimum number of antigenic determinants required to explain these reactions? Use the symbols A, B, C, etc., for antigenic determinants.

(b)   What analogies can you draw between these determinants and known cell-surface components?

6-5   (a)   Suppose you prepare an alloantiserum by immunizing an inbred mouse of strain A with cells "X" from an inbred mouse of a different strain. The absorption analysis of this serum is presented in Table 6-5.

How might you interpret these results in terms of the minimum number of antigenic determinants necessary to explain them? Use the symbols A, B, C, etc., as antigenic determinants.

(b)   Which of these antigens do the X cells have? Can the X cells have additional antigens? Which of these antigens are present on cells from the host in which the antiserum was raised?

(c)   Are the detectable antigens allelic forms of the same structural gene? How would your answer change if mice 1 through 4 were wild mice?

(d)   How might you raise an alloantiserum that is directed specifically against the product of a single genetic locus?

6-6   The rejection of tissue transplants is determined by multiple histocompatibility or H genes. Graft acceptance occurs if all the histocompatibility alleles present on the graft are also present in the host. The H alleles code for alloantigenic cell-surface molecules present on most tissues, which induce an immune response in an allogeneic or xenogeneic host. In an individual heterozygous at an H locus, both gene products are expressed on the cell surface. This phenomenon is termed *codominance*. From these simple generalizations and the following data, it is possible to deduce the five laws of transplantation first summarized in 1941 by the pioneer of mouse transplantation genetics, C. C. Little.

In the following problems, the different histocompatibility loci are represented by H-1, H-2, H-3, etc. Different alleles at one locus are indicated by H-1^a, H-1^b, H-1^c, etc. Suppose that two inbred strains of mice, A and B, with a single

Table 6-6 The Expected Outcome of Transplants Made from Strain A to Strain B, and to F_1, F_2, and Backcross Generations Produced by Crossing Strain A and Strain B (Problem 6-6)

Generations	Genotypes and Outcomes of Transplants*		
	Strain A	F_1	Strain B
Parental strains (P)	H-2^a/H-2^a(+)		H-2^b/H-2^b(−)
F_1		H-2^a/H-2^b(+)	
F_2	25% H-2^a/H-2^a(+)	50% H-2^a/H-2^b(+)	25% H-2^b/H-2^b(−)
Backcross of F_1 to Strain B		50% H-2^a/H-2^b(+)	50% H-2^b/H-2^b(−)

*A plus (+) sign indicates graft acceptance, a minus (−) graft rejection.
[From G. Snell and J. Stimpfling in *Biology of the Laboratory Mouse*, E. L. Green (Ed.), McGraw-Hill, New York, 1966, p. 457.]

histocompatibility difference at the H-2 locus, are crossed. The results of transplants to various generations are given in Table 6-6.

(a) Comment on the acceptance or failure of the following grafts and explain in molecular terms why failure or acceptance occurred: (1) From strain A to strain A individuals, (2) from strain A to strain B individuals, (3) from strain A to F_1 individuals, and from F_1 individuals to strain A, (4) from F_2 or subsequent generations to F_1 individuals, and (5) from strain A to F_2 individuals, and to individuals resulting from a backcross of F_1 individuals to strain B.

(b) When the parents differ at one H locus, what fraction of the F_1 generation is susceptible to tumor grafts from one of the parents? What fraction of the F_2 generation? What fraction of a backcross generation?

(c) Suppose the parents differ at two H loci. Answer the same questions as for part (b).

(d) Can you generalize from answers (b) and (c) to predict what fraction of F_1, F_2, and backcross individuals will be susceptible to a parental tumor if two inbred strains that differ at n histocompatibility loci are crossed?

(e) How could this prediction be used to estimate a lower limit for the number of H loci in various inbred strains of mice or in wild mice?

6-7 (a) Suppose that you have generated four congenic strains, three from mating inbred strains A and B [A.B(1), A.B(2), and A.B(3)] and the fourth from mating inbred strains A and C [A.C(4)]. Assume that each congenic strain differs from the background strain A at either the H-1 or H-2 locus. Pairs of the congenic lines are crossed, and the F_1 generation is challenged with a tumor transplant from the A strain (Table 6-7). This experiment is termed the *F_1 test*. What conclusions can you draw about the identity of the histocompatibility loci in various strains?

(b) Table 6-7 is an actual analysis of congenic strains by the F_1 test. What conclusions can you draw about the identity of the H loci in the two congenic strains?

(c) Given a known congenic strain A.B that carries the H-1^b allele in an A background, how can an F_1 test be used to determine whether the H-1 allele in a new congenic strain A.U is the same as or different from the H-1^a allele in the background strain?

Table 6-7 Analysis of CR Lines B10.C(41N) and B10.C(47N) by the F_1 Test[a] (Problem 6-7)

	Test F_1's				Simultaneous Controls	
Experiment	Known Parent	Difference from C57BL/10	Unknown Parent	Fraction Dying	Strain	Fraction Dying
					C57BL/10	50/50
					B10.C(47N)	0/27
1	B10.LP	H-3	B10.C(41N)	10/10	B10.LP	0/10
2	B10.BY	H-1	B10.C(41N)	0/10		
3	B10.129(5M)	H-1	B10.C(41N)	0/10	B10.129(5M)	0/10
4	B10.129(5M)	H-1	B10.C(47N)	10/10		
5	B10.C(41N)	H-1	B10.C(47N)	10/10	B10.C(41N)	0/10
6	B10.D2	H-2	B10.C(47N)	10/10		
7	B10.LP	H-3	B10.C(47N)	10/10	B10.LP	0/19
8	B10.129(21M)	H-4	B10.C(47N)	10/10	B10.129(21M)	0/19

[a]Strains run as controls with each group always include the susceptible congenic partner, C57BL/10, and usually one or both of the CR strains used as parents in any given cross. All mice were preimmunized with three injections of C57BL/10 thymus and challenged with a C57BL/10 transplantable leukemia. CR denotes congenic resistant. [From G. Snell and J. Stimpfling in *Biology of the Laboratory Mouse*, E. L. Green (Ed)., McGraw-Hill, New York, 1966, p. 457.]

6-8 Class I cell-surface molecules can be analyzed by serological techniques. For example, if cells from a mouse of background strain A (H-2a) haplotype are injected into mice congenic at the H-2 complex (A.B), the congenic mice make antibodies against the antigenic determinants encoded by the H-2a complex that are different from those encoded by the H-2b complex. Appropriate cross absorptions can then render the antiserum specific for one (monospecific) or a few H-2 determinants. This is one way that a series of specific alloantisera have been raised against various H-2 specificities. The antigenic determinants present on the most common H-2 chromosomes from inbred strains of mice are given in Table 6-3. With reference to the table, answer the following questions.

(a) Which H-2 chromosome encodes the most public antigenic determinants? The least? Which polypeptide (K or D) carries the most? The least?

(b) What explanation can you offer for the presence of multiple antigenic determinants on a single polypeptide?

(c) Explain the distinction between private and public H-2 specificities.

(d) What does the existence of identical or cross-reactive specificities shared between the D and K regions of the H-2 complex suggest about the evolution of these regions?

6-9 The H-2K and H-2D class I molecules are integral membrane proteins that are difficult to purify. These alloantigens constitute somewhat less than 1% of the protein in the membranes of mouse spleen cells. A partial purification has been achieved by *indirect immunoprecipitation*. This technique employs specific alloantisera to isolate alloantigens, as depicted in Figure 6-26. Class I molecules are radiolabeled by incubation of living spleen cells *in vitro* with tritiated fucose. The membranes of the radiolabeled cells are then solubilized by incubating with the nonionic detergent NP-40. This detergent solubilizes the membrane without destroying the antigenic de-

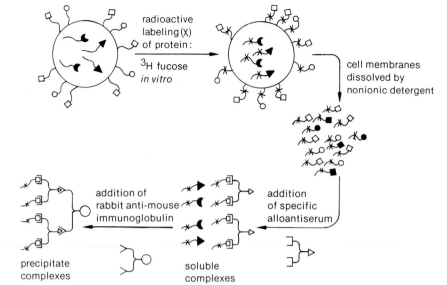

Figure 6-26

The isolation of specific membrane molecules by indirect immunoprecipitation (Problem 6-9).

terminants on the alloantigens. The soluble spleen cell extract is incubated with a specific unlabeled mouse alloantibody, for example, anti-H-2Kª. This alloantibody combines with its complementary alloantigen, but the complex does not precipitate. Precipitation is achieved by adding goat antimouse γ globulin, which combines with the mouse alloantibody and precipitates the entire complex. When the complex is run on SDS polyacrylamide gels, the specific H-2K or H-2D product appears as a single tritiated peak of about 45,000 daltons.

Consider the following experiment. Spleen cells from F_1 mice (H-2ª/H-2ᵇ heterozygous) are labeled with ³H-fucose. Alloantisera that detect private specificities of the four H-2 gene products present are used: (a) specificity H-2.4 to detect the H-2Dª gene product, (b) specificity H-2.11 to detect the H-2Kª gene product, (c) specificity H-2.33 to detect the H-2Kᵇ gene product, and (d) specificity H-2.2 to detect the H-2Dᵇ gene product (see Table 6-3). The ³H-fucose-labeled antigen preparation is solubilized with NP-40 and divided into five portions (*A–E*). *A* is reacted with a control antiserum that can detect none of the specificities known to exist in this heterozygous cell type. *B* is reacted with antiserum to H-2.2; *C* with an antiserum to H-2.4; *D* with an antiserum to H-2.11; and *E* with an antiserum to H-2.33. Goat antimouse γ globulin is added, and the precipitates that form are removed from the supernatant solutions. In the next phase of this experiment, the supernatant solutions from *A*, *B*, *C*, *D*, and *E* are each subdivided into five portions and retested for the presence of radioactive material reactive with the five antisera. The results of this second set of alloantigen–antibody precipitin assays are presented in Figure 6-27, which shows the polyacrylamide gel patterns obtained from these precipitates. With reference to this figure, answer the following questions.

(a) What can you deduce about the molecular structure of the various private alloantigens on the cell surface of spleen cells from a heterozygous mouse? Explain your reasoning.

(b) What does this finding indicate about the expression of the genes that code for these alloantigens in heterozygous mice?

Figure 6-27

The analysis by immunoprecipitation of antigen extracts solubilized with NP-40 (Problem 6-9). This figure shows the SDS-polyacrylamide gel patterns of precipitates from the reactions of test antisera (shown on the *left* of the figure) with the supernatant fraction remaining after reaction with the pretreatment antisera (shown across the *top* of the figure) and removal of the resulting precipitate. The counts per minute (cpm) of ^{3}H-fucose-labeled antigen are plotted along the ordinate of each graph. [From S. Cullen et al., *Proc. Natl. Acad. Sci. USA* **69**, 1394(1972).]

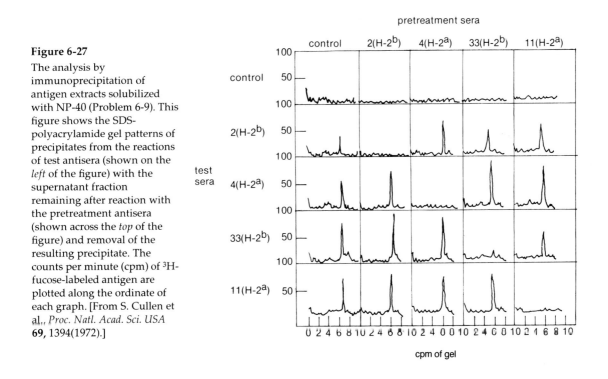

Table 6-8 H-2 Haplotypes of Various Recombinant Inbred Mouse Strains (Problem 6-10)

Strain	H-2 Haplotype	Region of H-2 Complex			
		K	I	S	D
A	a	k	k	d	d
B10	b	b	b	b	b
B10.D2	d	d	d	d	d
A.TH	th	s	s	s	d
A.TL	tl	s	k	k	d

6-10 (a) The techniques originally developed for the study of the H-2K and H-2D products of the MHC of the mouse can be employed to search for other cell-surface antigens (see Problem 6-9). For this purpose, inbred strains of mice that are recombinant at the H-2 complex have been particularly useful (Table 6-8). An antiserum was made by injecting spleen cells from A.TL mice into A.TH mice. These inbred strains are congenic at the H-2 complex. The haplotypes of these and other relevant inbred strains are given in Table 6-8. By indirect immunoprecipitation, the A.TH anti-A.TL antiserum was used to isolate cell-surface molecules radioactively labeled with ^{125}I from spleen cells of a B10.D2

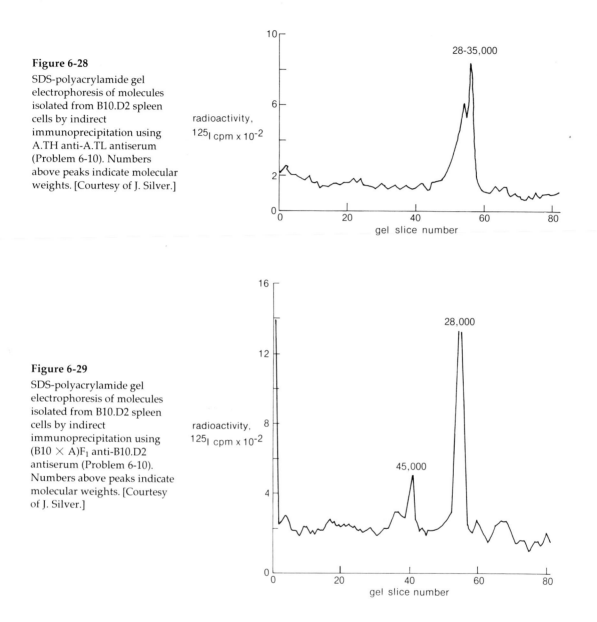

Figure 6-28

SDS-polyacrylamide gel electrophoresis of molecules isolated from B10.D2 spleen cells by indirect immunoprecipitation using A.TH anti-A.TL antiserum (Problem 6-10). Numbers above peaks indicate molecular weights. [Courtesy of J. Silver.]

Figure 6-29

SDS-polyacrylamide gel electrophoresis of molecules isolated from B10.D2 spleen cells by indirect immunoprecipitation using (B10 $\times$ A)F$_1$ anti-B10.D2 antiserum (Problem 6-10). Numbers above peaks indicate molecular weights. [Courtesy of J. Silver.]

mouse. The antigens isolated were electrophoresed on SDS polyacrylamide gels to separate molecules on the basis of their molecular weight. The gels were then cut into thin slices and counted for radioactivity, as shown in Figure 6-28. Suggest the probable identity of the peaks that range in molecular weight from 28,000 to 35,000.

(b) A second antiserum was made by injecting cells from B10.D2 mouse spleens into (B10 $\times$ A)F$_1$ hybrids. Figure 6-29 shows the gel pattern obtained when the antigens from radioactively labeled B10.D2 cell membranes were isolated using this antiserum. Against what antigens would you expect the (B10 $\times$ A)F$_1$ anti-B10.D2 antiserum to be directed?

Table 6-9 Absorption Experiments with Anti-H-2 Antisera and Cells from Three Different Haplotypes (Problem 6-11)

Antiserum	Haplotype of Cells Used for Absorption	Haplotype of "Target" Cells		
		b	d	k
d-anti-k	—	+[a]	0	+
	b	0	0	+
b-anti-d	—	0	+	+
	k	0	+	0
k-anti-b	—	+	+	0
	d	+	0	0

[a] + indicates a serological reaction; 0 indicates no reaction.

(c) How does your reasoning in part (b) check with the data in Figure 6-29?

(d) The technique of using antisera made in congenic strains to immunoprecipitate specific antigens requires awareness of some important limitations. Suggest several limitations in this technique.

6-11 Reciprocal immunizations of congenic mouse strains allow one to raise specific antisera with which to study the genetic organization of the H-2 complex. Three specific antisera raised in three congenic strains of C57BL mice carrying the H-2b, d, or k haplotypes, respectively, were tested against cells from each congenic strain as shown in Table 6-9. In some experiments, the antisera were first absorbed with lymphocytes carrying the indicated haplotype. With reference to the table, answer the following questions.

(a) What is the minimum number of specificities detected by these antisera?

(b) Which specificities are associated with each haplotype?

(c) Are specificities shared?

(d) Assume that these specificities all are present on K-region gene products. If so, how would you reconcile this fact with the immunochemical evidence that the K region of each haplotype codes for a single, distinct cell-surface molecule?

(e) Cells from (b × d)F$_1$ progeny reacted with both the b-anti-d antiserum absorbed with k cells and the k-anti-b antiserum absorbed with d cells. What does this result indicate about expression of these antigens?

(f) The (b × d)F$_1$ mice were backcrossed with d mice. Cells from half the backcross mice reacted with both absorbed antisera ("F$_1$-like" mice); cells from the other mice reacted only with the absorbed b-anti-d antiserum. Explain.

(g) One thousand backcross "F$_1$-like" mice received (b × d)F$_1$ skin grafts. Every mouse except one accepted the graft. The exceptional mouse, X, subsequently rejected another F$_1$ graft, this time even more vigorously. Suggest an explanation for these observations.

(h) Suggest a way to test your hypothesis in part (g).

6-12 Lethal irradiation of mice destroys primarily cells associated with the blood-cell system. The irradiated animals generally die within a period of weeks. However, lethally irradiated recipients can be "protected" by injection with bone-marrow cells; protected animals will survive for extended periods of time. If the protecting bone marrow comes from an F$_1$ donor (i.e., progeny of a cross between the recipient and

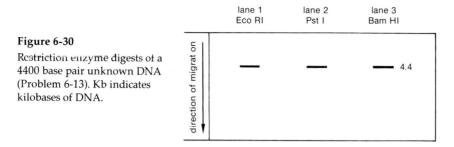

Figure 6-30
Restriction enzyme digests of a
4400 base pair unknown DNA
(Problem 6-13). Kb indicates
kilobases of DNA.

another inbred strain), the irradiated recipient is a hemopoietic chimera with blood
cells that express the phenotypes of both the donor's parents. Frequently such chimeras show permanent acceptance of skin grafts from either parental type.

Suppose that you carried out the following set of experiments. You protected lethally irradiated recipients of inbred mouse strain C57BL/6 with (C57BL/6 × A)F_1
hematopoietic cells. Animals grafted 1 week later with skin from either A or F_1
accepted the grafts. However, animals grafted similarly 11 weeks later all rejected the
grafts. Subsequent tests showed that the lymph node cells and erythrocytes in the
recipients were exclusively of the donor type. What would you suggest is the basis for
the graft rejection after 11 weeks? Propose an explanation for the finding that the F_1
hematopoietic cells are not tolerant to skin grafts of an identical genotype.

6-13   (a)   Your advisor decides that you, as a first-year graduate student, should begin in
the laboratory by tackling a simple problem. He gives you a cloned DNA molecule isolated from an invertebrate in which you hope to find MHC-like genes.
You are to generate a restriction enzyme map using restriction endonucleases of
your choice. The only facts you know in advance concerning this DNA is that it
is double stranded and approximately 4400 nucleotides long.

To begin, you digest separate samples of the DNA with the restriction enzymes Bam HI, Eco RI, and Pst I, which cut the DNA at particular sites. You
electrophorese the digested DNA on an agarose gel that separates all of the DNA
fragments according to their sizes. Then you stain the gel with ethidium bromide
to visualize the DNA fragments and obtain the results shown in Figure 6-30. You
estimate the molecular weights of the bands by comparing the band migration
distance to the migration distance of molecular weight standards; you approximate the length of fragments in kilobases. Because the molecular weight of the
DNA molecule appears to be the same after each restriction enzyme digestion,
you conclude that this DNA molecule lacks sites recognized by the three restriction enzymes that you have chosen. Your advisor insists that at least one restriction site exists for each restriction enzyme. Given this fact, what are two possible
explanations for the results that you have obtained?

       (b)   You decide to perform a series of double digests and obtain the results shown in
Figure 6-31. Which explanation in part (a) do the double enzyme digest results
support?

       (c)   Construct a map of the identified restriction sites for this DNA molecule.

6-14   Mutant transplantation antigens can be detected by reciprocal grafting. For example,
six sibling mice may be placed in a circle and skin from each transplanted to the
neighbor on either side (Figure 6-32). A transplantation antigen that has mutated can
be recognized as foreign by the T cells of the sibs on either side, leading to graft
rejections.

Figure 6-31

Restriction maps of a 4.4-kb DNA fragment treated with one or more restriction enzymes (Problem 6-13). Numbers indicate kilobases of DNA.

Eco RI	Eco RI + Bam HI	Eco RI + Pst I	Bam HI + Pst I
4.4	4.0	3.6	3.2
			1.2
	.4	.8	

direction of migration

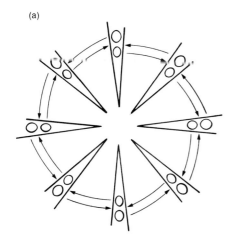

(a)

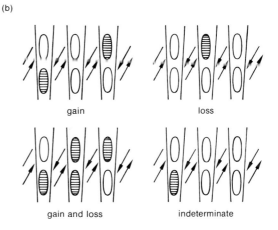

(b)

gain

loss

gain and loss

indeterminate

Figure 6-32

(a) Reciprocal circle system of skin grafting for detection of H mutations. Large Vs represent mouse tails, small ovals within the Vs represent grafts, and arrows indicate direction of grafting. (b) Different patterns of graft rejection expected in segments of the reciprocal circle when H mutation occurs. Shaded ovals represent rejected grafts; empty ovals represent permanently accepted grafts. [Taken from D. W. Bailey and H. I. Kohn, *Genetic Research* (Camb.) **6**, 330(1965). Copyright © 1965 by Cambridge University Press.]

A series of mutant transplantation antigens of the K locus, detected in this manner, have been analyzed at the amino-acid-sequence level. With reference to the results presented in Figure 6-33, answer the following questions.

(a) Two surprising observations emerge from these data, at least in comparison to the changes seen in the mutant hemoglobins. What are they?

(b) How would you explain these observations?

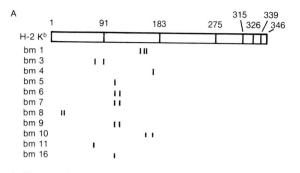

Figure 6-33   A diagram depicting how the sequences of the K^{bm} mutant class I molecules differ from their wild type K^b counterparts (Problem 6-14). The residue numbers indicate the boundaries of the eight class I exons. The vertical bars indicate the positions of mutations. [Taken from R. Nairn et al., *Ann. Rev. Genet.* **14**, 241 (1980).]

	145			150	152			155	156				160		165
	His	Lys	Trp	Glu Gln	Ala	Gly	Glu	Ala	Glu	Arg	Leu Arg	Ala Tyr	Leu	Glu Gly	Thr
K^b	CAC	AAG	TGG	GAG CAG	GCT	GGT	GAA	GCA	GAG	AGA	CTC AGG	GCC TAC	CTG	GAG GGC	ACG
K$_2^b$	——	——	——	— A ——	— G	——	——	— C ——	——	——	——	— A —	— A —	— A —	T
K^{bm-1}	——	——	——	——	CT	——	——	TAT — TA	——	——	——	——	——	——	——
L^d	–G —	——	——	——	CT	——	TAT	TA —	——	——	——	——	——	— GA–	
	Arg —	——	——	——	Ala	——	Tyr	Tyr	——	——	——	——	——	— Glu–	

Figure 6-34   The DNA and protein sequences for three wild type (K^b, K$_2^b$, and L^d) and one mutant (K^{bm1}) class I gene (Problem 6-14). The sequence spans residues 145–165 from the N terminus of the class I polypeptide. The amino acid sequence of the K$_2^b$ gene is not indicated. A horizontal line denotes homology with K^b. The K$_2^b$ gene is the second gene on the cosmid cluster containing the functional K^b gene (Figure 6-14). (The K$_2^b$ sequence is hypothetical.) [Data taken from E. H. Weiss et al., *Nature* **301**, 671 (1983).]

(c) A Boston research group has completed the DNA sequence of the Class I K^{bm1} gene, a spontaneous mutant derived from the K^b gene. The only DNA sequence differences between the two genes are contained within the 57-nucleotide sequence shown in Figure 6-34. What two features of the mutation event that generated the K^{bm1} gene are most striking?

(d) You notice that the L^d gene contains the same nucleotide sequence as the K^{bm1} gene in the region where the mutant allele differs from K^b. You therefore propose that a gene conversion event involving the K^b and L^d genes may have generated the mutant allele. Gene conversion leads to the correction or conversion of one DNA sequence against a second. If the mutant was generated in this way, what can we infer concerning the class I gene against which K^b was corrected? Where might this second gene be located? *Hint:* Look at the K$_2^b$ gene (Figure 6-34). What does this result indicate about the gene correction mechanism?

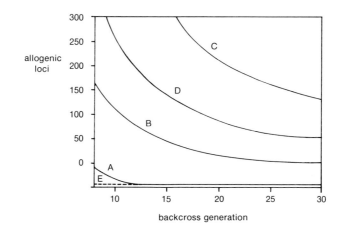

Figure 6-35 The number of heterozygous or allogeneic loci theoretically expected to remain after successive generations of backcrossing to construct a congenic strain (Problem 6-15). The calculations used to generate these curves assume that the two parental strains differ at 10,000 protein coding loci. Curve A represents the number of allogeneic loci unlinked to the differential marker locus. Curve B represents the allogeneic loci, both linked and unlinked, expected to remain during the construction of a congenic strain for which a marker has been selected. Curve C represents the upper 95% confidence limit for the number of allogeneic loci carried in the congenic strain. Curve D represents the number of allogeneic loci remaining if a second gene, unlinked to the marker, is carried along because it interacts with the marker to provide a trait essential for reproductive fitness. Curve E represents the mutational load. [Taken from D. Bailey, *Immunology Today* **3,** 213(1982).]

(e) Given the nucleotide sequence in Figure 6-34, what is the minimum length of DNA that must have been exchanged between L^d-like and K^b genes to generate the mutant? What is the maximum length?

(f) Besides gene conversion, what are two additional possible explanations for the generation of the mutant gene?

6-15 (a) Inbred and congenic strains of mice have been of enormous value to immunologists. However, as the following problem illustrates, some care must be employed when interpreting the results of experiments using these strains. Inbred mice are assumed to be homozygous at all loci. However, even mice inbred for many generations may have residual heterozygosity. Aside from mislabeling or other trivial errors, name two factors that can contribute to the persistence of heterozygous loci.

(b) Congenic strains of mice are created by backcrossing a strain with a selectable trait—for example, a particular MHC haplotype—to a second parental strain. Progeny that have the desired trait are then used for the next backcross. As an immunogeneticist interested in transplantation, you are attempting to create a congenic strain that differs from its partner at only a single minor transplantation locus. Thus, following a backcross, you select for the minor locus by testing for chronic rejection of the appropriate graft. You can also test for the presence of this particular minor locus using specific antisera. It has been estimated that any two inbred mouse strains may differ at 10,000 protein coding loci. Although congenic strains are often thought of as differing at only a single genetic locus, curve B in Figure 6-35 indicates that after ten backcross generations (often taken

mice	regions and subregions				
	K	I–A	I–E	S	D
H-2^a	k	k	k	d	d
H-2^b	b	b	b	b	b
3R	b	b	k	d	d
5R	b	b	k	d	d

Figure 6-36

Haplotypes of mice in Problem 6-15.

as the generation when the strain can be termed congenic), roughly 150 alloge-neic loci, in addition to the selected locus, will remain. However, if an unlinked gene from the second strain is essential for reproductive fitness in the presence of a marker, some 300 such loci may remain (curve B, Figure 6-35). Assume that the strains used to construct the congenic strain differ at a second minor histo-compatibility locus. Given differences in 10,000 protein coding loci for the two strains used, what is the chance of this second locus being present in the congenic mice after ten backcross generations for the cases in which 150 alloge-neic loci are present? 300 allogeneic loci?

(c) It has been estimated that the mouse genome may code for at least 50 minor transplantation loci. Thus it is not inconceivable that the two partner strains used to construct the congenic strain may differ by 15 minor transplantation loci. If this were true, what would be the chance that a second minor transplantation locus was still present after ten backcross generations? As in part (b), assume the existence of 150 and 300 residual allogeneic loci.

(d) In a separate experiment, you have generated a very large number of (H-2^a × H-2^b)F$_1$ mice. The H-2 haplotypes of these mice are shown in Figure 6-36. By testing the progeny of these F$_1$ mice for H-2K and H-2D, you are able to identify two new intra-H-2 recombinants with the haplotypes also indicated in Figure 6-36. Where did the crossovers that led to the formation of these two recombinants probably occur?

(e) To better study the recombinants, you create congenic strains by backcrossing the two recombinant MHC haplotypes onto a C57(H-2^b) background. The result-ing strains are called B10A.3R and B10A.5R. After further research, you discover that the two recombinant congenic strains differ for the newly defined I-J sero-logic determinant. B10A.3R has the I-J allele of the H-2^b parent, whereas B10A.5R has the I-J allele of the H-2^a parent. If, as many data suggest, the I-J specificity is encoded in the I region, draw the MHC haplotypes of the recombinant congenic strains. Include the map order and alleles of K, D, I-A, I-J, and I-E, as well as the most likely points of recombination.

(f) Given the method of construction of the recombinant congenic strains, where on chromosome 17 are the B10A.3R and B10A.5R mice almost certain to differ, in addition to the subregion just discussed?

(g) Assuming that the I-J gene is actually located in this second different region on chromosome 17, draw the MHC haplotypes and points of recombination as re-quested in part (e).

6-16 (a) To study the function of class I genes in T-cell antigen recognition, you have transformed thymidine kinase-negative (tk$^-$) L cells with the tk gene alone or with the tk gene together with cloned class I genes. You have obtained one cell line that expresses the L^d gene (line 1) and a second that expresses the K^d gene (line 2). L cells are homozygous for the H-2^k haplotype. What class I genes will be expressed by line 1 and line 2?

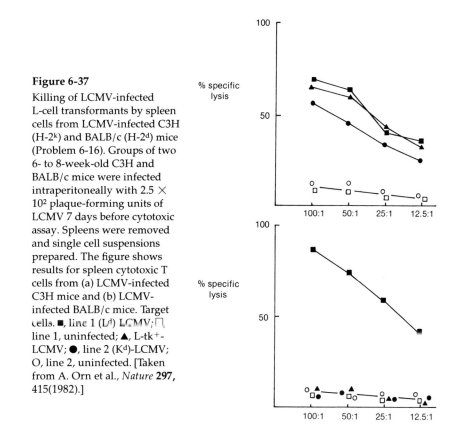

Figure 6-37

Killing of LCMV-infected L-cell transformants by spleen cells from LCMV-infected C3H (H-2^k) and BALB/c (H-2^d) mice (Problem 6-16). Groups of two 6- to 8-week-old C3H and BALB/c mice were infected intraperitoneally with 2.5 × 10^2 plaque-forming units of LCMV 7 days before cytotoxic assay. Spleens were removed and single cell suspensions prepared. The figure shows results for spleen cytotoxic T cells from (a) LCMV-infected C3H mice and (b) LCMV-infected BALB/c mice. Target cells. ■, line 1 (L^d) LCMV; ☐, line 1, uninfected; ▲, L-tk$^+$-LCMV; ●, line 2 (K^d)-LCMV; O, line 2, uninfected. [Taken from A. Orn et al., *Nature* **297**, 415(1982).]

(b) C3H(H-2^k) and BALC/c(H-2^d) mice were infected with lymphocytic choriomeningitis virus (LCMV) to generate cytotoxic T cells. Spleen cells from immunized mice were tested against various target cells using a 4-hour ^{51}Cr release assay. In this assay, transformed mouse L cells are loaded with radioactive ^{51}Cr which is taken up into the cytoplasm. This radiolabel is released when the L cells are lysed by appropriate cytotoxic T cells. Thus the amount of released label is proportional to the amount of killing. From the data in Figure 6-37, what structures can be recognized by the LCMV-immune C3H T cells?

(c) What structures are being recognized by the LCMV-immune BALB/c T cells?

(d) The results of experiments using antibody to block the cytotoxicity against LCMV-infected line 1 targets are presented in Figure 6-38. How do these results support your answer to part (c)?

(e) In Figure 6-37b, why don't the LCMV-immune BALB/c(H-2^d) spleen cells mount a cytotoxic response against the allogeneic C3H(H-2^k) target cells?

(f) Despite the fact that line 2 cells express the K^d gene, LCMV-immune BALB/c spleen cells do not kill LCMV-infected line 2 targets. However, BALB/c spleen cells immune to other viruses, such as vaccinia, can kill vaccinia-infected line 2 cells. Propose one explanation for the inability of LCMV-immune BALB/c T cells to kill LCMV-infected line 2 cells.

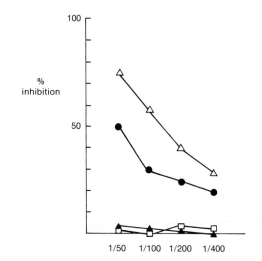

Figure 6-38 Inhibition of H-2-restricted, LCMV-specific cytotoxicity by antibodies directed against different H-2 antigens (Problem 6-16). Various antisera or monoclonal reagents were added at the start of the Cr-release assay in the dilutions shown. The cytotoxic reaction inhibited was that of LCMV-infected BALB/c spleen cells against LCMV-infected line 1 cells. Δ, 28-14-8S (anti-L^d monoclonal antibody); ●, 4-9.4 (anti-L^d monoclonal antibody); ▲, 34-2-12 (anti-D^d monoclonal antibody); and □, normal mouse serum. [From A. Orn et al., *Nature* **297**, 415(1982).]

(g) The MHC-encoded transplantation antigens are unusually polymorphic. How do the data presented in Figure 6-37 help to explain the evolution of this polymorphism?

6-17 (a) The Ia-encoded polypeptides influence the response levels to a number of antigens in a highly specific manner. To count the number of genes encoding Ia molecules, you have obtained cDNA clones for the human DR$_\alpha$ and DC$_\beta$ polypeptides (see Figure 6-9). These cDNA clones were used as hybridization probes to analyze Southern blots of Eco RI digested BALB/c DNA. The data are shown in Figure 6-39. You detect 6–7 bands with the DC$_\beta$ probe and 3 bands with the DR$_\alpha$ probe (Figure 6-39). However, you are concerned that the number of hybridizing restriction fragments may not correspond exactly to the number of genes encoding Ia polypeptides. Propose two reasons why the number of bands could be an underestimate of the number of genes. Propose two reasons why it might be an overestimate.

(b) When you use the DC$_\beta$ probe, the intensity of the hybridization signal varies greatly from band to band. Can you think of two explanations for this phenomenon aside from that of experimental artifact?

(c) The DC$_\beta$ cDNA clone contains the entire protein coding sequence. From this clone you purify a fragment that contains roughly 90 nucleotides coding for the β1 domain and a fragment coding for the transmembrane and cytoplasmic portions of the polypeptide. These two fragments give identical hybridization patterns on Southern blots of BALB/c DNA cut with any of six different restriction

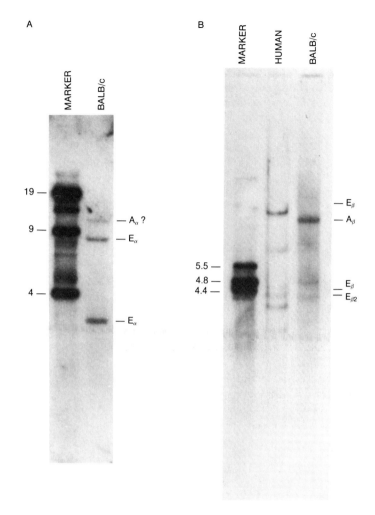

Figure 6-39

Southern blot analyses using (a) DR$_\alpha$ and (b) DC$_\beta$ cDNA clones (Problem 6-17). Sizes of molecular weight marker fragments are indicated in kilobases. [Taken from M. Steinmetz et al., *Nature* **300**, 35(1982).]

enzymes. Which explanation in question (a) for lack of correspondence between genes and bands does this result most likely rule out?

6-18 (a) The I-J serologic specificity is MHC-linked, polymorphic, and found mostly on suppressor cells and some soluble suppressor factors derived from those cells. However, the I-J protein has not been characterized. You have obtained clones containing 200 kb of contiguous DNA from the I region. You find that the right boundary of the I-A subregion and the left boundary of the I-E subregion are separated by no more than 3.4kb, and as much as 2.4 kb of this DNA is part of the E$_\beta$ gene (Figure 6-24). You use this 3.4 kb of DNA as a hybridization probe to test RNA from ten I-J positive suppressor T-cell hybridomas. Under conditions where one molecule per cell of RNA homologous to the probe could be detected, you find no I-J transcripts. Which of the six models (1a, 1b, 1c, 2a, 2b, 3) presented in Table 6-10 does this result argue against?

Table 6-10 Models for the Location of the I-J Gene

1. The I-J gene is encoded between the I-A and I-E subregions.
   (a) The I-J gene is the E_β gene product after special post-translational modification (e.g., glycosylation).
   (b) The I-J gene is formed via an alternative RNA splicing pattern that includes some but not all of the E_β exons.
   (c) The I-J gene is transcribed off the DNA strand complementary to that which encodes the E_β gene.
2. The I-J gene is not encoded between the I-A and I-E subregions.
   (a) Because of the occurrence of multiple recombination events, the map order I-A/I-J/I-E is incorrect.
   (b) The I-J subregion contains a control element that regulates the expression of I-J genes encoded elsewhere.
   (c) The I-J serologic specificities are anti-idiotypes directed against T-cell receptors for self-MHC molecules.

(b) A colleague points out that cosmid clones are derived from liver DNA while the I-J specificity is found on suppressor T cells. Why might this point be significant? How can you determine if it is?

(c) I-J has been precisely mapped in a number of strains but not in BALB/c mice. A second colleague suggests that the problem in identifying the I-J gene may have arisen because BALB/c mice have an inversion on chromosome 17. Draw the locations of the H-2K and H-2D genes and the I-A, I-E, I-J, and I-C subregions on a normal chromosome and on the putative inverted chromosome from BALB/c mice.

(d) How can you test for the presence of an inversion using the cosmid clones or parts of these clones as hybridization probes?

(e) Having determined that no inversion occurred, you are driven to a serious consideration of control element models (2b in Table 6-10). Given what we know about I-J polypeptides, what properties can we infer concerning this hypothetical control element and the genes that are controlled by it?

(f) T cells have dual specificity for antigen and MHC-encoded molecules. Some immunologists have therefore proposed that a functional T cell has two separate receptors: one for antigen and a second for self-MHC molecules. Another colleague suggests that the I-J serologic specificity is in fact present on the suppressor T-cell receptor for self-MHC. If this is the case, what molecule is probably being recognized as self by the suppressor cells? How does this model explain linkage of I-J to the MHC?

(g) T-cell specificity for self-MHC is apparently determined in the thymus (see Chapter 8). Briefly outline an experiment that tests your colleague's proposal in part (e) using thymus transplants.

6-19 (a) A very energetic research group has isolated a large collection (>30) of BALB/c ($H\text{-}2^d$) genomic DNA clones containing sequences homologous to murine class I genes. The products encoded by several individual cloned sequences have been determined by serologic analysis of L cells ($H\text{-}2^k$) transformed with individual clones. Surprisingly, a DNA sequence known to contain only a fragment of the K^d gene gave some transformants that were positive when tested with K^d-specific antisera. This curious result was investigated further using the BALB/c L^d

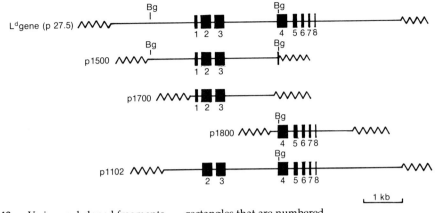

Figure 6-40 Various subcloned fragments of the L^d gene (Problem 6-19). The jagged line indicates plasmid vector DNA. The thin horizontal line denotes mouse DNA. The solid vertical rectangles that are numbered represent the L^d gene exons. Bg indicates Bgl II restriction enzyme sites. [Taken from R. Goodenow et al., *Nature* **301**, 388(1982).]

gene. Figure 6-40 shows the L^d gene and some truncated genes that were constructed. What features of the L^d gene are missing from the constructs p1500, p1700, p1800, and p1102?

(b) L cells were cotransformed with the tk gene and the truncated genes diagrammed in Figure 6-40. Transformants were selected for tk expression and were then analyzed using a radioimmunoassay. A monoclonal anti-L^d antibody was incubated with the transformed cells, followed by addition of radioactive protein A. Protein A binds to the F$_c$ region of mouse antibodies and, in this case, is a measure of the number of cell-surface molecules binding the mouse anti-L^d antibody. Figure 6-41 shows the amount of radioactive protein A bound to the transformed cell populations as a function of the micrograms of DNA used to transform the L cells. At all DNA concentrations tested, transformation with the complete L^d gene gave greater protein A binding (data not shown in the figure). What features of the L^d gene, as measured by the radioimmunoassay, appear most critical for expression of a serologically detectable product on the surface of transformed L cells?

(c) Provide two explanations for the large difference in protein A binding observed with transformants generated using the p1500 and p1700 constructs.

(d) The radioimmunoassay measures the number of L^d molecules present on an uncloned, transformed cell population. Only a fraction of the cells in the transformed population may actually be expressing the L^d antigenic determinant. Therefore, if transformation with a particular gene construct leads to increased protein A binding, it is not clear whether this increase is caused by increased levels of expression by a small subpopulation of cells or whether a larger fraction of the cells is expressing L^d. What experiment could distinguish between these possibilities?

(e) Outline two general mechanisms for expression of an L^d gene by L cells transformed with a truncated gene such as p1500.

(f) Cells transformed with p1500 were grown in the presence of ^{35}S-methionine to radiolabel the synthesized proteins. The radiolabeled cell extracts were

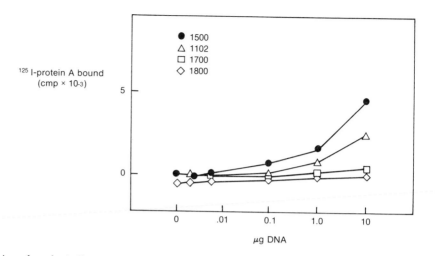

^{125} I-protein A bound
(cmp × 10-3)

Figure 6-41 Expression of serologically detectable L^d molecules by L cells transformed with truncated L^d genes. L cells cotransformed with the tk gene and various truncated L^d genes were first incubated with a monoclonal anti-L^d antibody followed by incubation with ^{125} I-radiolabeled protein A. The amount of protein A bound to the transformed cells is expressed as a function of the amount of L^d construct DNA used to transform the cells. The structures of the various truncated L^d genes used are shown in Figure 6-40. [From Goodenow et al., *Nature* **301**, 388(1982).]

immunoprecipitated with a monoclonal anti-L^d antibody, and the precipitate was analyzed on an SDS-polyacrylamide gel under reducing conditions. Polypeptides of 45,000 and 12,000 daltons were detected, whereas no peptides were present in immunoprecipitates of extracts from L-cell controls. What type of mechanism outlined in part (e) does this result tend to rule out?

(g) The same radiolabeled material as in part (f) was immunoprecipitated and electrophoresed on a two-dimensional gel. This gel separates proteins in one dimension by molecular weight and in the second dimension by isoelectric point. On such two-dimensional gels, the L^d protein derived from L cells transformed with p1500 was identical to the L^d protein precipitated from H-2^d spleen cells. Why is this surprising? How is this result best explained?

6-20 (a) When defined class I genes such as H-2K^d or H-2L^d are transferred into L cells (H-2^k), they are expressed at levels comparable to those found in normal H-2^d haplotype cells. In addition, the transformed cells express higher levels of B_2-microglobulin as measured by a cell-surface radioimmunoassay.

What do these observations suggest about the regulation of expression of B_2-microglobulin?

(b) Six BALB/c(H-2^d) class I genes have been identified by serologic assay of tk$^-$ L cells cotransformed with the tk gene and individual cloned sequences. The function of the other 25–30 class I genes is unknown, and many of these may be pseudogenes. Transformation with several of these genes leads to increased B_2-microglobulin expression compared to tk$^+$ L-cell controls. However, the transformed cells do not display any of the K, D, L, Qa, or TL serologic specificities characteristic of BALB/c mice. To investigate whether the increased B_2-microglobulin expression reflects synthesis of a novel H-2^d-encoded class I gene product, some California scientists attempted to make antisera against one of the transformed L-cell lines expressing increased amounts of β_2-microglobulin. Repeated attempts to make antibody against the transformed cell line in C3H (H-2^k) mice failed. What are three explanations for this result?

(c) Attempts to make antibody against the transformed cell line in four other inbred mouse strains with different H-2 haplotypes were also unsuccessful. Does this result make any of the explanations in part (b) unlikely?

(d) Finally, antisera are raised against the cell line by immunizing rabbits. Rabbit antiserum extensively absorbed with L cells or L cells transformed with the tk gene still reacts with the transformed line. This antiserum can kill the transformed L cells in the presence of complement, and it can immunoprecipitate a 45,000-dalton protein with a unique isoelectric point on two-dimensional gels. What explanations in part (b) are consistent with all the results just described?

(e) There is little or no detectable killing of BALB/c spleen cells in the presence of the specific rabbit antiserum just described and its complement. Explain this result. From the results presented, what can you conclude about the product of the class I gene used in these experiments? What location might you assign this class I gene in the MHC? Why?

6-21 You are interested in determining which domains of the class I molecule are recognized by specific antibody and by antigen-specific, MHC-restricted cytotoxic T cells. You decide on a strategy that uses recombinant genes constructed *in vitro* (exon shuffling) followed by transformation of tk⁻ L cells to assay the recombinants. However, after reading a paper published by a French research group, you realize that in some cases antigenic determinants may be very difficult to localize.

Nevertheless, you generate four cell lines generated by transformation using four separated, well-defined HLA heavy-chain genomic clones. You then test these transformants with various monoclonal antibodies using a cell-surface radioimmunoassay similar to the one described in Problem 6-19. With reference to the data you obtain (shown in Table 6-11), answer the following questions.

(a) What is the most surprising result? How can you explain this result?

(b) What is the likely antigenic determinant recognized by the B.1.G.6 monoclonal antibody?

(c) The C.23.24.2 monoclonal antibody was made using free β_2-microglobulin as antigen, while the B.1.G.6 monoclonal was made against intact human cells. How might this difference explain the difference in reaction patterns seen with these monoclonals?

(d) How might you explain the lack of reactivity of B.1.G.6 with TRH 42?

(e) Undaunted by these difficulties, you construct the L^d-D^d recombinant genes shown in Figure 6-42 and transform separate L cell lines with each of these genes. You test the transformants with four monoclonal antibodies: 30.5.7 and 28.14.8 directed against the L^d gene and 34.5.8 and 34.2.12 directed against D^d. The results are shown in Table 6-12. What parts of the appropriate class I molecule are recognized by the different monoclonal antibodies?

(f) When BALB/c mice (H-2^d) are infected with lymphocytic choriomeningitis virus (LCMV), most of the viral-specific cytotoxic T lymphocytes recognize LCMV in conjunction with L^d. A colleague has reported to you that this viral-specific killing can be blocked by the 28.14.8 monoclonal antibody. You infect BALB/c mice with LCMV and seven days later you remove the spleens of the infected mice. These spleen cell suspensions, which should contain many LCMV-specific T lymphocytes, are then tested against chromium-labeled, LCMV-infected T1.1.1, T4.8.3, T37.1.3, and T37.2.1 cell lines in a cytotoxic assay. Only T1.1.1 and

Table 6-11 Cell Surface Radioimmunoassay of Murine L(tk⁻) Cells Transformed with Purified HLA Class I Genes (Problem 6-21)

Cell Lines	Monoclonal Antibodies					
	B.9.12.1 (Anti-HLA class I)	B.1.23.2 (Anti-HLA class I)	B.1.G.6 (Anti-Human β_2-m)	C.23.24.2 (Anti-Human β_2-m)	10-3.6 (Anti-I-A$_k$)	11-4.1 (Anti-K$_k$)
L(tk⁻)	531 ± 130	573 ± 153	538 ± 80	957 ± 44	467 ± 14	38,188 ± 2,089
TRH 42	7,029 ± 1,377	12,553 ± 431	1,248 ± 1,515	2,253 ± 87	405 ± 151	55,025 ± 1,941
TRH 44	26,255 ± 397	685 ± 36	30,594 ± 1,515	1,162 ± 70	341 ± 35	70,184 ± 1,026
TRH 64	20,054 ± 1,373	810 ± 412	24,789 ± 420	1,257 ± 158	527 ± 10	63,041 ± 394
TRH 27	2,486 ± 577	345 ± 12	3,063 ± 529	ND	688 ± 190	18,061 ± 1,800
RAJI	31,732 ± 4,626	29,541 ± 152	32,363 ± 3,379	7,486 ± 1,086	573 ± 63	545 ± 14

Cells were incubated with selected monoclonal antibody. After washing, the cells were incubated with radiolabeled F(ab')₂ goat anti-mouse immunoglobulin. The cells were then washed again and the cell-associated radioactivity evaluated. Results are the mean of duplicates and are expressed in counts per minute ± standard error of the mean. The underlined values designate statistically significant binding above background. TRH 27, 42, 44, and 64 are four cell lines, each transformed with a different HLA cosmid clone. RAJI is a human lymphoblastoid line. β_2-m denotes β_2-microglobulin. B.9.12.1 and B.1.23.2 monoclonal antibodies both react with a wide variety of HLA molecules. [From Lemonnier et al., *J. Immunol.* **130**: 1432–1438(1983).]

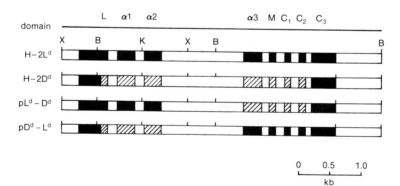

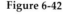

Figure 6-42 Construction of recombinant genes from the cloned H-2D^d and H-2L^d genes (Problem 6-21). The hybrid genes were combined at the Xba I site located within the 1.3-kb intervening sequence separating the exons encoding for the α2 and α3 domains. The hybrid H-2 gene carried on pL^d-D^d contains the first three exons, corresponding to the leader (L), α1, and α2 domains of H-2L^d and the following five exons of H-2D^d. The gene on pD^d-L^d contains the L, α1, and α2 coding regions of H-2D^d and the 3′ domains of H-2L^d. Cross-hatched areas represent the regions coding for H-2L^d; solid regions represent those coding for H-2D^d domains. L, α1, α2, α3, m, I1, I2, and I3 refer to the regions of the protein encoded by each exon. X, Xba I; B, Bam HI cleavage sites. [From G. Evans et al., *Nature* **300**, 755(1982).]

Table 6-12 Cell-Surface Radioimmunoassay of Murine L(tk⁻) Cells Transformed with L^d, D^d, and Recombinant Genes (Problem 6-21)[a]

Cell (Gene)	Antibody Reactivity[a]			
Monoclonal Antibody	30.5.7	28.14.8	34.5.8	34.2.12
Specificity	L^d	L^d	D^d	D^d
L	110	115	125	150
T1.1.1 (L^d)	2,925	2,335	107	116
T4.8.3 (D^d)	88	140	4,292	3,713
T37.1.3 (L^dD^d)	4,219	161	169	3,799
T37.2.1 (D^dL^d)	113	4,193	4,319	171

[a]T1.1.1, T4.8.3, T37.1.3, and T37.2.1 are L cell lines transformed with the indicated murine class I genes or *in vitro* generated recombinants. Methods are as described for Table 6-11.

T37.1.3 are killed by the immune BALB/c spleen cells. How can you explain the apparent discrepancy between this result and the data obtained using monoclonal antibody to block killing?

Answers

6-1   (a) True

     (b) True

     (c) False. It contains 2000–4000 kb of DNA, which is sufficient DNA to code for thousands of genes 600 nucleotides in length.

     (d) True

     (e) False. Acute graft rejection is an advanced immunological trait found only in some fish, some amphibia, birds, and mammals.

     (f) True

     (g) True

     (h) False. These genes are present on most chromosomes of the mouse.

     (i) True

     (j) False. The TL antigen is not highly polymorphic; the transplantation antigens are highly polymorphic.

     (k) True

     (l) True

     (m) True

     (n) False. The BALB/c mouse has at least 36 class I genes.

     (o) True

     (p) False. Novel class I gene products are associated with β_2-microglobulin.

     (q) True

     (r) False. At least the 5′ portion of the E_β gene lies in the I-A subregion.

     (s) True

(t) True
(u) False. A class III gene has not yet been localized.
(v) False. The location of the gene encoding the I-J determinant is unknown.
(w) False. Nine I region recombinants examined all appeared to have their crossover points within a region of 8 kb.
(x) True

6-2 (a) HLA, H-2
(b) Congenic
(c) haplotype
(d) recombination (or crossover)
(e) complement
(f) public
(g) suppressor factor
(h) homologous
(i) Complex
(j) class I, class II, and class III
(k) codominantly
(l) A_β, A_α, E_β, and E_α
(m) Ss and Slp
(n) transplantation antigens and hematolymphoid antigens
(o) transplantation-antigen
(p) eight; domain
(q) restriction enzyme site polymorphisms and DNA-mediated gene transfer
(r) gene conversion, gene duplication and deletion, and selection
(s) α and β
(t) five
(u) homologous
(v) ten

6-3 (a) The gene that specifies the S^+ antigen must be present in S^- as well as S^+strains of rats. Its phenotypic expression must be under the control of one (or more) additional gene(s) whose function is altered in certain S^- strain leukemias so that the S^+ antigen can be expressed.
(b) Apparently antibody specific to the S^+ antigen can modulate its expression so that, in the presence of antibody S^+, leukemias become S^-. When the anti-S antibody is removed, these same tumors can revert back to the S^+ phenotype. This process, called *antigenic modulation,* is observed in the TL system.

6-4 (a) Three classes of antigenic determinants on mouse RBCs are indicated. One class (A) is present on all test cells; a second class (B) is present only on RBCs and brain cells; and the third class (C) is present only on RBCs.
(b) The A antigens could be H-2 determinants. The C antigens could be blood-group antigens. There is no known cell-surface marker with the B distribution.

6-5 (a) The cells from mouse 1 have antigenic determinant A; the cells from mouse 2 have antigenic determinant B; the cells from mouse 3 have antigen determinants A and B; the cells from mouse 4 lack these antigenic determinants.
(b) The X cells have both determinants, A and B, because the antiserum was raised against X cells. The X cells could have additional antigens that could be detected by absorption tests with cells from other inbred strains of mice. The host has neither of these antigens; otherwise it could not have generated an immune response to them.
(c) These antigens cannot be alleles because both are present in inbred mouse 3, which presumably is homozygous for all genetic loci. Wild mice could be hetero-

zygous; hence it would be impossible to determine whether these antigens are alleles without breeding studies to follow their genetic segregation.

    (d) Construct a congenic mouse strain of the 1.2 type (i.e., with the locus of interest from inbred mouse 2 superimposed on the background of inbred mouse 1). Then immunize a number 1 mouse with 1.2 cells.

6-6 (a) (1) Grafts within inbred strains are successful. Syngeneic grafts between individuals of the same sex always succeed because the H-2 alleles are identical in the graft and in the host. Because all the graft antigens are self-antigens of the host, the host cannot mount an immune response to any of them. (2) Grafts between inbred strains with different H-2 alleles are not successful. Allogenic grafts always fail because the H-2 alleles are different in the graft and in the host. Consequently, the host will mount an immune response against the alloantigens of the graft. (3) Grafts from either inbred parent strain to the F_1 hybrid succeed, but grafts in the reverse direction fail. When the graft is from the parent to F_1, the H-2 determinants on the graft are all present in the host and, accordingly, are not immunogenic. In contrast, the F_1 graft has an H-2 allele, H-2^b, which is not present in strain A; therefore, the corresponding alloantigen is rejected. (4) Individuals from the F_2 and subsequent generations of mice can be heterozygous or homozygous for the H-2 alleles. In either case, a heterozygous F_1 recipient will have both of the H-2 alleles present in any F_2 graft and, therefore, will not reject it. (5) Grafts from (either) inbred parent strain are accepted by some members of the F_2 generation and rejected by others. The same is true for backcross individuals as recipients. In both cases, rejections occur in those homozygous recipients that lack the parental H-2 allele expressed in the graft. The foregoing five answers have been termed the five laws of transplantation.

    (b) All F_1 individuals are susceptible to a parental tumor graft. Three-quarters of the F_2 generations is susceptible to such a graft. One-half of a backcross generation is susceptible to such a graft.

    (c) F_1: all susceptible
F_2: $(\frac{3}{4})^2 = \frac{9}{16}$ susceptible
backcross: $(\frac{1}{2})^2 = \frac{1}{4}$ susceptible

    (d) F_1: all susceptible
F_2: $(\frac{3}{4})^n$
backcross: $(\frac{1}{2})^n$

    (e) To determine a lower limit on the number of H loci in a given population, one could cross two mice, raise a large F_2 generation, and then determine what fraction (x) of grafts from one parent are successful in the F_2 generation. Because $x = (\frac{3}{4})^n$, n can be readily evaluated. If this process is repeated with a number of inbred strains or with wild mice, one can estimate the number of H loci that differ in each parental combination.

6-7 (a) If the two congenic strains are identical, the F_1 generation reduplicates their genotype and likewise their resistance to tumors of the background strain (Table 6-7, Experiment 2). If the two congenic strains are not identical, the two genotypes complement each other and produce a susceptible hybrid (Table 6-7, Experiment 1). A special case arises when the two congenic lines come from different initial crosses. Here the two lines may differ from the common partner at the same locus but by different alleles. Accordingly, the hybrid will not have all of the A strain H alleles and, therefore, will be resistant (Table 6-7, Experiment 3). However, if A.B(3) and A.C(4) differed from strain A at different loci, the hybrid would be susceptible. The F_1 test is very useful for identifying shared H loci among congenic strains with the same background.

Table 6-13   Conclusions from the F_1 Tests in Table 6-7 (Answer 6-7)

(1) B10.C(41N) is not H-3	(5) B10.C(47N) is not H-1
(2) B10.C(41N) is H-1	(6) B10.C(47N) is not H-2
(3) B10.C(41N) is H-1	(7) B10.C(47N) is not H-3
(4) B10.C(47N) is not H-1	(8) B10.C(47N) is not H-4

(b) See Table 6-13.

(c) You have three strains of mice:

tissue donor	known parent	unknown parent
A	A.B	A.U
(A) H-1^a	(A) H-1^b	(A)H-1^u

Cross A.B $\times$ A.U. If u $=$ a, the F_1 will be susceptible to a tumor from A. If not, the F_1 will be resistant.

6-8   (a) The d chromosome encodes 21 known antigenic determinants. The z chromosome encodes 6. The D^d gene product has 14 antigenic specificities. The D^z gene product has just one.

(b) The K and D alleles encode gene products that differ from one another by multiple structural differences that can be detected serologically.

(c) In general, the private specificities are encoded only in either the D or K region of one of the known H-2 chromosomes, hence these specificities can be used to identify particular haplotypes. In contrast, the public specificities are encoded in more than one H-2 chromosome, and sometimes they are encoded in both the D and K regions (e.g., specificities 1, 3, 5, 35, and 36 in Table 6-3). The private specificities elicit very high titer antisera, whereas the public specificities tend to elicit less specific antisera of lower titer.

(d) The presence of shared serological specificities suggests that the K and D genes arose from a common ancestor by gene duplication. The alternative hypothesis to explain structural similarities, the convergent evolution of genes of independent origin, is considered less likely because of the requirement for parallel evolution.

6-9   (a) Precipitation of solubilized spleen cells from a mouse heterozygous at the H-2 complex with alloantisera to any one of the four private alloantigens completely removes that alloantigen but none of the other three. This observation suggests that each of the four alloantigens is present on a different glycoprotein, each about 45,000 in molecular weight.

(b) The K and D gene products are *codominantly* expressed in heterozygous individuals so that each cell carries four different H-2 gene products: two from the K locus and two from the D locus.

6-10   (a) The A.TH anti-A.TL antiserum should be directed only against I- and S-region cell-surface gene products, which represent the only known differences between the two congenic strains A.TH and A.TL (see Table 6-8). The S region does not encode any known cell-surface molecules. Therefore, the 28,000- to 35,000-molecular weight components are probably Ia molecules. Their precipitation with the A.TH anti-A.TL sera indicates that the I region of the d haplotype has serological specificities that cross-react with the I region of the k haplotype (see Table 6-8). Thus the Ia molecules of different haplotypes have cross-reacting serological specificities similar to those of the K and D gene products (Table 6-8).

(b) The (B10 × A) anti-B10.D2 antiserum should be directed against cell-surface molecules encoded by the K and I regions of the d haplotype because these molecules represent the only antigenic differences between a B10.D2 and a (B10 × A)F$_1$ hybrid mouse (Table 6-8).

(c) An Ia-like molecule (28,000) and a K molecule (45,000) are seen on the gel in Figure 6-29. Thus the experimental data agree very well with theoretical expectations.

(d) Several precautions must be considered when defining the specificities of antisera produced with congenic pairs of mice. First, the number of genes in the H-2 complex almost certainly exceeds the number of available genetic markers. This means that independently derived recombinants that appear identical by the limited number of genetic markers currently available may differ in genes for which no genetic markers are available. Accordingly, the antiserum raised against the lymphocytes of one recombinant may have antibodies directed against cell-surface molecules that are absent in a second apparently identical recombinant strain. Second, congenic strains may retain genes that are outside the H-2 complex, but closely linked to it, and for which there are no genetic markers. Therefore, the use of lymphocytes from such a strain may result in antisera that are directed against the products of a non-H-2 gene. Third, one must be careful of antisera raised against cell-surface molecules encoded by viruses present in the immunizing cells. Fourth, one may raise antibodies to differentiation antigens expressed only on a subset of cells (e.g., B$_\alpha$ cells), and their detection depends on the concentration of these cells in the test sample. Finally, one must be certain that the immunoprecipitate contains cell-surface molecules detected by the primary antiserum, rather than aggregated γ globulins in general, and that the cell-surface antigens detected are actually coded by the H-2 genes in question.

6-11 (a) The data in Table 6-9 can be explained by three antigenic specificities that can be designated A, B, and C.

(b) If the A and B specificities are assigned to the k haplotype, then the d haplotype has B and C specificities and the b haplotype has A and C specificities.

(c) Each specificity is shared by two haplotypes.

(d) These antigens appear to be public specificities that are present on the K gene products of several haplotypes (Table 6-3).

(e) The absorbed antisera are specific for the K gene products of the b and d haplotypes, respectively. Hence the gene products must be codominantly expressed on the cells of F$_1$ hybrid mice.

(f) Half the backcross mice should be b/d heterozygotes and the other half should be d homozygotes. Cells from the heterozygotes should react with both absorbed antisera, whereas cells from the homozygotes should react only with absorbed b-anti-d antiserum.

(g) The X mouse must have had a mutation in the H-2 complex of one chromosome that led to alteration of a cell-surface class I molecule. Thus this mouse would reject as foreign (b × d)F$_1$ skin grafts because it differs from the donor mouse in one of its b or d haplotype class I gene products.

(h) One approach to testing the hypothesis in part (g) is the following. Construct a congenic C57B1.X mouse strain. Attempt to raise alloantiserum against the mutant gene product. If you are successful, use this antiserum with the indirect immunoprecipitation procedure to isolate the mutant molecule. Do peptide-mapping and microsequencing studies on the K molecules from the x, b, and d haplotypes to determine whether the K gene product from X differs from its counterparts in either d or b by a single amino acid substitution.

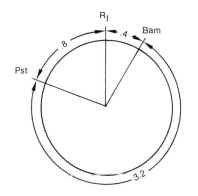

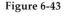

Figure 6-43

A restriction map of the circular DNA molecule (Problem 6-13). Numbers indicate kilobases of DNA.

6-12   The skin from the A or F donors apparently contains cells that express a differentiation antigen that is not recognized as self by the hemopoietic cells. This skin antigen must be quite antigenic because the chimeras reject A skin almost as rapidly as if there were an H-2 incompatibility. The rejection must be carried out by donor cells (F_1), for there is no evidence that any recipient cells survive. Therefore, the donor cells must have lost tolerance to their native skin alloantigen during residence for 11 weeks in the new host, which lacks that allele. This observation implies that the immune system can remain tolerant to differentiation alloantigens expressed in the same animal only as long as these alloantigens are continuously exposed to the immune system. Removal of the immunocompetent cell population to another host may result in the termination of self-tolerance to alloantigens not expressed on the hemopoietic cells. Accordingly, this approach may be used to demonstrate new types of differentiation alloantigens.

6-13   (a)   The DNA may be a circular molecule containing one site for each enzyme. A single cut in a circular DNA molecule just leads to a linear DNA molecule. It is also possible, although rather unlikely, that the DNA is a linear molecule that contains restriction sites for these enzymes located very near (probably within 100 base pairs from) the termini of the molecule. If this is the case, then the large fragment generated by restriction enzyme cleavage will not migrate much differently from the uncut 4.4-kb molecule, and the small fragment(s) (<100 base pairs) are not likely to be detected because they stain very poorly and may in fact have been electrophoresed off the gel.

(b)   The double enzyme digests support the hypothesis that the DNA is circular.

(c)   See Figure 6-43.

6-14   (a)   (1) Mutations at the same position occur multiple times (e.g., Figure 6-33, bm6, bm7, and bm9). (2) Seven of eleven mutants show two or more amino acid substitutions that are close to one another in the chain. Most hemoglobin mutants have single substitutions. The few mutants with two substitutions have them widely spaced.

(b)   (1) Perhaps certain antigenic sites on class I molecules require multiple changes before they can be seen as foreign by the T-cell system. Furthermore, perhaps there are relatively limited numbers of sites involved in T-cell recognition. This is an ad hoc and admittedly unsatisfactory explanation. (2) Perhaps an unusual genetic mechanism can, in a single event, lead to multiple clustered nucleotide changes in a gene.

(c)   There are a relatively large number of differences between the two alleles. All the differences between the alleles are confined to a very short sequence.

Figure 6-44

Answer to Problem 6-15d. The vertical lines indicate the likely position of the crossover.

	K	I – A	I – E	S	D
3R	b	b	k	d	d
5R	b	b	k	d	d

Figure 6-45

Answer to Problem 6-15e. Vertical line indicates likely position of the crossover.

	K	I – A	I – J	I – E	D
B10. A 3R	b	b	b	k	d
B10. A 5R	b	b	k	k	d

(d) Obviously the mutant mouse must have contained both the K^b gene and a class I gene identical to the L^d gene in this region. As to the location of the second gene, there are several possibilities. Because the K_2^b gene, the only other known class I gene in the K region, cannot be the correction partner, the second gene must be elsewhere in the MHC because all the class I genes are in the MHC. The gene correction could be intrachromosomal or it could be interchromosomal. Because the K^b gene is approximately 0.5 cM from the other known class I genes, it appears that the gene conversion can occur across large chromosomal distances and even across different gene families (class II and class III). Another possibility is that the mouse was an F_1 with the K^b gene on one chromosome 17 and the D^d gene on the second. In this case, the gene correction would be interchromosomal.

(e) Thirteen nucleotides is the minimal length and 52 nucleotides is the maximal length for gene conversion in the K^{bm1} mutant gene.

(f) Either mutation and selection or a double crossing-over event might generate the K^{bm1} mutant gene.

6-15 (a) There may be a very strong reproductive advantage for mice that are heterozygous at a few selected loci. In addition, there is a continuous low level of spontaneous mutation generating new alleles.

(b) The probabilities are $150/10,000 = 1.5\%$ and $300/10,000 = 3.0\%$.

(c) Assume that the probabilities of carrying along any one of the 15 unselected minor histocompatibility loci through ten backcross generations is independent of the probability of carrying a second unselected locus. For the case where 150 allogeneic loci remain, the probability of not carrying one of the unselected allogeneic minor histocompatibility loci is $1 - 150/10,000$ or 98.5%. The probability of not carrying any of the 15 unselected allogeneic minor histocompatibility loci is $(0.985)^{15} \cong 80\%$. Therefore, $1 - (1 - 150/10,000)^{15} = 20\% =$ the probability of a second unselected locus being present. If there are 300 unselected allogeneic loci, then the probability of a second unselected minor histocompatibility locus being present is $1 - (1 - 300/10,000)^{15} \cong 37\%$. These calculations indicate that there may be substantial difficulties in trying to obtain congenic mouse strains that differ only at a single minor histocompatibility locus.

(d) See Figure 6-44.

(e) See Figure 6-45.

(f) B10.A3R and B10.A5R are almost certain to differ at the right end of the MHC, distal to H-2D. Both congenic recombinant strains have the H-2D^d allele that has been backcrossed onto the C57(H-2)^b background. In generating the congenic recombinants, the actual points of recombination between the H-2^d and H-2^b chromosomes in the two strains are likely to be quite different. For a quantitative illustration of this point, compare curves B and C in Figure 6-35.

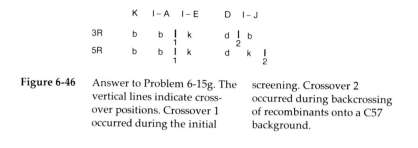

Figure 6-46 Answer to Problem 6-15g. The vertical lines indicate crossover positions. Crossover 1 occurred during the initial screening. Crossover 2 occurred during backcrossing of recombinants onto a C57 background.

(g) See Figure 6-46.

6-16 (a) Line 1 will express H-2K^k, H-2D^k, and H-2L^d. Line 2 will express H-2K^k, H-2D^k, and H-2K^d. C3H mice do not express an L^k molecule.

(b) LCMV antigens and H-2K^k and/or LCMV antigens and H-2D^k may be recognized by the immune T cells.

(c) LCMV antigens and H-2L^d are being recognized by the cytotoxic T$_C$ cells because only the L^d molecule functions as a restricting element.

(d) Monoclonal antibody directed against H-2L^d blocks killing of line 1 targets, whereas monoclonal antibody against an irrelevant specificity has no effect.

(e) The BALB/c spleen should certainly contain effector T cells specific for H-2^k-encoded alloantigens. However, no lymphocytes immunized against those antigens should be present in the spleens from virus-infected mice that were used as a source of effector cells. While a primary response requires several days before specific T-cell-mediated cytotoxicity can be generated, the ^{51}Cr release assay requires only 4 hours.

(f) This question is one of the central and most controversial ones in immunology today. Several kinds of explanations have been offered to account for this type of phenomenon. It is possible that the T cells in BALB/c mice do not contain the gene(s) required to synthesize the receptor(s) that bind(s) to LCMV and H-2K^d. It also is possible that BALB/c mice are tolerant to the combination of LCMV and H-2K^d molecules. Finally, some immunologists feel that close interaction between a class I molecule and antigen is required to stimulate cytotoxic T cells. In this case, LCMV antigen and H-2K^d may somehow be unable to interact appropriately closely with one another.

(g) Clearly a hypothetical mouse expressing only a single class I molecule, namely H-2K^d, would be very vulnerable to infection with LCMV. Because there are many other cases of viral-specific, class I gene-specific low responsiveness similar to the situation described for H-2K^d and LCMV, it is believed that an MHC heterozygous mouse would have selective advantage in responding to pathogens when compared to an MHC homozygote. A strong selection for heterozygosity could lead to the presence of a multiallelic or highly polymorphic locus.

6-17 (a) There are several reasons why counting bands on Southern blots may lead to an underestimate of the number of genes. First, some genes encoding Ia antigens may not be homologous enough to hybridize detectably with the probe. Under commonly used hybridization conditions for genomic blots, greater than 80–85% nucleotide sequence identity is required. Second, two or more genes may be located on the same restriction fragment. Third, two genes may be located on different restriction fragments that have the same molecular weight. The number of genes will be overestimated if a restriction enzyme cuts one or more times

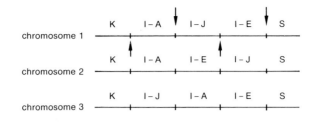

Figure 6-47 Answer to Problem 6-18c. Short vertical lines indicate boundaries between subregions. Chromosome 1 is a normal chromosome. Arrows above the line indicate breakpoints to form inversion chromosome 2, whereas arrows below the line indicate breakpoints required to form inversion chromosome 3.

in the middle of the gene, generating several fragments homologous to different parts of the probe. In addition, because of inframe stop codons or other defects, some homologous sequences may not actually encode Ia polypeptides. These defective sequences, or pseudogenes, have been found in many multigene families.

(b) Different sequences may have different degrees of homology with the probe sequence. Differences in homology will affect both the rate of hybridization and the T_m or stability of the resulting hybrid. Therefore, as the homology between the radioactive probe and a filter-bound sequence decreases, the hybridization signal decreases. In addition, the length of sequence homologous to the probe will affect the hybridization signal. A restriction fragment containing only one exon homologous to the probe will give a lower hybridization signal relative to a fragment containing a fully homologous gene. Finally, the hybridization signal may be sensitive to the amount of hybridizing sequence present. A restriction fragment containing two or more homologous sequences or two different fragments with the same molecular weight, each containing a homologous sequence, will give an increased signal for a particular band on the Southern blot.

(c) This result most likely rules out the possibility that the number of genes was overestimated due to the presence of a restriction enzyme site in the middle of one or more of the genes. However, it is conceivable (but unlikely) that a very long intervening sequence between two exons would contain restriction enzyme sites for all the restriction endonucleases tested.

6-18 (a) Models 1a and 1b are ruled out because they require RNA transcripts that are encoded between the I-A and I-E subregions. Model 1c also is ruled out if a double-stranded hybridization probe is used.

(b) It is possible that the I-J gene is formed through rearrangement of sequences into the region between I-A and I-E. Southern blots of DNA made from cloned suppressor T cells and from livers of the same inbred strain can be hybridized with the 3.4-kb probe to determine whether a DNA rearrangement has occurred.

(c) See Figure 6-47.

The hypothetical inversion breakpoints do not have to occur precisely at the subregion boundaries so long as part of the I-A subregion is brought into close proximity with part of the I-E subregion.

(d) Around the inversion breakpoint, BALB/c mice should have a unique restriction enzyme map. Farther away from the breakpoint ($>$20–25 kb), there should be few differences except for the normal restriction enzyme site polymorphisms found between strains. Thus Southern blots of BALB/c DNA hybridized with subclones from the cosmids can be compared to blots of other DNAs to determine if there are any gross differences in BALB/c. Note that one of the hypothetical inversion breakpoints should be at or near the I-A/I-E boundary.

(e) The control element should be polymorphic because many I-J alleles have been defined. Furthermore, recombination in the control element located between I-A and I-E can affect the expression of genes that are encoded elsewhere, even in MHC congenic strains having identical background genes. Therefore, it is probable that each inbred strain has several I-J genes, only one of which is selected for expression by the control element.

(f) Because of the molecular and genetic map of the MHC, it is likely that E_β or exons very close to E_β are being recognized as restriction elements by suppressor T lymphocytes. This model would propose that T-cell receptors that recognize a different I-J allele as self would have different antigenic determinants or idiotypes. As long as the genes for these T-cell receptors are similar in different inbred mouse strains, then differences in MHC haplotype should completely determine the T-cell receptor idiotype, and hence the serologic specificity will map to the MHC even though the genes are encoded elsewhere.

(g) You can obtain nude homozygous mice (nu/nu) that are heterozygous (H-2^a/H-2^b) for the MHC. Nude mice have very little ability to promote T-cell differentiation. These mice can then receive a transplant of either an H-2^a or an H-2^b irradiated thymus. If I-J is similar to other class II molecules, then the I-J specificity should be a function of the genotype of the host lymphocytes (H-2^a/H-2^b). On the other hand, if I-J is a serologic determinant on the T-cell receptor for self-MHC, then the genotype of the transplanted thymus will determine the I-J specificity.

6-19 (a) Clone p1500 is missing exons encoding most of the third external domain (α3), the transmembrane domain, the cytoplasmic domains, and the 3' untranslated sequences. Clone p1700 is probably missing the 5' control sequences and exons coding for the entire α3 domain, the transmembrane domain, the cytoplasmic domains, and the 3' untranslated sequences. Clone p1800 is missing the 5' control sequences and exons for the leader and the first three external domains. Clone p1102 is missing the exon coding for the leader. It may also be missing 5' control sequences. However, it is not clear from the figure how large a deletion was used to construct p1102.

(b) The first and second external domains (α1 and α2) are necessary for expression of the anti-L^d serological determinants, but they may not be sufficient. The small portion of the α3 domain present in p1500 but absent from p1700 may be required as well.

(c) It is possible that the 5' or left-hand portion of the α3 domain present in p1500 may be required to generate the L^d antigenic determinant. It is also possible that 5' control sequences that may be missing from p1700 are required to give a relatively high level of L^d expression.

(d) A number of serologic techniques could be employed, but probably the best way to distinguish between these possibilities would be to analyze the transformed cell populations using fluorescence-labeled antibody and a fluorescence-activated cell sorter. This kind of analysis will allow you to determine the fraction of cells expressing any given amount of the L^d antigen.

(e) The gene fragment may be transcribed and translated. The resulting truncated protein, which lacks a transmembrane domain, may then be present at the cell surface via noncovalent interaction with some other integral membrane protein.

Alternatively, a complete 45,000-dalton polypeptide may be synthesized. This would most likely occur if the truncated gene integrated into the chromosome adjacent to the proper class I transmembrane and cytoplasmic exons. Such an integration event could occur as a result of either homologous recombination or gene conversion. Finally, it is possible, although unlikely, that fusion of RNA or protein molecules derived from the truncated and endogenous genes leads to cell-surface expression of L^d.

(f) This result rules out any mechanism involving expression of a truncated L^d polypeptide at the cell surface.

(g) The result is surprising because there are more than 30 class I genes, and many of these probably have $\alpha 3$, transmembrane, and cytoplasmic domains that would allow expression of the L^d determinants if a recombination had occurred. Because these genes are polymorphic, especially for the transmembrane exons, it seems unlikely that the protein product resulting from the recombinant gene would have the same isoelectric point as the intact L^d polypeptide.

The most likely explanation for the result is that the p1500 construct recombined with the class I gene most homologous to itself. This is somewhat surprising because the L cell does not express an L product. Alternatively, the charge in the C-terminal half of class I polypeptides appears to be highly conserved even though the sequence is not. Thus perhaps the charge differences among class I molecules are determined primarily by the $\alpha 1$ and $\alpha 2$ domains.

6-20 (a) The data suggest that the amount of β_2-microglobulin expressed at the cell surface is a function of either the number of different class I genes or the amount of class I protein expressed by the cell.

(b) It is possible that the increased β_2-microglobulin expression may not actually reflect the presence of a new class I gene. It also is possible that the new class I gene expressed is not very polymorphic, and there are no differences in the H-2^d- and H-2^k-encoded alleles for this gene. Finally, it is possible that the new class I gene expressed is actually formed via homologous recombination or gene conversion between the transforming H-2^d gene and endogenous H-2^k class I genes. In this case, most of the new class I sequences expressed could be H-2^k encoded and, therefore, C3H mice would be tolerant to it.

(c) This result makes it unlikely that the novel class I gene expressed is a recombinant between the transforming gene and cellular DNA that contains a large amount of H-2^k sequence because at least one of the other inbred mouse strains should make antibody against a polymorphic H-2^k-encoded molecule.

(d) This result demonstrates that the transformation event did lead to expression of a new class I gene that presumably exhibits very little polymorphism among the inbred mice used in this experiment.

(e) It is likely that the novel class I molecule is expressed on only a small subpopulation of spleen cells. Cytotoxic reactions of this kind have a significant background of cell killing in the presence of complement alone, so that a small subpopulation could be easily missed. Alternatively, this molecule may not be expressed on spleen cells at all. From the limited data presented, the novel class I molecule appears to be not highly polymorphic and not ubiquitously expressed. Therefore, it is unlike transplantation antigens and appears to be more like the differentiation antigens encoded in the Tla region of the MHC. This gene may well be encoded in the Tla complex.

6-21 (a) It is very surprising that three L cell lines that express human class I genes have acquired a human β_2-microglobulin serologic specificity.

(b) Several explanations are possible. For example, the mouse may harbor a cryptic β_2-microglobulin gene, related to human microglobulin, which is expressed only in the presence of HLA genes. A number of experiments not described in the problem argue against this unlikely possibility. It is most likely that the B.1.G.6 monoclonal antibody recognizes an antigenic determinant, on human β_2-microglobulin, which is also present on murine β_2-microglobulin only if the mouse β_2-microglobulin is associated with an HLA polypeptide. Therefore, normal mouse cells will not express this conformational determinant.

(c) Because C23.24.2 was raised against free human β_2-microglobulin, it might not be expected to detect antigenic determinants of murine β_2-microglobulin which depend on interaction with HLA heavy chain. By contrast, B.1.G.6 was raised against β_2-microglobulin, which was presumably associated with HLA molecules.

(d) The $\alpha3$ domain interacts with β_2-microglobulin. It is therefore possible that the genomic clone used to generate the TRH 42 transformant has differences in the $\alpha3$ domain when compared to the other clones. These $\alpha3$ differences may not permit the mouse β_2-microglobulin associated with this HLA heavy chain to attain the proper conformation required to react with B.1.G.6.

(e) It is safe to assume that the antigenic determinants are not located on the leader, on the transmembrane domain, or on the cytoplasmic domains. Therefore, 30.5.7 recognizes determinants located on either $\alpha1$, $\alpha2$, or both domains of the L^d gene, whereas 28.14.8 recognizes determinants on $\alpha3$ of L^d. 34.5.8 must recognize determinants on $\alpha1$, $\alpha2$, or both $\alpha1$ and $\alpha2$ of H-2D^d, and 34.2.12 recognizes determinants on the $\alpha3$ domain of H-2D^d.

(f) When the 28.14.8 monoclonal binds to L^d on the surface of an LCMV-infected cell, it inhibits killing of that cell. However, the antibody may not be binding directly to determinants recognized by the cytotoxic T lymphocytes. Because the antibody molecule is relatively large compared to a class I molecule, it may interfere with T-cell recognition by steric hindrance. Thus definition of the critical determinants for T-cell recognition by gene transfer is more accurate than trying to define these determinants using antibody blocking.

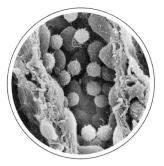

CHAPTER 7

Development of the Immune System

Chapter Outline

Immune responses are initiated in lymphoid organs, which are constructed to receive circulating lymphocytes from the bloodstream, to channel them into pathways of interaction with antigen-charged accessory cells, and to aid in the generation of effective immune responses. These secondary lymphoid organs depend for their function on virgin B and T lymphocytes that are produced in the bone marrow and thymus—the primary lymphoid organs. To understand the cellular interactions involved in immune responses, it is useful to know the structure and developmental origins of the immune system. This chapter considers the architecture and the developmental biology of the immune system.

Concepts

7-1 The structure of the lymphoid system allows lymphocytes to recognize their cognate antigens efficiently

Overview of the lymphoid system

The lymphoid system is composed of the primary lymphoid organs, the bone marrow and the thymus, the B and T lymphocytes they produce, and a collection of secondary lymphoid organs that are the sites where immune responses are initiated. The secondary lymphoid organs are interconnected by a circulatory system composed of two circulatory networks, the bloodstream and the lymphatic system (Figure 7-1). B and T lymphocytes are carried throughout most of the tissues and organs of vertebrates by this circulatory system. Lymphocytes make up 20–80% of the nucleated cells in the blood and more than 99% of the nucleated cells in the lymphatic fluid (lymph). This circulatory system has three principal functions: (a) to filter and trap antigens from all parts of the body into a few secondary lymphoid organs; (b) to circulate the lymphocyte population through these organs so that every antigen is exposed to the organism's repertoire of antigen-specific lymphocytes in a short period of time; and (c) to carry the products of the immune response, antigen-specific effector T cells and humoral antibodies, to the bloodstream and the tissues.

Lymphatic circulation

The lymphatic system is an extensively branched and widely dispersed network of thin-walled vessels with one-way valves and interspersed filtering organs called *lymph nodes* (Figure 7-1). The lymphatic vessels originate in the interstitial spaces of the tissues. The interstitial fluid (*lymph*), which bathes the cells in a tissue, is pulled into and pumped through the lymphatics by osmotic pressure and muscular contraction. The lymph is transported from the tissues to the lymph nodes through *afferent lymphatic vessels*. It enters a node through a series of cavities (sinusoids), percolates through the tissues of the

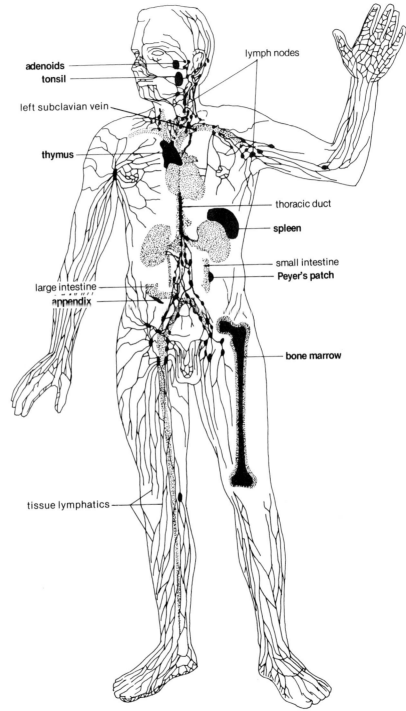

Figure 7-1

A diagram of the human lymphoid system. The system consists of circulating lymphocytes and the lymphoid organs, which include the tree of lymphatic vessels and the lymph nodes stationed along them, the bone marrow (in the long bones, only one of which is illustrated), the thymus, the spleen, the adenoids, the tonsils, the Peyer's patches of the small intestine, and the appendix. The lymphatic vessels collect the lymphocytes and antibody molecules from the tissues and lymph nodes and return them to the bloodstream at the subclavian veins. [Adapted from N. K. Jerne, *Sci. Am.* **229,** 52(1973). Copyright © 1973 by Scientific American, Inc. All rights reserved.]

Figure 7-2

The pathway of lymphocyte circulation. (a) Blood lymphocytes enter lymph nodes, adhere to the walls of specialized postcapillary venules, and migrate to the lymph-node diffuse cortex. Many lymphocytes then migrate to T- or B-cell domains and percolate through lymphoid fields to medullary lymphatic sinuses and then to efferent lymphatics, which in turn collect into major lymphatic ducts in the thorax, which then empty into the neck veins leading to the heart. (b) The gut associated lymphoid tissues (Peyer's patches and mesenteric lymph nodes are shown here) also possess specialized postcapillary venules active in lymphocyte migration. The mesenteric lymph node also receives lymphocytes draining from the Peyer's patch efferent lymphatics. (c) The spleen receives lymphocytes and disburses them mainly via the blood vascular system, although it is possible that splenic efferent lymphatics also play a role in lymphocyte circulation through the spleen.

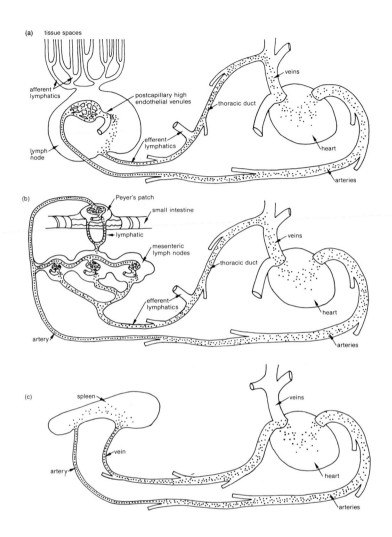

lymph node, and exits through *efferent lymphatic vessels.* Several efferent lymphatics join together into larger lymphatic ducts that in turn empty into the venous system. The interstitial lymphatic fluid is replaced by diffusion of water, ions, and selected proteins through the walls of blood capillaries in the tissues, thereby completing the lymphatic circulatory network (Figure 7-2).

Structure of peripheral lymphoid organs

The secondary lymphoid organs include the lymph nodes, spleen, tonsils, adenoids, Peyer's patches, and appendix. These organs are the sites where immune responses are initiated. All are analogous in

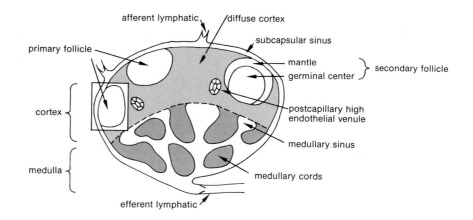

Figure 7-3 The general structure of a lymph node. The cortical subcapsular sinus lies beneath the capsule of the node and communicates extensively with the sinuses of the medulla. The subcapsular sinus drains the extracellular space via afferent lymphatics and is lined with phagocytic cells. The primary follicle, lying directly under the subcapsular sinus in the cortex, is an ovoid accumulation of small lymphocytes lying in a meshwork of dendritic reticular cells. The secondary follicle is composed of the mantle—the components of which are similar to those of the primary follicle—and the germinal center, which contains small and large lymphocytes, many large blast cells with abundant cytoplasm, macrophages (containing phagocytized cell debris), and dendritic reticular cells. The diffuse cortex includes many small lymphocytes, macrophages, interdigitating reticular cells, and postcapillary venules. The medullary sinus is lined by phagocytic cells. This sinus constitutes the route of emigration of circulating T and B lymphocytes, as well as blast cells after antigen stimulation. The medullary cords are close-packed, interconnected spaces containing cords of cells, particularly plasma cells and large lymphocytes.

structure in that they have specialized ports through which lymphocytes can enter from the bloodstream, discrete domains that are specific for B cells or T cells, and an elaborate architecture that maximizes interaction of lymphocytes with antigen-charged accessory cells.

A typical lymph node is a bean-shaped organ that consists of an outer layer, the *cortex*, and an inner core called the *medulla* (Figure 7-3). The cortex is divided into discrete B-cell domains, called the *primary follicles*, and a surrounding T-cell domain, called the *diffuse cortex* (Figure 7-4). A fibrous tissue network (*reticulum*) throughout the lymph node supports large phagocytes, called *macrophages* (Figure 1-2c), and extensively branched *interdigitating cells* and *dendritic reticular cells*. The reticulum and its adherent cells trap antigen and provide passageways and specialized niches for lymphocytes and their progeny (Figure 7-5).

Lymphocytes enter a lymph node from the bloodstream via arterioles and capillaries to reach postcapillary venules in the diffuse cortex. Both T and B cells, but not other blood cells, adhere specifically to large, specialized endothelial cells in the venule walls and then

(a)

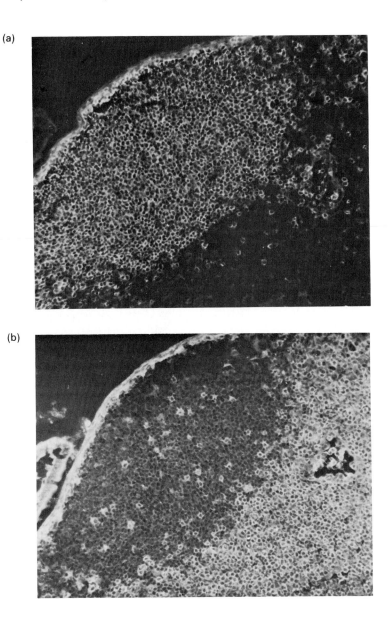

Figure 7-4

Localization of T cells and B cells in a lymph node. A lymph node was frozen rapidly, and sections of the node were stained with antibodies coupled to a fluorescent tracer. Photomicrographs were taken to locate bound fluorescent antibodies. (a) Anti-B-cell fluorescent antibodies were used to stain the cortex of a node containing a primary follicle (top left) and its adjacent diffuse cortex (bottom right) containing a postcapillary venule. B cells predominate in the primary follicle; they are also found in the lumen and wall of the postcapillary venule, presumably just having entered via the bloodstream. (b) A serial section adjacent to the one in (a), stained with anti-T-cell fluorescent antibodies. T cells predominate in the diffuse cortex and are also found in the postcapillary venule. [Photomicrographs by G. A. Gutman and I. Weissman.]

(b)

traverse these walls to enter the node (Figure 7-6). Upon entering, B cells migrate specifically to the primary follicle and T cells remain in the diffuse cortex. After slowly traversing their specific cortical domains, B and T cells enter the medulla, which serves primarily as a collection point for the sinusoids that lead to the efferent lymphatic vessels. From the nodes, the lymphocytes are carried via the main lymphatic ducts back to the bloodstream to begin the cycle again. Circulating B and T cells take more than 6 hours to traverse the lym-

Figure 7-5

Microscopic anatomy of a lymph node. (a) Scanning electron micrograph of the subcapsular sinus; the flattened bodies with long branching processes are part of the reticulum, and the adherent cells with multiple globular protrusions are macrophages. Notice the large intercellular spaces in the sinus. (b) Scanning electron micrograph of the medullary sinus; again a flattened reticulum with adherent macrophages is evident. The smaller round cells with or without filamentous protrusions are lymphocytes, and a biconcave red blood cell is seen at the left. (c) An electron microscopic view of a cross section of the medulla. The clear space is the medullary sinus with a few large pale macrophages and many small dark lymphocytes. The highly cellular portions are medullary cords that contain dividing lymphocytes and plasma cells. (d) Scanning electron micrograph view of the diffuse cortex, where a fine meshwork of reticulum and interdigitating cells surrounds many lymphocytes. (e) Light microscopic view of a standard histological section of a lymph node from a thymus-deprived mouse. The only region containing large numbers of small, dark, round lymphocytes is the primary follicle at top. (f) Scanning electron micrograph view of a primary follicle; dendritic reticular cells with long lacy processes surround densely packed small lymphocytes. [Electron micrographs (a) to (d) and (f) courtesy of W. van Ewijk; photomicrograph (e) by I. Weissman.]

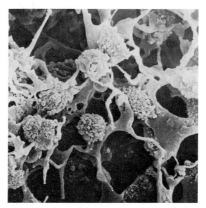
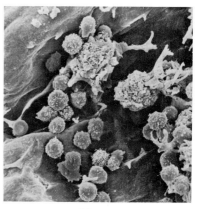

(a)

(b)

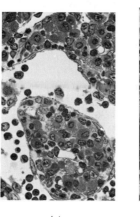
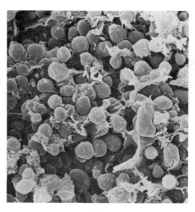

(c)

(d)

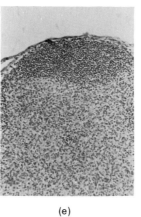

(e)

(f)

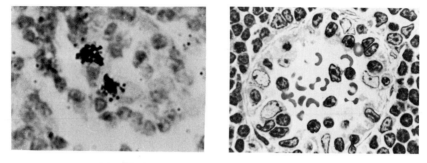

(a)   (b)

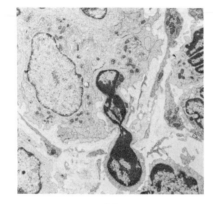   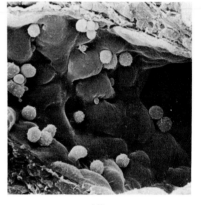

(c)   (d)

Figure 7-6   Microscopic views of lymphocytes traversing postcapillary venules. (a) An autoradiograph of labeled lymphocytes in the walls of a postcapillary venule within minutes after their injection into the bloodstream [G. A. Gutman and I. Weissman, *Transplantation* **16**, 621(1973)]. (b) A thin section of a postcapillary venule under high power, showing lymphocytes in different stages of passage with several red blood cells in the vessel lumen. [Photomicrograph courtesy of G. Levine.] (c) An electron microscopic view of a lymphocyte (lower right) squeezing through a narrow passageway in a postcapillary venule. Lymphocyte nuclei stain densely, whereas endothelial nuclei stain lightly with a dark rim just inside the nuclear membrane. [Electron micrograph courtesy of G. Levine and G. A. Gutman.] (d) A scanning electron microscopic view of several lymphocytes in contact with the inner surface of postcapillary venule endothelial cells. [Electron micrograph courtesy of W. van Ewijk.]

phoid fields of a lymph node. On the average, lymphocytes have a total circulation time of about 24 hours.

The spleen serves a dual function as a lymphoid organ and a hematopoietic organ. The spleen is differentiated into two types of tissue called *lymphoid white pulp* and *erythroid red pulp* (Figure 7-7). The white pulp, which forms a bumpy sheath that surrounds the

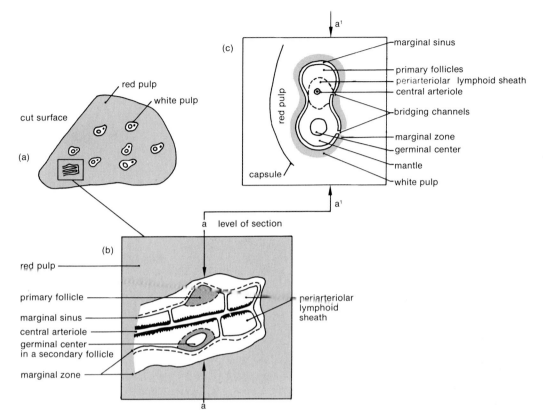

Figure 7-7 General structure of a spleen. (a) A cross section of the spleen. (b) Enlargement of an area of white pulp. (c) Cross section of an area of white pulp. *White pulp:* The central arteriole, a branch of a *trabecular* artery, has branches that empty into the marginal zone, marginal sinus, and red pulp. The periarteriolar lymphoid sheath is an accumulation of small lymphocytes surrounding the central arteriole. The primary follicles, mantle, and germinal center are similar to those described for the lymph node (Figure 7-3). *Marginal area:* The marginal sinus separates the white pulp from the marginal zone and red pulp. The marginal areas, including the sinuses, receive much of the blood entering the spleen. These areas are major sites of entry of T and B cells. Bridging channels appear to interrupt the marginal area and form connections between the white and red pulp. *Red pulp:* In addition to hematopoietic cells, plasma cells appear in this site and are particularly prominent after antigenic stimulation.

small splenic arteries (arterioles) from their origin as arterial branches to their termini, is analogous in structure and function to the cortex of a lymph node. The bumps on the sheath are primary follicles, that is, B-cell domains, whereas the rest of the sheath is the T-cell domain (Figures 7-8 and 7-9). The red pulp is involved in scavenging old red blood cells and is a reserve site for hematopoiesis.

In contrast to the pathway taken by lymphocytes through other secondary lymphoid organs, most lymphocytes enter and leave the spleen directly via the bloodstream. The lymphoid white pulp is separated from the red pulp by the marginal zone, which receives blood from a specialized venule called the *marginal sinus.* This sinus arises at

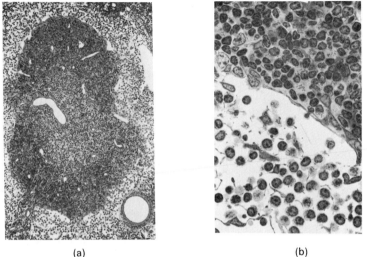

(a)   (b)

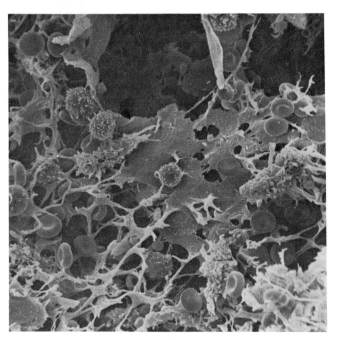

(c)

Figure 7-8   Microscopic anatomy of the spleen. (a) A light micrograph of a section of the spleen. The structures have the same relationship to each other as diagrammed in Figure 7-7c. (b) An electron microscopic view of a primary follicle (top) and the marginal zone (right). One cell appears to be traversing the boundary. (c) A scanning electron microscopic view of the marginal zone. The dendritic reticulum and its adherent macrophages surround the space containing lymphocytes and red blood cells. [Electron micrographs courtesy of W. van Ewijk.]

(a)

(b)

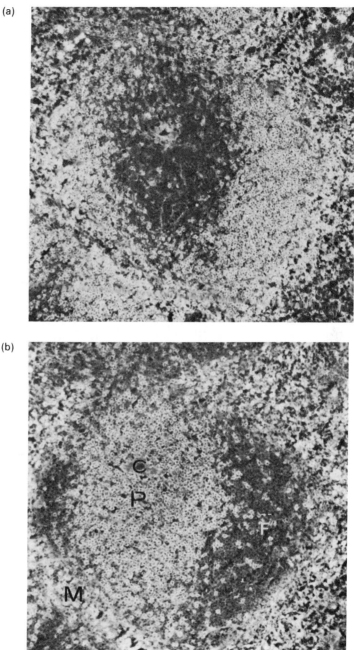

Figure 7-9

Localization of B cells and T cells in the spleen. Photomicrographs are of sections stained as in Figure 7-4. (a) Anti B-cell stain of a spleen. The central arteriole (C) is immediately surrounded by a fluorescent-negative periarteriolar lymphoid sheath (P). B cells predominate in the eccentric follicles (F) and are interspersed around the marginal zone (M). (b) Anti-T-cell stain of an adjacent serial section. T cells predominate in the periarteriolar lymphoid sheath and are interspersed around the marginal zone. [Micrographs by G. A. Gutman and I. Weissman.]

the termination of the arteriole ensheathed by white pulp and curves back to envelop the white pulp. B and T cells, but no other blood cells, enter the white pulp by traversing the walls of the marginal sinus and then migrate slowly through their respective domains. Circulating B and T cells take about 6 hours to traverse the lymphoid fields of the spleen. Most lymphocytes then cross the marginal zone via so-called bridging channels from the white pulp to the red pulp, where they are taken up by veins that leave the spleen. However, some lymphocytes appear to flow into the efferent lymphatics that drain the spleen and are carried via the lymphatic ducts back to the bloodstream.

Antigen trapping in lymphoid organs

Antigens are trapped by different lymphoid organs depending on their route of entry into the body (Figure 7-1). Antigens that enter the intercellular spaces of any tissue are swept into the lymphatic system by the lymph and collect in the local lymph nodes that drain the region of entry. Antigens that enter the body via the upper respiratory and gastrointestinal tracts are trapped in local lymph nodes as well as in the tonsils, adenoids, Peyer's patches, and appendix. Antigens that enter the bloodstream collect in the spleen. Blood-borne antigens also are filtered out by macrophages in the liver and lungs, but only the spleen is capable of mounting an immune response against them.

Antigens are trapped in lymphoid organs by macrophages, which bind the antigen at their surface. Some of the antigen is taken up by pinocytosis, digested, and returned to the surface in a "processed" form. Surface-bound forms of antigen on accessory cells are recognized efficiently by circulating lymphocytes as the first step in initiating an immune response (Concept 8-3).

7-2 The bone marrow produces precursor lymphocytes

Migration of primordial precursors

During mammalian development, the primordial hematolymphoid precursors initially appear at the head end of the embryo. They then migrate successively to the blood islands of the yolk sac, to the embryonic liver, and finally to the bone marrow. Throughout the remainder of the organism's lifetime, the bone marrow produces blood-forming (hematopoietic) stem cells, which have lymphocyte precursors among their progeny.

Maturation pathways for hematolymphoid cells

All cells of the hematolymphoid system follow analogous maturation pathways (Figure 7-10). A common stem cell produces distinct sets of progeny cells that each are programmed to interact with sessile cells in a particular tissue microenvironment. That interaction causes the

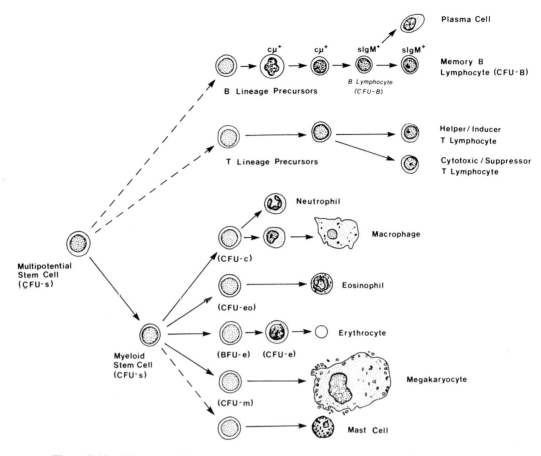

Figure 7-10 Maturational phases in the hematolymphoid system. A common hematopoietic stem cell may give rise to all elements in the blood and in the lymphoid system. Within particular maturational microenvironments, progeny of that stem cell progress along specific differentiation pathways. The branched pathways shown here represent current knowledge or best estimates of specific lineage relationships; additional cellular intermediates almost certainly exist. [Courtesy Dr. P. Kincade.] The precise lineage of natural killer cells is unclear. Although these cells are not shown in Figure 7-10, they share some characteristics with T cells, myelomonocytic cells, and mast cells.

cells to undergo commitment to their specific developmental lineages. These committed cells bear surface receptors that enable them to recognize specific cell-bound or soluble molecular structures. A recognition event triggers their differentiation through intermediate and terminal stages to effector cells with defined functions. At each stage of differentiation, the hematolymphoid precursors appear to be freely mobile cells. Except for erythrocytes, all the committed and differenti-

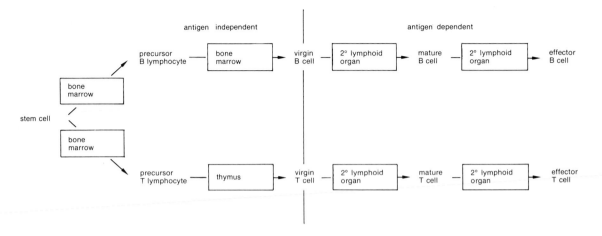

Figure 7-11   Antigen-independent and antigen-dependent phases in maturation of B and T cells. Maturation of virgin cells to mature cells is probably antigen dependent.

ated cells that arise from hematolymphoid precursors (Figure 7-10) are involved in host defense mechanisms.

Maturation time of the lymphoid system

The ontogenic maturation times of the immune system relative to birth differ from species to species. As measured by the onset of immune responsiveness as well as by the appearance of peripheral B and T lymphocytes, mice and birds develop their immune systems just before and after birth, whereas sheep and humans develop functional immune systems early in gestation, well before birth. However, in all species the immediate postnatal period is marked by dramatic differentiative changes in the immune system, reflecting the sudden exposure to environmental antigens.

7-3   Maturation of B and T lymphocytes includes antigen-independent and antigen-dependent phases

Overview of maturation

During the maturation of both B and T cells, the antigen-independent phase of differentiation always precedes the antigen-dependent phase (Figure 7-11). The differentiation steps that occur in the fetus or in organs like the bone marrow and thymus, which do not filter foreign antigens, are considered to be antigen-independent. Lymphocytes that differentiate in these environments become *immunocompetent;* that is, they acquire antigen-specific cell-surface receptors and the cellular machinery to respond to antigen stimulation. These cells are called *virgin lymphocytes.* Antigen-dependent differentiation of these lymphocytes results eventually in the generation of memory cells and effector cells, probably through an intermediate class of immunocompetent cells, termed *mature lymphocytes.* It has not yet been demonstrated that the steps leading from virgin to mature lymphocytes are antigen-driven, but the differentiation of mature lymphocytes to effector cells definitely requires stimulation by antigens.

Differentiation markers

Each phase in the differentiation of B and T lymphocytes may involve several steps, each of which yields cells at a defined maturational stage. Each stage is characterized by a distinct set of cell-surface antigens. Although in most cases the functional significance of these antigens is not understood, they are extremely useful as *differentiation markers.*

7-4 B cells develop immunocompetence in the bone marrow

Overview of B-cell development

In fetal mammals, the antigen-independent maturation of precursor B lymphocytes to immunocompetent virgin B cells occurs in the hematopoietic portions of the liver and spleen. *After birth* this process takes place exclusively in the bone marrow. Virgin B cells migrate to the B-cell domains of peripheral lymphoid organs. These cells are thought to be short-lived and probably require antigenic stimulation for further differentiation to mature, long-lived, circulating B cells. Mature B cells respond to antigenic stimulation by proliferating and differentiating to memory B cells and antibody-secreting plasma cells.

B-cell developmental lineage

The earliest identified cells in the B-cell lineage are found in the bone marrow (or fetal liver). They contain internal μ chains but no detectable light chains, and they carry no detectable cell-surface immunoglobulins. These precursor cells differentiate in the bone marrow to virgin B lymphocytes that carry IgM on their cell surface. Because they express IgM, they are referred to as B_μ cells. During the development of precursor B cells, heavy-chain gene rearrangements normally precede light-chain gene rearrangement. Later in development, perhaps in response to antigens, a new class of B cells appears in lymphoid organs. These mature $B_{\mu+\delta}$ cells express both IgM and IgD on their cell surface. Although $B_{\mu+\delta}$ cells probably differentiate directly from B_μ cells, it is possible that they arise instead by an independent pathway from a common precursor cell. Throughout life, $B_{\mu+\delta}$ cells

Table 7-1 Cell-Surface Markers for Mouse B Cells

	Marker Name									
	B220	ThB	Lyb-2	Lyb-3	Lyb-4	Lyb-6	Ia	FcR	C3R	Pc-1
Molecular weight[a]	220	?	45	70	45	45	28,33	20	?	70
Cell type										
Pre-B	+	+	±	−	−	−	−	−	−	−
B_μ	+	+	+	?	+	+	+	+	+	−
$B_{\mu+\delta}$	+	+	+	+	+	+	+	+	+	−
Plasma cells	+	+	?	?	?	?	?	−	−	+

[a]Molecular weights are expressed in kilodaltons.

are the predominant class of B cells, but other classes, such as B_α, B_ϵ, and $B_{\gamma 1}$ cells, appear with time. These cells express other classes of immunoglobulin on their cell surface (e.g., B_α cells express IgA) and are thought to arise from $B_{\mu+\delta}$ cells by heavy-chain gene rearrangements known as class switching (Concepts 4-8 and 8-6).

B-cell differentiation markers

Several other cell-surface antigens and receptors have been identified on B cells; however, their relationship to the functionally defined classes of B cells is not clear (Table 7-1). Several surface markers are found on B-cell precursors, B cells, and plasma cells. In all vertebrate species examined, different classes of B cells express one or both of two receptors for immunologically significant molecules: one for the Fc region of IgG and the other for the activated form of serum complement component C3b (Figure 7-12). The functional significance of these receptors is still unknown, but they provide useful markers for the identification of B cells in humans and may represent stage-specific differentiation markers.

Bursa of Fabricius

In birds, the development of B cells but not T cells can be prevented by exposing the embryo to the male hormone testosterone. The *bursa of Fabricius*, a lymphoid pouch that connects with the intestinal lumen, fails to develop in these birds, and B cells and plasma cells do not appear. The lack of a bursa and the developmental failure of the B-cell system are probably linked. Consequently, many immunologists believe that the bursa is the site for the generation of virgin B cells in birds; in fact, this belief gave rise to the designation "B" for bursal cells. However, there is still no definitive proof that avian B cells develop solely in the bursa and not in the hematopoietic tissues, as in mammals.

Figure 7-12
A diagram of four classes of B cells with differing combinations of B-cell-specific surface receptors. It is not known whether these B cells result from distinct pathways of differentiation or whether they represent different stages along a single differentiation pathway.

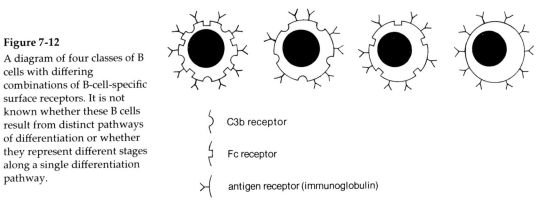

C3b receptor

Fc receptor

antigen receptor (immunoglobulin)

7-5   T cells develop immunocompetence in the thymus

Overview of T-cell development

The antigen-independent maturation of precursor T lymphocytes to immunocompetent virgin T cells occurs in the bone marrow and thymus. Stem cells in the bone marrow differentiate into precursor T lymphocytes that may be committed already to becoming a particular functional class of T cells. Precursor T cells further differentiate into immunocompetent, virgin T cells in the thymus. These cells then migrate to the T-cell domains of peripheral lymphoid organs. Virgin T cells, like virgin B cells, are thought to be short-lived. Probably as a result of antigenic stimulation, a small fraction of virgin T cells is converted to mature, long-lived, circulating T cells. Mature T cells possess surface receptors for antigens and, upon stimulation, proliferate and terminally differentiate into effector T cells and probably into memory T cells as well.

Developmental aspects of the thymus

The thymus originates embryologically with the movement of cells from one embryonic germ layer, the endoderm, into another layer, the mesoderm. The third and fourth pouches of the anterior endoderm with attached ectoderm penetrate the surrounding mesoderm to initiate formation of the thymus and parathyroid (Figure 7-13). The thymus rudiment then detaches and migrates down into the chest cavity. For a brief interval just after its downward migration, the thymus rudiment actively collects T-cell precursors from the blood. Thereafter, the hematopoietic tissues of the bone marrow provide only a low level of T-lymphocyte precursors to the thymus, but they can serve as a reservoir for massive thymic regeneration, if necessary. During thymus development, the precursor T cells organize into an

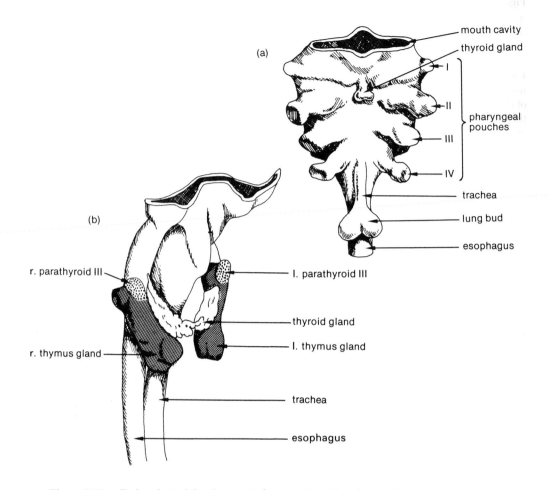

Figure 7-13 Embryological development of the thymus. (a) The third and fourth endodermal pharyngeal pouches with attached ectoderm migrate into surrounding mesoderm and then split. The portions that remain in the neck (b) form the parathyroids, whereas the portions that migrate down into the chest cavity form the thymic lobes. [Adapted from G. L. Weller, *Contrib. Embryol. Carneg. Inst.* **24**, 93(1933).]

outer cortical layer from 2 to 10 cells thick, enlarge, and begin to divide (Figures 7-14 and 7-15). These thymic lymphoblasts give rise to all the types of lymphocytes of the thymus. At maturity, the thymus is more than 99% lymphocytes. Under normal conditions, the large dividing lymphocytes account for about 5% of the thymic lymphocytes; the deeper cortical small lymphocytes account for about 85%; and the medium-sized medullary lymphocytes account for about 10%.

At puberty the thymus shrinks considerably in size in response to repeated release of both sex and adrenal steroid hormones. Cortical lymphocytes (but not the medullary lymphocytes) lack the enzyme

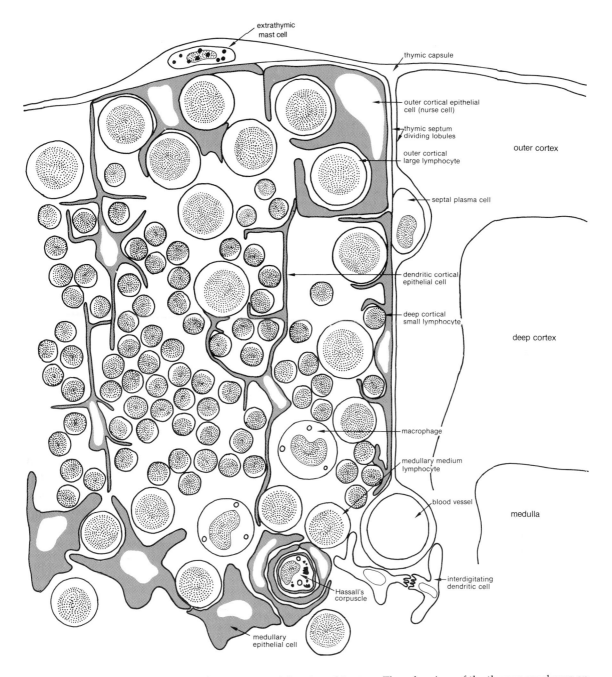

Figure 7-14 (a)   General diagram of thymic architecture. The subregions of the thymus are shown on the right, with their cellular constituents on the left.

Figure 7-14 (b)

A thymus with nonadherent lymphocytes removed by perfusion, stained with anti-I-A^k antibodies. The dendritic cortical epithelial cells stain darkly, whereas the adherent thymic lymphocytes do not. (Photomicrograph provided by R. Rouse.)

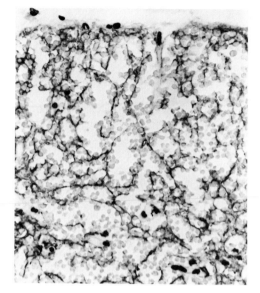

20-α-hydroxyl-steroid dehydrogenase, which is involved in steroid hormone catabolism. As a result, cortical cells are particularly sensitive to circulating levels of testosterone and adrenal steroid hormones. Despite this reduction in size, the thymus remains functional and continues to produce virgin T cells throughout life.

Virgin T cells

The immunocompetent, virgin T cells that migrate from the thymus represent only a very small fraction of the lymphocytes produced in the thymus. For example, in the mouse, the outer cortical cells produce nearly 10^8 lymphocytes per day, but not more than 2×10^6 lymphocytes per day leave the thymus. The reason for such a massive overproduction of lymphocytes is unknown, but many immunologists believe that the emigrants are the only cells that have matured appropriately to virgin T cells and thereby have gained "exit visas." The sites of intrathymic cell death are also not known, but the medullary Hassall's corpuscles are likely sites for destruction; these prominent structures include macrophages, medullary epithelial cells, and cell debris (Figure 7-14a).

The relationships among the subpopulation of thymic lymphocytes and virgin T cells are not clear, in part because such a small fraction of thymic lymphocytes become T cells. Ultimately, of course, the virgin T cells are mainly derived from the large cortical lymphocytes, but the relationship of these T cells to the small cortical lymphocytes and the medullary lymphocytes is not known. Virgin T cells emigrating from the thymus mainly derive from deep cortical precursors, but they share many surface properties and size with medullary lymphocytes.

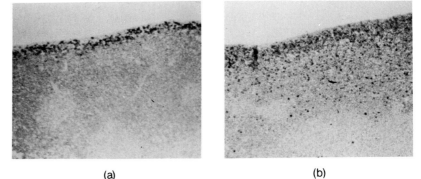

(a)

(b)

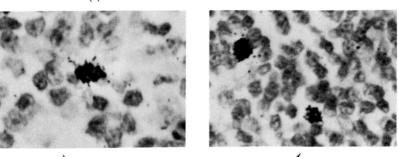

(c)

(d)

Figure 7-15
Autoradiographs of thymus cells. A radioactive DNA precursor, tritiated thymidine, was applied to the thymus surface at time zero. Within an hour, the layer of dividing thymus cells beneath the surface had incorporated this label into their DNA (a). One day later these labeled cells had migrated from the thymus surface to deeper areas of the cortex and to the medulla (b). By the second or third day, labeled cells were found in the lymph nodes (c) and the spleen (d). [Adapted from I. Weissman, *J. Exp. Med.* **126**, 291(1967) and **137**, 504(1973). Copyright © 1973 by The Rockefeller University Press.]

Epithelial cells in the development of T cells

The thymus contains several types of nonlymphoid cells that may play key roles in the proliferation, differentiation, and selection of developing thymic lymphocytes (Figure 7-14a). Specialized thymic epithelial cells known as *nurse cells* are associated with the large outer cortical lymphocytes. When released from the thymus by treatment with proteolytic enzymes, these nurse cells contain the large cortical lymphocytes in cytoplasmic vesicles. Because such relationships are difficult to identify in the intact thymus by electron microscopy, it is unknown whether these lymphocytes are normally inside the nurse cells. The epithelial cells of the deep cortex have highly branched dendritic processes whose surfaces are particularly rich in MHC Ia antigens (Figure 7-14b). These *dendritic cells* interconnect with one another via desmosomes to form a network through which cortical lymphocytes must pass on their way to the medulla (Figure 7-16g). Some of the spaces between these cells appear as lakes of lymphocytes that span the boundary between the cortex and medulla. Although some of these lakes connect directly to perivascular lymphatics, it is not known whether virgin T cells leave the thymus via the lymphatic system or via the bloodstream.

The epithelial cells of the medulla have broader processes that interconnect to form a loose webbing (Figure 7-14a). These *medullary epithelial cells,* in contrast to the cortical epithelial cells, express most if not all MHC antigens in abundance. The differential expression of

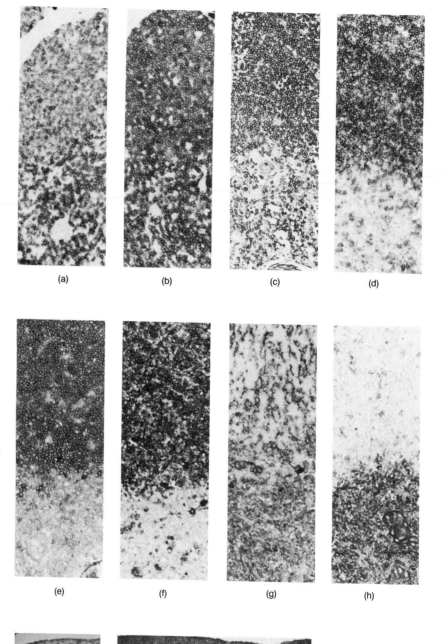

(a)   (b)   (c)   (d)

(e)   (f)   (g)   (h)

(i)   (j)

Figure 7-16

Immunohistochemical identification of human (a–h) and mouse (i, j) thymic cell subpopulations. (In all sections, the cortex is on the top and the medulla is on the bottom.) (a) Anti-T1 (leu-1), (b) anti-T3 (leu 4), (c) anti-T4 (leu 3), (d) anti-T8 (leu 2), (e) anti-cortical thymocytes (antibody 12E7), (f) PNA, (g) anti-Ia, (h) anti-HLA-A2, (i) PNA, (j) anti-homing receptor (Mel 14) reveals the location of rare cortical cells, which include virgin T cells. [(a–h) courtesy of Dr. Robert Rouse; (i, j) courtesy of Roger Reichert.]

Table 7-2 Purified Thymic Polypeptide "Hormones"

Name	Size (Number of Amino Acids)	Distinctive Structural Features	Bioassay
Thymopoietins			
TP I	49	I–III differ in their amino termini	TP I, TP II, and TP 5 all induce T-cell markers on a subset of bone-marrow cells; augment several T-cell functions
TP II	49		
TP III	49		
TP 5	5	Amino acids 32–36 of II	
Thymosins (at least 25 polypeptides)			
α1	28	—	Induces T-cell markers; augments mitogen response
β4	43	—	Augments expression of the thymic DNA synthesis enzyme terminal transferase
α7	MW = 2500	—	Augments T_S activity
Thymulin	9	Requires Zn > Ga > Al >>> other metallic cations for activity	Induces T-cell markers; augments effector T-cell functions; decreases terminal transferase expression
Thymic humoral factor	31	Not yet sequenced	Augments thymocyte → T-cell maturation assayed by alloreactivity and mitogen reactivity

self-MHC antigens by these epithelial cells and other nonlymphoid cells in different maturational layers of the thymus implies functionally distinct microenvironments for the maturation of T cells that recognize self-components. This subject of self-recognition by T cells is discussed in more detail in Chapter 8. In addition to providing differential sets of MHC antigens, the thymic epithelial cells are thought to produce several polypeptide "hormones" that are involved in the maturation of T cells (Table 7-2). It is not yet known which cells produce which of the maturation factors.

Other classes of nonlymphoid cells—*macrophages* and two types of nonphagocytic dendritic cells, the *dendritic reticular cells* and the *interdigitating dendritic cells*—are present at specific locations within the thymus. Both cell types are derived from hematolymphoid precursors in bone marrow, and both have been implicated as accessory

Table 7-3 Cell-Surface Differentiation Markers for Mouse T Cells

Marker Name	Lyt-5 (T200)	Thy-1	TL	L3T4	Lyt-1	Lyt-2	Lyt-3	Qa-1	I-J
Molecular weight[a]	180,200	25–28	45	55–62	65	34,38[b]	30[b]	45	?
Cell type									
Bone-marrow pre-T	+	−	−	−	−	−		−	−
Natural killer	+	+	−	−	−	−		−	−
Thymic lymphoblast	+	+	+(70–90)[c]	+	+	+(80–85%)		−	−
Thymic small lymphocyte	+	+	+(70–90)	+	+	+(80–35%)		−	−
Medullary lymphocyte	+	+	−	+	+	+(50%)		+(<50%)	−
Thymus emigrants	+	+	−	+	+	+(30–40%)		+(<50%)	−
Helper T cells	+	+	−	+	+	−		+(<50%)	− or +
Cytotoxic T cells	+	+	−	−	±	+	+	−	−
Suppressor T cells	+	+	−	−	±	+	+	+	+ or −

[a]Molecular weights are expressed in kilodaltons.
[b]Lyt-2 and Lyt-3 are linked to each other by disulfide bonds to form larger molecular weight oligomers.
[c]Percentages indicate the fraction of the cell population that expresses the marker; if unstated the fraction is 100%. The fractions arise because the population is a mixture of precursors to the different functional T-cell classes.

Table 7-4 Cell-Surface Differentiation Markers for Human T Cells

Marker Name (Alternative Name)	E Rosettes (Leu-5 or T11)	T1 (Leu-1)	T3 (Leu-4)	T4 (Leu-3)	T5/8 (Leu-2)	T6	T9	T10
Molecular weight[a]	55	67–69	19	55–62	30,32,43[b]	49	94[b]	45
Cell type								
Thymus cortex	+	−	−	+	+(80%)[c]	+(20%)	+(10%)	+
Thymus medulla	+	+	+	+	+	−	−	+
Helper T	+	+	+	+	−	−	−	+
Suppressor T	+	+	+	−	+	−	−	+
Cytotoxic T	+	+	+	−	+	−	−	+
Mouse homologue	−	Lyt-1	−	L3T4	Lyt-2,3	TL(?)	−	−

[a]Molecular weights are expressed in kilodaltons.
[b]The molecular weights of the reduced subunits are given; however, disulfide-linked oligomers are the predominant form in cells.
[c]Percentages are explained in Table 7-3.

cells involved in antigen presentation in secondary lymphoid organs (Concept 8-3). The dendritic cells contribute primarily to the loose webbing in the medulla, whereas the thymic macrophages are located (like sentinels) on both sides of the corticomedullary junction in the center of the lymphocyte streams.

T-cell developmental lineage

At different stages in their development, T lymphocytes express characteristic sets of gene products on their surface. These surface molecules include receptors for cell-specific interactions and for antigen recognition, as well as serologically defined antigens of unknown function that serve as useful differentiation markers for cells in the T-lymphocyte lineage. The differentiation markers for T-cell development in mice and humans are shown in Tables 7-3 and 7-4, and the putative maturation scheme for mouse T cells is shown in Figure 7-17.

In mice there are two distinct subclasses of T cells that appear to be separate at all stages of T-cell development. Cells in one subclass have both the Lyt-2 and Lyt-3 markers (Lyt-2,3), whereas cells in the other class lack both markers. In mature cells, these antigenic subclasses correlate with functional T-cell subclasses: cytotoxic (T_C) and suppressor (T_S) cells usually have the Lyt-2,3 markers, but T cells in the helper class (T_H, T_A, and T_D) usually do not. This correlation implies that the decision to express the Lyt-2,3 markers usually represents a commitment to an eventual T-cell function. This commitment is made at the earliest stages of T-cell maturation because bone-marrow-derived precursor T cells develop into Lyt-2,3 positive or negative cells within hours after their entry into the thymus.

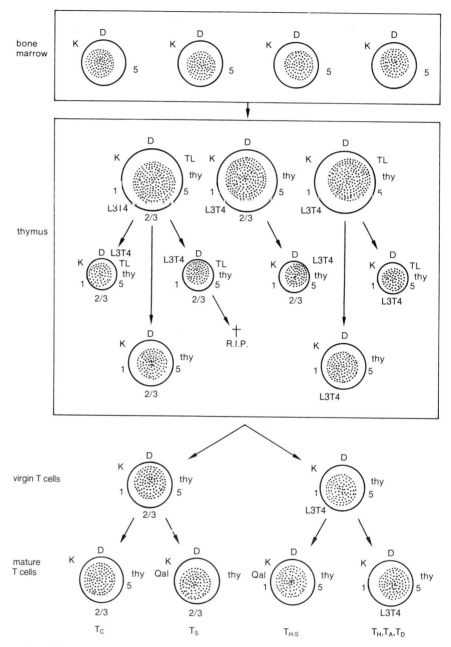

Figure 7-17 Putative maturational lineages for mouse T cells. Bone-marrow T-cell precursors lack any specific T-cell markers, but they express the Ly-5 marker, which distinguishes lymphocytes from other hematopoietic cells. Outer cortical lymphoblasts, which are already divided into Lyt-2,3 defined subpopulations, divide to give rise to progeny in the deep cortex, the medulla, and the emigrating virgin T-cell pool. A high proportion of deep, cortical, small thymic lymphocytes die; they are unusual because they do not express detectable levels of the class I MHC marker, H-2K. The emigrant pool is phenotypically identical to the medullary pool, and it lacks the early thymic lymphocyte marker TL. Mature peripheral T cells of defined function (T_S, T_C, T_H, T_A, T_D) are usually identifiable by their expression of the Lyt-2,3 markers.

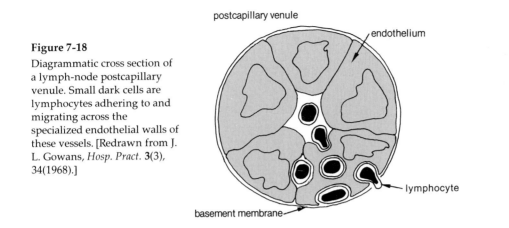

Figure 7-18
Diagrammatic cross section of a lymph-node postcapillary venule. Small dark cells are lymphocytes adhering to and migrating across the specialized endothelial walls of these vessels. [Redrawn from J. L. Gowans, *Hosp. Pract.* **3**(3), 34(1968).]

7-6 B cells and T cells home to specific lymphoid organs

Both virgin and mature B and T cells carry on their surfaces receptors that target them for preferential entry into particular lymphoid organs, such as peripheral lymph nodes, spleen, and Peyer's patches. This homing tendency is controlled by lymphocyte receptor interactions with complementary receptors on the large, specialized endothelial cells of the postcapillary venules. The interactions between these receptors permit immunocompetent B and T cells (but neither their precursors nor any other blood cells) to bind and traverse the venule walls (Figure 7-18). The selectivity of homing implies that the endothelial cells of postcapillary venules in different lymphoid organs display distinctive receptors. In mice at least two distinct lymphocyte receptor types exist; one governs homing to lymph node postcapillary venules, and the other governs homing to Peyer's patch postcapillary venules. These receptor interactions govern the tendency of lymphocytes in a particular lymphoid organ to return to that organ and, in addition, govern the characteristic ratio of T to B cells in different lymphoid organs (2.5 for lymph nodes, 0.5 for spleen, and 0.4 for Peyer's patches). Because this interaction is virtually the only mechanism for the selective entry of lymphocytes into lymphoid organs, it is critical for the embryogenesis of these organs and for the continuing maintenance of their lymphocyte populations. Thus it is also critical for the immune response itself.

A monoclonal antibody has been raised against a determinant at or near the lymphocyte receptor for lymph node postcapillary venule high endothelial cells, but it does not react with molecules at or near the Peyer's patch homing receptor. Staining of lymphoid organs with this antibody reveals the architectural localization of cells capable of migrating to lymph nodes when released into the bloodstream. For

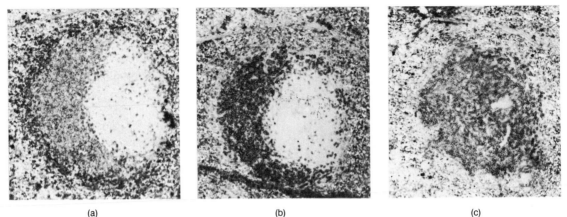

(a)   (b)   (c)

Figure 7-19   Localization of B-cell subsets in the spleen by immunoperoxidase staining. (a) All B cells in the follicles and the marginal zone are stained by anti-μ chain reagents, whereas only follicular B cells also stain with anti-δ chain reagents (b). Staining with a monoclonal antibody to lymph-node homing, receptor-associated antigens in (c) reveals that follicular T and B cells stain positively, whereas B_μ cells in the marginal zones do not. [Photos courtesy of Roger Reichert.]

example, several experiments have implied that virgin B cells are newly developed in the bone marrow, are B_μ, and can home to spleen but not lymph nodes. Figure 7-19 demonstrates that lymph node, homing receptor negative B_μ cells are localized to the splenic marginal zones, whereas mature lymph node, homing receptor positive $B_{\mu+\delta}$ spleen cells are concentrated in the splenic primary follicles.

7-7   Lymphoid tumors provide clonal cell populations at particular developmental stages

Cancers of the lymphoid system

Cancers of the lymphoid system are among the best-studied animal and human malignancies. In animals they appear to be induced by DNA or RNA tumor viruses, which may be either rapidly transforming or slowly transforming agents (Concept 13-3). If a lymphoid cancer is localized to a lymphoid organ, it is called a *lymphoma*. However, if the cancer cells reside primarily in the blood and bone marrow or spill into the blood, they are called *leukemias*. The etiology of lymphomas and leukemias and the host immune responses to them are discussed in Chapter 13. These tumors are experimentally useful because they make available for study clonal populations of cells at particular stages of B-cell and T-cell development.

Usefulness of mouse B- and T-cell lymphomas

Leukemias and lymphomas in mice represent some of the best-studied examples of lymphoid tumors. The use of inbred mouse strains with specific properties of tumor susceptibility, immune responsiveness, and viral infectivity has provided several important experimental systems. Lymphoid tumors occur in mice spontaneously, or they can be induced by X irradiation, chemical carcinogens, or viruses. However, the nonviral induction of these tumors almost always involves the activation of an intracellular RNA leukemia virus. Many B-cell and T-cell lymphomas and leukemias have been induced and examined; they represent many different stages in the development of B and T cells. The usefulness of such clonal tumor lines is illustrated by studies on the homing of B cells and T cells.

B-cell lymphomas may show particular homing patterns that correlate with the stage of cell maturation they represent. For example, one $B_{\mu+\delta}$ cell lymphoma with high surface IgM and low surface IgD was found predominantly in bone marrow and spleen. These lymphoma cells homed selectively to the spleen and were absolutely dependent on the spleen for growth. Subsequent analysis of normal B cells with high IgM to IgD ratios indicated that they, too, were found predominantly in bone marrow and spleen, whereas normal cells with low IgM to IgD ratios were found predominantly in lymph nodes. Thus this tumor provides a clonal model for the study of one subset of B cells.

Similarly, T-cell lymphomas can be used to study the homing of subsets of T cells. For example, some T-cell lymphomas, although still restricted to a thymic stage of development, nonetheless possess cell-surface receptors for the specialized endothelial cells in the postcapillary venules of particular lymphoid organs, such as Peyer's patches or peripheral lymph nodes. Interestingly, their pattern of homing appears to correlate with their pattern of *metastasis* (formation of secondary cancers at a distance from the primary cancer; see Concept 13-2). Thus the study of homing of these T-cell lymphomas, as well as some B-cell lymphomas, may provide information for both the chemistry and biology of the receptors on the specialized endothelial cells, as well as for the understanding of how and why particular tumors metastasize.

Selected Bibliography

Origins and development of the hematolymphoid system

Dexter, T. M., Allen, T. D., Lajtha, L. G., Knizsa, F., and Testa, N. G., "*In vitro* analysis of self-renewal and commitment of hematopoietic stem cells," in *Differentiation of Normal and Neoplastic Hematopoietic Cells*, Eds. Clarkson, B., Marks, P. A., and Till, J. E., p. 433(1978).

Ford, C. E., Micklem, H. S., Evans, E. P., Gray, J. G., and Ogden, D. A., "The inflow of bone-marrow cells to the thymus. Studies with part body-irradiated mice injected with chromosome-marked bone marrow and subjected to antigenic stimulation," *Ann. N.Y. Acad. Sci.* **129**, 283(1966).

LeDouarin, N. M., and Jotereau, F., "Tracing of cells of the avian thymus through embryonic life in interspecific chimeras," *J. Exp. Med.* **142**, 17(1975).

Moore, M. A. S., and Owen, J. J. T., "Experimental studies on the development of the thymus," *J. Exp. Med.* **126**, 715(1967).

Till, J. E., and McCulloch, E. A., "A direct measurement of the radiation sensitivity of normal mouse bone marrow cells," *Radiat. Res.* **14**, 213(1961).

Weissman, I., Papaioannou, V., and Gardner, R., "Fetal hematopoietic origins of the adult hematolymphoid system," Cold Spring Harbor Meeting on *Differentiation of Normal and Neoplastic Hematopoietic Cells*, pp. 37–47(1978).

Wolf, N. S., and Trentin, J. J., "Hemopoietic colony studies V: Effect of hemopoietic organ stroma on differentiation of pluripotent stem cells," *J. Exp. Med.* **127**, 205(1968).

Wu, A. M., Till, J. E., Siminovitch, K., and McCulloch, E. A., "Cytological evidence for a relationship between normal hematopoietic colony-forming cells and cells of the lymphoid system," *J. Exp. Med.* **127**, 455(1968).

The preceding papers describe research that helped put hematolymphoid differentiation on an experimental and quantitative cellular basis. The experiments by Till's and Ford's groups deal with the total differentiative potential of hematopoietic stem cells. The paper by Wolf and Trentin describes the microenvironmental induction of a particular differentiation pathway. The papers by LeDouarin's and Owen's groups demonstrate that hematopoietic precursors seed the developing thymus in a nonrandom fashion.

The thymus and T lymphocytes

Cantor, H., and Boyse, E. A., "Functional subclasses of T lymphocytes bearing different Ly antigens I: The generation of functionally distinct T cell subclasses is a differentiative process independent of antigen," *J. Exp. Med.* **141**, 1375(1975).

Miller, J. F. A. P., "Immunological function of the thymus," *Lancet* **ii**, 748(1961).

Weissman, I. L., "Thymus cell migration," *J. Exp. Med.* **126**, 291(1967).

Weissman, I. L., Rouse, R. V., Kyewski, B. A., Lepault, F., Butcher, E. C., Kaplan, H. S., and Scollay, R. G., "Thymic lymphocyte maturation in the thymic microenvironment," in *Behring Institute Mitteilungen*, "The Influence of the Thymus on the Generation of the T Cell Repertoire." Presented at the International Workshop, Rudesheim, September 16–19, 1981. (F. R. Seiler and H. G. Schwick, Eds.), pp. 242–251(1982).

The preceding papers define the role of the thymus in immunological maturation, the cellular basis for the development of peripheral T cells, and the division of peripheral T lymphocytes into functional subpopulations.

Development of B lymphocytes

Moller, G. (ed.), "B cell differentiation antigens," *Immunol. Rev.* **69**, (1982).

Szenberg, A., and Warner, N. L., "Dissociation of immunological responsiveness in fowls with a hormonally arrested development of lymphoid tissues," *Nature* **194**, 146(1962).

Weissman, I. L., "Development and distribution of immunoglobulin-bearing cells in mice," *Transplant. Rev.* **24**, 159(1975).

Whitlock, C. A., and Witte, O. N., "Long-term culture of B lymphocytes and their precursors from murine bone marrow," *Proc. Nat. Acad. Sci. USA* **79**, 3608(1982).

The preceding sources describe the development of B-cell lines, the controversy as to their sites of development, their functional subpopulations, and some preliminary research into their maturational sequences.

Physiology of the lymphocyte and compartmentalization in lymphoid organs

Butcher, E. C., Kraal, G., Stevens, S. K., and Weissman, I. L., "A recognition function of endothelial cells: Directing lymphocyte traffic," in *Pathobiology of the Endothelial Cell*, Academic Press, New York, 1982, pp. 409–424.

Gowans, J. L., and Knight, E. J., "The route of recirculation of lymphocytes in the rat," *Proc. R. Soc. Lond.* [Biol.] **159**, 257(1964).

The preceding papers define the types of antigen-independent cellular interactions, between lymphoid and nonlymphoid cells, that result in the establishment and maintenance of lymphocyte migration pathways in peripheral lymphoid organs.

Additional concept presented in the problems

Chromosomal, radioactive, and cell-surface antigenic markers to study hematolymphoid cell lineages. Problems 7-5, 7-6, 7-7, and 7-8.

Problems

7-1 Indicate whether each of the following statements is true or false. Explain the error in each statement you consider to be false.
(a) T cells first appear in humans prior to the sixth month of gestation.
(b) B cells that enter the spleen home to the lymphoid white pulp of the periarteriolar sheath.
(c) Antigenic stimulation of macrophages in the thymus will trigger their differentiation into T cells.
(d) T cells are derived from hematopoietic stem cells.
(e) Monocytes and T and B lymphocytes all possess surface receptors that enable them to home to particular lymphoid organs by recognition of specialized endothelial cells in those organs.
(f) Pre-B lymphocytes express cytoplasmic μ chains prior to expressing surface IgM molecules.
(g) T_H and T_C lymphocytes share a common postthymic ancestor.

7-2 Supply the missing word or words in each of the following statements.
(a) Antigen enters lymph nodes via _____ , whereas it enters the spleen via _____ _____ .

(b) _____ are the blood counterparts of tissue mast cells.
(c) During embryogenesis, hematopoietic stem cells are first found in the _____ ; then later they are found in the _____ and _____ . Finally they are limited to the _____ _____ in late gestation and throughout postnatal life.
(d) In mice, effector T_C cells express Lyt antigens _____ and _____ , whereas in humans $_C$ cells express _____ and _____ antigens.
(e) Lymphocytes leaving most lymph nodes first enter _____ _____ , and then collect into a major _____ _____ before reentering the venous system.
(f) An infection that develops in the skin causes a local immune response in the _____ _____ _____ , whereas an infection of the blood induces an immune response in the _____ .
(g) Maldevelopment of the third and fourth anterior endodermal pouches will lead to a deficiency in the development of _____ lymphocytes.

7-3 Choose the specified surface determinants from column B that best characterize each of the specific subpopulation of mouse cells from column A.

Table 7-5 Distribution of Labeled Cells Following Infusion of ^{3}H-Nucleosides into the Thymus (Problem 7-5)

Organ and Tissue	Percentage Thymus-Derived Cells[a]			
	Adult		Newborn	
	Adenosine Label	Thymidine Label	Adenosine Label	Thymidine Label
Thymus	100	100	100	100
Splenic white pulp	2.9	0.024	9	18
Splenic red pulp	0	—	0	—
Mesenteric node, whole	0.51	—	19	12
Mesenteric node, diffuse cortex	2.7	0.12	—	—
Cervical node, whole	0.44	—	—	—
Cervical node, diffuse cortex	1.6	—	—	—
Bone marrow	0.017	—	0	—
Intestinal mucosa	0	—	0	—

[a]Measured by autoradiograph of tissue slices 24 hours after administration of labeled nucleoside; normalized to 100% for whole thymus. (—) indicates not measured.
[From I. L. Weissman, *J. Exp. Med.* **126,** 291(1967). Copyright © 1967 by The Rockefeller University Press.]

Column A:
(1) All T cells
(2) Mast cells
(3) Epidermal Langerhans cells, macrophages, thymic epithelial cells, and subsets of B and T cells
(4) Most if not all nucleated cells in the mouse
(5) B cells
(6) A functional subset of T cells involved in helper functions (T_H and T_A)

Column B:
H-2K and H-2D antigens
Ia antigens
Thy-1

Lyt-1$^+$ Lyt-2,3$^-$

Immunoglobulin receptors for antigen
Receptors for the Fc portion of IgE

7-4 A mouse heterozygous for H-2 haplotype and immunoglobulin allotype has the following genotype: H-2$^{b/d}$ and Ig$^{a/c}$. What combination of these alleles will be expressed on the surface of a B cell? On the surface of a T cell?

7-5 (a) A cellular immunologist wished to trace the fate of thymocytes in adult and newborn mice. He labeled thymus cells in living animals by infusing ^{3}H-adenosine or ^{3}H-thymidine into the thymus with a microneedle, and then 24 hours later

Table 7-6 Antibody Staining of Lymphocytes from Mice Whose Thymus Was Infused with Fluorescein Isothiocyanate 2 Hours Earlier (Problem 7-5)

Rhodaminated Antibody Used for Counterstain	Percentage Cells Stained			
	Thymocytes		Lymph-Node Cells	
	All Cells	Green Cells	All Cells	Green Cells
Monoclonal anti-dextran (control)	<0.5	<0.5	<0.5	<0.5
Monoclonal anti-κ light chain	<2	<0.5	28	<0.5
Monoclonal anti-Thy-1	99	98	68	98
Monoclonal anti-Lyt-1	97	98	69	99
Monoclonal anti-Lyt-2	85	84	20	29

[From R. Scollay, E. Butcher, and I. L. Weissman, *Eur. J. Immunol.* **10,** 210(1980).]

he measured the percent of thymus cell migrants among the cells of various tissues. From the data shown in Table 7-5, what can you conclude about the homing specificity of thymus cell migrants?

(b) How might you explain the differences between the results of adenosine and thymidine labeling in adults?

(c) Compare the results obtained with adults and newborns, and propose an hypothesis to explain any differences you observe.

(d) Fifteen years later that same cellular immunologist had another idea, and he infused the mouse thymus with a green fluorescent marker (fluorescein isothiocyanate) that conjugates to living cells. Cells emigrating from the thymus were stained green when examined with a fluorescent microscope. When he counterstained such cells with antibodies conjugated with a red fluorochrome (tetramethylrhodamine isothiocyanate), he obtained the distribution of stained cells shown in Table 7-6. What are the phenotype and percent representation of the major class of cells emigrating from the thymus?

(e) What are the phenotype and percent of the minor class of cells emigrating from the thymus?

(f) Do these results support the hypothesis that all T_H and T_C cells are derived from Lyt-1^+,2^+,3^+ postthymic precursors?

(g) Why is there such a discrepancy in the staining of migrants versus all cells when the antibody is anti-κ?

(h) What are the comparative frequencies of Lyt-1^+,2^+ cells in all node T cells versus node T-cell migrants?

(i) Table 7-7 shows the results of a total accounting of fluorescein labeled cells 24 hours after thymic infusion. Previous studies had shown that ~85% of thymus cells that are labeled *in situ* remain as nondividing cells in the thymus for 3–5 days and then disappear. What percent of cells in the thymus emigrate per day?

(j) What is the fate of most thymic lymphocytes?

Table 7-7 Distribution of Green Cells 24 Hours after Thymic Infusion with Fluorescein Isothiocyanate (Problem 7-5)

Organ Examined	Number of Stained Cells/Organ
Thymus	8×10^7
Spleen	2×10^5
All lymph nodes combined	4×10^5
Blood	1×10^4
Liver, kidney, heart combined	$< 1 \times 10^3$
Brain	$< 1 \times 10^3$
Lung	$\sim 1 \times 10^3$
Muscle	$< 1 \times 10^3$
Intestines (excluding Peyer's patches)	$< 1 \times 10^3$
Bone marrow	2×10^3

[From R. Scollay, E. Butcher, and I. L. Weissman, *Eur. J. Immunol.* **10**, 210(1980).]

7-6 (a) CBA/H T6/T6 mice have a pair of very small metacentric chromosomes, called T6, which arise from fusion of two telocentric chromosomes at their centromeres. CBA/H mice have 20 pairs of telocentric chromosomes, with no metacentric T6 chromosomes. F_1 progeny of matings between these strains (CBA/H T6/T6 × CBA/H)F_1 have one T6 chromosome. The T6 chromosome is used as a convenient marker to follow cells of different origin in the following experiments.

Fifty-day-old CBA/H mice that had been neonatally thymectomized were grafted with thymus from newborn (CBA/H T6/T6 × CBA/H)F_1 mice and injected intraperitoneally with 10^6 CBA/H T6/T6 cells from various hematopoietic organs. The cells containing T6 are scored as percentage of metaphase cells with metacentric chromosome(s). Why is there a delay in the appearance of T6/T6 cells in lymph nodes? (See Figure 7-20.)

(b) In another experiment, the host mice were either given donor cells alone (without thymus graft) or grafted with a thymus contained in a diffusion chamber. No T6/T6 cells could be found in the lymph nodes although a small but significant reconstitution of T-cell functions was restored in these mice. What is the effect of a thymus on migration of T6/T6 cells to lymph nodes? How might this effect be operating?

(c) The thymus graft in the first experiment was excised after 25 days and regrafted into another neonatally thymectomized CBA/H host. The percentage of T6/T6 cells in the metaphase cell population in lymph nodes was scored after the following different treatments, which stimulate particular subpopulations of lymphoid cells.

	No treatment	PHA	LPS	MLR
Percent of T6/T6 cells in metaphase population	18	13	0	14

PHA = Phytohemagglutinin
LPS = Salmonella lipopolysaccharides
MLR = Mixed lymphocyte reaction using C57BL/6 cells as stimulator

What conclusions can you draw from this experiment?

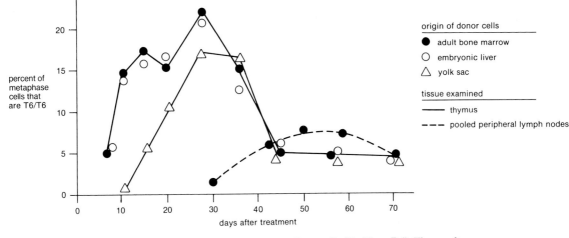

Figure 7-20 Percentage of metaphase cells with T6/T6 karyotype in two tissues at various times after intraperitoneal injection of three types of T6/T6 donor cells (Problem 7-6). The results shown are based on several experiments by C. E. Ford, J. E. Harris, and H. S. Micklem.

(d) What cell-surface marker(s) would you expect to find on the T6/T6 cells in the thymus and in the lymph node, respectively?

(e) If the grafted thymus in the first experiment were transferred to a second host along with a normal CBA/H thymus, T6/T6 cells could later be found in lymph nodes but not in the normal CBA/H thymus. What does this result tell you about the migration route of T cells?

(f) Looking back at Figure 7-20, why does the percentage of T6/T6 cells in the thymus decrease after 30 days? What might you expect to happen if the host mice were lethally irradiated before grafting?

(g) Why does yolk sac repopulate the thymus more slowly than adult bone marrow or embryonic liver in the first experiment and not at all in this experiment?

(h) Whenever a thymus is grafted, there is a massive necrosis of resident lymphocytes because of a lack of a functional blood vessel supply for 2–3 days. Thus these experiments are open to some question because one is not studying a physiological preparation. In addition to this methodological problem, can you think of another potential error concerning the analysis of cell traffic patterns using T6 markers?

7-7 When 10^4 to 10^5 viable bone-marrow cells are injected into lethally irradiated mice, distinct nodules appear in the host spleen, representing foci of cell proliferation. Each nodule consists of the clonal progeny of one cell called a *colony forming unit* (CFU), and it can be of either erythropoietic, granulocytic, or mixed type.

To study the relationship of CFUs to cells of the lymphoid system, genetic markers were introduced into normal bone-marrow cells using gamma irradiation. This method produces a variety of chromosomal aberrations that are useful as markers, each of which is unique to a given clone of cells. Following irradiation, the bone-marrow cells were injected into *unirradiated* W/W^v congenitally anemic mice (which have defective stem cells unable to form spleen colonies). After 2–6 months, the thymus and lymph nodes were examined for the presence of chromosomal markers. Simultaneously, bone-marrow cells from these same animals were injected into irradiated mice, and the resulting spleen colonies were examined for cells with the same chromosomal aberrations. The results of one such experiment are presented in Table 7-8. Answer the following questions with reference to the table.

(a) Is there a direct correlation between spleen CFU stem cells and thymus-repopulating stem cells? Discuss your answer in terms of a scheme of hematolymphoid maturation.

(b) Does mouse number 5 represent evidence for a common lymphoid (B and T) and hematopoietic stem cell? Discuss your answer.

(c) Devise an experiment that tests for the presence or absence of pluripotent stem cells, lymphoid stem cells, and thymic stem cells using the approach described in this problem and any antibody reagents already discussed.

7-8 It is possible to extract factors in crude form from various lymphoid organs and assess their effect *in vitro* on undifferentiated cells—for example, cells from bone marrow or embryonic liver in the mouse.

Table 7-9 shows data generated by one group of researchers who incubated bone-marrow cells from normal mice with a series of factors isolated from thymus and spleen and then studied the cells for both the *de novo* appearance of cell-surface antigens and for functional capability.

(a) Why were the preceding surface markers chosen as criteria in evaluating the effects of the factors tested? How might one assay for the presence of a surface marker on a population of cells?

(b) What is the significance of the data generated when treated cells were used as a source of helper activity in an *in vitro* response to sheep red blood cell antigens?

(c) Only the thymus, and not the spleen, is a good source of inductive factors. Why might this be true?

Table 7-8 Presence of Chromosomally Marked Bone-Marrow Cells in Spleens of Injected Congenitally Anemic Mice (Problem 7-7)

| Mouse No. | Time Interval After Injection (Days) | Chromosomal Aberration (Marker) | Percent of Cells with Marker | | Number of CFU Spleen Colonies with Marker |
			Lymph Nodes	Thymus	
1	65	Long (type 1)	0	56	2/25
2	65	Minute (type 1)	0	80	24/24
3	84	Metacentric	0	76	13/13
4	83	Long (type 2)	0	80	12/15
5	174	Minute (type 2)	65	84	7/7

[Data from Wu et al., *J. Exp. Med.* **127**, 455(1968).]

Table 7-9 Effects of Lymphoid Organ Factors on *in Vitro* Differentiation of Bone-Marrow Cells (Problem 7-8)

Material Tested	Percent of Cells Expressing:		Helper Activity of Treated Cells: Antibody-Forming Cells per Culture
	Thy-1	TL	
Untreated cells	0	0	1,3
Medium only	1%	0	2,2
Mouse thymus factor	23%	20%	184,223
Mouse spleen factor	<5%	1%	0,12

The data in column three represent number of plaque-forming cells producing antibody to sheep red blood cells as measured in the Jerne plaque assay. Results of two independent experiments are shown in each line.

Answers

7-1 (a) True
     (b) False. B cells that enter the spleen home to follicles on the outside of the sheath.
     (c) False. Macrophages do not belong to the lymphocyte lineage and never differentiate into T cells.
     (d) True
     (e) False. Monocytes do not possess such receptors; only T and B lymphocytes possess them.
     (f) True
     (g) False. Current evidence places the separation of the T_C and the T_H lineages at a prethymic or early thymic developmental stage.

7-2 (a) Lymphatics, blood vessels
     (b) Basophiles
     (c) yolk sac, liver, spleen, bone marrow
     (d) 2 and 3, T5 and T8
     (e) efferent lymphatics, thoracic duct
     (f) draining lymph node, spleen
     (g) T

7-3 Column   Column
     A   B
     1   Thy-1
     2   Receptors for the Fc-portion of IgE
     3   Ia antigens
     4   H-2K and H-2D antigens
     5   Immunoglobulin receptors for antigen
     6   Lyt-1$^+$, Lyt-2$^+$, 3$^-$

7-4 All B cells will express both H-2 haplotypes b and d, but each B cell will express only one of the two Ig allotypes, a or c, because of allelic exclusion. T cells also will express H-2$^{b/d}$, but neither Ig^a or Ig^c, because T cells do not express immunoglobulins.

7-5 (a) Thymus cell migrants home to lymph nodes and spleen but not to intestine. In spleen, they home to white pulp, and in lymph nodes, to diffuse cortex. White pulp and diffuse cortex contain the thymus-dependent areas (domains) of spleen and lymph nodes, respectively.

(b) Thymus cells labeled *in situ* with ^{3}H-adenosine migrate rapidly to the periphery, whereas cells labeled with ^{3}H-thymidine migrate much more slowly. Because ^{3}H-adenosine is incorporated into both DNA and RNA, it probably labels all thymus cells. ^{3}H-thymidine labels only cells that are in the process of dividing and are synthesizing DNA. These cells must apparently undergo some thymic maturation prior to migration.

(c) A higher proportion of peripheral lymphocytes are thymus cell migrants in newborns as compared to adults. Moreover, most of these migrants appear to be cells that were in the process of DNA synthesis and division during the labeling period because they are labeled approximately equally by adenosine or thymidine. The higher proportion of migrants in newborns could be explained either by a higher rate of thymus cell production and migration or by entry of migrants into a smaller pool of preexisting cells. It is not yet known which of these explanations is correct.

(d) Thy-1$^+$ Lyt-1$^+$ Lyt-2$^-$ Ig Kappa$^-$ ($\sim$70%)

(e) Thy-1$^+$ Lyt-1$^+$,2$^+$,3$^+$ Ig Kappa$^-$ ($\sim$30%)

(f) No; the two major classes of functional T cells are mainly defined by Lyt markers—T_H = Lyt-2$^-$,3$^-$, and T_C = Lyt-1$^-$,2$^+$,3$^+$. Thymus cell migrants are already divided into these two classes.

(g) B cells represent $\sim$30% of the total lymph node population but less than 0.5% of the thymus cell migrant (T-cell) population.

(h) All lymph-node T cells: Lyt-1$^+$,2$^+$ = 29%. Lymph-node thymus cell immigrants: Lyt-1$^+$,2$^+$ = 29%.

(i) $\sim$1%

(j) They disappear and probably die in the thymus.

7-6 (a) Because T6/T6 cells appear earlier in the thymus than in lymph nodes, the cells presumably have to pass through the thymus before migrating to the lymph nodes.

(b) The thymus is required for these T6/T6 cells to acquire the ability to migrate to lymph nodes. Diffusible factors released from the thymus are not sufficient, suggesting a requirement for a cell-cell contact (or "short-range" factor) in the thymus microenvironment.

(c) These T6/T6 cells in lymph nodes are T cells. (With LPS, B cells of the host origin are stimulated to proliferate, obscuring the presence of T6/T6 T cells.) With the T-cell mitogen, you stimulate T cells of both host origin and of T6/T6 donor origin. Their proportions after and before stimulation are roughly equal.

(d) Thymus thymocytes: TL$^+$, Thy-1$^+$, Lyt-1$^+$,2$^+$,3$^+$, some Lyt-1$^+$,2$^-$3$^-$. Lymph node T cells: TL$^-$, Thy-1$^+$, Lyt-1$^+$,2$^+$,3+ (30%), Lyt-1$^+$,2$^-$3$-$ (70%).

(e) The T cells that have migrated out of the thymus do not return.

(f) In the grafted thymus, there will be a *fixed* number of T6 cells present at the time of transplantation, a *fixed* number of T6/T6 cells that migrated in after the thymus transplantation, and a *continuous* source of non-T6 cells from the host. As the T6/T6 cells mature and migrate out, their percentage in the mitotic population decreases. If the host were irradiated before grafting, the continuous source of host non-T6 cells would be lost, and the percentage of T6/T6 metaphase cells would initially go up to a maximum higher than that in the first experiment. Assuming that the immigrant T6/T6 and T6 populations behave in the same way, their relative percentages would be maintained. If the host bone marrow were seeded by injected T6/T6 hemopoietic cells, then the thymus would be repopulated with T6/T6 cells (approaching 100%).

(g) The thymus-seeking hematopoietic cells are themselves generated by bone-marrow hematopoiesis, presumably from yolk sac pluripotential stem cells that settled into a bone-marrow inductive microenvironment. These progenitors of T cells are apparently lacking in the yolk sac, induced efficiently in the bone marrow, and induced inefficiently in the spleen.

(h) T6 markers can be detected only in dividing cells at metaphase. Because only primitive thymic lymphocytes and antigen- or mitogen-activated lymphocytes divide, one is sampling only a small percentage of the total population, and a nonrandom subset at that. It would be better to use a marker that is easily detected on all cells and does not compromise the acceptability or differentiation of the marked cells.

7-7 (a) No. Pluripotential stem cells that can give rise to spleen colonies appear *not* to be the direct progenitors of T-cell precursors. T-cell precursors are generated in the bone-marrow microenvironment and are self-sustaining thereafter. Thus there can be a large discrepancy between the frequencies of spleen colony-forming stem cells and thymic progenitors in the same marrow, as shown in the experiment.

(b) Not necessarily. Unfortunately the lymph-node cells showing the minute marker chromosome were not analyzed for their T- or B-cell status in these experiments, which were done in the same year that T and B cells were first recognized as distinct lineages.

(c) Such a test could be made by preirradiating the bone-marrow donor as done previously but then isolating cells from the W/W^v recipient by the presence of B-cell and T-cell surface markers *before* doing the chromosome spread to check for chromosome markers. It is also possible to use irradiated marrow from mice whose Lyb-2, IgM, IgD, Lyt-1,2,3, and Thy-1 alleles are different from the W/W^v host. One could then analyze *only* those B or T cells expressing donor allotypic markers.

7-8 (a) Thy-1 is expressed on all T cells but not on bone-marrow precursors of T cells; TL is expressed only on immature thymocytes. One can use the antibodies to define individual cells—for example, by immunofluorescence—and in that way detect conversion of even a small percent of cells from marker positive.

(b) This experiment shows that bone-marrow cells are not induced only to express markers of the first stage of T-cell development (pre-Tthymocyte); it also shows that at least some cells complete their maturation (thymocyteT_H cell). It is now believed that several distinct thymic factors are involved in this multistep differentiation pathway.

(c) If the factors are produced by thymic epithelial cells, the spleen lacks them.

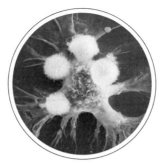

CHAPTER 8

The Immune Response

Chapter Outline

8-8 Associated recognition appears to be a general property of T cells
Associated recognition
Function of associated recognition
What is the nature of T-cell receptors?

8-9 MHC genes control immune responsiveness
Nature of high and low immune responsiveness
Possible controlling mechanisms

Entry of antigen into the body triggers an amazing defensive system. The antigen is trapped by accessory cells, and its antigenic determinants are presented efficiently to B and T lymphocytes. Antigen-stimulated B and T cells interact specifically with one another to trigger proliferation and differentiation into effector cells. These terminally differentiated cells and their products combine with the antigen and initiate several overlapping mechanisms for its elimination. The immune system, with its genetic control of cellular diversity, its elaborate architecture that promotes cellular interactions, its intricate patterns of antigen-specific cellular associations, its precise elimination mechanisms, and its cell-based memory for antigen, rivals the central nervous system in sensitivity, specificity, and complexity. This chapter considers the cellular biology of the vertebrate immune response.

Concepts

8-1 Immune responses to foreign antigen result from cascades of cellular interactions

Immune response cascade

Vertebrates react to foreign antigen with a cascade of molecular and cellular associations that leads to the humoral and cellular immune responses (Figure 8-1). Upon entry into the body, foreign antigen is trapped by accessory cells and concentrated in lymphoid organs (Concept 7-1). Two classes of mature T cells, *helper* T_H cells and *amplifying* T_A cells, interact with antigen presented by accessory cells, proliferate, and differentiate to their effector forms. Effector T_H cells specifically interact with mature B cells in the presence of antigen, thereby inducing these B cells to proliferate and differentiate into plasma cells, which are responsible for antibody secretion and humoral immunity. In an analogous fashion, effector T_A cells stimulate proliferation and differentiation of T_C cells. The resulting effector T_C cells are cytotoxic for antigen-bearing target cells and are responsible in part for cellular immunity. An additional aspect of cellular immunity is provided by effector T_D cells (*delayed hypersensitivity*), which help to wall off and to contain antigen at its site of entry by initiating inflammatory responses. A fifth class of T cells, *suppressor* T_S cells, which is involved

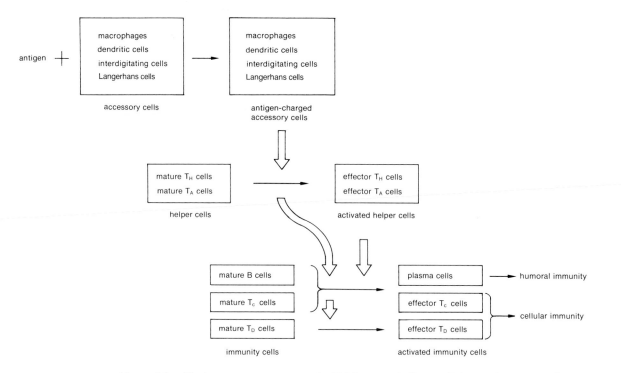

Figure 8-1   The immune response cascade. Thick arrows indicate cellular participation in the transitions indicated by the thin arrows.

in tolerance and regulation of the immune response, is discussed in detail in Chapter 10. Each of the cellular interactions in the immunity cascade is governed by the gene products of the MHC. Although the major pathways for immune responses have been worked out, the molecular details are far from clear.

Changes in lymphoid organs

Immune responses are initiated in the lymphoid organs. Antigen is first taken up by macrophages at the site of entry. Within a day or two, adherent or processed antigen appears on the surface of other accessory cells in the B-cell and T-cell domains of lymphoid organs. Circulating mature B and T cells, which are small cells with dense nuclei surrounded by a thin layer of cytoplasm, enter the lymphoid organ via specialized postcapillary venules (Concept 7-1). Upon encountering cognate antigen bound to accessory cells, first T cells and subsequently B cells enlarge, initiate DNA synthesis, proliferate, and differentiate into effector cells. During the first 2 days following antigenic stimulation, antigen-specific lymphocyte clones are retained within the lymphoid organ that contains the antigen, and these clones are largely depleted from the circulating lymphocyte population.

The proliferation and differentiation of activated B and T cells are associated with changes in the morphology of the lymph organ (Fig-

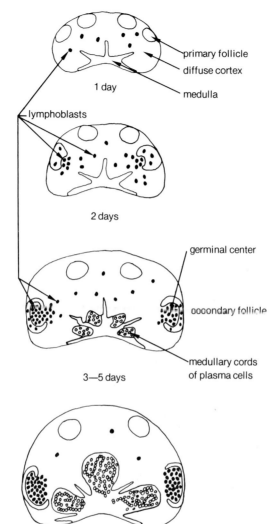

Figure 8-2
Morphological changes in a lymph node after stimulation with antigen. The diagram depicts the time course of antigen-dependent changes in multicellular structures, and it emphasizes changes in size and shape of the separate lymphoid compartments, caused largely by selective proliferation and altered movement patterns of lymphocyte subclasses. Analogous changes occur in antigen-activated spleen.

ure 8-2). The wave of T-cell division in the diffuse cortex is followed closely by B-cell division in the primary follicles. Some T cells migrate into the follicle where a focus of dividing B and T cells, as well as active macrophages, builds up to form a *germinal center*, which compresses the follicle into a crescent around it. Follicles with germinal centers, which are known as *secondary follicles*, appear 4–5 days after antigen stimulation and may remain for several days (Figure 8-3). At the same time, plasma cells (effector B cells) begin to settle between the sinusoids of the medulla to form medullary cords. Memory B cells and memory and effector T cells percolate through the lymph node and eventually reenter the general circulation. Although most plasma

Figure 8-3

Microscopic views of antigen and germinal centers in antigen-draining lymph nodes. (a) Labeled antigen detected by autoradiography inside a digestive vacuole or phagolysosome (p1) of a macrophage. [Courtesy of J. J. Miller III.] (b) An autoradiogram of labeled antigen adhering to the processes of follicular dendritic reticular cells. [Courtesy of J. J. Miller III and G. J. V. Nossal.] (c) The distribution of antigen within a primary follicle 1 to 2 days after immunization, shown by immunofluorescence. [Courtesy of J. J. Miller III.] (d) Immunofluorescence of antigen bound to follicular dendritic reticular cells that have been compressed into a crescent by the development of a germinal center. [Courtesy of J. J. Miller III.] (e) Immuno-histochemical identification of Lyt-1 T cells in the upper pole of a germinal center. [Photomicrograph by R. Rouse and I. Weissman.] (f), (g), (h) Views of an antigen-stimulated lymph node with abundant germinal centers. The germinal center large B cells lack terminal sialic acids on cell-surface glycoproteins and are then stainable with the terminal galactose-specific lectin, PNA (linked to horseradish peroxidase for this immunohistochemical stain) in (f). These germinal center B cells also lose their lymphoid organ homing receptors, and

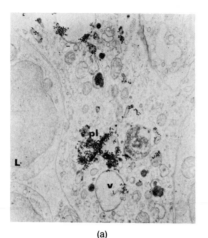

(a)

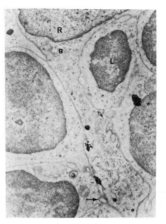

(b)

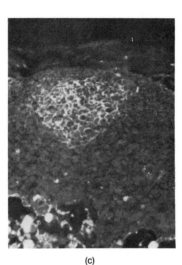

(c)

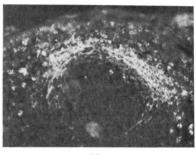

(d)

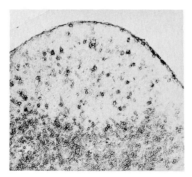

(e)

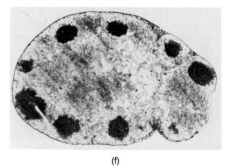

(f)

in (g) they are unstained (in contrast to surrounding small B and T cells) with a peroxidase-conjugated monoclonal antibody (MEL14) directed against a homing receptor. (h) Peroxidase-conjugated monoclonal antibodies to a determinant on the δ heavy chain do not stain germinal center B-cell lymphoblasts, but they do stain the surrounding mantle of follicular B cells. The germinal center B cells are B_μ in a primary response and B_γ in a secondary response. (i) and (j) Views of actively stimulated Peyer's patches with large germinal centers, (i) with PNA and (j) with MEL14. Peyer's patch germinal center B cells are B_α. [Courtesy of R. A. Reichert, W. M. Gallatin, I. L. Weissman, and E. C. Butcher.] [From *J. Exp. Med.* **157**, 813, (1983).]

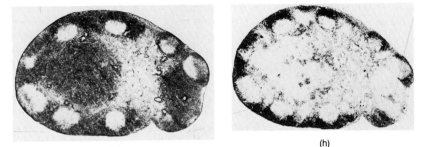

(g)　　　　　　　　(h)

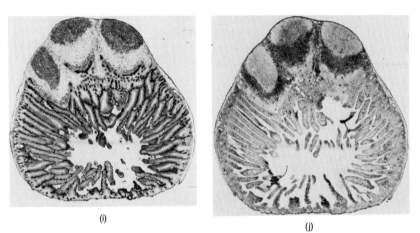

(i)　　　　　　　　(j)

cells are retained in the lymph node, the antibody molecules they secrete enter the general circulation.

Following antigenic stimulation of a lymphoid organ, activated B and T cells release soluble factors that attract macrophages and other phagocytes and cause local vessel dilation, which allows leakage of plasma fluids into the lymphoid organ. The combination of retention of normally circulating lymphocytes, specific cellular proliferation, increased fluid in the tissues (edema), and increased numbers of nonlymphoid cells causes the lymphoid organ to enlarge rapidly, resulting in the typical "swollen glands" of infection. The organs return to their original size only as the response to infection abates.

Affinity maturation and immunologic memory

Following a primary immunization, effector T cells and antibodies—first of the IgM class and then of the other secreted classes—appear in the bloodstream (Figure 8-4). The average affinity of these antibodies increases with time in a "learning" process termed *affinity maturation*. Following secondary immunization with the same antigen, large amounts of high affinity antibodies appear, mainly of the IgG classes (Figure 8-4). In cell-mediated immunity, secondary immunization leads to the rapid appearance of large numbers of effector T cells. Both

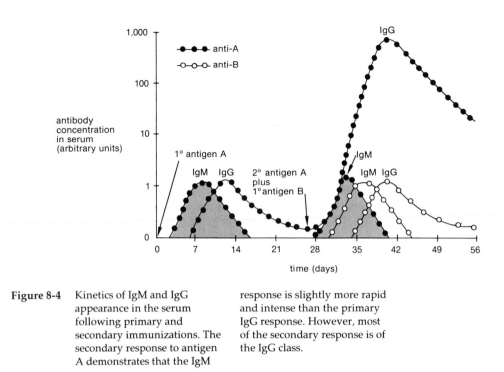

Figure 8-4 Kinetics of IgM and IgG appearance in the serum following primary and secondary immunizations. The secondary response to antigen A demonstrates that the IgM response is slightly more rapid and intense than the primary IgG response. However, most of the secondary response is of the IgG class.

the memory of previous antigenic exposure and the maturation of antibody affinity have a cellular basis—memory by increased clone size of cells responding to the antigen and affinity maturation by the competition for limiting amounts of antigen by T and B lymphocytes possessing the most avid receptors for the antigen (Figure 8-5).

8-2 The cellular basis of the immune response usually is studied under artificial conditions

Difficulties of experimentation

Because of the complexity of the cellular interactions that underlie the immune response, immunologists have had to develop model systems to study the roles of the individual cell types involved. The basic requirement for these systems is that relatively well-defined cell populations can be studied under conditions that provide both metabolic support and an appropriate environment for antigen recognition and response. This requirement was met first by the development of inbred strains of experimental animals for cell-transfer studies and later by various cell and tissue culture techniques. Immunologists continue to make more and more clever refinements of these systems. Such modifications often make the system less phys-

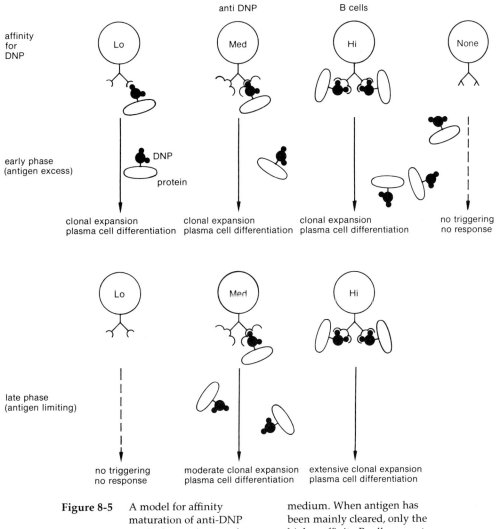

Figure 8-5   A model for affinity maturation of anti-DNP antibodies with time after antigenic stimulation. When antigen is abundant, all cognate clones respond, and the average affinity is low to medium. When antigen has been mainly cleared, only the higher affinity B cells compete for antigen and undergo full responses, and the resultant average antibody affinity is high.

iological, but they nevertheless lead to new and valid information. However, the potentially artifactual nature of these systems makes conflicting claims and observations difficult to evaluate, so that progress has been slow and cautious.

Adoptive transfer in inbred strains

Inbred strains of animals—produced by repeated brother–sister mating—allow transfer of cells and tissues between individuals of the same strain and sex without inducing transplantation immunity (Chapters 6 and 11). Using inbred strains, the immune status of a donor can be transferred to a recipient by injection of viable cells. However, to distinguish clearly between donor and recipient immune responses, such *adoptive transfer* experiments are usually performed with recipients whose lymphocytes have been removed or inactivated. These immunodeficient hosts must retain the essential cells and structures for antigen delivery and processing as well as the essential microenvironments for productive cellular collaboration, proliferation, and differentiation. Although a few genetically immunodeficient hosts are available, their rarity and difficulty of maintenance through successive breeding cycles limit their usefulness for adoptive transfer experiments. More commonly immunodeficient hosts are created artificially by X irradiation, removal of circulating lymphocytes, or prevention of T-cell development.

X irradiation is the method most widely used to prepare immunodeficient hosts for adoptive transfer of immunity. Small lymphocytes are exquisitely sensitive to X irradiation and undergo a unique cell death, which is termed *interphase death* because its expression does not require cell division. Almost all other cells in the body, including cells that assist in the immune response, sustain potentially lethal X-ray damage to their DNA but do not die until the first or second postradiation mitosis (*mitotic death*). Because the survival curve for interphase death is much steeper than for mitotic death (Figure 8-6) and because cells that are susceptible to mitotic death can function perfectly well unless stimulated to divide, it is possible to render a host relatively immunodeficient by administering a dose of whole-body irradiation that is just sublethal. After irradiated hosts have been injected with viable lymphocytes and with antigen, the specificity, magnitude, and type of immune response depend on the type of cells injected and on the antigenic experience of the donor (Figure 8-7).

A more direct way to eliminate lymphocytes selectively is to drain them externally via a plastic cannula inserted into the thoracic duct. Drainage removes all circulating lymphocytes over an interval of 5 to 8 days and produces a profound B-cell and T-cell immunodeficiency that can be corrected by adoptive transfer of viable lymphocytes (Figure 8-7).

Finally, an absolute lifelong absence of T lymphocytes can be produced by removing the thymus prior to emigration of virgin T cells (Concept 7-5). Such hosts are ideal for studying the properties of injected T cells. A comparable experimental system for B-cell depletion does not exist in mammals.

Cell and tissue culture techniques

Cell and tissue culture techniques are extremely useful for dissecting immune responses. Not only are the cultured cells much more accessible to manipulation, but *in vitro* experiments typically require from

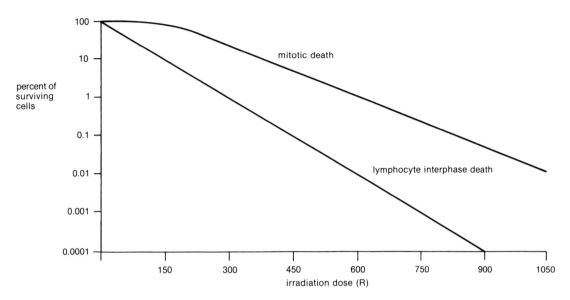

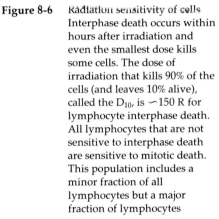

Figure 8-6 Radiation sensitivity of cells. Interphase death occurs within hours after irradiation and even the smallest dose kills some cells. The dose of irradiation that kills 90% of the cells (and leaves 10% alive), called the D_{10}, is ~150 R for lymphocyte interphase death. All lymphocytes that are not sensitive to interphase death are sensitive to mitotic death. This population includes a minor fraction of all lymphocytes but a major fraction of lymphocytes recently activated by antigen. Doses of irradiation under 100–150 R are insufficient to cause mitotic death. The D_{10} for mitotic death in the linear portion of the curve is ~300 R. Thus a dose of 600 R should kill ~99.99% of the major population of lymphocytes (reducing their numbers in a mouse from ~3×10^8 cells to ~3×10^4 cells), but it should reduce the number of mitotic death-sensitive cells by only ~97%.

10- to 100-fold fewer cells than do adoptive transfer experiments. Many lymphoid cells can be grown *in vitro* in rich medium supplemented with serum and growth hormones. Under appropriate culture conditions, these cells retain the ability to function in an immune response. For example, early *in vitro* studies of antibody production by unfractionated spleen or lymph node cells suggested that three distinct cell types were required for a response. Selective culturing (or killing) of particular cell types allowed reconstitution of the normal response and identification of the cell types as accessory cells such as macrophages, T_H cells, and B cells. As the growth requirements for specific classes of lymphoid cells become defined, as they already are for many T_H and T_C cell clones, it becomes possible to study the interactions of pure populations of defined cells.

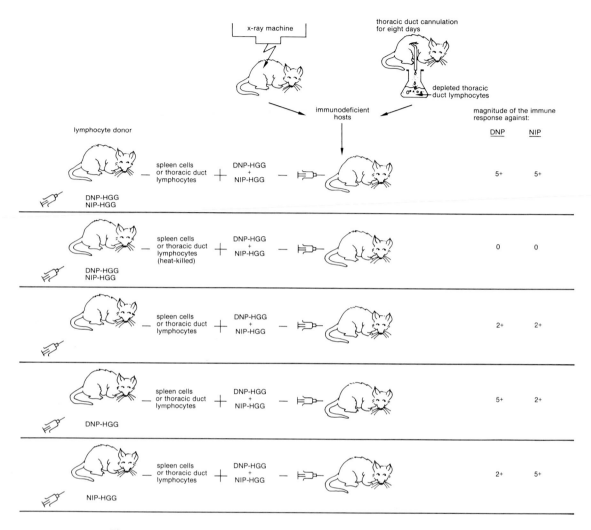

Figure 8-7   Adoptive transfer of immunity to irradiated hosts or to lymphocyte-depleted hosts.

Quantitation of responses

Adoptive transfer and cell culture techniques are most informative when the magnitude of the overall response and the fraction of the responding cells (or other unit) can be quantitated (Figure 8-8). Most sophisticated studies using adoptive transfer and cell culture require cell sorting so that known numbers of defined cells can be tested. Lymphocytes can be sorted by size, density, surface charge, adherence to various solid substrates alone or substrates coated with specific ligands (such as antigens), or by attaching fluorescent ligands to the cells and passing them through a fluorescence-activated cell sorter (Concept 3-7).

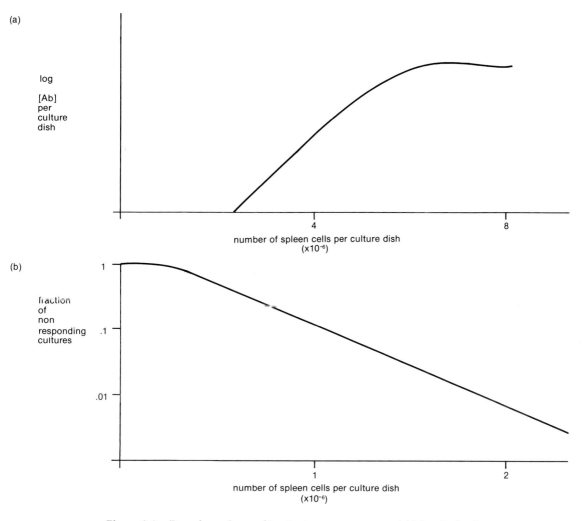

Figure 8-8   Dose dependence of *in vitro* immune responses. (a) Magnitude of response. (b) Frequency of responding units.

8-3 Antigen uptake by accessory cells is the first step in the immune response cascade

Within minutes after infection or injection, free antigen is bound by the macrophages in lymphoid organs. Most of this surface-bound antigen is internalized by phagocytosis and digested after fusion with lysosomes, which contain hydrolytic enzymes that degrade most of the antigens to nonantigenic components. However, the macrophage

Figure 8-9

Macrophage processing of antigen leading to antigen presentation to a T_H cell. An antigen-bearing bacterium (O-O-O) binds to the macrophage surface (1); it is enveloped by extensions of the macrophage membrane (2); it is endocytosed along with the adherent membrane to form a phagosome (3); the phagosome unites with a lysosome (4) to form a phagolysosome; part of the endocytosed membrane (—) is recycled to the surface away from the lysosome. Much of the bacterial structure is broken down and digested, leaving some fragments of macromolecules undigested and adherent to the inner surface of the phagolysosomal membrane (5), which again becomes cell-membrane surface-bound antigen (6) when the phagolysosome fuses with the plasma membrane to release soluble digestion products and complete the endocytotic cycle. A helper T cell recognizes and responds most likely to surface-bound processed antigens, but it may possibly respond also to surface-retained undigested bacteria.

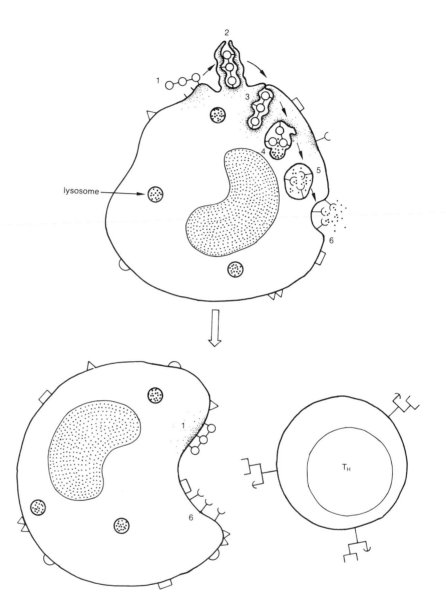

either retains some of the unmodified antigen at its surface or more likely returns some partially digested antigen (processed antigen) to its surface so that antigenic determinants can be "presented" efficiently to antigen-specific lymphocytes (Figure 8-9).

Three kinds of nonphagocytic dendritic cells also bind antigen to their surfaces although this antigen may be processed first by other cells. Two of these cell types are found in lymphoid organs: *interdigitating cells* in T-cell domains and *dendritic reticular cells* in B-cell domains. The dendritic reticular cells begin to display antigen on their

Figure 8-10

Antigen-induced activation of T cells. (a) The appearance of a T cell (lymphoblast) activated *in vitro* and surrounded by resting T cells. (b) The appearance of an activated T cell in the tissue. The peculiar morphology of this cell is emphasized by using a dye (pyronin Y) that stains RNA intensely. [Photographs courtesy of R. Rouse.]

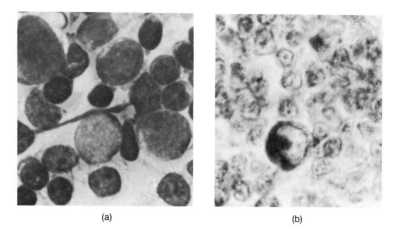

(a)   (b)

surface 1–2 days after antigen entry. The third cell type, *Langerhans cells*, is found in the epithelial linings of the skin and parts of the gastrointestinal tract. Antigen that penetrates these epithelial surfaces adheres to the dendritic processes of Langerhans cells and is carried by these cells to the draining lymph node, especially to T-cell domains. Skin depleted of Langerhans cells can neither initiate an immune response in the draining lymph node nor support skin-localized, delayed hypersensitivity.

All these antigen-presenting cells, including macrophages, are derived from circulating bone-marrow precursors and express high concentrations of cell-surface Ia as well as MHC class I antigens. These gene products of the MHC restrict interactions between accessory cells and lymphocytes.

8-4 Mature T$_H$ and T$_A$ cells interact with antigen-charged accessory cells to become effector cells

Blast transformation

Upon stimulation by antigen-charged accessory cells, mature T$_H$ and T$_A$ cells undergo a general activation, called *blast transformation*, in which the cell enlarges, the nucleolus swells, microtubules and polysomes form, and rates of macromolecular synthesis increase markedly (Figure 8-10). The activated cells (blast cells) proliferate and differentiate, giving rise to effector T$_H$ and T$_A$ cells. Effector T$_H$ cells interact with mature B cells to promote antibody formation. Effector T$_A$ cells secrete growth factors that aid in T$_C$ development and cellular immunity.

MHC restriction

Stimulation of T_H and T_A cells by antigen-charged accessory cells normally occurs only if the T cells and the accessory cells share MHC antigens. Genetic studies with T cells and accessory cells from congenic mice reveal that the requirement for compatibility correlates mainly with Ia antigens encoded by the I-A and I-E regions and only rarely with the D or K regions. Supporting this notion is the observation that anti-Ia antibodies can mask the Ia determinants on accessory cells to interfere selectively and specifically with T-cell stimulation. It is thought that responding T cells co-recognize specific foreign antigenic determinants and self-Ia molecules and that both components must be present on the accessory cell surface at the same time for full expression, proliferation, and differentiation of T_H and T_A cells. This phenomenon of *associated recognition* of cell-surface self-MHC markers and exogenous antigens extends to other classes of T cells as well and is considered in detail in Concept 8-8. The phenomenon is also called *MHC restriction* to signify that T cells are restricted to interact with cells bearing the particular MHC gene products they recognize.

8-5   Mature B cells interact with effector T_H cells and antigen to become antibody-secreting plasma cells

T_H-cell function

T_H cells are essential for all IgG, IgA, and IgE immune responses, whereas they are important for only certain IgM responses. Stimulation of mature B cells by effector T_H cells usually requires an antigen that carries at least two different antigenic determinants, suggesting that the antigen functions as a bridge. In many immunizations with a hapten conjugated to a carrier, T_H cells specific for carrier determinants cooperate with B cells specific for hapten components. Additionally, effector T_H cells also require accessory cells, perhaps macrophages or dendritic cells, to trigger specific B cells. Finally, many T_H cells can stimulate only those B cells with which they share MHC Ia determinants. This class of MHC-restricted effector T_H cells will be designated T_{H-MHC} cells. MHC restriction in the interaction with B cells coupled with requirements for multivalent antigens and accessory cells suggests a three-cell model for the triggering of mature B cells by effector T_{H-MHC} cells (Figure 8-11).

Several experiments suggest the existence of another class of effector T_H cells that can trigger only those mature B cells that express particular isotypic, idiotypic, or allotypic determinants. For example, one can identify effector T_H cells that selectively trigger antigen-spe-

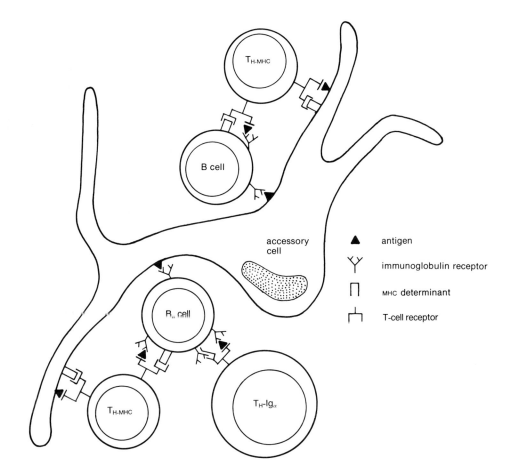

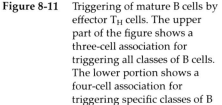

Figure 8-11 Triggering of mature B cells by effector T$_H$ cells. The upper part of the figure shows a three-cell association for triggering all classes of B cells. The lower portion shows a four-cell association for triggering specific classes of B cells—a B$_\alpha$ cell in this case. The antigen and MHC-specific portions of the T-cell receptor here are shown combined for illustrative purposes; the true nature of the T-cell receptor is just now being determined.

cific B cells to become IgE-secreting plasma cells, while leaving unstimulated other classes of B cells specific for the same antigen. Because this class of T$_H$ cells is not MHC restricted in its interaction with B cells and does not recognize MHC determinants on accessory cells, it is designated T$_{H\text{-Ig}}$ to indicate its *immunoglobulin restriction*. Several experiments suggest that selective triggering of B-cell classes may require the simultaneous action of more than one type of effector T$_H$ cell (Figure 8-11).

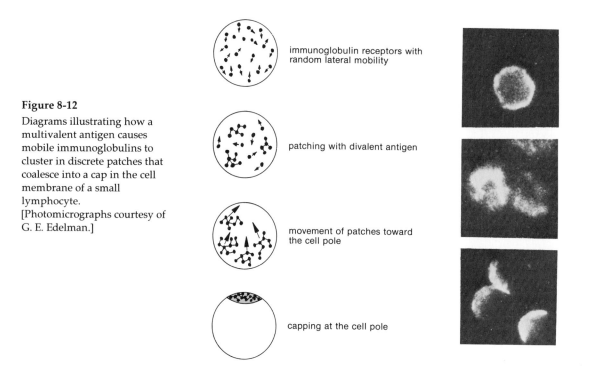

immunoglobulin receptors with random lateral mobility

patching with divalent antigen

movement of patches toward the cell pole

capping at the cell pole

Figure 8-12
Diagrams illustrating how a multivalent antigen causes mobile immunoglobulins to cluster in discrete patches that coalesce into a cap in the cell membrane of a small lymphocyte.
[Photomicrographs courtesy of G. E. Edelman.]

Triggering mechanism of B cells

Antigen binding to B-cell surface receptors in the presence of effector T_H cells activates B cells, but the molecular mechanism is not yet understood. The triggering event is difficult to study directly with antigens because only 1 in 10^4 to 10^5 cells will bind antigen strongly enough to initiate a primary immune response. Even in a secondary response following clonal expansion of antigen-specific cells, less than 1% of the lymphocyte population has the capacity to bind the antigen and be stimulated. However, progress is being made in studies of two presumably closely related processes: (a) the response of cell membranes to the binding of surface molecules in general and (b) the action of substances called *mitogens* that induce many kinds of cells to divide by binding to their surfaces.

Cross-linking and rearrangement of cell-surface antibody receptor molecules could be among the events that trigger changes in the nucleus. Because receptor proteins in the cell membrane are often mobile, many of them can be cross-linked by specific divalent reagents, such as antibody molecules, to form areas of two-dimensional precipitation that are termed *patches*. These patches coalesce into a polar *cap*, most of which is shed from the cell or endocytosed (Figure 8-12). Different surface molecules can usually be capped independently, suggesting that they are not normally physically associated. Cap formation is an energy-requiring process that involves contractile microfilament activity. These microfilaments could play a role in transmitting the binding signal from the membrane to the nucleus (Concept 5-4).

The possibility that receptor cross-linking triggers cellular differentiation is supported by the observation that a number of general mitogens also bind to cell-surface molecules and induce capping. Certain mitogenic agents stimulate a large fraction of a lymphocyte population in an antigen-independent manner to proliferate and differentiate into effector cells. These agents include the mitogenic *lectins*, which are plant proteins that bind specifically to various carbohydrate groups. Such agents also include lipopolysaccharides, which are large sugar polymers linked to lipid A in the cell walls of gram-negative bacteria, and a few chemical reagents such as periodate.

Although mitogens interact with specific carbohydrate groups that are about equally represented on the glycoproteins of B-cell and T-cell surfaces, they often affect the two cell types differently. The lectins, phytohemagglutinin and concanavalin A, stimulate differentiation of subsets of T cells only; pokeweed mitogen stimulates differentiation of both B and T cells; and lipopolysaccharides selectively stimulate subsets of rodent B cells.

Mitogenic stimulation requires that the surface binding signal somehow be transduced to the cell interior in order to initiate the sequence of metabolic events that precede proliferation and differentiation. These events include changes in cyclic nucleotide levels, in the methylation and turnover of membrane lipids, in transport of ions and small molecules, and in nucleic acid metabolism. The binding events occur in seconds to minutes, whereas the metabolic changes take minutes to hours. If mitogen is removed prior to the metabolic changes, proliferation and differentiation do not occur.

Recent studies suggest that the cross-linking of surface molecules is a critical event in B-cell activation. In principle the normal activating signal could result from cross-linking of immunoglobulin receptors, from cross-linking of distinct mitogen receptors subsequent to antigen binding, or from cross-linking of both kinds of receptors. Because normal activation of mature B cells occurs in the presence of T_H cells and accessory cells, either cell type could be the source of a multivalent array of antigens or mitogenic signals. Recent studies using cultured T_H cell lines have suggested that they may secrete antigen-specific helper factors (perhaps the T-cell antigen receptor) as well as B-cell growth and differentiation factors that are not antigen specific (Figure 8-13).

IgM response not T-cell dependent

Whereas most humoral immune responses are T-cell dependent, IgM responses to antigens made up of repeating, identical determinants (e.g., polysaccharides or proteins with identical subunits) can occur in the apparent absence of T cells (Figure 8-14). These antigens stimulate primarily IgM synthesis (and, in mice, IgG_3) and do not generate synthesis of the other IgG subclasses or memory B cells characteristic

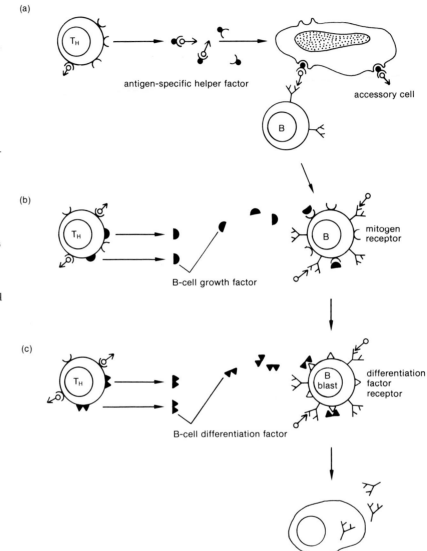

Figure 8-13

T-cell factor models of T_H-cell–B-cell interactions. (a) T cells may release antigen-specific factors that bind to accessory cells and/or (b) other factors that act directly as mitogens specific for B cells that bind antigen. Activated B cell blasts then express surface receptors (c) for B-cell differentiation factors, also secreted by T_H cells. In this figure, the symbol for antigen is ⚬→ , with T_H cells recognizing the ◯ determinants and B cells recognizing → determinants on the same antigen.

of a normal T_H-cell-dependent response. Therefore, the function of effector T_H cells in other responses is not simply to convert a monovalent determinant to a multivalent surface array. The unusual features of these IgM responses are not understood. However, IgM-secreting plasma cells are derived from B_μ or $B_{\mu+\delta}$ cells; B_μ cells are thought to be virgin cells. Perhaps antigenic stimulation of virgin cells is relatively T-cell independent and does not generate memory cells. Other possibilities are that polymeric antigens promote suppression of the

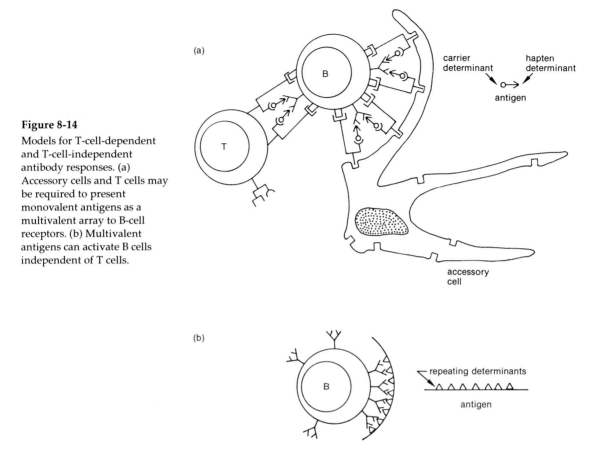

Figure 8-14

Models for T-cell-dependent and T-cell-independent antibody responses. (a) Accessory cells and T cells may be required to present monovalent antigens as a multivalent array to B-cell receptors. (b) Multivalent antigens can activate B cells independent of T cells.

IgG response and B-cell memory or that these antigens are selectively mitogenic for defined subsets of B cells.

8-6 The antibodies produced in an immune response usually are heterogeneous in specificity and immunoglobulin class

Heterogeneity of antibody affinity

An individual mature B cell activated by effector T_H cells and cognate antigen proliferates and differentiates to form plasma cells that secrete identical antibodies with a single specificity at a rate of about 10,000 molecules per cell per second. However, an organism's total response to even the simplest antigens is usually heterogeneous with respect to antibody specificity. This heterogeneity arises because most antigens have multiple antigenic determinants, and each determinant gener-

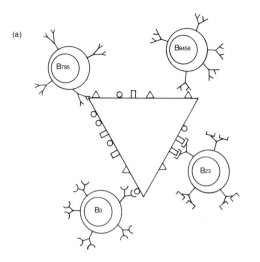

(a)

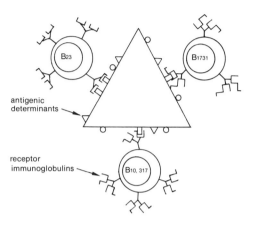

(b)

antigenic
determinants →

receptor
immunoglobulins →

Figure 8-15   Two sources of heterogeneity in an antibody response to an antigen. (a) Different antigenic determinants on the same antigen trigger B cells with different receptors. (b) The same antigenic determinant triggers B cells with similar but nonidentical receptor immunoglobulins.

ally activates several different B cells with similar but nonidentical receptor specificities (Figure 8-15). Consequently, the serum of any vertebrate contains an extremely heterogeneous collection of immunoglobulin molecules whose specificities reflect the organism's past antigen exposure.

Heterogeneity of antibody class

Different classes of antibodies (isotypes) with the same antigenic specificity (idiotype) are produced in response to antigenic stimulation. As explained in Chapter 4, the phenomenon of class switching occurs by joining the same heavy-chain variable segment, which controls idiotype, to different heavy-chain constant genes, which control isotype. A given plasma cell secretes antibody of a single isotype class. The isotype of the secreted antibody is generally the same as the isotype of antibody receptors expressed on the mature B-cell precursor of the secreting plasma cell. As mentioned in Chapter 4, mature B cells, memory B cells, and plasma cells are designated by a Greek letter that corresponds to the isotype of the membrane receptor or secreted antibody. For example, B_μ cells carry monomeric receptor IgM molecules, B_γ cells carry receptor IgG molecules and the corresponding plasma cells, PC_μ and PC_γ, secrete IgM and IgG antibodies, respectively.

Mature and memory B cells are usually restricted to producing plasma cells of the same isotype. However, $B_{\mu+\delta}$ cells give rise primar-

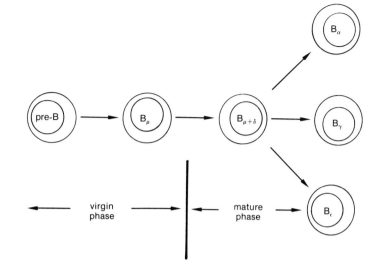

Figure 8-16

Probable lineage of B cells. No direct evidence indicates that $B_{\mu+\delta}$ cells derive from B_{μ} cells; the two cell types could arise by independent pathways from a common precursor.

ily to PC_{γ} cells and very rarely to PC_{δ} cells. This exception helps to explain two puzzling quantitative features of humoral immune responses. B_{γ} cells represent a minority of circulating B cells, yet IgG is the major class of antibody produced in an immune response. Conversely, IgD is a common receptor on B-cell surfaces, and yet only minute concentrations of IgD antibodies are produced in an immune response.

How are isotype-defined classes generated?

Although the transition from mature B cells to plasma cells is fairly well understood in terms of effector T_H requirements, antigen dependence, and isotype expression, very little is known concerning the generation of isotype-specific classes of mature B cells. Experimentally, the problem has been studied by the injection of anti-isotype antisera into animals or by adding the antisera to spleen cells *in vitro*. Anti-γ, anti-ϵ, or anti-α antiserum causes the disappearance of B cells bearing the corresponding isotype marker and prevents antigen-driven generation of the corresponding plasma cells. Interestingly, anti-μ antiserum prevents the expression of all immunoglobulin classes, and anti-δ antiserum prevents the expression of all but IgM. These experiments suggest the order for B-cell isotype generation shown in Figure 8-16. This model is also consistent with the developmental order of appearance of isotype classes of B cells: first B_{μ}, then $B_{\mu+\delta}$, and finally B_{γ}, B_{ϵ}, and B_{α} (Concept 7-4). However, there is no direct evidence indicating that $B_{\mu+\delta}$ cells derive from B_{μ} cells; that is, the two cell types could arise by independent pathways from a common precursor. In addition, it should be noted that T_S cells are generated in these experiments, and thus they could be responsible for suppression of some classes of B cells (Chapter 10). Because of the potential "hidden" effects of T_S cells, it is difficult to distinguish the model in Figure 8-16 from other plausible models.

Is class switching internally programmed or externally induced?

The final stage of class switching could be programmed internally or induced by an external influence, such as a particular tissue microenvironment. If the switch is programmed internally, then B cells must be sorted into particular microenvironments because isotype-specific plasma cells and their immediate blast-cell precursors are located preferentially in characteristic lymphoid organs. During a primary response, the B blast cells in newly developing *germinal centers* express only IgM receptor immunoglobulin. During a secondary response, the splenic and peripheral lymph node germinal centers contain B blast cells expressing only IgG receptor immunoglobulin, whereas most of the B blast cells in Peyer's patches express only IgA receptor immunoglobulin. Thus this intermediate stage of differentiation is already committed to isotype-specific, heavy-chain expression.

Either the induction of the switch or the selection of B cells that have already switched is apparently controlled by immunoglobulin-restricted T_H cells. The addition of $T_{H\text{-}MHC}$ cells alone to an appropriate culture of B cells results in the appearance of plasma cells of all isotypes. However, the simultaneous addition of presumptive $T_{H\text{-}IgA}$ cells (from antigen-activated Peyer's patches) selectively increases the appearance of PC_α cells.

How are memory cells generated?

The stage at which memory B cells are generated is still undefined. Some are represented among the progeny of germinal center B blast cells, but others might be derived from a common precursor along a parallel line of development.

8-7 Mature T_A, T_C, and T_D cells cooperate with one another and with accessory cells to provide cellular immunity

Differentiation of T_A and T_C cells

Mature T_A and T_C cells are small lymphocytes that undergo blast transformation upon contact with antigen-charged accessory cells (Figure 8-17). Most mature T_A cells co-recognize antigens and MHC Ia molecules, whereas most mature T_C cells co-recognize antigens and MHC D or K molecules. Continued proliferation and differentiation of T_A blast cells to effector T_A cells depend on repeated contact with antigen-charged accessory cells. By contrast, T_C blast proliferation is not controlled directly by antigen recognition. Instead, T_C blast cells express a new surface receptor for a *T-cell growth factor* called *interleukin 2*, which is produced and secreted by effector T_A cells. Interleukin 2 is not antigen specific and stimulates all activated T_C cells and perhaps other T cells, such as pre-T cells and immature thymic lymphocytes, as well. Thus mature T_C cells respond to antigen recognition by blast transformation, expression of interleukin 2 receptors, and maturation of killer functions. Most effector

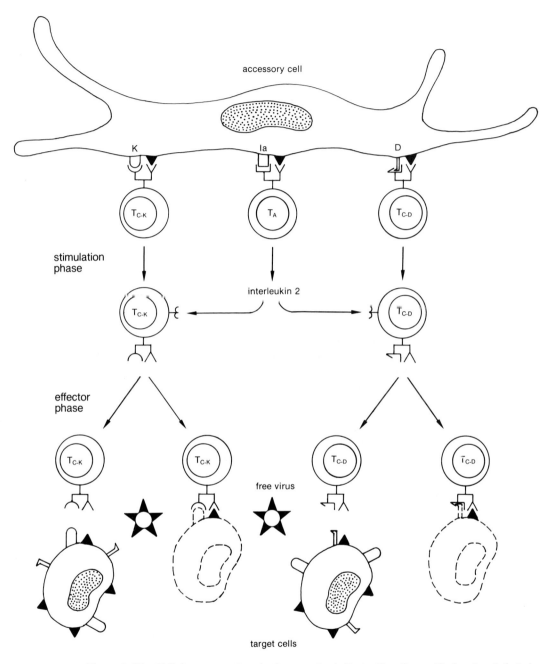

Figure 8-17 Cellular cooperations in the genesis of effector T_C cells specific for virus-infected target cells. Dotted figures represent lysed cells.

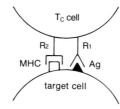
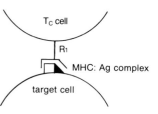

Figure 8-18 Two models for T-cell receptors. In altered self-recognition (right), the complex of MHC and antigen could result from covalent or noncovalent association. A covalent complex would predict that the cell surfaces of macrophages, accessory cells, and target cells will carry antigenically modified MHC gene products and that only these molecules will be recognized by cognate T cells. A noncovalent complex might form on the target cell surface in the absence of T cells, or it might form only when the association was stabilized by interaction with the T-cell receptor.

T_C cells recognize target cells bearing cognate antigen and MHC D or K surface molecules and kill them (Figure 8-17).

Differentiation of T_D cells

Mature T_D cells co-recognize cognate antigen and self-Ia molecules on antigen-charged accessory cells in lymphoid organs and undergo blast transformation. Following proliferation and differentiation to effector T_D cells, they enter the circulation to be carried to sites of peripheral antigen deposition. Effector T_D cells recognize antigen-charged, Ia-bearing Langerhans cells in the skin and initiate local inflammatory responses and elimination reactions (Concept 9-4).

8-8 Associated recognition appears to be a general property of T cells

Associated recognition

In addition to their dependence on cognate antigen, cellular interactions in the immune response cascade are generally restricted by gene products of the MHC. Mature T_H, T_A, and mature and effector T_D cells interact predominantly with antigen-charged accessory cells that bear self-Ia determinants (Concepts 8-4 and 8-7); effector T_{H-MHC} cells interact with mature B cells that bear self-Ia determinants (Concept 8-5); mature T_C cells interact mainly with accessory cells that bear self-D and K determinants (Concept 8-7); and effector T_C cells interact mainly with target cells that bear self-D and K determinants. Even effector T_{H-Ig} cells, which are not restricted by MHC determinants, are restricted by surface immunoglobulin determinants in their interaction with B cells (Concept 8-5). Thus the phenomenon of associated or dual recognition by T cells is quite general. Another way of describing this phenomenon is to say that T_H, T_A, and T_D

cells recognize foreign antigen in the *context* of Ia determinants, whereas T_C cells recognize foreign antigen in the *context* of D and K determinants.

The stage of T-cell differentiation at which the capacity for associated recognition develops is not clear. Some experiments suggest a thymic stage of differentiation, whereas others suggest a postthymic stage. For MHC-restricted T cells, a thymic stage would seem quite natural given the differential expression of MHC determinants on the epithelial cells of the cortex and medulla (Concept 7-5). However, resolution of this question awaits further experimentation.

Function of associated recognition

Although the biological function of associated recognition is not yet established, a plausible suggestion is that MHC determinants serve as a cellular identification system. Ia determinants—which are found almost exclusively on macrophages, accessory cells, B cells, and some T cells—could restrict the interactions of T_H, T_A, and T_D cells to functionally significant cellular contacts. Similarly, D and K determinants—which are on nearly all cells of the body—could permit T_C cells to provide surveillance for all cells while avoiding inappropriate interaction with free-floating antigens. For example, T_C cells must identify and eliminate cells that carry viral antigens and yet not be inappropriately triggered by free viral antigens (Figure 8-17, bottom). Similar arguments could be made for the other classes of T cells.

What is the nature of T-cell receptors?

Identification and characterization of T-cell receptors for antigen and MHC determinants would clarify the mechanism of associated recognition and perhaps provide insight into its biological function. However, the molecular nature of the T-cell receptor has proven elusive. It is not even clear whether T cells have distinct receptors for MHC and antigenic determinants or single receptors that have both specificities combined. T-cell receptors are usually discussed in terms of dual recognition or altered self-recognition models as shown in Figure 8-18. Throughout this book, the T-cell receptor is represented schematically as two distinct binding specificities located in one molecule. This representation combines elements of both models and emphasizes the duality of the recognition process.

The nature of the T-cell receptor will not remain mysterious for much longer. T-cell antigen receptors have now been isolated from clonal T-cell populations using monoclonal and monospecific antibodies. The isolated T-cell receptors are heterodimeric aggregates (90,000 daltons) composed of one α and one β chain of similar size, which are linked together in the cell membrane by a disulfide bond.

Recently, the genes encoding the α and β chains have been cloned. Although these genes are distinct from immunoglobulin genes, they contain V, D, J, and C gene segments, which are rearranged and expressed only in T cells. The family of β gene segments is located on chromosome 6 in mice and chromosome 7 in humans. Each of the two identified C_β gene segments is associated with a cluster of

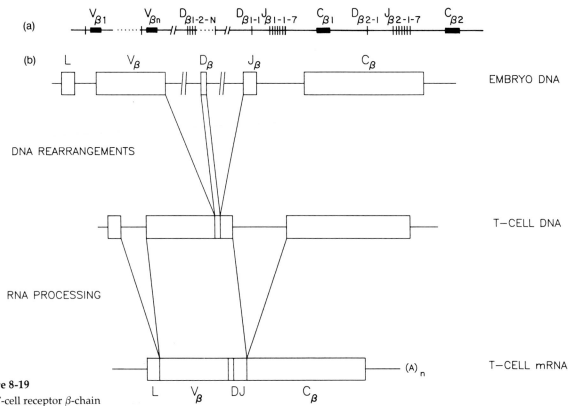

Figure 8-19

The T-cell receptor β-chain gene. (a) Diagrammatic representation of the organization of the T-cell receptor β-chain gene segments. (b) The DNA rearrangements and RNA processing events necessary for the expression of the mRNA for the β-chain of the T-cell antigen receptor. The C_β gene segment has three introns that are not indicated.

seven J_β gene segments and one or more D_β gene segments. These gene segments are linked to an unknown number of V_β gene segments (Figure 8-19). The arrangement of α gene segments is being determined. Diversity in T-cell receptor specificity apparently is generated much the same as for antibodies: by combinatorial joining of gene segments in the α and β clusters, by combinatorial association of α and β chains, and by somatic mutation.

The immunoglobulin light and heavy chain genes, the T-cell receptor α- and β-chain genes, and the class I and class II gene families of the MHC have all evolved from a common ancestral gene family and together constitute a supergene family encoding the receptor molecules that participate in the vertebrate immune response (Figure 4-23).

In addition to the T-cell antigen receptor other T-cell-specific glycoproteins appear to be involved in T-cell recognition. For the most part, T_H cells carry Lyt-1 and L3T4 polypeptides and recognize Ia determinants, whereas T_C cells carry Lyt-2,3 and recognize D and K determinants. The few exceptions to these relationships between cell function, surface phenotype, and MHC restriction are instructive. A few T_H cells that carry Lyt-2,3 have been isolated; they recognize K and D determinants. Similarly, a few T_C cells that carry L3T4 have been found; they recognize Ia determinants. Thus Lyt phenotype correlates more closely with MHC restriction than with cell type, as might be expected if the Lyt determinants were part of the recognition apparatus. Antibodies to Lyt-2,3 determinants are very potent inhibitors of antigen-stimulated blast transformation of Lyt-2,3 bearing mature T_C and T_H cells and antigen-stimulated cytolysis by effector T_C cells. Similarly, antibodies to L3T4 determinants block recognition by T_H cells. In humans, antibodies to T8 and to T4 determinants block functions dependent on antigen recognition by the T cells bearing these determinants. In addition, the T3 molecule is associated in the cell membrane with the T-cell receptor candidates, and antibodies to T3 block T-cell recognition of targets. The Lyt-2,3, L3T4, T3, T4, and T8 molecules do not vary from cell to cell. Thus, the actual recognition and signal delivery by T cells probably involves a complex of constant and variable recognition molecules in an array on the T-cell membrane.

8-9   MHC genes control immune responsiveness

Nature of high and low immune responsiveness

Immune response genes were originally defined by genetic differences in the responsiveness of the immune system to particular antigens. Most of these genes were subsequently shown to be located in the MHC and to affect only T-cell-dependent immune responses. In general, the immune responses controlled by different alleles of these genes can be classified as high or low. In a humoral immune response in mice, *high responders* typically synthesize 10 to 20 times as much antigen-specific antibody as *low responders*. Response genes that affect T_H-cell functions in humoral immunity map in the I region. Response genes that affect T_A-cell functions in cellular immunity also map in the I region, whereas those that affect T_C-cell functions map in the D or K regions. Therefore, immune response genes are probably simply genes that code for class I and class II MHC surface determinants, and responsiveness somehow depends on associated recognition by T cells. The following observations are consistent with the view that low responsiveness results from inefficient associated recognition of a particular MHC determinant and a particular antigen; that is, the population of T cells is partially blind to particular combinations of MHC and antigenic determinants.

Immune response genes do not affect general immune responsiveness because mice that are high responders to some antigens can be low responders to others. Also, the lack of responsiveness to a particular antigen is not due to an absence of B cells that are specific for the antigen because mice that are low responders to a particular antigen can give a high response if that antigen is linked to an immunogenic carrier (Figure 8-20a). As might be expected from this observation, high or low responsiveness can generally be demonstrated only for simple antigens. However, even highly complex multideterminant antigens can be made to show the phenomenon if

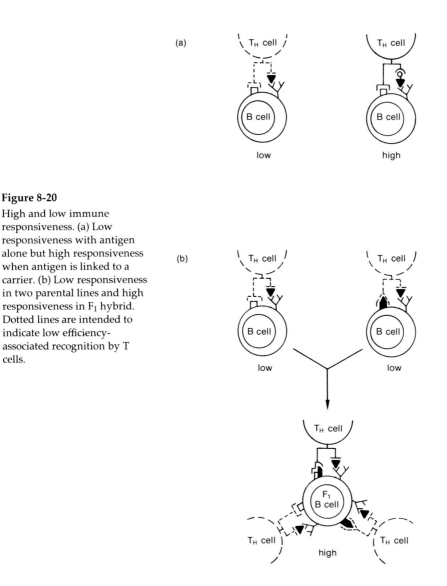

Figure 8-20

High and low immune responsiveness. (a) Low responsiveness with antigen alone but high responsiveness when antigen is linked to a carrier. (b) Low responsiveness in two parental lines and high responsiveness in F_1 hybrid. Dotted lines are intended to indicate low efficiency-associated recognition by T cells.

they are injected at barely immunogenic doses where one particular antigenic determinant is immunodominant.

In some cases, two strains of mice that each are nonresponsive to one particular antigen will give F_1 hybrids that are responsive to that antigen. Thus a high responder phenotype can arise by complementation between two low responder genotypes. This result suggests that the critical MHC determinant is composed of two gene products (Figure 8-20b).

The molecular basis for such complementation is now clear. Ia antigens are dimers composed of α chains and β chains, the genes for which are located in the I-A and I-E regions of the MHC (Concept 6-7 and Figure 8-21). The I-A region product is an $A_\alpha A_\beta$ dimer and the I-E region product is an $E_\alpha E_\beta$ dimer. In outbred populations where virtu-

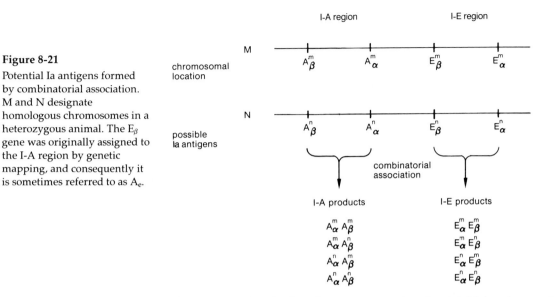

Figure 8-21

Potential Ia antigens formed by combinatorial association. M and N designate homologous chromosomes in a heterozygous animal. The E_β gene was originally assigned to the I-A region by genetic mapping, and consequently it is sometimes referred to as A_e.

ally every individual is heterozygous for the highly polymorphic MHC locus, there are at least eight different possible Ia antigens that can arise by combinatorial association (Figure 8-21). Such diversity is probably important in ensuring high immune responsiveness to a large number of diverse antigens. Thus complementation between low responder genotypes occurs when combinatorial association in the hybrid gives rise to a more functional $A_\alpha A_\beta$ or $E_\alpha E_\beta$ dimer.

The immune response genes that are K or D linked were discovered in studies of the T_C-cell response to viral infections. For example, the population of effector T_C cells that arises after infection of mouse strain $AKR(K^k D^k)$ with influenza virus can kill infected strain AKR cells, but usually it cannot kill cells from other strains $(K^x D^x)$ infected with the same virus. One can create recombinant strains that carry the k haplotype at only the K or D locus by mating. Sometimes the population of T_C cells induced by the original infection is found to kill infected cells that are $K^k D^x$ but not those that are $K^x D^k$. Thus strain AKR, when infected with influenza virus, produced no effector T_C cells that associatively recognized D^k and antigen. There are several examples of such *precluded pairs* of viral or cell-surface antigens and MHC K or D alleles, in which the latter behave as immune response genes.

The I-region immune response genes affecting T_H- and T_A-cell functions express their effects primarily at the level of antigen presentation by accessory cells. T_H or T_A cells from the F_1 mice of a mating between low and high responders will respond to the antigen if it is presented on accessory cells from the high responder strain, but will not if it is presented on accessory cells from the low responder strain. Blockade of Ia molecules on the high responder cells by Ia-specific monoclonal antibodies renders these accessory cells unable to stimulate T_H or T_A cells. In an analogous fashion, the D and K immune response genes affecting T_C-cell function express their effects primarily at the level of antigen presentation by target cells. In matings between a mouse strain that exhibits a precluded K or D allele for a particular cell-surface antigen and one that does not, T_C effector cells from the F_1 progeny can lyse target cells from the parent bearing the nonprecluded MHC–antigen pair, but not from the parent bearing the precluded MHC–antigen pair. Blockade of the nonprecluded K or D determinant on the target cells by monoclonal antibodies prevents T_C-cell lysis of that target cell.

Possible controlling mechanisms

The foregoing observations are consistent with the idea that low responsiveness and precluded pairs arise because T cells co-recognize particular MHC–antigen pairs with low efficiency. Such a defect in recognition could result from any of several causes. The cognate T-cell receptors might not be produced. The cognate T-cell receptors might be produced, but cells bearing such receptors might be eliminated specifically during development. The defect could reside in an inability of certain MHC–antigen combinations to associate in a manner appropriate for T-cell recognition. Alternatively, particular MHC–antigen pairs could interact most efficiently with cells in the T_S pathway, thereby leading to suppression of cognate T_H- and T_A- or T_C-cell clones. Interestingly, low responder mice often are found to have strong T_S suppression. However, whether this suppression is the cause of low responsiveness or merely a secondary effect is unclear.

Selected Bibliography

Lymphocytes as specific elements of the immune system

Billingham, R. E., Brent, L., and Medawar, P. B., "Quantitative studies on tissue transplantation immunity II: The origin, strength, and duration of actively and adoptively acquired immunity," *Proc. R. Soc. Lond.* [Biol.] **143**, 58(1954).

Gowans, J. L., McGregor, D. D., Cowen, D. M., and Ford, C. E., "Initiation of immune responses by small lymphocytes," *Nature* **196**, 651(1962).

The preceding two germinal papers introduced the concept of afferent, central, and efferent limbs of the immune response; the concept of specific and nonspecific cellular elements in the immune response; and the concept that primary, secondary, and tolerance responses are properties of immuno-specific lymphocytes.

The uptake and processing of antigen by accessory cells

Möller, G. (Ed.), "Accessory cells in the immune response," *Immunological Reviews* **53**(1980).

Nieuwenhuis, P., van der Brock, A. A., and Hanna, M. G. (Eds.), *In Vivo Immunology: Histophysiology of the Lymphoid System*, Plenum Press, New York (1982).

Steinman, R. M., and Cohn, Z. A., "Identification of a novel cell type in peripheral lymphoid organs of mice. II. Functional properties *in vitro*," *J. Exp. Med.* **139**, 380(1974).

Unanue, E. R., and Rosenthal, A. S. (Eds.), *Macrophage Regulation of Immunity*, Academic Press, New York (1980).

Lymphocyte interactions in immune responses

Cantor, H., and Asofsky, R., "Synergy among lymphoid cells mediating the graft-versus-host response III: Evidence for interaction between two types of thymus-derived cells," *J. Exp. Med.* **135**, 764(1972).

Claman, H. N., Chaperon, E. A., and Triplett, R. F., "Thymus-marrow cell combinations. Synergism in antibody production," *Soc. Exp. Biol. & Med.* **122**, 1167(1966).

Mitchell, G. F., and Miller, J. F. A. P., "Cell-to-cell interaction in the immune response II: The source of hemolysin-forming cells in irradiated mice given bone marrow and thymus or thoracic duct lymphocytes," *J. Exp. Med.* **128**, 821(1968).

The foregoing three papers describe the initial experiments proving that immune responses required lymphoid cell interactions.

MacDonald, H. R., "Differentiation of cytolytic T lymphocytes," *Immunology Today* **3**, 183(1982).

Melchers, F., Andersson, J., Corbel, C., Leptin, M., Lehnhardt, W., Gerhard, W., and Zeuthen, J., "Regulation of B lymphocyte replication and maturation," *J. Cellular Biochemistry* **19**, 315(1982).

Möller, G. (Ed.), "Interleukins and lymphocyte activation," *Immunological Reviews* **63**(1982).

Current reviews of cells and factors mediating lymphocyte interactions in the immune response.

Associated recognition by T cells and the role of Ir genes

Bevan, M. J., "Killer cells reactive to altered-self antigens can also be alloreactive," *Proc. Natl. Acad. Sci. USA* **74**. 2094(1977).

Doherty, P. C., Blanden, R. V., and Zinkernagel, R. M., "Specificity of virus-immune effector T cells for H-2K or H-2D compatible interactions, implications for H-antigen diversity," *Transplant. Rev.* **29**, 89(1976).

Fathman, C. G., and Fitch, F. W. (Eds.), *Isolation, Characterization, and Utilization of T Lymphocyte Clones*, Academic Press, New York, 1982.

Fink, P. J., and Bevan, M. J., "H-2 antigens of the thymus determine lymphocyte specificity," *J. Exp. Med.* **148**, 766(1978).

Matzinger, P., "A one-receptor view of T-cell behaviour," *Nature* **292**, 497(1981).

Zinkernagel, R. M., Callahan, G. N., Althage, A., Cooper, S., Klein, P. A., and Klein, J., "On the thymus in the differentiation of 'H-2 self-recognition' by T cells: Evidence for dual recognition?" *J. Exp. Med.* **147**, 882(1978).

T-cell antigen receptor genes

Hedrick, S., Nielsen, E., Kavaler, J., Cohen, D., and Davis, M., "Sequence relationships between putative T-cell receptor polypeptides and immunoglobulins," *Nature* **308**, 153(1984).

Malissen, M., Minard, K., Mjolsness, S., Kronenberg, M., Goverman, J., Hunkapiller, T., Prystowsky, M. B., Yoshikai, Y., Fitch, F., Mak, T. W., and Hood, L., "Mouse T-cell antigen receptor: Structure and organization of constant and joining gene segments encoding the β polypeptide," *Cell* **37**, 1101(1984).

Siu, G., Clark, S. P., Yoshikai, Y., Malissen, M., Yanagi, Y., Strauss, E., Mak, T. W., and Hood, L., "The human T-cell antigen receptor is encoded by variable, diversity, and joining gene segments that rearrange to generate a complete V gene," *Cell* **37**, 393(1984).

Siu, G., Kronenberg, M., Strauss, E., Haars, R., Mak, T. W., and Hood, L., "The D_β gene segments of the murine T-cell antigen receptor: Structure, rearrangement and expression," *Nature*, September 1984(in press).

Yanagi, Y., Yoshikai, Y., Leggett, K., Clark, S., Aleksander, I., and Mak, T., "A human T cell-specific cDNA clone encodes a protein having extensive homology to immunoglobulin chains," *Nature* **308**, 145(1984).

Additional concepts introduced in the problems

1. The role of the thymus in transplantation rejection. Problem 8-4.
2. Idiotypic determinants in common on T and B cells. Problem 8-6.
3. The carrier effect. Problems 8-8 and 8-9.
4. H-2 restriction of T cells and of antibodies. Problems 8-10, 11, 12, 13, 14, and 15.

Problems

8-1 Indicate whether each of the following statements is true or false. Explain the error in each statement you consider to be false.

(a) Blast transformation is an antigen-driven differentiation process that occurs in B and T cells.

(b) When triggered by a cognate antigen, B_γ lymphocytes may differentiate to give plasma cells that secrete IgM antibody.

(c) Some antigens can evoke an antibody response in B cells that do not require T-cell cooperation.

(d) Mice that show a low immune response (low responders) to artificial polypeptides lack the genes for the corresponding antibody molecules.

(e) The typical antibody response to a single antigen is heterogeneous.

(f) In the presence of antigen, a purified population of T and B cells may cooperate *in vitro* to produce a B-cell immune response.

(g) Genes that code for antibody combining-site specificities, and thereby control the immune response to specific antigens, are linked to MHC genes.

8-2 Supply the missing word or words in each of the following statements.

(a) The major class of antibody synthesized in a _____ immune response is IgG.

(b) _____ is the process whereby a lymphocyte undergoes an antigen-driven differentiation.

(c) The process whereby antigens and receptors coalesce into a single aggregate at one pole of the lymphocyte is termed _____ .

(d) The B-cell response usually requires the cooperation of _____ , _____ , and _____ .

(e) T-cell-independent antigens evoke the synthesis of antibody of the _____ class.

(f) Genes that regulate the antibody response to many antigens and are linked to the major histocompatibility genes of the mouse are called _____ genes.

(g) Accessory cells involved in antigen processing include _____ and _____ .

(h) The _____ of anti-hapten antibodies increases late in an immune response, after peak titers are reached.

(i) In the three-signal model of T-cell-dependent B-cell triggering, antigen binds to B-cell surface _____ , and T cells secrete factors that signal B-cell _____ and _____ receptors.

8-3 What markers can be used to distinguish the following cells in mice? Suppressor T cell, killer T cell, the precursor of an IgM plasma cell, the precursor of an IgG plasma cell, macrophage, dendritic reticular cell?

8-4 (a) For many years, the function of the thymus was unknown. Although the gland was found to consist of a mass of rapidly dividing lymphocytes within an epithelial meshwork, no antibody synthesis could be detected in the thymus, nor did it display any histological changes upon antigenic challenge. Surgical removal of the thymus (thymectomy) had no effect on the immune capabilities of adult animals. However, in 1960 an Australian scientist, J.F.A.P. Miller, thymectomized some mice within 16 hours of birth. Within 3 months, most of these mice began to lose weight, suffer from chronic diarrhea, and become "runted" or "wasted" in appearance, and eventually all died. A strictly germ-free environment, however, prevented this wasting. What inferences can you draw about the

Table 8-1 Survival of Allogeneic Skin Grafts in Mice Thymectomized in the Neonatal Period (Problem 8-4)

Group	Age at Operation	Strain of Mice	Skin Graft Donor Strain	Number of Grafts	Number of Grafts Accepted	Median Survival Time of Graft (Days)
A Thymectomized	1–16 hours	C3H	Ak	7	5	45–101[a]
		Ak	C3H	6	4	41–90[a]
		(Ak × T6)F₁	C3H	8	8	50–118[a]
B Thymectomized	5 days	C3H	Ak	5	0	11 ± 0.7
C Thymectomized and thymus-grafted 3 weeks later	5 hours	C3H	Ak	5	0	11–15
D Sham thymectomized	1–16 hours	C3H	Ak	6	0	11 ± 0.6
		Ak	C3H	3	0	10 ± 0.8
E Intact		C3H	Ak	61	0	11 ± 0.6
		Ak	C3H	45	0	10 ± 0.9
		(Ak × T6)F₁	C3H	10	0	11 ± 0.1

[a]These figures apply only to mice that accepted the foreign transplant.
[From J.F.A.P. Miller, *Lancet* **2**, 749(1961).]

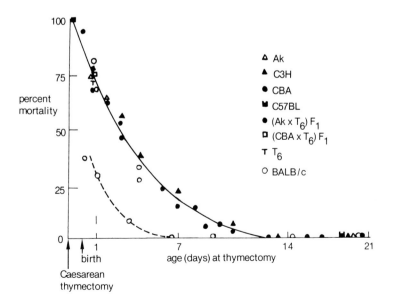

Figure 8-22

Mortality from wasting disease in thymectomized mice of several different strains (Problem 8-4). [From J. F. A. P. Miller, A. H. E. Marshall, and R. G. White, *Adv. Immunol.* **2**, 111(1962).]

Figure 8-23

Plaque-forming cells (PFC) produced in the spleens of neonatally thymectomized CBA mice at various times after injection of sheep red blood cells (SRBC) and syngeneic thymus or thoracic duct cells (Problem 8-5). □-□, sham-operated controls given SRBC only; ○-○, neonatally thymectomized mice given SRBC only; ●-●, neonatally thymectomized mice given 10 million CBA thymus cells and SRBC; ▲-▲, neonatally thymectomized mice given 10 million thoracic duct cells and SRBC. [From J. F. A. P. Miller and G. F. Mitchell, *J. Exp. Med.* **128**, 801(1968). Copyright 1968 by The Rockefeller University Press.]

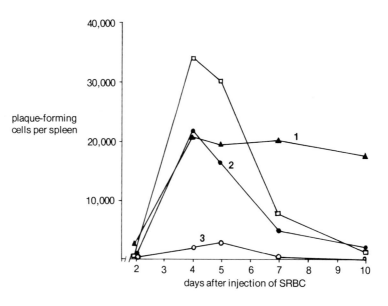

nature of the wasting disease? What other experiments could you do to investigate your inferences further?

(b) Table 8-1 gives data showing the survival of foreign skin grafts on normal and thymectomized mice. Sham thymectomized mice are controls that were subjected to the same surgical procedures as thymectomized mice except that their thymuses were not removed. *Allogeneic grafts* are those exchanged between individuals that are not genetically identical; *syngeneic grafts* are those exchanged between individuals that are genetically identical.

Compare the median survival time of allogeneic skin grafts on normal mice and on neonatally thymectomized mice. What seems to be the effect of neonatal thymectomy? What other immunologic functions would you expect to be impaired in neonatally thymectomized mice?

(c) Compare groups A, B, and E in Table 8-1. What do you infer from these data about the timing of the role of the thymus in the development of cellular immunity? Now consider Figure 8-22, which shows cumulative percent mortality as a function of age at thymectomy for several strains of mice. Suggest explanations both for the shape of the curve and for the difference between BALB/c mice and the other strains. Suppose Miller had used BALB/c mice originally; what might he have thought?

8-5 (a) In experiments related to those in Problem 8-4, Miller tested the effect of neonatal thymectomy on humoral antibody formation and the ability of various lymphoid cells to substitute for the missing thymus-derived cells. Rather than measure directly the amount of specific antibody produced in response to antigenic challenge, he chose to measure the number of spleen lymphocytes that could be induced to secrete antibody specific for sheep red blood cells (SRBC) injected into the mice. To quantitate these spleen cells, he used the Jerne plaque assay. Figure 8-23 shows the results of this experiment. What do you conclude about antibody production in mice subjected to these procedures? What do

Figure 8-24

PFC produced in the spleens of heavily irradiated CBA mice injected after irradiation, with SRBC alone (△), SRBC and 1 million syngeneic thoracic duct cells (●–●), SRBC and 10 million syngeneic bone-marrow cells (▲ . . . ▲), or SRBC and a mixed inoculum of 1 million syngeneic thoracic duct cells and 10 million syngeneic bone-marrow cells ○–○ (Problem 8-5). Vertical bars indicate the magnitudes of the standard errors. [From J. F. A. P. Miller and G. F. Mitchell, *J. Exp. Med.* **128**, 801(1968). Copyright 1968 by The Rockefeller University Press.]

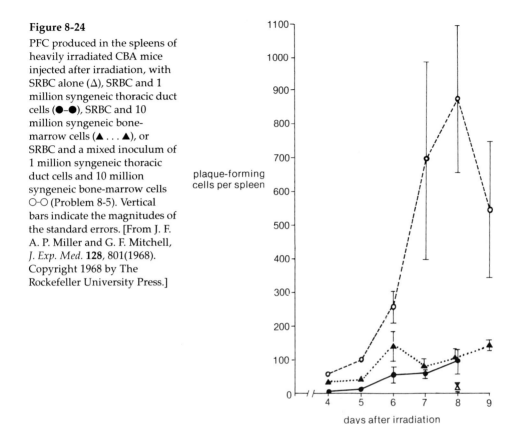

curves 1, 2, and 3 in Figure 8-23 indicate? Given that thymic lymphocytes do not synthesize antibody, how can you explain the experimental data?

(b) Figure 8-24 illustrates the response to SRBC of heavily X-irradiated mice, some of which were reconstituted with various lymphoid cells. Heavy X irradiation kills a high proportion of lymphoid cells of all classes. What is the basic difference between the experimental protocol here and the protocol in part (a) of this problem? What do you infer from the cell types required for an antibody response? Does this modify your conclusions from part (a)?

8-6 Immunization of Lewis rats with Brown Norway (BN) rat fibroblasts elicits a T-cell response as well as production of antibodies specific for those antigens that distinguish Lewis rat cells from BN rat cells. Following such an immunization experiment, the specific anti-BN antibodies were isolated by adsorbing the Lewis antiserum with BN cells and then eluting the specifically bound antibodies. These Lewis anti-BN antibodies were then injected into $(L \times BN)F_1$ rats. The F_1 rats should have reacted against any antigenic determinants that were present on the Lewis anti-BN antibodies and that are not normally present on $(L \times BN)F_1$ immunoglobulins. These immunized F_1 rats and nonimmunized F_1 control rats were then injected in one footpad with either L or BN parental lymphocytes, and the resulting graft-versus-host response (GVHR) was measured by determining the weight of the lymph node that drains the foot after several days, as a function of the number of cells injected. The data are shown in Figure 8-25.

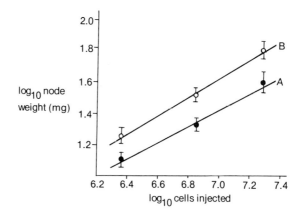

Figure 8-25 The local popliteal node GVHR produced by Lewis and BN spleen cells in (L × BN)F$_1$ hosts (Problem 8-6). The response (the weight of the nodes in milligrams) is plotted against the number of cells injected. Curve A shows the response produced by Lewis cells in immunized F$_1$ hosts. Curve B shows the response produced by Lewis cells in nonimmunized hosts; these responses were all equivalent (p > 0.4). Curve A differs significantly from curve B (p < 0.02). The points plotted are means ± standard error of mean. [From T. McKearn, *Science* **183**, 93(1974). Copyright 1974 by the American Association for the Advancement of Science.]

Can you explain the differences in GVHR generated by Lewis lymphocytes in immunized versus nonimmunized hosts? Can you explain the differences in the GVHR of Lewis and BN lymphocytes in immunized hosts? What do these results suggest about the similarity of T-cell-surface receptors?

8-7 You have decided to study the histology of lymphoid tissues of mice in various reactive situations. Assuming that you have available to you fluorescein-labeled antibodies that are directed against various cell populations, answer the following questions.

(a) What antigenic targets could your antibodies be directed against to stain B cells selectively? What about T cells?

(b) You look at a tissue section of a "normal resting" lymph node. What areas would you expect to stain for B cells? T cells?

(c) You look at a lymph node involved in a primary response to an antigen. Do you expect to see any differences compared to the resting lymph node? If so, what are they?

(d) You then look at a lymph node involved in a secondary response to an antigen. What kind of staining patterns do you see?

(e) You then decide to look at the spleen. Where are the B and T cells found? What route of antigenic challenge could selectively stimulate the lymphoid tissue of the spleen?

8-8 Research with hapten-carrier conjugates has revealed a curious phenomenon termed the *carrier effect*. An animal immunized with Hapten A attached to carrier B and then challenged with the same A-B conjugate will produce copious anti-hapten (and anti-carrier) antibody. However, if the same animal is challenged instead with Hapten A attached to a different carrier, C, it will produce little anti-hapten antibody in the

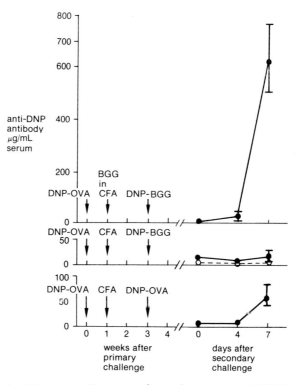

Figure 8-26 A study of the carrier effect in inbred guinea pigs (Problem 8-8). Primary immunization with DNP-OVA was performed at week 0. One week later supplemental immunization was carried out with either 50 μg of BGG emulsified in CFA or with a saline-CFA emulsion. Four weeks after primary immunization, the animals were challenged with either DNP-BGG or DNP-OVA. The figure shows serum anti-DNP antibody concentrations just prior to challenge and on days 4 and 7. In the middle panel, the results indicated by O-O were observed in animals that were passively immunized with anti-BGG serum 24 hours before administration of DNP-BGG. [From D. Katz, W. Paul, E. Goidl, and B. Benacerraf, *J. Exp. Med.* **132,** 261(1970). Copyright 1970 by The Rockefeller University Press.]

secondary response. Figure 8-26 shows the results of experiments using 2,4-dinitrophenol (DNP) as a hapten and ovalbumin (OVA) and bovine gamma globulin (BGG) as carrier. (CFA designates complete Freund's adjuvant. Adjuvants are usually oily substances which, when mixed and injected with antigen, serve both as a tissue depot that slowly releases the antigen and also as a lymphoid system activator, which nonspecifically enhances the immune response.) With reference to the figure, answer the following questions.

(a) What is the significance of the results shown in the lower panel?

(b) What is the difference between the experimental protocols shown in the upper and middle panels? What sorts of cell populations appear to be necessary for a secondary anti-hapten response? If the first immunization with DNP-OVA were omitted, what sort of anti-DNP response do you think would result?

(c) In the experiment shown in the upper panel, the animals are actively immu-

Table 8-2   Responses of Spleen Cells from Bone-Marrow Chimeras to a Hapten-Carrier Complex (Problem 8-10)

Experiments	Responder Spleen Cells	PFC/Culture[a]	
		TNP-KLH	No Antigen
	B10	180	0
	B10.A	120	0
	(B10 × B10.A)F$_1$	180	2
(1)	B10→(B10 × B10.A)F$_1$	100	0
(2)	B10.A→(B10 × B10.A)F$_1$	130	1
(3)	(B10 × B10.A)F$_1$→B10	250	5
(4)	(B10 × B10.A)F$_1$→B10.A	140	0
(5)	B10→B10.A	1	1
(6)	B10.A→B10	1	1

[a]Geometric means of triplicate cultures.

nized against BGG. In the experiment shown in the middle panel, the animals are passively immunized with antiserum against the heterologous carrier. What does the difference in the two results imply? What result would you expect if the animals had been adoptively immunized by transfer of lymphocytes from a donor that had been immunized with BGG?

8-9   Another approach toward the analysis of the carrier effect uses a procedure termed *adoptive transfer* to place hapten-specific and carrier-specific lymphocytes derived from different mice together in a third mouse. The procedure employs inbred mice, all of whose genes and surface antigens are identical, so that cellular transplants will not be subject to graft rejection. The recipient mice are heavily irradiated so that a high proportion of their own lymphocytes are destroyed. The irradiated mice can then be reconstituted immunologically by transfer of spleen lymphocytes from normal mice. In the experiment, lymphocytes from one mouse immunized with DNP-OVA and lymphocytes from a second mouse immunized with BGG are transferred into the same irradiated host. Such reconstituted mice give a large secondary anti-hapten response to a DNP-BGG conjugate. Pretreatment of the DNP-OVA-primed lymphocytes with anti-Thy-1 antiserum and complement has no effect on the response of the reconstituted mice. However, pretreatment of the BGG-primed lymphocytes with anti-Lyt-1 antiserum and complement before transfer into the irradiated host destroys the host's ability to respond to the DNP-BGG conjugate. What do these experiments reveal about the nature of the carrier-specific cells and the hapten-specific cells in this immune response?

8-10   H-2 restriction is often studied using radiation and bone-marrow chimeras. In the following problems, chimeras are designated as follows: bone-marrow donor → irradiated recipient. Thus, a chimera made by reconstituting an irradiated B10 mouse (H-2^b) with B10.A (H-2^a) bone-marrow cells would be designated B10.A → B10.

Recipient mice were irradiated with 950 rad (X ray), and chimeras were produced by reconstitution with 15 × 10^6 bone-marrow cells that had been treated with anti-Thy-1 plus complement to remove T cells. Spleen cells were obtained from each chimera no earlier than 2 months postirradiation. The spleen cells were individually

Table 8-3 Responses of Mixed Spleen Cells from Bone-Marrow Chimeras to a Hapten-Carrier Complex (Problem 8-10)

| | PFC/Culture | |
Responder Spleen Cells	TNP-KLH	No Antigen
B10→B10.A	9	0
B10.A→B10	8	2
(B10→B10.A)+(B10.A→B10)	330	0

typed by indirect immunofluorescence using H-2-specific reagents. The typing showed that spleen cells from each chimera were of donor origin without detectable cells of host origin.

Unfractionated spleen cells were removed from each chimera and tested for their ability to generate responses to soluble TNP-KLH (TNP = trinitrophenyl, the hapten; KLH = keyhole limpet hemocyanin, the carrier).

The responses were primary responses and were dependent on T_H cells. The number of plaque-forming cells (PFC) was measured to determine the number of B cells secreting anti-TNP antibody. The data obtained are shown in Table 8-2. With reference to the table, answer the following questions.

(a) Using your understanding of H-2 restriction, predict which H-2 haplotype would be recognized as self by the spleen cells in experiment (1). Do the same for the spleen cells in experiments (2), (3), (4), (5), and (6).

(b) Why are the spleen cells in experiments (5) and (6) unable to generate a primary response to soluble TNP-KLH? You should be able to come up with three alternative explanations.

(c) Spleen cells from B10.A → B10 and B10 → B10.A chimeras were mixed and tested for their ability to generate an *in vitro* anti-TNP-KLH primary response. The results are shown in Table 8-3. Based on this additional information, which of your possible explanations in part (b) is most likely to be correct?

8-11 In a second chimera experiment, recipient mice were irradiated with 950 rad (X ray) and reconstituted with 10×10^6 syngeneic bone-marrow cells and 20×10^6 allogeneic bone-marrow cells that had been pretreated with anti-Thy-1 and complement. Spleen cells were obtained from each double donor chimera 2 months after irradiation and were individually typed by indirect immunofluorescence using H-2-specific reagents. Peripheral blood lymphocytes were also obtained and typed by indirect immunofluorescence to ascertain that each chimera was balanced; that is, the chimeras contained equal proportions of syngeneic and allogeneic lymphocytes. No discrepancy between the typing of peripheral blood lymphocytes and spleen cells was observed, and the chimeras were found to be balanced.

As in the preceding problem, unfractionated spleen cells from the double donor chimeras were tested for their ability to generate T_H-dependent primary *in vitro* anti-hapten PFC responses to soluble TNP-KLH. The results are shown in Table 8-4. Next, the adherent accessory cells were removed from the spleen cells of double donor chimeras by passing the unfractionated spleen cells over a G-10 Sephadex column, which retains splenic adherent cells but allows T and B cells to pass through. The T_H-dependent primary anti-hapten PFC responses to TNP-KLH were then reconstituted by the addition of varying amounts of splenic adherent cells from B10 or B10.A. The

Table 8-4 Responses of Spleen Cells from Double Donor Bone-Marrow Chimeras to a Hapten-Carrier Complex (Problem 8-11)

Responder Spleen Cells	PFC/Culture	
	TNP-KLH	No Antigen
B10+B10.A→B10	150	0
B10+B10.A→B10.A	130	1

Figure 8-27

Restricted recognition of lymphocytes from double donor chimeras of accessory cells. Graded numbers of splenic adherent cells from B10 (○) or B10.A (△) were added to cultures containing TNP-KLH and 5 × 10⁵ Sephadex G-10-passed spleen cells from (B10 + B10.A) → B10 chimeras (panel A) or (B10 + B10.A) → B10.A chimeras (panel B). In the absence of antigen, <5 PFC/culture were obtained.

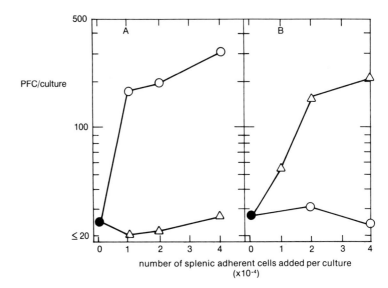

results are shown in Figure 8-27. The population of splenic adherent cells in this case provides antigen-processing accessory cells but not T or B lymphocytes. With reference to the figure, answer the following questions.

(a) Which H-2 haplotype(s) does T cells from (B10 + B10.A) → B10 chimeras recognize as self?

(b) Which H-2 haplotype(s) does T cells from (B10 + B10.A) → B10.A chimeras recognize as self?

(c) Which H-2 determinants (i.e., H-2 antigens of which haplotypes) were present in the recipient thymus of (B10 + B10.A) → B10 chimeras while the T cells were maturing?

(d) Which H-2 antigens were present in the recipient thymus of (B10 + B10.A) → B10.A chimeras while the T cells were maturing?

(e) Which cells in the chimeras could have dictated self-recognition to the maturing T cells? Which cells definitely did not?

8-12 The following series of experiments was performed to study the mechanism of H-2-restricted T-cell help. I-region and H-2 haplotypes of the mouse strains used are shown in Table 8-5.

About 10⁸ (CBA × B6)F₁ T cells were injected intravenously into (CBA × B6)F₁ mice that had been exposed to 900 rad 2 days earlier. At the same time as the T cells were injected, some of the mice received 0.5 mL of sheep erythrocytes. The T-cell

Table 8-5 I-Region and H-2 Haplotypes of Five Mouse Strains (Problem 8-12)

Strain	I-A	I-E	H-2 Haplotype
CBA	k	k	$H\text{-}2^k$
B6	b	b	$H\text{-}2^b$
B10.BR	k	k	$H\text{-}2^k$
B10	b	b	$H\text{-}2^b$
B10.A(4R)	k	b	$H\text{-}2^{k/b}$

Table 8-6 H-2 Restriction of T-Cell Help in Irradiated (CBA × B6)F_1 Mice Reconstituted with T Cells from (CBA × B6)F_1 Mice and B Cells from Other Inbred Strains (Problem 8-12)

Antibodies Added During Selection	SRBC Added During Selection?	Source of Primed B Cells for Measuring T_H Function	Relative Numbers of Anti-SRBC PFC/Spleen in Irradiated F_1 Mice[a]	
			IgM	IgG
(a) None	yes	B10.BR	+++	+++
		B10.A(4R)	+++	+++
		B10	+++	+++
(b) None	no	B10.BR	+	−
		B10.A(4R)	+	−
		B10	+	−
(c) Anti-Ia^k antiserum	yes	B10.BR	−	−
		B10.A(4R)	−	−
		B10	+++	+++
		(CBA × B6)F_1	+++	+++
(d) Three monoclonal anti-I-A^k antibodies	yes	B10.BR	−	−
		B10.A(4R)	+++	+++
		B10	+++	+++

[a] +++ = secondary response level of anti-SRBC PFC
    + = primary response level of anti-SRBC PFC
    − = no response—essentially no PFC/spleen

recipients were injected intraperitoneally with large doses of one of the following three sera: normal mouse serum, an antiserum that reacts with all H-2^k I-region molecules, or a mixture of three monoclonal antibodies that react with A_α^k, A_β^k, and E_β^k determinants. The latter mixture is referred to later as anti-I-A^k. Half the dose was given 2–4 hours before the T-cell injection; the other half was given 1 day later.

T cells were recovered from the spleen and mesenteric lymph nodes of the hosts 5 days after injection and washed twice. Small doses of T cells plus sheep red blood cells (SRBC) were transferred intravenously with B cells from SRBC-primed mice into

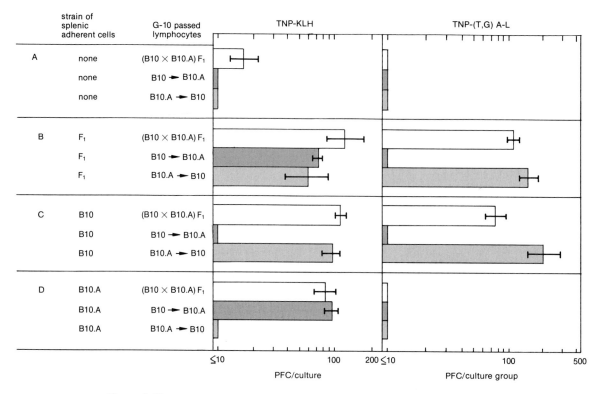

Figure 8-28 Influence of the differentiation environment on the Ir gene phenotype expressed by lymphocytes (Problem 8-13). 2×10^4 splenic adherent cells from (B10 × B10.A)F$_1$ (B), B10 (C), or B10.A (D) were added to cultures containing either TNP-KLH or TNP-(T,G)-A–L and 5×10^5 Sephadex G-10-purified spleen cells from (B10 × B10.A)F$_1$, B10 → B10.A, or B10.A → B10. In the absence of antigen, <5 PFC/culture were obtained.

irradiated (CBA × B6)F$_1$ mice. The direct (IgM) and indirect (IgG) plaque-forming cells (PFC) were measured in the spleen 1 week later. The results are shown in Table 8-6. With reference to the table, answer the following questions. (*Hint*: It is helpful to diagram the experimental design.)

(a) To which H-2 haplotype(s) should the (CBA × B6)F$_1$ T cells transferred into the irradiated recipients be restricted?

(b) Explain why the anti-Ia^k antiserum should abolish the generation of (CBA × B6)F$_1$ T$_H$ cells for B10.BR and B10.A(4R) B cells but allow the generation of (CBA × B6)F$_1$ T$_H$ cells for B10 and (CBA × B6)F$_1$ T cells (Table 8-6c).

(c) Explain why the monoclonal anti-I-A^k antibody abolishes the generation of (CBA × B6)F$_1$ T$_H$ cells that can help B10.BR cells but allows the generation of T$_H$ cells that can help B10.A(4R) cells.

(d) At minimum, based on your answers to parts (b) and (c), how many subpopulations of T$_H$ cells (based on their H-2-restricted response) must there be in your (CBA × B6)F$_1$ T$_H$ population?

8-13 This problem also involves chimeric mice and assays similar to those in the two preceding problems. The *in vitro* primary responses to the antigen TNP-(T,G)-A–L

Table 8-7 Specificity of Target Cell Lysis by H-2-Restricted Cytotoxic T Cells (Problem 8-14)

Virus Immune Spleen Cells (H-2 Type)	Specific ^{51}Cr Release from Humongo-Infected Target Cells (Percent of Total Release)		
	B10.D2 H-2^d Cells	B10 H-2^b Cells	B10.BR H-2^k Cells
B10 (H-2^b)	0	64	2
B10.D2 (H-2^d)	48	3	0
BALB/c (H-2^d)	46	4	2
BALB/b (H-2^b)	8	60	1

are regulated by autosomal dominant H-2-linked Ir genes, such that H-2^b mice are responders whereas H-2^a mice are nonresponders. B10 → B10.A and B10.A → B10 chimeras were assessed for the *in vitro* responsiveness of spleen lymphocytes to TNP-(T,G)-A–L by measurement of *in vitro* PFC formation in the Jerne plaque assay. Spleen cell populations from normal (B10 × B10.A)F$_1$ and chimeric B10 → B10.A and B10.A → B10 mice were depleted of adherent accessory cells by passage through G–10 Sephadex and reconstituted with (B10 × B10.A)F$_1$ splenic adherent cells. These reconstituted populations were then tested for their ability to generate significant responses to TNP-KLH and TNP-(T,G)-A–L. Results are shown in Figure 8-28. With reference to the figure, answer the following questions.

(a) Which H-2 haplotype do the lymphocytes that respond to TNP-(T,G)-A–L possess? Which H-2 haplotype do the lymphocytes that do not respond to TNP-(T,G)-A–L possess?

(b) To which H-2 haplotype are the TNP-(T,G)-A–L responding lymphocytes in panel B restricted? To which H-2 haplotype are the lymphocytes that do not respond to TNP-(T,G)-A–L restricted?

(c) From the information in panel B, is the Ir phenotype of a lymphocyte a consequence of the genotype of the lymphocyte or of the environment in which it differentiates?

(d) Based on your understanding of cell-cell cooperation in the generation of T-cell help and the information in the figure, describe a model to explain how this MHC-linked Ir gene might function at a molecular level.

8-14 (a) Cytotoxic T cells (T$_C$) can be generated *in vivo* by inoculating mice with certain viruses. Spleen cells from virus-primed animals can be tested for *in vitro* cytotoxicity against virus-infected target cells internally labeled with ^{51}Cr (chromium). The release of ^{51}Cr into the medium can be used as a relative measure of target cell lysis.

Assume that mice on a space shuttle returning from the planet Humongo become ill with a humongo virus fever. In a study on the specificity of cell-mediated cytotoxicity, H-2^b and H-2^d congenic mice were inoculated with humongo virus and sacrificed 6 days later. Spleen cells from these animals were used in a chromium release assay against a panel of humongo-infected target cells. The results are shown in Table 8-7. Background (spontaneous) release of ^{51}Cr from target cells in the presence of nonimmune spleen cells has been sub-

Table 8-8 Cytotoxic T-Cell Lysis of Target Cells Coated with Various Anti-MHC Antibodies (Problem 8-14)

Virus Immune Spleen Cells (H-2 Type)	Antibodies Used to Coat Targets	Specific ^{51}Cr Release from Humongo-Infected Target Cells (Percent of Total Release)		
		B10.D2(d)	B.10(b)	B10.BR(k)
B10	anti-Ia^b	0	60	5
	anti-K^b	1	30	2
	anti-D^b	0	32	1
	anti-K^b, D^b	2	1	2
	anti-Ia^d, K^d, D^d	1	62	1
B10.D2	anti-Ia^d	45	2	0
	anti-K^d	2	1	2
	anti-D^d	42	3	0
	anti-K^d, D^d	2	0	2
	anti-Ia^b, K^b, D^b	48	5	2

tracted. The total amount of ^{51}Cr released by complete cell lysis is determined by freeze-thawing humongo-infected ^{51}Cr-labeled spleen cells. What do these data suggest about the restrictions on the interaction between T_C and target cells?

(b) When the same killers and targets were incubated together after precoating the target cells with various monospecific anti-MHC antibodies, the results shown in Table 8-8 were obtained. (Because the experiments shown in Table 8-7 and 8-8 were done simultaneously, it is legitimate to consider them as one experiment.) What two conclusions can you draw from this experiment?

(c) To investigate further the restrictions on T_C-target cell interactions, chimeric mice were produced by injecting adult spleen cells or mature T-cell-depleted bone-marrow cells into lethally irradiated hosts. Parental cells were injected into F_1 recipients, or F_1 cells were injected into parental recipients. After 6–12 weeks, the recipient host immune systems had been fully reconstituted by the donor cells, and the animals were immunocompetent. These host mice were challenged with humongo virus. Six days later, the mice were sacrificed and the virus-specific T_C cells (donor derived) were tested against humongo virus-infected target cells in a ^{51}Cr-release assay. With reference to the results shown in Table 8-9, answer questions (c)–(f). Considering first the bone-marrow chimeras in line 1, what do these data suggest about the way in which T_C restriction is determined?

(d) What differences are there between the T_C restriction of adult spleen and bone-marrow chimeras of lines 1 and 2? How do you account for these differences?

(e) Comment briefly on the differences between T_C restriction for parent → F_1 and F_1 → parent chimeras (lines 1 and 3).

(f) Do these results alter your answer to question (a)? If so, why?

(g) To study the effect of the thymus on T_C restriction, thymic chimeras were prepared by implanting irradiated donor thymuses into irradiated, thymectomized and bone-marrow reconstituted hosts (ATXBM). Irradiation of the donor thymus

Table 8-9 Specificity of Target Cell Lysis by Mouse Cytotoxic T Cells from Bone-Marrow Chimeras (Problem 8-14)

Chimeras[a]		Specific ^{51}Cr Release from Humongo-Infected Target Cells (Percent of Total Release)		
Donor Cells Injected	Recipient	H-2^d	H-2^b	H-2^k
1. H-2$^{b/d}$ bone-marrow cells	H-2^d	40	0	0
2. H-2$^{b/d}$ spleen cells	H-2^d	55	30	0
3. H-2^b bone-marrow cells	H-2$^{b/d}$	40	24	0
immune controls				
H-2$^{b/d}$		62	42	0
H-2^d		60	0	0
H-2^b		0	27	0

[a]All donors and hosts were congenic B10 mice of the H-2 genotype indicated.

Table 8-10 Specificity of Target Cell Lysis by Cytotoxic T Cells from Thymectomized, Bone-Marrow-Reconstituted Mice (Problem 8-14)

BM Donor	Thymus Donor	Thymectomized Recipient	^{51}Cr Release from Humongo-Infected Target Cells		
			H-2^d Cells	H-2^b Cells	H-2^k Cells
H-2$^{d\times b}$	H-2^d	H-2$^{d\times b}$	50	0	0
H-2$^{d\times b}$	H-2^b	H-2$^{d\times b}$	4	57	1
H-2$^{d\times b}$	H-2$^{d\times b}$	H-2$^{d\times b}$	43	55	0

was necessary to prevent donor thymic lymphocytes from proliferating and repopulating the peripheral lymphoid tissues. Following challenge of these ATXBM mice with humongo virus, immune T$_C$ cells were tested in a chromium release assay, with the results shown in Table 8-10. What effect does the donor thymus have on T$_C$ restriction in this experiment? What cell type or population in the thymus is most likely to be responsible for this effect?

8-15 (a) Immunologists have long believed that B-cell receptors (antibodies) mainly see native antigenic determinants on proteins (such as influenza virus envelope HA hemagglutinin glycoproteins), whereas T cells have receptors that mainly see such antigens in the context of particular cell-surface allotypic MHC determinants. Two papers have tested that assumption [D. E. Wylie and N. R. Klinman, *J. Immunol.* **127**, 194(1981); D. E. Wylie, L. A. Sherman, and N. R. Klinman, *J. Exp. Med.* **155**, 403(1982)]. They injected mice intravenously with strain PR8 influenza virus-infected fibroblasts, removed their spleens, isolated tiny fragments containing clones of antibody-forming cells, and scored for those antibodies

Table 8-11 Binding of Monoclonal Antibodies Raised Against PR8-Infected Fibroblasts

Target Cell	H-2K Allele	H-2D Allele	Percent of Monoclonal Antibodies Binding to Cells
	Immunogen = PR8-BALB/H-2^k fibroblasts		
Experiment 1			
PR8-BALB/H-2^k	k	k	100*
PR8-BALB/c	d	d	30
PR8-C57BL/6	b	b	29
Experiment 2			
PR8-BALB/H-2^k	k	k	100*
PR8-C3H.OH	d	k	86
PR8-B10.A(4R)	k	b	19
	Immunogen = PR8-EL4/H-2^b cells		
Experiment 3			
PR8-BALB/H-2^b	b	b	100*
PR8-D2.GD	d	b	27†
PR8-B10.A(5R)	b	d	100
H-2K^b mutants‡			
bm1	bm1	b	18
bm4	bm4	b	12
bm8	bm8	b	55
bm9	bm9	b	69
bm10	bm10	b	82
bm11	bm11	b	67

*Only antibodies reactive to these cells were analyzed further.
†These include antibodies reacting to both PR8-D2.GD and PR8-B10A(5R); none reacted to PR8-D2.GD but not to PR8-B10.A(5R).
‡These are mutants of the H-2K^b gene.

which bound to influenza HA antigens on the isolated PR8 viruses and on PR8-infected cells. While 36% of the HA-binding monoclonal antibodies detected the antigens on free virions, 64% detected HA antigens only on the original virus-infected cells. Give two hypotheses to explain this result.

To test these hypotheses, they infected several different fibroblast lines with PR8 and screened them with the PR8-infected cell-specific monoclonal antibodies (Table 8-11).

(b) Explain the data in experiments 1 and 2.
(c) Explain the data in experiment 3.
(d) What do these results imply about T-versus-B-cell receptor repertoires?

Analysis of H-2 restriction by T_C cells raised against syngeneic influenza-infected cells shows that most H-2^k T_C cells are mainly H-2K^k restricted.

(e) Discuss these results in terms of the models described in Concept 8-9.

Answers

8-1 (a) True

      (b) False. B_γ cells are committed to give rise to IgG-secreting plasma cells only.

      (c) True

      (d) False. In low responder mice, a normal spectrum of antibodies to artificial polypeptides is synthesized, but in low amounts.

      (e) True

      (f) False. Macrophages or other antigen-presenting accessory cells are also required for a B-cell immune response.

      (g) False. The genes that code for antibody combining-site specificities (variable-region genes) are linked to allotypic markers that represent antibody constant-region genes. Ir genes are linked to the MHC.

8-2 (a) secondary

      (b) Blast transformation

      (c) capping

      (d) T cells, B cells, and macrophages

      (e) IgM

      (f) immune response (Ir)

      (g) macrophages and dendritic reticular cells

      (h) affinity

      (i) immunoglobulins; growth factor; differentiation factor

8-3

Cell	Distinctive markers
T_S	Lyt-2$^+$,3$^+$, I-J$^+$
T_C	Lyt-2$^+$,3$^+$, I-J$^-$
IgM plasma cell precursor	Surface IgM$^+$, IgG$^-$
IgG plasma cell precursor	Surface IgG$^+$
Macrophage	Ia$^+$, phagocytic
Dendritic reticular cell	Ia$^+$, nonphagocytic

8-4 (a) The protective effect of a sterile environment clearly indicates that the symptoms of the thymectomized mice are caused by external microbial agents rather than by internal causes (spontaneous cancers, hormonal deficiencies, histological damage, etc.). This increased susceptibility to infections suggests that the immune system may have been impaired. To test this suggestion further, you could survey the immunologic status of these mice by testing for transplant rejection, delayed hypersensitivity, and antibody production and by examining the histology of the lymphoid organs.

      (b) The extended survival of allogeneic skin grafted onto neonatally thymectomized mice demonstrates a marked depression of cellular immunity in these mice. Therefore, delayed hypersensitivity responses should also be diminished. Even if thymectomy affects only cellular immunity, antibody formation should nevertheless be reduced in accordance with the requirements for T-cell and B-cell cooperation.

      (c) By 5 days after birth, the thymus has fulfilled a major part of its role in the development of the cellular immune system. Thus adult thymectomy has little effect. The shape of the curve can best be explained by assuming that the immune system needs a population of cells that differentiate in the thymus. Over a period of days, these cells leave that organ and migrate elsewhere to proliferate and develop further. The effect of thymectomy decreases with age as an increasing number of differentiated cells leave the thymus and become established in peripheral organs. There is no satisfactory explanation as to why this developmental process seems to occur several days earlier in BALB/c mice than in most other strains. If Miller had used BALB/c mice in his original experiments, he might have concluded that the thymus was less important because the effects he saw would have been much reduced. This observation points up the possibility that even closely related organisms may vary, and it illustrates the possible role of luck in the choice of an experimental system.

8-5 (a) Spleen cells from neonatally thymectomized mice are unable to produce antibodies specific for SRBC. Intravenous injection of thymus cells, or thoracic duct lymphocytes, can restore this ability. Because thymic lymphocytes do not synthesize antibody (at least while in the thymus), there are two possible explanations: (1) the thymic lymphocytes make anti-SRBC antibody only after they have migrated from the thymus to peripheral organs; and (2) thymus-derived cells must cooperate, in some undefined manner, with antibody-producing lymphocytes before those cells can actually make antibody. In either case, a high proportion of thoracic duct lymphocytes seems to be thymus derived.

(b) In part (a), the lymphocytes in the bone marrow, nodes, and spleen were unaffected; only the thymus-specific component of the immune system was ablated. X irradiation ablates the entire system. The data show an impressive synergistic interaction between bone-marrow and thymus cells, but thymus cells alone are ineffective. This result excludes the first explanation offered in the answer to part (a). Because antibody formation by bone-marrow-derived lymphocytes is well known, it can be inferred that these cells produce antibody only following some sort of cooperative interaction with thymus-derived lymphocytes.

8-6 BN lymphocytes generate GVHR of similar magnitude in immunized and nonimmunized F_1's. The reaction generated in nonimmunized hosts by Lewis lymphocytes is also similar. However, in immunized hosts, the Lewis lymphocyte GVHR is significantly inhibited. Consider exactly what antibodies are elicited in the F_1 host by immunization with the Lewis anti-BN antibodies. The only antigenic determinants on these antibodies not normally found on the F_1 immunoglobulins should be their idiotypic determinants—that is, those of the actual antigen-binding site. Thus the F_1 rats are making antibodies against those particular antigen-binding sites on Lewis immunoglobulins that are specific for BN antigens. Those Lewis rat T cells that are specific for BN histocompatibility antigens probably have receptors (either antibodies or other molecules) whose active sites closely resemble the antigen-binding sites on the anti-BN antibodies, and hence they cross-react with the antibodies raised in the F_1's. Thus, when Lewis lymphocytes are injected into an immunized F_1, the F_1 antibodies could combine with those Lewis anti-BN receptors and presumably block the triggering process. This would not happen in nonimmunized F_1's, and the BN lymphocytes—carrying noncross-reactive receptors for Lewis antigens—would not be affected in immunized or nonimmunized hosts.

These results suggest that the same antibodies in F_1 hosts recognize both Lewis anti-BN idiotypes and Lewis anti-BN T-cell-surface receptors. Thus receptors on B cells and T cells that are specific for the same antigens could be very similar in a portion of their structure.

8-7 (a) B cells can be stained by anti-immunoglobulin. T cells can be stained by antibodies to specific T-cell membrane differentiation antigens such as Thy-1 (mouse) or T11 (man).

(b) The primary follicles will stain for B cells; the diffuse cortex will stain for T cells.

(c) You will see development of germinal centers with large B cells expressing IgM but not IgD; expansion of medullary cords with many IgM plasma cells and a few IgG and IgA plasma cells.

(d) You will see the same patterns as in part (c) except that the germinal center cells are IgG$^+$IgD$^-$, and the plasma cells are predominantly IgG$^+$.

(e) T cells are found in the periarteriolar sheath, and B cells are found in eccentric follicles on the sheath. Intravenous or intraarterial injections of antigens give preferential responses in the spleen.

8-8 (a) This experiment is a control that illustrates the normal secondary response when animals immunized with DNP-OVA are challenged with DNP-OVA.

(b) The middle panel of Figure 8-26 shows the absence of a secondary response when animals immunized with DNP-OVA are challenged with DNP-BGG. The upper panel shows the result of preimmunizing with the heterologous carrier. Preimmunization generates a population of BGG-immune ("BGG-primed") lymphocytes. Consequently, both hapten-primed cells (generated by the first immunization with DNP-OVA) and carrier-primed cells seem necessary for a secondary anti-hapten response. Without the first DNP-OVA immunization, there would be no DNP-primed cells; therefore only a primary anti-DNP response would be expected.

(c) An animal can be immunized passively by transfer of humoral antibodies—either purified or as an unfractionated antiserum—or by transferring lymphocytes. Because passive immunization with antibody against heterologous carrier did not increase the secondary anti-hapten response (middle panel, Figure 8-26), the carrier effect appears to be a manifestation of cellular immunity. This notion could be tested by adoptively immunizing with BGG-primed lymphocytes, which would be expected to enhance the secondary anti-hapten response. The results of these experiments support the conclusion that T$_H$ cells specific for carrier determinants somehow cooperate with B cells specific for hapten determinants to produce the secondary anti-hapten response.

8-9 Treatment with anti-Lyt-1 antiserum plus complement lyses thymus-derived lymphocytes that express the Lyt-1 antigen on their surfaces. Because the DNP-primed cells are unaffected by this treatment, they must be B cells. This result is expected because these cells actually produce the anti-hapten antibody. The destruction of BGG-primed cells by the antiserum provides additional evidence that these BGG-primed specific cells are T cells.

8-10 (a) The following H-2 haplotypes would be recognized as self in experiments (1)–(6):

(1) H-2^b, H-2^a
(2) H-2^b, H-2^a
(3) H-2^b
(4) H-2^a
(5) H-2^a
(6) H-2^b

Remember that the spleen cells differentiated in the recipient mice: thus they will recognize the H-2 haplotype of the recipient as self.

(b) Three alternative explanations would be as follows:

1. Failure occurs in cell-cell cooperation because the T cells are restricted to a different haplotype than that expressed by the antigen-presenting cells and B cells (which are of donor origin and thus express donor H-2 molecules).

2. Failure occurs in development, differentiation, or survival of one or more of the cell populations needed for a response in the recipient.

3. The immune response is suppressed.

(c) The first explanation is the only one consistent with the results.

8-11 (a) H-2^b
(b) H-2^a

(c) H-2^a, H-2^b

(d) H-2^a, H-2^b

(e) Remember that there were donor cells (i.e., the developing lymphocytes) expressing donor H-2 antigens in the recipient mouse during T-cell differentiation. The developing lymphocytes definitely did not dictate self-recognition to each other, despite the fact that they express donor-type H-2 antigens; therefore, recipient tissues, such as thymic epithelium, must have dictated self-recognition to the maturing T cells.

8-12   This experiment illustrates the generation of H-2-restricted helper T cells. In the recipient mouse, "virgin" T cells are exposed to antigen in an environment where none, some, or all H-2^k Ia molecules have been blocked by antibodies. Only those T cells that recognize unblocked Ia molecules (i.e., H-2^b Ia molecules) in the presence of antigen will be stimulated to proliferate and become effector T_H, capable of helping B cells. The PFC assay measures the number of B cells helped to secrete anti-SRBC antibody, and thus it indicates the number of T_H cells generated.

(a) The injected (CBA $\times$ B6)F$_1$ T cells should be restricted to haplotypes H-2^b and H-2^k.

(b) The anti-Ia^k antiserum blocks all Ia^k molecules in the T-cell-recipient mouse: thus only T cells that recognize Ia^b molecules in conjunction with SRBC are stimulated to proliferate.

(c) The three anti-I-A^k monoclonal antibodies prevent activation of T_H cells that recognize as restricting elements $A_\alpha^k A_\beta^k$, $A_\alpha^b A_\beta^k$, $A_\alpha^k A_\beta^b$, $E_\alpha^k E_\beta^k$, or $E_\alpha^b E_\beta^k$. However, $E_\alpha^k E_\beta^b$ is unblocked (remember that E_α^k is encoded in the I-E subregion).

(d) There must be a minimum of two subpopulations, and there are probably eight.

8-13   (a) The haplotype of the responders is genetically either H-2^a or H-2^a/H-2^b. The haplotype of the nonresponders is genetically H-2^b.

(b) The responders are restricted to haplotype H-2^b. The nonresponders are restricted to haplotype H-2^a.

(c) The Ir phenotype of a lymphocyte is a consequence not of its genotype but of the environment in which it differentiates.

(d) One plausible explanation for these results is that Ir genes code for Ia antigens so that a T_H cell's Ir phenotype reflects simply its Ia haplotype and therefore its potential for MHC-associated recognition in carrying out helper function.

8-14   (a) T_C cells raised against humongo virus by *in vivo* immunization recognize and destroy humongo-infected target cells only if they share H-2 haplotypes. This recognition could occur through like-like interactions or receptor-ligand recognition events.

(b) The following two conclusions can be drawn. First, B10 killer T cells include T_C cells that recognize humongo-infected cells with H-2K^b as the restricting determinant as well as others that recognize H-2D^b as the restricting determinant, but few if any that recognize Ia^b as a restricting determinant. B10.D2 T_C cells use only H-2K^d as a restricting determinant with humongo viral antigens; H-2D^d-humongo antigens are a *precluded* pair.

(c) T_C restriction is determined by the environment in the irradiated host, not by the H-2 type of the injected donor cells.

(d) Whereas spleen cells from bone-marrow chimeras are host restricted, spleen cells from spleen cell chimeras are donor restricted. This phenomenon occurs because T cells from the donor spleen have already gone through their early maturation in an F$_1$ (H-2^b $\times$ H-2^d) environment.

(e) Again, H-2 restriction is dependent on the H-2 determinants in the microenvironment in which the bone-marrow cells mature to peripheral T cells, and not, in this case, on the bone-marrow donor environment.

(f) Based on this result, the possibility of like-like interactions is unlikely; therefore, H-2 restriction probably involves T-cell receptor recognition of target cell H-2 restricting elements.

(g) The microenvironment that dictates H-2 restriction of developing T cells in bone-marrow chimeras appears to be in the irradiated thymus. Because the thymic lymphocytes, macrophages, and dendritic cells are derived from bone marrow, whereas the thymic epithelial cells are derived from the thymus, the evidence points to thymic epithelial cells as being responsible for the development of specific H-2 restriction. As a cautionary note, however, these experiments are highly artificial, involving irradiation, bone-marrow transplantation, and thymus transplantation, so that the potential for artifact is great in drawing conclusions about the physiological development of H-2 restriction.

8-15 (a) The two most likely hypotheses are (1) that the influenza HA antigen reveals on the cell surface antigenic determinants that are hiding in the close packing of HA proteins on the virion and (2) that the cell-surface antigenic determinants involve some interaction complex between HA molecules and cell-surface molecules.

(b) The anti-H-2^k PR8-infected cell antibodies appear to be H-2 restricted in their binding, mainly to the H-2D^k allele. These experiments rule out model (1) and favor model (2).

(c) The anti-H-2^k PR8-infected cell antibodies appear to be H-2 restricted in their binding and to bind exclusively to the H-2K^b allele. The mutants of the H-2K^b allele quite often lost that restricting specificity.

(d) These experiments show that antibodies, like T cells, may be H-2 restricted in their recognition of antigens. Thus a single combining site (in this case V_H-V_L bounded) can detect an H-2-restricted antigen, and T-cell receptors could theoretically do so also. Obviously, these B cells did not undergo thymus "education" like their T-cell counterparts, and if self-MHC-directed education is required for self-MHC restriction, the educating elements for these B cells are likely to be extrathymic.

(e) In essence, these data apparently demonstrate that T_C-recognized *precluded pairs* are not necessarily precluded for antibody combining sites. All combinations of PR8 HA antigens and H-2^k or H-2^b gene products are susceptible to associated recognition, and preclusion is apparently at the level of the antigen receptor. These findings make difficult the simple hypothesis that, for example, influenza HA and H-2K^b are a precluded pair for T_C cells because they cannot associate in the cell membrane of an infected target cell; they are easily recognized by a single combining site. Rather, they are not capable of forming an appropriate antigenic complex for the repertoire of available T-cell receptors on competent T_C cells in mice. Thus these findings weaken the simplest hypotheses that put Ir gene function and the phenomenon of preclusion at the level of failure of particular precluded pairs to form a complex antigen (or altered self), and they require more complicated models of MHC and nominal antigen interactions at the cell surface if these models are to survive. These data do *not* weaken the arguments that preclusion is due to the lack of production of cognate T-cell receptors, or of survival of cells bearing those receptors, or that such precluded pairs selectively stimulate suppressor cell pathways.

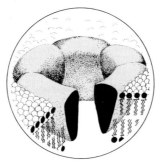

CHAPTER 9

Immune Effector Mechanisms and the Complement System

Chapter Outline

Immune responses provide several overlapping mechanisms for eliminating foreign macromolecules, microorganisms, and cancer cells. The humoral immune system is most effective for surveillance of extracellular pathogens, whereas the cell-mediated immune system

Table 9-1 Physiological Properties of the Five Immunoglobulin Classes in Humans

Class	Mean Adult Serum Level (mg/mL)	Serum Half-Life (Days)	Physiological Functions
IgM	1.0	5	Complement fixation; early immune response; stimulation of ingestion by macrophages
IgG	12	25	Complement fixation; placental transfer; stimulation of ingestion by macrophages
IgA	1.8	6	Localized protection in external secretions
IgD	0.03	2.8	Function unknown
IgE	0.0003	2	Stimulation of mast cells; parasite expulsion

is most effective for surveillance of infected or antigenically foreign cells. Both the antibody-mediated and the cell-mediated immune responses initiate elimination reactions by recognition of antigenic targets. Antigen recognition triggers containment, neutralization, and cleanup operations. Containment of antigen at its point of entry is accomplished by walling off the area by localized inflammation. Neutralization of free antigen targets such as toxins or viruses occurs by antibody binding, whereas neutralization of antigen-bearing target cells is accomplished by direct cell lysis or by phagocytosis and internal killing. Antigen–antibody complexes and any remaining debris are cleaned up by phagocytosis. This chapter considers the variety of effector mechanisms utilized by the vertebrate immune system.

Concepts

9-1 The function of an antibody is determined by its heavy chains

Properties of antibody classes

Although all immunoglobulin molecules probably bind antigen in a similar fashion, the five different antibody classes serve different physiological functions (Table 9-1). These functional differences reflect the structural differences in their heavy-chain constant regions, which comprise the effector domains of all immunoglobulin molecules. Antibodies of the five classes are produced in different relative amounts in primary and secondary immune responses (Figure 8-4), are present in normal human serum at very different concentrations, and differ significantly in normal serum half-life (Table 9-1).

IgM

IgM, the first antibody produced in response to an immunogen, is a pentamer of antibody structural units held together by the so-called J (for joining) chain polypeptide (Figure 2-5). IgM is principally an antibody of the blood. Because of its large size, it enters the interstitial fluid slowly, if at all, and it does not cross the placenta to enter fetal circulation. IgM is particularly effective against invading microorganisms. Although the affinity of each IgM active site for a cognate antigenic determinant may be low, the overall avidity of the IgM pentamer for a complex antigen is very high because of the presence of repeating determinants on many complex antigens and most cell-membrane antigens. Because it is pentameric, IgM is about 1000 times more effective on a molar basis at agglutinating cells by cross-linking than are monomeric divalent antibodies. IgM bound to an antigenic target stimulates its ingestion by macrophages and its destruction by complement fixation (Concept 9-2).

IgG

IgG is a monomeric antibody produced later in an immune response than IgM (Figure 8-4). Low doses of antigen stimulate IgM production only; higher doses are required to stimulate IgG appearance. The several subclasses of IgG are collectively the most prevalent antibodies in the blood. Of the five classes of antibody, IgG can traverse blood-vessel walls and enter the interstitial spaces most efficiently. Typically about half of an organism's IgG antibodies are found in the bloodstream and about half in the interstitial spaces. Certain subclasses of IgG are the only antibodies that can cross the placenta to provide immunity for a developing fetus. The prevalence of IgG in the bloodstream makes it a major trigger of complement fixation, although on a molar basis it is many times less effective than IgM. IgG bound to an antigenic target stimulates its ingestion by macrophages.

IgA

IgA is also produced later in an immune response than IgM, and it can be made in both monomeric and dimeric forms. The dimers are composed of two monomers held together by J chain protein produced by IgA-secreting plasma cells. IgA is found predominantly in the gastrointestinal tract, in saliva, in sweat and tears, and it is the major immunoglobulin in milk and colostrum where it may function to protect the gastrointestinal tracts of nursing infants. IgA antibodies protect epithelial surfaces by combining with microorganisms to prevent their attachment. Failing attachment, these organisms are swept out by local motive forces (Figure 9-1).

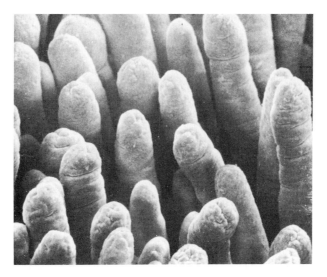

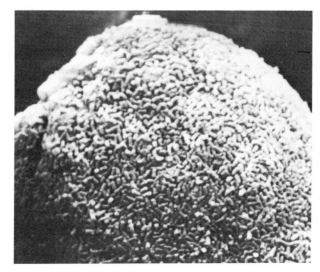

Figure 9-1

Scanning electron micrographic view of neonatal pig intestinal epithelium (a) devoid of bacterial attachment and (b) with bound enterotoxigenic *E. Coli.* Figure (b) is a closeup of a single intestinal villus packed with the rodlike bacilli, a state which can occur in IgA-deficient individuals. [Photo courtesy of Richard E. Isaacson.]

IgA is directed to specific epithelial sites by a two-step process. Antigen-activated B_α blast cells home selectively to these sites and there complete their maturation into IgA-secreting plasma cells. Epithelial cells at these sites produce a membrane-bound protein called SC_m (secretory component, membrane form) that has a high affinity for immunoglobulin-bound J chains (Figure 9-2). SC_m·J·Ig complexes are endocytosed by the epithelial cells and transported via intracellular vesicles to the luminal (apical) cell surface. There a membrane fusion event and a proteolytic cleavage release soluble SC·J·Ig com-

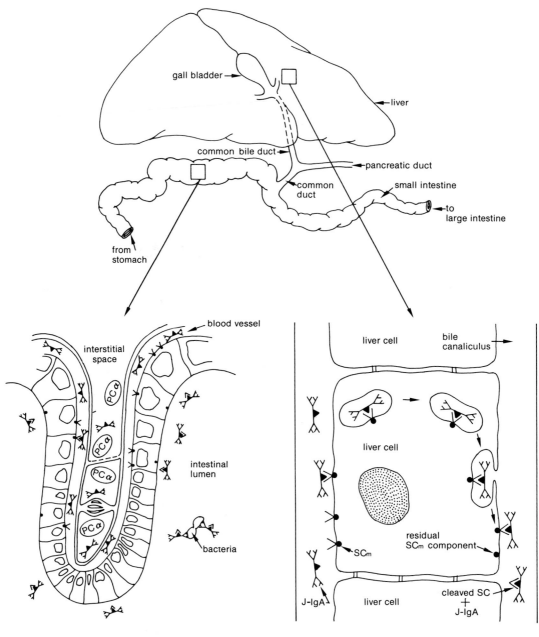

Figure 9-2   Production and transport of IgA antibodies to epithelial surfaces. Symbols: ▲ = J chain; 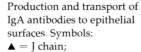 = J · IgA (dimer); 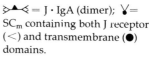 = SC$_m$ containing both J receptor (<) and transmembrane (●) domains.

plexes, leaving the transmembrane portion of SC_m in the membrane. IgM, which also contains a J chain, can be secreted by this mechanism as well. However, because the local concentration of IgA is much higher than that of IgM at these epithelial sites, the concentration of IgA in extracellular fluids bathing epithelial cells is also much greater. IgA-deficient vertebrates have significant concentrations of IgM in these fluids.

IgD, IgE

IgD, a monomeric antibody whose function is unknown, is normally present in the blood only in minute concentrations. IgE, a monomeric, heat-labile antibody, is also normally present in the blood in minute concentrations. Blood IgE levels rise significantly in allergic individuals (Concept 12-8) and in individuals with gastrointestinal parasites. IgE antibodies bind tightly via their Fc regions to blood basophiles and to *mast* cells in connective tissues.

9-2 Antigen-bound IgM and IgG antibodies initiate complement fixation

Opsonization

The phagocytes of the blood—monocytes, macrophages, and polymorphonuclear leukocytes (Figure 1-3)—bind and ingest foreign substances even prior to an antibody response. However, the rate of binding and phagocytosis increases by an order of magnitude if the foreign substance is coated with IgM or IgG antibodies. This process of preparing foreign particles for ingestion by phagocytes is called *opsonization*, and the specifically bound antibodies are called *opsonins*. Phagocytic cells bear multiple low affinity receptors for the constant regions of IgM and IgG antibodies. A particulate antigen coated with these antibodies binds with high avidity to the receptors and triggers phagocytosis. First, Fc receptors on a small area of the macrophage surface interact with the Fc regions of antibody molecules bound to the particle. Then additional Fc receptors on the macrophage interact with the remaining antibody molecules by extension of membrane leaflets over the surface of the particle in a zippering process that results in membrane fusion on the opposite side, forming a phagosome (Figure 9-3). This receptor-ligand binding leads to a highly local phagocytic response; antigens bound experimentally (for example, by lectins) to other regions of the macrophage membrane at the same time are not phagocytosed (Figure 9-4).

Complement fixation

IgM and most subclasses of IgG antibodies activate the *complement system* when they bind to foreign antigens. The complement system is a set of proteins that constitutes about 10% of the globulins in the

Figure 9-3

A diagram of an experiment to show that IgG-Fc receptor-mediated phagocytosis is a local, segmental response on the macrophage membrane. Macrophages bearing lectin-binding sites and Fc receptors are bound to target red blood cells either via Fc receptors or via lectin cross-linking. Only Fc-receptor binding triggers phagocytosis, and only membrane areas with IgG-coated red blood cells participate in the formation of a phagosome. Red blood cells bound by lectin cross-links stay on the macrophage surface. Attachment, engulfment, and membrane zippering lead to formation of the phagosome. [Adapted from F. M. Griffin Jr., J. A. Griffin, J. E. Leider, and S. C. Silverstein, *J. Exp. Med.* **142,** 1263(1975).]

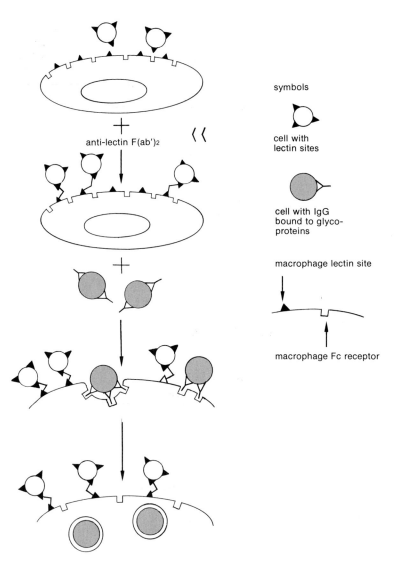

anti-lectin F(ab')₂

symbols

cell with lectin sites

cell with IgG bound to glyco-proteins

macrophage lectin site

macrophage Fc receptor

normal serum of humans and other vertebrates (Figure 9-5). Complement proteins are not immunoglobulins, and their concentrations are not affected by immunization. At least three complement components—C2, C4, and B—are coded for or regulated by genes in the MHC. The so-called *classical pathway* of the complement activation is triggered by antigen–antibody complexes to initiate a cascade of proteolytic cleavage and protein-binding reactions with at least three important consequences for host defense (Figure 9-6). First, if the antigen–antibody complex is on the surface of a foreign cell, activated complement components attack the cell membrane to cause lysis and cell death. The utilization of complement components in this process is called *complement fixation.* Second, a cleavage product of comple-

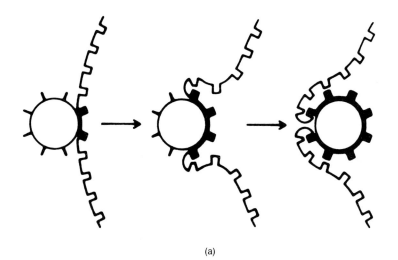

(a)

Figure 9-4
The formation of a phagosome in a macrophage interacting with IgG-coated red blood cells via the Fc receptor on the macrophage plasma membrane. (a) Diagram of the zippering of macrophage membrane leaflets around IgG-coated red blood cells. (b) - (e) Sequential scanning electron micrographs of the process. [Electron micrographs courtesy of J. Orenstein and E. Shelton.]

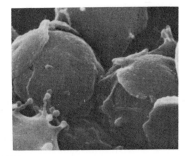

(b)

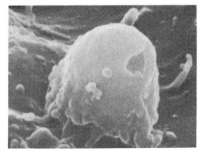

(c)

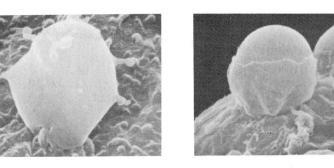

(d)

(e)

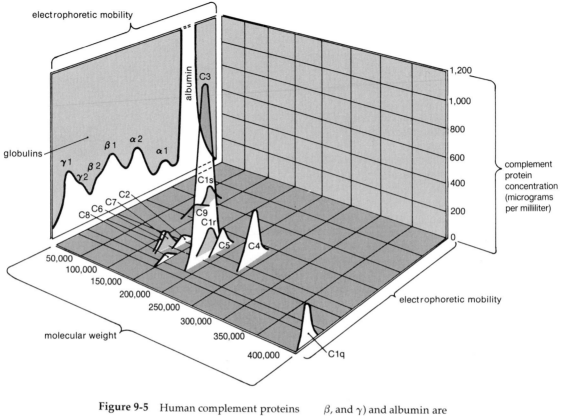

Figure 9-5 Human complement proteins characterized by molecular weights, electrophoretic mobilities at pH 8.6, and concentrations in the blood serum. For purposes of comparison, the mobilities and concentrations of globulins (α, β, and γ) and albumin are shown as well. [From M. Mayer, "The Complement System," *Sci. Am.* **229,** 54(1973). Copyright 1973 by Scientific American, Inc. All rights reserved.]

ment component C3 binds to foreign particles that have complexed with antibodies. The attached C3 fragment (C3b) interacts with C3b-specific receptors on phagocytic cells to promote the process of *immune adherence*, which is similar to opsonization. Third, release of other cleavage products results in the development of a local, acute inflammatory reaction (Concept 9-4) that walls off the area and attracts large numbers of phagocytic polymorphonuclear leukocytes. These cells carry Fc receptors and, like macrophages, can engulf and digest IgG antibody-coated particles. They also release several acid hydrolases that catalyze digestion of extracellular macromolecules and activation of the blood-clotting system.

The complex sequence of events in the classical pathway of complement fixation is diagrammed in Figure 9-7. Complement activation

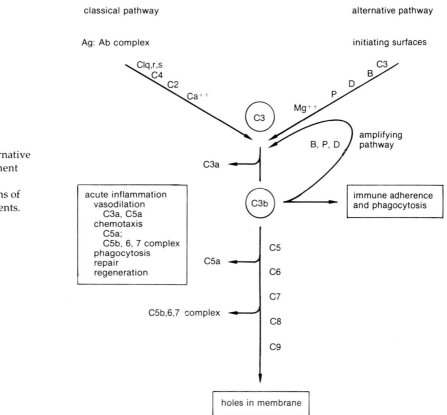

Figure 9-6

The classical and alternative pathways of complement activation and the physiological functions of complement components.

is initiated by the binding of one IgM or several IgG molecules—perhaps as few as two in close proximity—to an antigen on a foreign cell surface. This interaction exposes complement-binding sites on the Fc regions of the antibody molecules. Complement component C1, a heat-labile complex of three proteins, binds to the antigen–antibody complex via its C1q subcomponent, which has six binding sites specific for IgM and IgG Fc regions (Figure 9-8). In the presence of Ca^{2+}, this interaction activates C1s, another subcomponent with proteolytic activity, to cleave C4. The larger of the two C4 fragments, in association with C1, then specifically cleaves C2. The larger fragments from C4 and C2 combine on the membrane to form a specific protease that cleaves C3. The two resulting fragments of C3—C3a and C3b—have distinct activities. C3a (molecular weight 7000) causes local blood-vessel dilation and may also attract polymorphonuclear leukocytes; a subfragment of C3a is a potent immunosuppressant of lymphocyte activation. C3b is a metastable molecule with an internal thiolester bond which becomes labile following cleavage of the intact C3 molecule. The thiolester bond opens, and the activated carbonyl either interacts with H_2O to form a fluid-phase C3b, or it attacks a cell-

Figure 9-7

Diagrammatic representation of the sequence of events in complement activation on a cell membrane. (a) When two IgG molecules bind to adjacent sites on a foreign cell, they can activate complement factor C1. C1 consists of three subunits, C1q, C1s, and C1r, that are held together by a calcium ion. (b) C1 is inactive until it binds antibody through the C1q subunit. Then C1s, a serine esterase, becomes activated (shading). (c) C4 is cleaved into two parts, C4a and C4b. (d) C4b binds to the cell surface nearby. (e) C2 is split by the activated C1s. (f) The C2a fragment combines with C4b to form a proteolytic enzyme that splits C3. (g) The C3b fragment binds to the surface. *(Figure continues on next page.)*

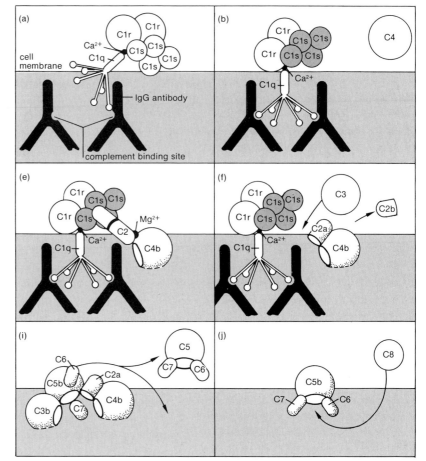

surface R-OH group to form a covalent bond. C3b attaches over the entire cell membrane, promotes opsonization, and combines with the C4–C2 complex to initiate cleavage of C5. The smaller of the resulting C5 fragments (molecular weight 15,000) is vasoactive like C3a, and it may attract polymorphonuclear leukocytes. The larger C5 fragment binds to the cell membrane and combines with C6 and C7 to form a trimolecular complex—C5,6,7—which in turn can bind C8 and C9. In addition, free forms of the C5,6,7 complex are strong chemotactic attractants for polymorphonuclear leukocytes. Upon binding of C8 and C9, the *membrane attack complex* (C5–9) is completed, and the cell membrane develops characteristic circular lesions (Figure 9-9a) that permit cell contents to leak out. The lesions probably do not result from direct enzymatic attack but rather from hydrophilic channels in the membrane formed by insertion of C8 and C9 into the membrane. In this remarkable process, water-soluble C9 monomers polymerize,

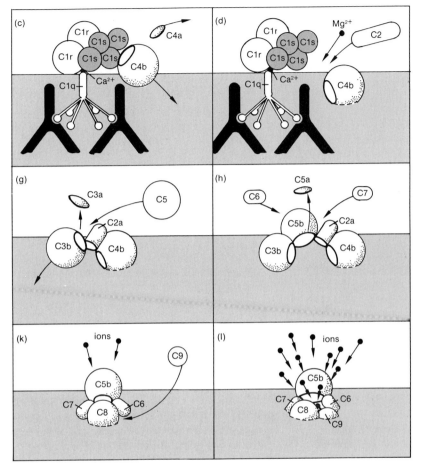

(h) If C3b is near the C4b,2a complex, they bind together and cleave C5. (i) C5b then binds to C6 and C7. (j) The C5b,6,7 complex can act as an inflammatory mediator, or it can bind to the surface at a new site where it complexes with C8. (k) These components form a small hole in the membrane through which a few ions can pass. (l) The addition of C9 greatly enlarges the hole and speeds up the flow of water and ions, leading to osmotic lysis. The C3a, C5a, and C5b,6,7 fragments mediate various aspects of the inflammatory response (see text). [From M. Mayer, "The Complement System," *Sci. Am.* **229**, 54(1973). Copyright 1973 by Scientific American, Inc. All rights reserved.]

altering their conformation to expose hydrophobic domains that allow stable incorporation into the lipid bilayer.

The *alternative pathway (properdin pathway)* of complement activation is an important host defense against gram-negative bacteria that inhabit the gastrointestinal tract (Figure 9-6). Lipopolysaccharides in the cell walls of these organisms, which are *endotoxins* in their free form, trigger the alternative pathway by providing a surface that protects C3b from its normal inactivation by serum factor H. A low level of C3b is produced continuously through the actions of serum factors B and D in the presence of Mg^{++}. Serum factor B, when complexed with C3, is cleaved at a low rate by serum factor D. The resulting BbC3 complex acts as a low efficiency C3 convertase to produce some C3b. Surface-stabilized C3b complexes with B to promote its cleavage by D to Bb. In the presence of another crucial serum component, properdin (P), a ternary complex forms and efficiently cleaves C3 to C3b. From

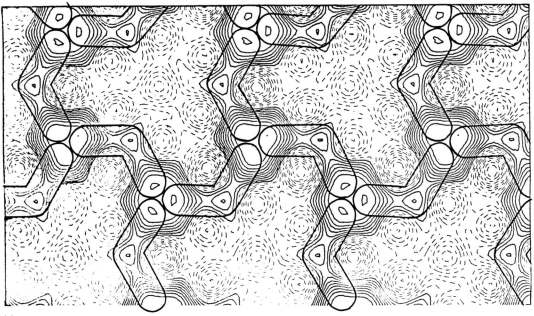

(a)

10nm

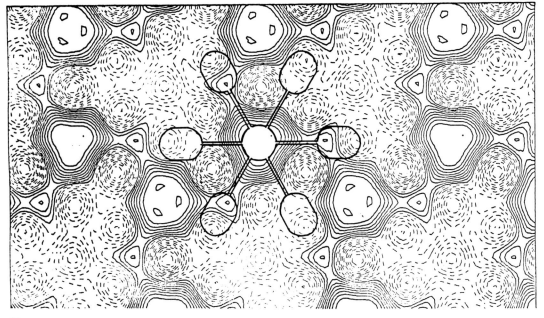

(b)

10nm

◄ **Figure 9-8**

The proposed interaction of antibodies (a) and C1q molecules (b) on a lipid-linked hapten in a monolayer that has formed a crystalline array. Monoclonal antibodies to DNP-phosphatidyl ethanolamine were allowed to diffuse laterally on a planar lipid monolayer, forming a crystalline lattice. The antibodies form a hexagonal array and their distribution was inferred by image analysis of electron micrographs. The proposed arrangement of antibodies is shown in (a) as inverted V-shape structures, whereas the proposed arrangement of C1q molecules is shown in (b) as a hexavalent molecule. [Courtesy of Dr. Roger Kornberg.]

(a)

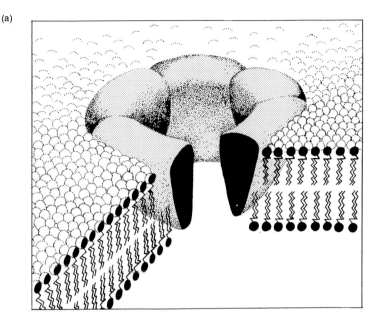

Figure 9-9

(a) A hypothetical model of a cell-membrane pore created by complement action. [From M. Mayer, "The complement system," *Sci. Am.* **229,** 54(1973). Copyright 1973 by Scientific American, Inc. All rights reserved.] (b) Model for the circular polymerization of C9 on a membrane. 1. Binding of monomeric C9 molecules to the membrane. 2. Polymerization of C9 monomers is associated with a conformational change leading to the exposure of hydrophobic domains that insert into the membrane's lipid bilayer. 3. Circular polymerization continues to form a membrane channel. [Adapted from J. Schopp et al., *Nature* **298,** 537(1982).]

(b)

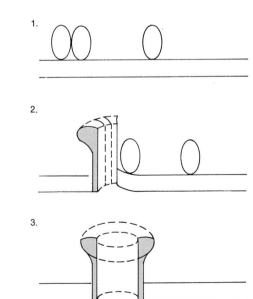

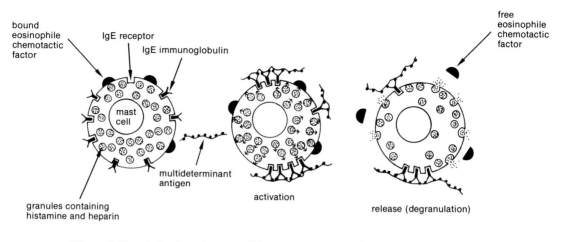

Figure 9-10   Activation of a mast cell by multivalent antigen bound to passively acquired IgE. Activation leads to the exocytosis of granules containing heparin and histamine and to their release into the extracellular fluid.

this point on, the sequence of events is the same as in the classical pathway.

The alternative pathway bypasses the need for antibody, C1, C4, and C2 and allows the complement system to be activated acutely in response to some infections. This pathway can probably be crucially important as a mechanism by which a local invasion of gastrointestinal gram-negative bacteria can activate a local protective response. However, if endotoxin enters the bloodstream, a catastrophic activation of the alternative pathway can rapidly lead to shock (massive vasodilation) and death. Endotoxin-induced shock is a late and common event for many patients with other primary disorders. The alternative pathway also serves an *amplifying* function for classical initiation of the complement cascade in that C3b combines with factors D, B, and P to amplify the further cleavage of C3.

9-3   Antigen-bound IgE antibodies trigger degranulation of mast cells

IgE antibodies on the surfaces of mast cells bind antigens from multicellular parasites and trigger mast cells to degranulate—that is, to release the contents of their intracellular vacuoles (Figures 9-10 and 9-11). IgE antibodies bind with high affinity ($K_A \sim 10^{11}$) to a special receptor complex on the surface of mast cells and basophiles. Intermolecular cross-linking of IgE receptors by bound multivalent antigens is required for and initiates mast cell triggering (Figure 9-12).

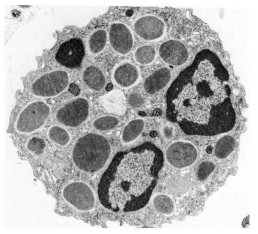

(a)

Figure 9-11

Stages of guinea pig basophile degranulation by sequential membrane fusion events. Figure (a) shows an intact basophile with numerous membrane-bound cytoplasmic vesicles, most containing an electron-dense granule. In (b) antigen combination with surface-adherent IgE has resulted in the release of all cytoplasmic granules into a central degranulation sac by multiple vesicle membrane fusions. The degranulation sac has also fused with the plasma membrane, and four granules are at the communicating pore to the extracellular environment. [Photos courtesy of Dr. Ann Dvorak.]

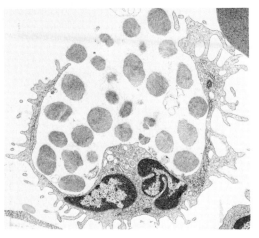

(b)

Degranulation releases several substances, including histamine, a sulfated polysaccharide called *heparin,* and leukotrienes C4, D4, and E4 (formerly known as the slow-reacting-substances of anaphylaxis, SRS-A). These molecules cause vasodilation and both rapid and prolonged smooth muscle contraction. Although the full functional significance of the IgE system is still a mystery, vasodilation and muscle contraction probably promote the expulsion of parasites from organs that are surrounded by smooth muscle, such as the gastrointestinal tract and the uterus. Individuals with gastrointestinal parasites usually have high concentrations of intestinal mast cells coated with IgE. The degranulation of mast cells also releases a chemotactic factor for eosinophiles, which enter the site of infection, bind to the parasites, and in some manner damage them.

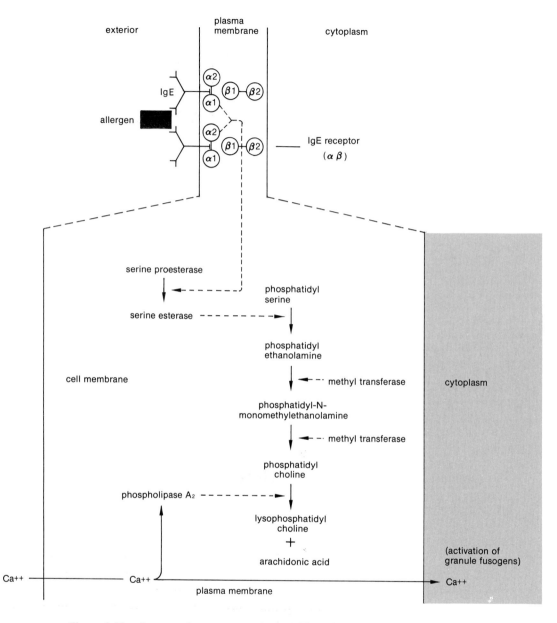

Figure 9-12 Intramembranous events in a mast cell leading to degranulation following triggering of the IgE receptors by allergen–IgE interaction. The enzymatic cascade leads to Ca influx, the activation of phospholipase A2, and the generation of arachidonic acid and lysophosphatidyl choline.

Figure 9-13

Photomicrographs of (a) *acute* and (b) *chronic* inflammation. Polymorphonuclear leukocytes predominate in acute inflammation, whereas lymphocytes and macrophages predominate in chronic inflammation. [Photomicrographs by R. Rouse and I. Weissman.]

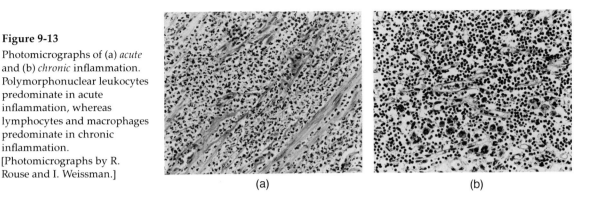

(a)   (b)

9-4 Inflammatory responses wall off sites of infection

Acute inflammatory response

Acute inflammatory responses, induced by antigen-complement complexes or by injury, involve a rapid set of events at the affected site. Local vessel dilation allows an influx of plasma proteins and polymorphonuclear leukocytes into the tissue spaces to cause swelling (Figure 9-13a). Activation of polymorphonuclear leukocytes by antigen–antibody complement complexes can trigger two reactions. If large numbers of complexes attach to the leukocytes, or if the complexes are too large to be digested, the phagolysosomal contents are released into the extracellular spaces where they can cause considerable tissue injury. In addition, the membranes of activated polymorphonuclear leukocytes initiate another set of events that results in the secretion of highly potent lipid mediators of inflammation. Membrane phospholipids are cleaved by phospholipases to form arachidonic acid, the precursor of prostaglandins, thromboxanes, and leukotrienes (Figure 9-14). Various of these substances are highly active in constriction of blood vessels and bronchiolar smooth muscles, in vasodilation, and in attracting eosinophiles and more polymorphonuclear leukocytes. Collectively, these events account for the four cardinal signs of inflammation: *heat* (calor) and *redness* (rubor) from local vessel dilation, *swelling* (tumor) from influx of proteins and cells, and *pain* (dolor) from the triggering of local nerve endings due to vasoactive products and increased tissue pressure.

If the acute response rids the host of the agents that induced inflammation, then repair and regeneration ensue. If not, the continued influx of polymorphonuclear leukocytes and serum proteins leads to cell death and, in some instances, to the formation of an abscess. Such a swelling is typically bounded by cells involved in phagocytosis and repair and by fibrin from clotted blood, and it has a central cavity of

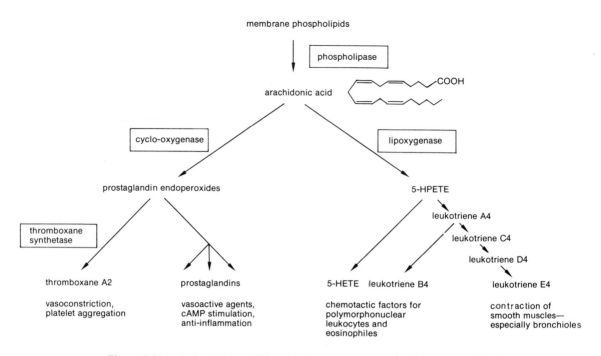

Figure 9-14   A simple view of the activation of membrane lipid mediators of inflammation.

live and dead polymorphonuclear leukocytes, tissue debris, and the injurious or infectious agents. The center of an abscess is said to be *purulent,* and the liquid it contains is commonly known as pus.

Chronic inflammatory response

Continuing acute inflammatory responses may become *chronic* inflammatory responses with the same four cardinal signs, but with different cellular and soluble protein participants. Chronic inflammatory responses are characterized by an infiltration of T lymphocytes and macrophages (Figure 9-13b). Effector T_D cells (and perhaps other T cells as well), when stimulated by cell-bound antigens at the affected site, are thought to release a variety of polypeptides, called *lymphokines,* to initiate the chronic inflammatory response.

Lymphokines have diverse activities on cells (Table 9-2). One set of lymphokines attracts macrophages to the site of antigen stimulation, activates them to a phagocytic state, and prevents their departure. Lymphokines also include agents that nonspecifically damage all cells except lymphocytes, and other agents, such as γ interferon, that prevent intracellular virus multiplication. γ interferon also activates natural killer cells, thereby increasing the number of killer cells in the region. Which of these agents are most important in inflammation is not yet known, but lymphokines induced in tissue culture will initiate inflammatory responses if injected into the skin, and antibod-

Table 9-2   Characteristics of Some T-Cell Lymphokines

Lymphokine	Properties
Macrophage chemotactic factor	Attracts macrophages *in vitro*
Macrophage migration inhibition factor	Inhibits macrophage movement *in vitro*
Macrophage aggregation factor	Agglutinates macrophages *in vitro*
Lymphocyte growth factors (e.g., IL2, BCGF, IL3)	Induce hematolymphoid cell DNA synthesis (IL2 for T cells; BCGF for B cells; IL3 for many myeloid stem cells and mast cells)
Lymphotoxin	Acts *in vitro* as a slow general cytotoxin that spares lymphocytes
γ interferon	Prevents viral replication in target cells; activates natural killer cells and macrophages
Transfer factor	Transfers delayed hypersensitivity to specific antigens from one person to another; dialyzable factor

ies against lymphokines will prevent chronic inflammatory responses if injected together with antigen.

Immediate and delayed hypersensitivity

Both acute (antibody-induced) and chronic (T-cell-induced) inflammations may occur in the skin, where they are called *immediate* and *delayed hypersensitivity*, respectively (Table 9-3). Immediate hypersensitivity, which is mediated by complement activation, begins within hours of antibody-induced immunological injury, usually peaks in intensity in 24 hours, and subsides in 48 hours. A special case of immediate hypersensitivity—induced by antigen, IgE, and mast cells, but not mediated by complement—arises within minutes of antigen–IgE binding and subsides several hours later. Delayed hypersensitivity first appears 24–48 hours after T-cell-induced immunological injury, peaks in intensity at 48–72 hours, and subsides thereafter.

9-5   Host cells destroy antigenically foreign cells by phagocytosis and by contact lysis

Phagocytosis

Phagocytic cells, such as macrophages and polymorphonuclear leukocytes, efficiently endocytose antigenically foreign cells that are coated

Table 9-3 Hypersensitivity Reactions in the Skin

Class	Subclass	Interval to Peak Reaction	Immune Effectors	Soluble Intermediates	Cellular Infiltrates
Immediate	(1) Anaphylactic	15–30 minutes	IgE + mast cells	Histamine Heparin Eosinophile Chemotactic factors Leukotrienes C4, D4, and E4	Mast cells, eosinophiles
	(2) Complement dependent	6–18 hours	IgM, IgG + complement	Anaphylotoxins (C3a, C5a) chemotactic factors (C5b, C6, C7 trimolecular complex)	Polymorpho-nuclear leukocytes
Delayed	(1) Cutaneous basophile hypersensitivity	24–48 hours	Sensitized lymphocytes	?	Lymphocytes, basophiles
	(2) Classical delayed hyper-sensitivity	48–72 hours	T_D cells T_C cells	Lymphokines	Lymphocytes, macrophages

with antibody. The phagocytosed cells are inactivated by reaction with toxic concentrations of oxygen radicals and by reaction with the halogenated oxides, hypochlorite, and hypoiodite (Figure 9-15). Soon after inactivation, the phagosomes fuse with lysosomes, thus exposing the phagocytized material to lysosomal hydrolytic enzymes, including lysozyme, lactoferrin, and acidic and neutral proteases.

Some microorganisms can exist in an intracellular infectious phase that protects them from the effector functions of the antibody system. Most of these agents infect macrophages but somehow avoid inactivation and incorporation into phagolysosomes. These microorganisms include several bacteria (Salmonella, Listeria monocytogenes, Brucella, and Mycobacteria), certain fungi (Candida, Cryptococcus, Histoplasma, and Coccidioides), and some protozoans (Plasmodium, Toxoplasma, Trypanosomes, Pneumocystis, and Leishmania). The immune system can respond to intracellular phagocyte infections through activation of the phagocytes by effector T_D cells or effector T_A cells. Phagocyte activation requires T-cell co-recognition of foreign antigen and MHC Ia molecules on the phagocyte cell surface. Acti-

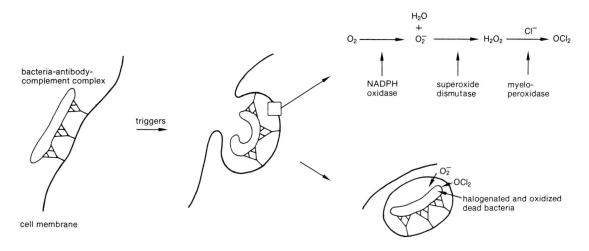

Figure 9-15   Activation of toxic oxygen products in polymorphonuclear leukocytes.

vated phagocytes convert arachidonic acid to prostaglandin E, activate the cyclic nucleotide systems, enlarge, and increase their rates of phagocytosis and intracellular production of peroxidases and hydrolases. Additionally, the release of proteases and plasminogen activators stimulates inflammatory responses that tend to isolate the infected cells. The net effect of such activity is to halogenate the intracellular microorganisms and digest them.

Contact lysis

Recognition of antigen-bearing target cells by effector T_C cells results in lysis of the target cells (Figure 9-16). This process requires that the T_C cells, but not the target cells, be metabolically active; however, it does not require new synthesis of DNA, RNA, or proteins. An individual T_C cell can carry out repetitive lytic cycles. Nontarget bystander cells are unaffected. Lysis of the target cell is initiated at the site of contact with the T_C cell, where interaction of the T_C-cell receptor with target antigen probably leads to formation of a lytic channel in the target cell membrane by an unknown mechanism.

In addition to killer T lymphocytes, a variety of other defensive cells can destroy foreign cells by contact lysis. These cells include socalled *killer cells, natural killer cells,* and *natural cytotoxic cells.* Both killer and natural killer cells have Fc antibody receptors and may acquire specificity for a target antigen by passive attachment of circulating antibodies. Killer cells are nonphagocytic members of the monocytemacrophage lineage and do not bear either T-cell or B-cell-specific surface markers. Cell lysis by killer cells is dependent on antibodies, but it is not dependent on the complement system. Natural killer cells and natural cytotoxic cells can recognize and kill in the absence of antibodies and are distinguished from each other only by differences in their activities against a variety of tumor cells. Both natural killer

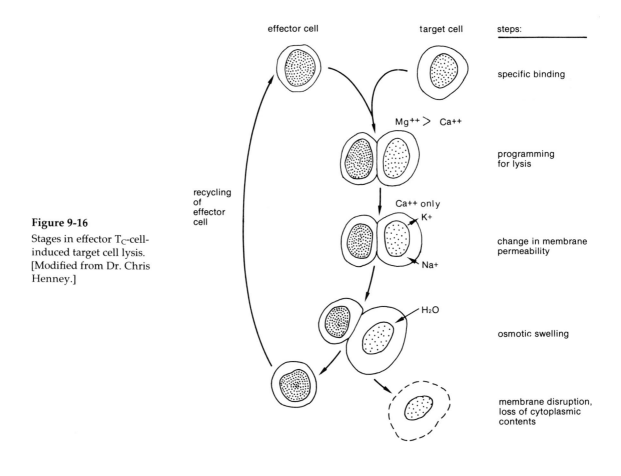

Figure 9-16

Stages in effector T$_C$-cell-induced target cell lysis. [Modified from Dr. Chris Henney.]

and natural cytotoxic cells are particularly active against transformed cells of virus-induced leukemias. Natural killer cells appear morphologically as large granular lymphocytes (Figure 1-3), and they express Ly-5 and Thy-1 cell-surface markers that are characteristic of T cells (Table 7-3). Thus these cells may be closely related to T cells.

The combined action of effector T$_C$ cells and other defensive cells to destroy virus-infected cells, coupled with the action of antibodies to inactivate extracellular virus and γ interferon to inhibit intracellular viral replication, usually provides an effective defense against viral infections.

9-6   Immunity against potential pathogens can be transferred passively or induced actively

Protection against first exposure

Effective immunity to a pathogen can be provided medically either by passive transfer or by active induction. *Passive immunity*, which is produced by injection of antibodies, confers short-term protection. *Active immunity*, which is usually induced by injection of an innocuous form of the pathogen, confers long-term protection by stimulating the host's immune system. These procedures are used to protect individuals from first exposure to potential pathogens, either because the normal primary immune response is not effective or because the individual possesses a defective immune system. (Some immunodeficiency diseases are considered in detail in Chapter 12.) The importance of such "first-strike" protection against human diseases has been underscored recently by the effective eradication of smallpox. Smallpox virus, whose only host is human beings, was contained and eliminated efficiently at each new site of appearance by immunizing the circle of individuals in contact with the site.

Passive immunity

Short-term protection can be transferred passively by intramuscular injection of purified concentrates of antibody. The duration of protection depends on the amount injected and on the half-life of the class of immunoglobulins introduced (Table 9-1). Although passive immunization does not confer long-term protection, it has the advantage of requiring neither identification nor isolation of the offending antigen. Immunoglobulins for injection are usually pooled from a large number of donors to provide maximum effectiveness. Any contaminating infectious agents are eliminated by purification or inactivation. Nevertheless, repeated injections of immunoglobulin are potentially hazardous in immune-competent individuals because of possible immune responses against allotypic markers.

Two natural analogs of passive transfer occur in mammals. During pregnancy, IgG antibodies, which have the longest serum half-life of the immunoglobulin classes, are passively transferred from the mother to the fetus to provide humoral immune protection. After birth, the mother passes on IgA antibodies in colostrum and milk to protect the infant's upper gastrointestinal tract.

Active immunity

Active immunity can be induced in an immune-competent individual by stimulating the immune system directly with an appropriate antigen. Immunization (vaccination) with an innocuous form of the antigen induces both an immediate immune response and immunological memory and thus provides long-term protection. Inactivated, nonpathogenic, or attenuated forms of an infectious agent are used in vaccines. These agents elicit effective immune responses because they share common antigenic determinants with the infectious pathogen. For example, the Salk poliovirus vaccine uses formalin-inactivated poliovirus as the immunizing agent, whereas the Sabin vaccine uses an attenuated strain of the virus. In a similar way, *toxins* can be converted to *toxoids* for vaccines by inactivating them in a way that preserves their antigenicity. These procedures are generally effective, but they require careful quality control and a close monitoring for side effects of vaccination.

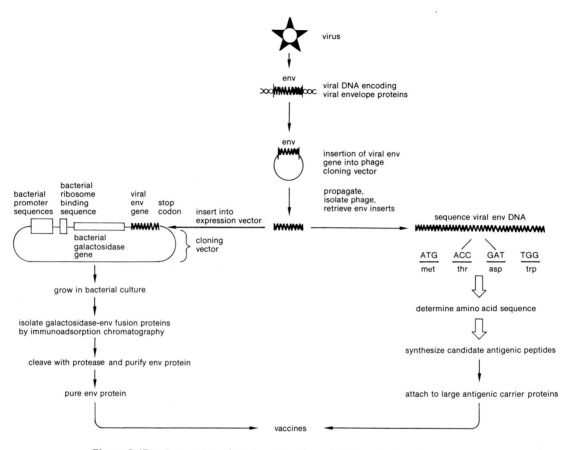

Figure 9-17   Preparation of viral vaccines free of viral contaminants.

A new method for creating safe vaccines has recently emerged from basic research. For example, if the nucleotide or amino acid sequence for a virus protein is known, a short viral polypeptide can be synthesized chemically or produced from a coding segment of DNA by recombinant DNA techniques (Figure 9-17). When injected, such a polypeptide elicits an immune response primarily against one or a few antigenic determinants of the virus. Perhaps vaccines of the future will contain an appropriate collection of antigenic polypeptides. Such a vaccine would be incapable of causing the disease it was meant to protect against.

The prevention of infection by active immunization is an ancient art and is called *vaccination* after the triumphant work of Jenner in the 18th century. Jenner induced immunity to smallpox virus by inoculation with cowpox virus (*vaccinia* virus), which carries antigenic determinants in common with smallpox virus, but produces only a mild infection in humans. Prior to the introduction of antibiotics, vaccina-

Table 9-4 Routine Vaccination Schedule (United States)

Age	Vaccine
3 months	Diphtheria-tetanus-polio and trivalent oral polio
4 months	Diphtheria-tetanus-polio and trivalent oral polio
5 months	Diphtheria-tetanus-polio and trivalent oral polio
15 months	Measles, mumps, rubella
18 months	Diphtheria-tetanus-polio and trivalent oral polio
4–6 years	Diphtheria-tetanus-polio and trivalent oral polio
14–16 years	Tetanus and low-dose diphtheria

tion was the major hope for protecting populations against infectious microorganisms. Vaccines are currently used for protection against viral infections, against antibiotic-resistant bacterial infections, and against rapid acting toxins like diphtheria and tetanus. The routine vaccination schedule for the United States is shown in Table 9-4.

Selected Bibliography

Non-antibody serum components involved in native and adaptive immunity

Fearon, D. T., and Wong, W. W., "Complement ligand-receptor interactions that mediate biological responses," *Ann. Rev. Immunol.* **1**, 243(1983).

Gewurz, H., Mold, C., Siegel, J., and Frede, B., "C-reactive proteins and the acute phase response," *Adv. Intern. Med.* **27**, 345(1982).

Larsen, G. L., and Henson, P. M., "Mediators of inflammation," *Ann. Rev. Immunol.* **1**, 335(1983).

Muller-Eberhard, H. J., and Schreiber, R. D., "Molecular biology and chemistry of the alternative pathway of complement," *Adv. Immunol.* **29**, 1(1980).

Pillemer, L., Blum, L., Lepow, I. H., Ross, O. A., Todd, E. W., and Wardlow, A. C., "The properdin system and immunity, I. Demonstration of isolation of a new serum protein and its role in immune phenomenon," *Science* **120**, 279(1954).

Reid, K. B. M., and Porter, R. R., "The proteolytic activation systems of complement," *Ann. Rev. Biochem.* **50**, 433(1981).

Antibody classes and their functions in immunity

Davies, D. R., and Metzger, H., "Structural basis of antibody function," *Ann. Rev. Immunol.* **1**, 87(1983).

Metzger, H., Goetze, A., Kanellopoulos, J., Holowka, D., and Fewtrell, C., "Structure of the high affinity mast cell receptor for IgE," *Federation Proceedings* **41**, 8(1982).

Spiegelberg, H. L., "Biological activities of immunoglobulins of different classes and subclasses," *Adv. Immunol.* **259**, 19(1974).

Killer cells, phagocytic cells, and inflammation

Fantone, J. C., and Ward, P. A., "Role of oxygen-derived free radicals and metabolites in leukocyte-dependent inflammatory reactions," *Am. J. Pathology* **107,** 397 (1982).

Griffin, F. M., Griffin, J. A., and Silverstein, S. C., "Studies on the mechanism of phagocytosis," *J. Exp. Med.* **144,** 788(1976).

Herberman, R. B., "Natural killer cells," *Hospital Practice* **17** (#4), 93(1982).

Karnovsky, M. L., and Bolis, L. (Eds.), *Phagocytosis, Past and Future,* Academic Press, New York(1982).

Nabholz, M., and MacDonald, H. R., "Cytolytic T lymphocytes," *Ann. Rev. Immunol.* **1,** 273(1983).

Active and passive immunity to microorganisms

Anderson, R. M., and May, R. M., "Directly transmitted infectious diseases: control by vaccination," *Science* **215,** 1053(1982).

Lerner, R. A., "Tapping the immunological repertoire to produce antibodies to predetermined specificity," *Nature* **299,** 592(1982).

Möller, G. (Ed.), "Immunoparasitology," *Immunological Reviews* **61**(1982).

Additional concepts introduced in the problems

1. Pathological consequences of complement activation. Problems 9-7, 8, 9.

2. How mast cells are triggered. The Prausnitz-Küstner reaction. Problem 9-10.

3. Immunity to gonorrhea. Problem 9-11.

Problems

9-1 Indicate whether each of the following statements is true or false. Explain the error in each statement you consider to be false.
  (a) The fixation of complement is triggered by the interaction of antibody with antigen.
  (b) The polypeptide called *secretory component,* which mediates the transport of IgA from blood to epithelial surfaces, is a T-cell lymphokine.
  (c) Activation of the third component of complement, C3, occurs only when an antigen interacts with specific antibody of a class that can fix complement.
  (d) Delayed hypersensitivity lesions contain cellular infiltrates composed of lymphocytes and macrophages.
  (e) Killer cells may derive from either T-cell or macrophage lineages.
  (f) In mice, T cells that mediate delayed hypersensitivity (T_D cells) may undergo antigen-driven maturation to killer T (T_C) cells.

9-2 Supply the missing word or words in each of the following statements.
  (a) The effector functions of an immunoglobulin are defined by the class of its _____ chains.
  (b) The _____ subcomponent of complement binds to the Fc portion of IgG in IgG-antigen complexes.
  (c) C8 and C9 effect the _____ function of the complement pathway.
  (d) Mast cells possess surface receptors for _____ antibodies.

9-3 How does activation of the complement enzymatic cascade contribute to the inflammatory response to bacterial infection? Describe two ways that gram-negative bacteria might cause activation of the complement system.

9-4 Name three distinct cell types involved in direct cell killing and comment briefly on the specificity of their recognition.

9-5 Allergic dermatitis, an example of a delayed-type hypersensitivity reaction, is one of the most common skin diseases in humans. List at least three characteristics of delayed-type hypersensitivity that distinguish it from immediate-type (antibody-mediated) hypersensitivity, and indicate the differences.

9-6 For each of the following toxins, pathogens, or disorders, indicate the primary immune response(s) and effector mechanism(s) involved (defensive or pathological). Be specific about the types of cells and/or humoral factors implicated.
(a) tetanus toxin
(b) fungal infection
(c) influenza virus infection
(d) tuberculosis infection
(e) bee sting
(f) heart graft rejection
(g) pollen allergy
(h) poison ivy dermatitis
(i) staphylococcal infection

9-7 A transient leukopenia is associated with hemodialysis, and it appears to result from the sequestration of leukocyte aggregates in lung capillaries. When plasma from a normal individual has been incubated with dialyzer cellophane (a complex polysaccharide), the plasma will induce leukocyte aggregation in an *in vitro* polymorphonuclear leukocyte activation assay. Speculate on the possible mechanism for this effect.

9-8 In laboratory animals, inappropriate activation of the complement system can result in aggregation of granulocytes, leading to occlusion of small vessels by leukoemboli. A clinical investigator suspects that a similar mechanism may be responsible for the tissue damage associated with certain human ischemic syndromes (deficient blood supply). To test this hypothesis, she designs an *in vitro* assay system in which polymorphonuclear leukocytes are incubated with various sources of plasma, and the degree of granulocyte aggregation is determined by the light-scattering properties of the cell suspension. The results of one such experiment are presented in Figure 9-18.
(a) Why was heat aggregated horse immunoglobulin added to the plasma?
(b) What do these findings suggest about the molecular identity of the granulocyte aggregating factor?

9-9 *Purtscher's retinopathy* is a syndrome characterized by sudden blindness due to microembolism of the small retinal vessels. One cause of this syndrome is reported to be acute pancreatitis, an inflammatory disease in which many pancreatic enzymes are liberated. Figure 9-19 illustrates the results of polymorphonuclear leukocyte aggregation assays using plasma from a patient with acute pancreatitis. With reference to the figure, answer the following questions.
(a) What do these data suggest about the pathogenesis of Purtscher's syndrome?
(b) What is the significance of the increased aggregation in the presence of added trypsin?
(c) What is the next appropriate experiment?

9-10 (a) Tissue mast cells (and blood-borne basophiles) possess receptors for the Fc portions of IgE molecules. When antigen binds to the membrane-bound IgE of sensitized mast cells, a sequence of events that results in the release of a variety of chemical mediators occurs. To study the mechanism of this IgE-mediated de-

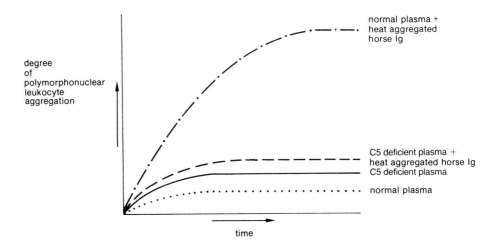

Figure 9-18   Aggregation of granulocytes in the presence of plasma from various sources and heat aggregated horse immunoglobulin (Problem 9-8).

granulation, an investigator prepares an antiserum that reacts specifically with the exposed Fc portion of membrane-bound IgE. When he adds the anti-IgE serum to previously sensitized mast cells, degranulation occurs. Suggest a mechanism for this mast-cell triggering.

(b) Would you expect any effect when this antiserum is added to normal mast cells that have not been previously sensitized?

(c) He prepares a second antiserum that reacts specifically with the Fc *receptor* for IgE on mast cells. When he adds this antiserum to nonsensitized mast cells, degranulation occurs. Propose a mechanism for the action of this antiserum.

(d) When he tests $F(ab)_2$ fragments prepared from the anti-Fc-receptor antibodies, degranulation still occurs, whereas when he tests Fab fragments, no degranulation occurs. What does this result suggest about the mechanism of mast-cell triggering?

(e) Given that a calcium ionophore (A23187) also induces mast-cell degranulation, propose a simple molecular model for mast-cell triggering by antigen.

9-11   *Gonococci* are believed to infect susceptible hosts by attaching to genital tract epithelial cells by both pilus proteins and outer membrane proteins of the class pII. The virulence of an infecting organism may thus be related to whether or not it is piliated, to the type of pII protein it expresses, and to its ability to produce an IgA-specific protease. Two observations concerning the transmission of gonorrhea may provide clues to the role of the immune system in protection against this widespread disease. First, no species other than man is known to support gonococcal infections. Second, not all individuals exposed to gonococci develop gonorrhea. Assume that all nonimmunological explanations for these observations have been ruled out (although in fact, they have not). Suggest an immunological explanation for each of the two observations, and describe an experimental approach to test each hypothesis.

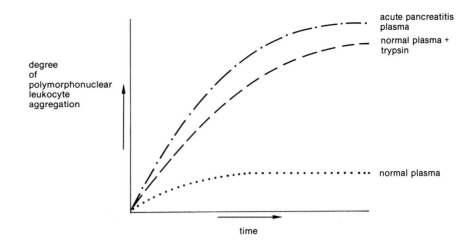

Figure 9-19 Polymorphonuclear leukocyte aggregation in the presence of various plasma preparations (Problem 9-9).

Answers

9-1 (a) True
    (b) False. The SC piece is synthesized by epithelial cells, not by T cells.
    (c) False. C3 also can be activated by the alternative (properdin) pathway.
    (d) True
    (e) True
    (f) False. T_D cells (Ly-1) and T_C cells (Ly-2,3) represent separate lineages that do not interconvert.

9-2 (a) heavy
    (b) C1q
    (c) lytic
    (d) IgE

9-3 Activation of complement leads to the stepwise cleavage of complement proteins. Some of the cleaved peptides are highly vasoactive, causing leakage of fluids into the region of their release, whereas others are highly chemotactic for polymorphonuclear leukocytes, causing their influx into the region of the complement activation.

    Gram-negative bacteria can activate the complement sequence directly via the alternative pathway, or they can use the classical pathway in the presence of IgM or IgG antibodies directed against them.

9-4
Cell type	Recognition specificity
T_C	Recognizes target-cell-surface antigen in the context of host MHC (mainly class I) determinants.
K	Recognizes the Fc region of antibody bound to a target cell; the actual target cell antigen is recognized by the bound antibody.
NK/NC	Target specificity is unknown, but target cell prototypes are well known. Killing of prototype target cells is *not* MHC restricted and does *not* require the presence of antibodies.

9-5

Characteristic	Delayed hypersensitivity	Immediate hypersensitivity
1. Initiating antigen-specific effector	T_D cells	Complement-fixing antibody
2. Major infiltrating cells	lymphocytes, macrophages	Polymorphonuclear leukocytes
3. Peak reaction time	48–72 hr	24 hr

9-6   (a) Humoral response; neutralizing antibodies.

(b) Cellular response; killer cells and macrophages.

(c) Cellular response; T_C and T_D cells destroy and wall off infected cells. Humoral response; neutralizing, opsonizing, and complement-fixing antibodies.

(d) Cellular response; T_D cells activate (but don't destroy) TB-infected macrophages.

(e) Humoral response; IgE antibodies lead to local or systemic release of heparin, histamine, and leukotrienes, leading to anaphylactic shock.

(f) Cellular response; T_D cells wall off and T_C cells kill graft.

(g) Humoral response; local IgE response.

(h) Cellular response; massive T_D and T_C response to poison ivy sensitizer attached to skin cells.

(i) Humoral response; mainly complement-fixing antibodies.

9-7   The observed effect almost certainly results from complement activation via the alternative pathway in the incubated plasma. Another formal possibility is that bacterial contaminants from the dialyzer could also bind C-reactive protein, which can activate the classical complement pathway. In either case, polymorphonuclear leukocyte recruitment, activation, and aggregation are induced by cleaved complement peptides C5a and C5b,6,7.

9-8   (a) Aggregation of IgG in the horse plasma mimics antigen–antibody complex formation and activates complement.

(b) The granulocyte activating factor appears to be C5, a component of C5, or dependent upon C5. The best data currently attribute this activity to C5a.

9-9   (a) Inappropriate proteolytic cleavage of some serum proteins could lead to microembolism as a result of polymorphonuclear leukocyte aggregation. Patients with acute pancreatitis could initiate this syndrome by release of their proteases into the circulation.

(b) Normal plasma plus trypsin can mimic the effect of acute pancreatitis plasma; this result supports the hypothesis in part (a). Interestingly, several complement cleavages are catalyzed by enzymes with trypsinlike activity.

(c) The next appropriate experiment might be to identify the proteolytically cleaved serum component that aggregates polymorphonuclear leukocytes in trypsin-treated normal plasma and to compare it with the component that is activated or selectively depleted, or both, in those patients with the disease.

9-10 (a) If the antibody binds only to the IgE molecules on the mast-cell membrane, then several explanations could be suggested. (1) The antibody cross-links surface IgE molecules, and the cross-linking changes the state of IgE-Fc receptors in a way that signals degranulation. (2) The binding of antibody to any IgE molecule (with or without cross-linking) induces a conformational change in the IgE that signals degranulation. (3) The anti-IgE antibody itself is brought into close proximity with the mast-cell membrane, and other mast-cell receptors specific for the Fc region of another isotype (e.g., IgG_{2a}) are filled, signaling degranulation.

(b) The antiserum could also possibly affect nonsensitized cells. The affinity of IgE for the mast cell is very high ($\sim 10^{11}$), and the turnover rate of the filled IgE mast-cell-receptor complex is very slow. Thus any normal mast cells taken recently from an animal are likely to have a fraction of their Fc-IgE receptors filled. If that fraction is sufficiently high, triggering by anti-IgE could occur. The high affinity of this interaction and the long residence time of the filled receptors on mast cells *in vivo* is the basis for the experiment that identified allergy as first an antibody-mediated and then an IgE antibody-mediated reaction. Injection of serum from an allergic patient into the skin of a nonallergic patient confers in that injection site donor-type specific allergy that lasts up to 6 weeks—the so-called *Prausnitz–Küstner* reaction.

(c) This experiment indicates that the receptor can be activated directly by reaction with cognate antibody in the absence of IgE, supporting the view that conformational change or cross-linking, or both, could be involved.

(d) This result indicates that cross-linking is required for activation, thereby arguing against the second and third mechanisms suggested in part (a).

(e) Events triggered by interactions between antigen, IgE, and Fc-IgE receptors on the mast-cell membrane might eventually lead to the activation of a Ca^{++} pump or development of a Ca^{++} channel, and the increase in cytoplasmic Ca^{++} concentration could be a sufficient signal to cause granule fusions and the degranulation that follows.

9-11 Several explanations can be suggested. Susceptible humans may lack the ability to produce antibodies to the determinants on gonococcal pili and class pII outer membrane proteins that recognize target cell-surface receptors. This explanation seems unlikely, but it could be tested by determining whether exposed susceptible and nonsusceptible humans (and any other nonsusceptible species) develop antibodies that block attachment phase of gonococci to target cells in the presence of inhibitors of the gonococcal IgA proteases. If such antibodies are missing from susceptible hosts, one could check whether the deficiency is genetically correlated with any HLA-D (Ir gene) determinant, immunoglobulin allotype (IgH, Igκ, Igλ), or idiotypic markers.

Another possible explanation is that gonococcal IgA proteases are active only on IgA molecules from susceptible hosts. This hypothesis could be easily tested by direct proteolysis assays.

A third possible explanation is that susceptible individuals can release only IgA into their secretions, whereas nonsusceptible individuals can also secrete IgM, IgG, or IgE neutralizing antibodies. This hypothesis could be tested by isotyping antibodies specific to gonococcal pili and outer membrane protein pII in oral and genital secretions of susceptible and nonsusceptible individuals.

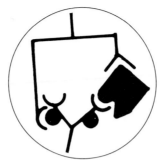

CHAPTER 10

Tolerance and the Regulation of Immunity

Chapter Outline

When presented with an antigen, the immune system normally responds positively to develop immunity and eliminate the antigen, or negatively to tolerate it, depending on whether the antigen is recognized as self or nonself. Both immunity and tolerance are active re-

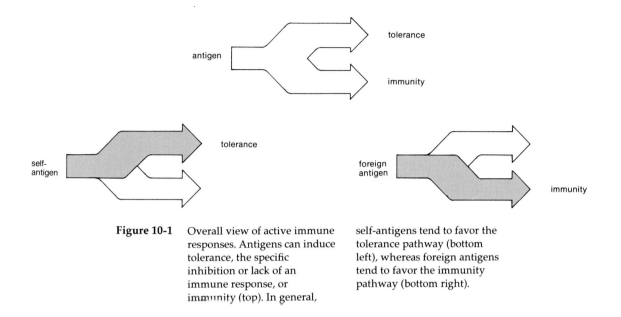

Figure 10-1 Overall view of active immune responses. Antigens can induce tolerance, the specific inhibition or lack of an immune response, or immunity (top). In general, self-antigens tend to favor the tolerance pathway (bottom left), whereas foreign antigens tend to favor the immunity pathway (bottom right).

sponses of the immune system and must be controlled reliably. An immunity response to self-antigens or a tolerance response to foreign antigens can have equally disastrous consequences. The concept that the immune system must discriminate continually between self and nonself is a cornerstone of all immunological theory. An analysis of responses to foreign antigens indicates that the immune system is linked through antibodies and MHC gene products into a network of potential responses. Tolerance for self-antigens is apparently accomplished by the continual suppression or deletion of newly developing, self-reactive lymphocytes. The resulting modified network is unable to mount an immune response to self-antigens. This chapter considers the regulation of immunity and the development of tolerance.

Concepts

10-1 The immune system reliably discriminates self from nonself

When the immune system encounters an antigen, the response can take either of the two general pathways represented in Figure 10-1. A foreign antigen usually elicits a positive response that leads to differentiation of effector B cells and T cells, antibody synthesis, antigen elimination, and immunologic memory. A self-antigen usually elicits a negative response that leads to inactivation or deletion of specific lymphocytes and to immunologic tolerance. Immunity and tolerance are active responses of the vertebrate immune system. Both immunity and tolerance are specific for individual antigens; both are acquired through appropriate antigenic exposure; and both are mediated by lymphocytes.

The ability to discriminate between self and nonself is a hallmark of the immune system. The developmental basis for this discrimination was revealed by Owen's pioneering studies on the immunogenetics of bovine blood groups. In observations on freemartins (nonidentical twins that share embryonic vasculature), Owen demonstrated that fetal exposure to cells from another individual produced tolerance to subsequent adult exposure to the same cells. Normally such an exposure is met with immunity. Thus foreign antigens that are present continuously from a time before the immune system develops are treated as self. How this developmental alteration of the immune system is accomplished remains unclear. However, some insights into the mechanism of tolerance have been gained by examining the regulation of normal immune responses to foreign antigens.

10-2 Cellular interactions in the immune response are regulated

Entry of a foreign antigen into the body initiates a cascade of cellular interactions that leads to humoral immunity, cellular immunity, or both (Figure 10-2). Both branches of the immune response are initiated by the interaction of an antigen-charged accessory cell with a T cell of the helper class (T_H cells for antibodies; T_A cells for cytotoxic cells). The interacting cells communicate with each other by contact, through soluble factors, or both, to form a two-cell *circuit* that leads to helper cell activation. The activated helper cells then form additional circuits of three or more cells with antigen-charged accessory cells and virgin or mature B or T_C cells. Some examples of such circuits are shown in Figure 10-3. These circuits trigger the differentiation and proliferation of effector T_C cells and antibody-secreting plasma cells for immediate use and memory T and B cells for future protection. Such circuits are maintained as long as antigen is present in the system.

Both the cellular and humoral immune response pathways are regulated at the first step by the action of their end products. The elimination functions of antibodies and effector T_C cells remove antigen from the system (Chapter 9). In addition, high affinity IgG antibodies feedback inhibit the immune response by complexing with antigen bound to accessory cells. Natural killer cells, activated by T-

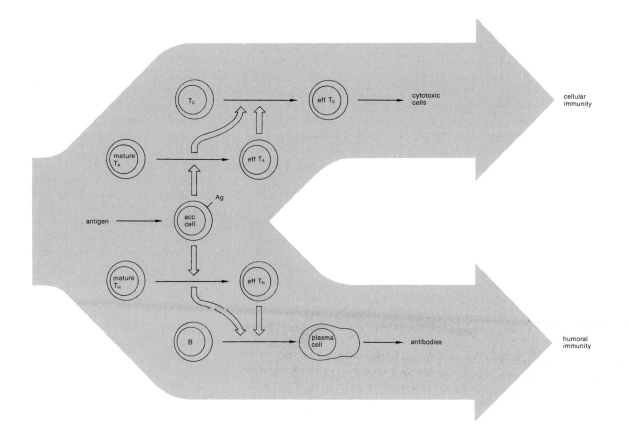

Figure 10-2   Pathways for the cellular (top) and humoral (bottom) immune responses. This diagram represents two possible paths in the immune response and indicates the types of cellular interactions.

cell lymphokines, congregate in germinal centers, where they may act as negative regulators by eliminating antigen-charged accessory cells. Removal or masking of antigen breaks the cell circuits and stops production of new effector cells. Unlike their long-lived precursors, effector cells typically have short lifespans of hours to days. Consequently, antigen elimination rapidly terminates both the cellular response and the synthesis of new antibody molecules. The subsequent persistence of serum antibodies depends on their half-lives (Table 9-1).

To a first approximation, the kinetics of the immune response can be understood in terms of the pathways shown in Figure 10-2. The proliferation phases of plasma cells and T_C cells account for the logarithmic nature of immune response curves, which closely resemble bacterial growth curves. Additional details of the response that are not predicted by these simple pathways can be accounted for in terms of the *network theory* of immune responses proposed by Jerne.

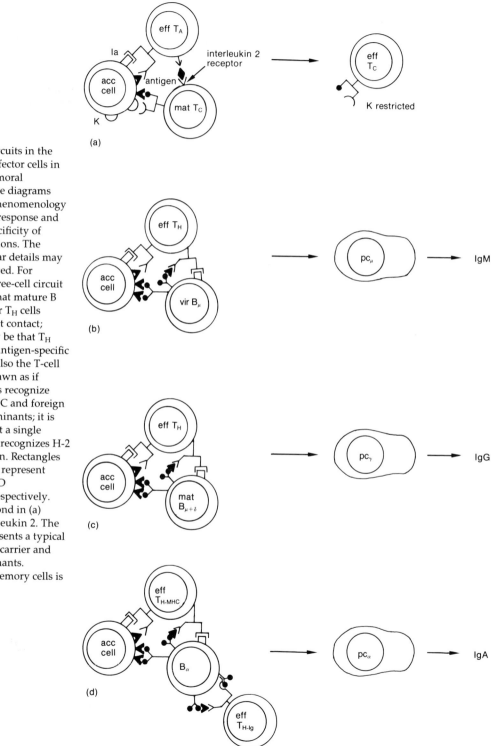

Figure 10-3

Multicellular circuits in the generation of effector cells in cellular and humoral immunity. These diagrams represent the phenomenology of the immune response and indicate the specificity of cellular interactions. The precise molecular details may not be as indicated. For example, the three-cell circuit in (c) suggests that mature B cells and effector T_H cells interact by direct contact; however, it may be that T_H cells secrete an antigen-specific soluble factor. Also the T-cell receptors are drawn as if discrete portions recognize unmodified MHC and foreign antigenic determinants; it is just as likely that a single receptor crevice recognizes H-2 restricted antigen. Rectangles and semi-circles represent MHC Ia and K/D determinants, respectively. The black diamond in (a) represents interleukin 2. The ▲ symbol represents a typical antigen with its carrier and hapten determinants. Production of memory cells is not shown.

Figure 10-4

Several idiotopes make up an immunoglobulin idiotype. Two antibodies are shown for comparison. They bind different antigens and are derived from independent V_H and V_L genes. All but one of the idiotopes shown are thus *private* to one of the two antibodies shown. However, one portion of the V_H region away from the antigen combining site has an idiotope in common between the two; it is a *public* idiotope. It should be noted that only a few of the indicated idiotopes are at or near the antigen combining sites, and therefore not all anti-idiotope antibodies will affect antigen binding by competition for the binding site. Collectively, the idiotopes on each antibody can be considered to be written letters, and the idiotype of that antibody is as individual as one's signature.

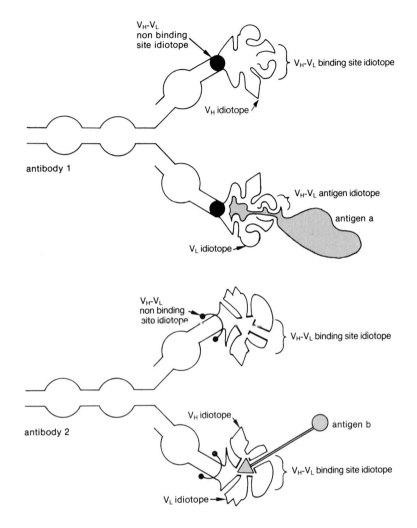

10-3   Antibodies can act as antigens to create a network of related responses

Antibodies carry new antigenic determinants

The key factor behind the network theory is that antibodies produced during an immune response will carry unique new antigenic determinants to which the organism is not tolerant. In general, these determinants, called *idiotopes*, are located in and around the antigen combining site (Figure 10-4). The set of idiotopes on an individual antibody molecule defines the *idiotype* of that antibody. The idiotopes present on the antibodies produced in the first wave of an immune response can then behave as antigens to trigger a second response.

Because these second-wave antibodies are directed against the idiotypes of the first-wave antibodies, the second-wave population is generally referred to collectively as *anti-idiotype antibodies.* However, these antibodies also possess a collection of idiotopes, and individual molecules have particular idiotypes. Therefore, they in turn can behave as antigens to induce a third wave of antibodies, and so on (Figure 10-5). The antibodies produced in such a response cascade are related by a *network* of interactions that could potentially involve the

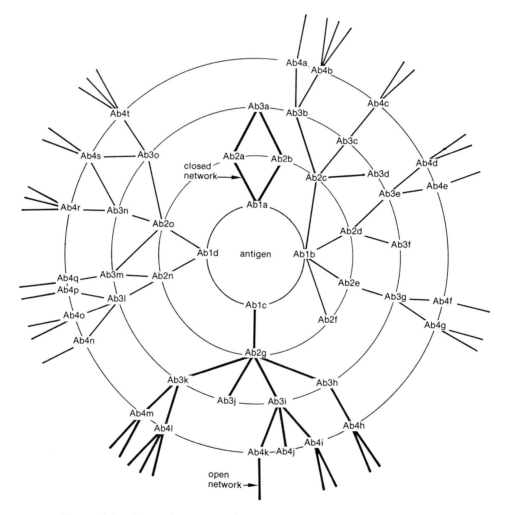

Figure 10-5 Potential expansion of the immune response through successive waves of an idiotype–anti-idiotype network. Such networks could be completely open and therefore expansive (shown in lower portion of figure), or they could result in self-contained, closed networks or circuits (shown in the upper portion of the figure).

entire immune system. The connections between individual antibodies in the network could be either open ended or closed; one example of each possibility is highlighted in Figure 10-5.

The network theory: Internal images and anti-images

The antibodies produced in successive waves should be complementary to each other by the following assignment. If properly arranged, the antigen combining sites represented in the population of first-wave antibodies would form a fragmentary surface complementary to the antigen (Figure 10-6). As just described, this "negative" or *anti-image* of the antigen can induce a new population of antibodies, a few of which are the complement to its collective antigen-binding surface (Figure 10-6). Because this complement of a complement corresponds to the original antigen, it has been termed by Jerne the *internal image* of the antigen. As indicated along the upper line in Figure 10-6, the internal image in the second-wave antibodies can reinduce the internal anti-image in the third wave. Thus, as an immune response proceeds along its path, the immune system alternately produces images and anti-images of the antigen. Because only the anti-image antibodies are antigen reactive, these expected oscillations in the network may account for the cyclical variations in reactive antibody levels that sometimes occur late in an immune response (Figure 10-7).

In addition to antigen-related determinants, the first wave of antibodies will almost certainly contain idiotopes that lie outside the antigen combining site. These idiotopes will induce a collection of anti-idiotypic antibodies that are unrelated to the antigen (Figure 10-6, lower lines). These antibodies will in turn induce antibodies that are idiotypically related to the first-wave antibodies but do not recognize the original immunizing antigen.

In support of the network theory, this prediction has been verified experimentally. Late in an immune response there appear newly synthesized immunoglobulins that carry idiotopes in common with the first-wave antibodies, but they do not themselves bind to the original antigen (Figure 10-8). Further support comes from observations that in some responses, synthesis of (first-wave) antibodies is followed by appearance of anti-idiotypic T cells as well as B cells, as would be required to form a network. Also, T cells bearing idiotypic or anti-idiotypic determinants have been found in the helper and suppressor classes, and there is strong evidence that such cells interact with other cells through these determinants.

Relevance of the network to regulation of immune responses

Most immunologists now agree that the immune system is indeed linked by antibodies into a network of potential responses and that some portion of the network is actually induced by each foreign antigen. However, two major unresolved questions that may be related remain. First, what prevents any immune response from continuing to expand in successive waves until the entire immune system is in-

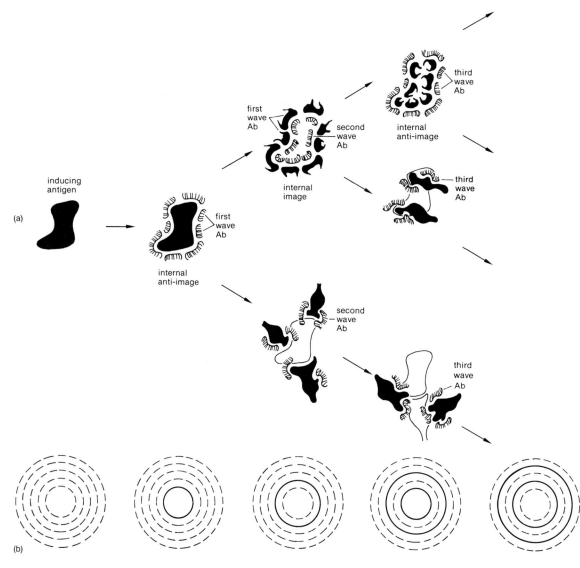

Figure 10-6 Internal anti-image and internal image of a foreign antigen. (a) The shaded segments represent the antigen combining sites of reactive antibodies, and the blackened surfaces represent the antigens or idiotopes to which they are complementary. (b) In the lower portion of the figure is a diagram of the oscillation between internal anti-images and internal images in the progress of an immune response. Each ring of antibodies at the next oscillation will induce two rings of antibodies—one ring just inside it and one just outside it.

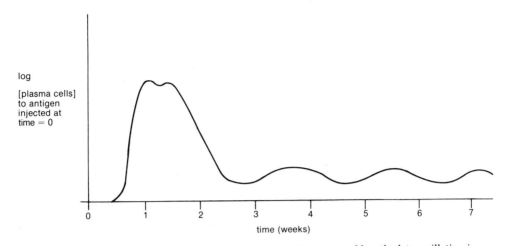

Figure 10-7   An example of the time course of an antibody response. Note the late oscillation in levels of antigen-reactive antibodies.

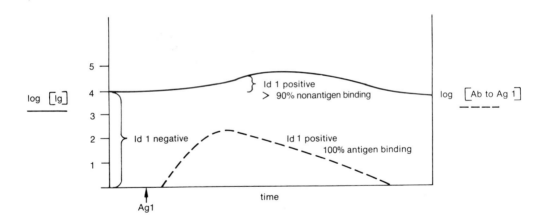

Figure 10-8   Appearance of idiotype-positive, but nonantigen-binding antibodies during an immune response to antigen.

volved? Second, are networks simply a trivial consequence of idiotope-anti-idiotype interactions, or are they the basis for regulation of immune responses? Answers to both these questions will probably require a more complete understanding of suppressor T cells, which are discussed in the following section.

The potentials for both positive and negative controls mediated through network interactions are enormous, not only for responses to foreign antigens but also in the development of the immune system itself. As pointed out by Jerne, the network theory includes the expectation that the immune system contains among its diverse receptors internal images of all external antigens. Conceivably these fragmentary internal images could participate during development in the generation of expanded clones of responsive lymphocytes. If so, then the notions of antigen-independent and antigen-dependent phases of lymphocyte maturation will have to be modified (Concept 7-3).

10-4   Suppressor T_S cells are regulatory elements of the immune system

Activation of effector T_S cells

In a typical immune response, effector cells of the T_H, T_A, T_D, and T_C classes are induced early, and effector T_S cells are induced somewhat later. The details of T_S-cell induction are not clear. However, all T_S cells appear to be induced by interaction with effector T_H cells, which in turn are induced by antigen-specific interactions with charged accessory cells. As in other pathways for effector cell induction, antigen-charged accessory cells also seem to be required at additional stages in the induction of effector T_S cells. By analogy with other pathways, this fragmentary information can be arranged into a tentative pathway for T_S-cell induction (Figure 10-9). In this pathway, the cellular interactions involving T_S cells appear to be MHC-restricted to I-J region gene products. It has not yet been established whether the T_H cells required for generating effector T_S cells are generally the same as those involved in B-cell induction ($T_{H\text{-}MHC}$ and $T_{H\text{-}Ig}$) or form a separate subclass ($T_{H\text{-}S}$) of helper cells. In mice, it has been demonstrated that at least one type of T_H cell can help either B cells or T_S cells.

During the course of an immune response, the predominant population of T_S cells changes in several ways, including surface phenotype and targets of suppression. These new species of T_S cells are probably induced through antibody linkages in the immune network. Antibodies produced in the first wave of an immune response can serve as antigens to induce a second wave of antibodies as described in Concept 10-3. Presumably these antibodies can also serve as antigens in the pathway in Figure 10-9 to induce new species of T_S cells. In support of this notion, considerable evidence indicates that multistep induction pathways for T_S cells involve multiple species of effector T_H cells.

Function of effector T_S cells

Nearly all early studies indicated that effector T_S cells act directly or via secreted suppressor proteins to suppress immune responses by inhibiting antigen-specific T_H cells, thereby preventing production of antigen-specific plasma cells and antibody secretion. However, current studies indicate that the potential targets for suppression by T_S

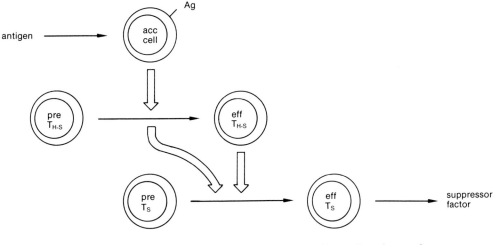

Figure 10-9   Tentative pathway for induction of effector T$_S$ cells. In the suppressor cell circuit, the relevant Ia determinants are each encoded in one of three subregions of the putative I-J region complex; the exact position of these determinants on accessory cells, T$_{H-S}$ cells, and T$_S$ cells is still unclear, and therefore it is not depicted. Suppressor-effector cells secrete suppressor-effector factors that contain antigen-binding regions, I-J determinants, and, in some cases, idiotypic determinants.

cells may include most, if not all, classes of T cells and B cells. One such study is instructive. Myeloma tumors contain proliferating B stem cells that differentiate into plasma cells at high cell density and begin to secrete antibodies. Animals that develop immunity to the tumors do so by recognizing the idiotype of the secreted antibody. In these animals, two classes of suppression mediated by T$_S$ cells have been found: in one class, T$_S$ cells directly inhibit proliferation of the B stem cells and, in the other, an idiotype-specific suppressor protein binds to plasma cells and to cells in transition to plasma cells and inhibits the synthesis of immunoglobulin. Thus T$_S$ cells may act even at the level of terminally differentiated effector cells.

The broad target specificity of effector T$_S$ cells raises the possibility that they might suppress one another and suggests that suppression could be relieved by the action of other suppressors. A class of T lymphocytes that fulfills this expectation has recently been discovered. These *contrasuppressor* T cells do not affect the generation of effector T$_S$ cells, but rather they interfere with their suppression of target cells. Contrasuppressor cells are induced to their effector stage by effector T$_H$ cells; however, the conditions and restrictions required for their activation are not yet known.

The multitude of potential targets and the possibility for both positive and negative regulatory effects makes investigation of T_S cells an especially challenging area of current immunological activity. However, the number, type, and lineage relationships of cells involved in suppression are still incompletely characterized. Cell-surface differentiation markers are being used to define developmental aspects of the system. In addition, it has recently become possible to clone some cells in the suppressor pathway and to purify their antigen-binding suppressor proteins. These two approaches may permit dissection of suppressor pathways *in vivo* and *in vitro* by use of differentiation markers, suppressor factors, and antibodies specific to them. For example, at least one type of suppressor protein consists of an antigen-binding domain and a suppressor-effector domain. Following binding to antigen, the suppressor-effector portion can separate and diffuse to act locally on its targets.

Mechanisms of suppression by T_S cells

In the absence of detailed information about suppressor proteins and T_S-cell receptors, the molecular basis for suppression remains speculative. However, the concept of internal images and anti-images developed from network theory provides a useful way of thinking about the problem. B cells, as well as T_H, T_A, T_D, and T_C cells, all appear to interact directly with determinants on the inducing antigen. Consequently, the antigen-specific portions of their receptors represent a fragmentary internal anti-image of the antigen (Concept 10-3). In an immune response, this internal anti-image is ultimately amplified into a population of antigen-reactive antibodies and T_C cells.

If the critical portion of the T_S-cell receptor binds not to the antigen but rather to the internal anti-image carried on the receptors of effector T_H cells, a subset of T_S cells that would carry fragments of the internal image of the antigen would be among the population of these anti-idiotope T_S cells (Figure 10-10). The potentials for complementary interactions between the internal image carried on T_S cells and suppressor factors and the internal anti-image carried on B cells and the other classes of T cells could provide a natural explanation for the broad target specificity of T_S cells.

The role of antigen-charged accessory cells in the immune response cascade has not yet been defined completely. It is possible that distinct subsets of accessory cells induce preferentially or exclusively effector T cells of different functions (T_{H-MHC}, T_{H-S}, T_S, etc.). Alternatively, a common set of accessory cells may localize several different cells at a common site as the immune response progresses. For example, it is conceivable that a single accessory cell (or a local cluster of accessory cells) simultaneously presents cell-surface antigen, antibodies directed to the antigen, and anti-idiotypic antibodies. In principle, such a cell could focus the various classes of T cells and B cells with specific receptors for antigenic determinants, for immunoglobulin determinants, or for cross-reactive idiotypic determinants, as shown in

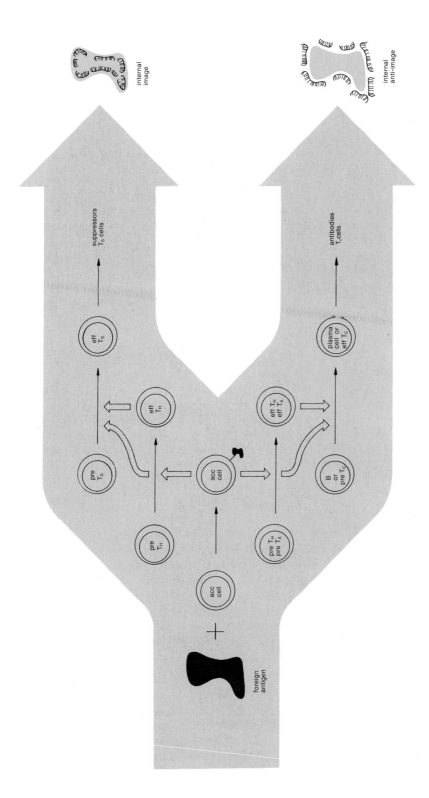

Figure 10-10 A model for the induction (bottom) of the immunity pathway—plasma cells and effector T$_C$ cells, and (top) of the suppression pathway—T$_S$ cells. In this model, the immunity pathway results in the production of antibodies and receptors complementary to the antigen image, whereas the T$_S$ recognition molecules would be complementary to the anti-image molecules and could construct an internal image

Figure 10-11. The binding of a T_S cell to such an accessory cell could result in the secretion and cleavage of a suppressor protein to release its suppressor-effector subunit to act locally on the entire cell cluster.

It has recently become evident that other types of suppressor T cells exist. For example, several classes of T cells can be demonstrated to express receptors for the Fc region of specific isotypes (e.g., $T_{Fc\gamma2}$, $T_{Fc\mu}$, $T_{Fc\alpha}$, and $T_{Fc\epsilon}$). The number of these cells rises as serum levels of the particular isotype rise, and it has been shown that these cells do not change Fc receptor specificity. Purified populations of $T_{Fc\alpha}$ cells suppress IgA responses and, likewise, isotype-specific suppression exists for $T_{Fc\gamma(subclass)}$ and $T_{Fc\epsilon}$ cells. Surprisingly, $T_{Fc\mu}$ cells *augment* IgM responses. T_{Fc} cells could act as antigen-specific, isotype-specific, and even idiotype-specific helper or suppressor cells if they were available to participate in circuits such as the one described in Figure 10-11. It is

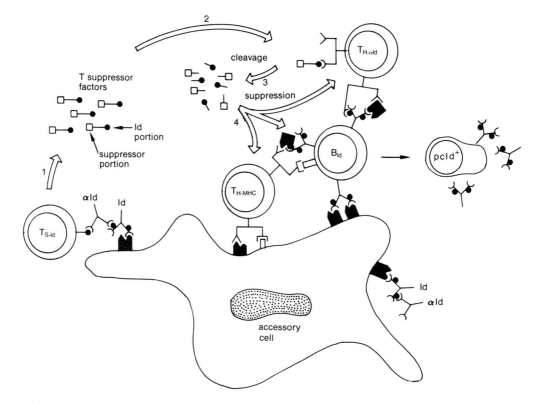

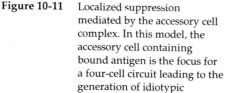

Figure 10-11 Localized suppression mediated by the accessory cell complex. In this model, the accessory cell containing bound antigen is the focus for a four-cell circuit leading to the generation of idiotypic antibody, as well as a site for the collection of idiotype and anti-idiotype antibodies and suppressor T cells. In the case shown on the left, idiotype-positive T_S cells secrete (1) idiotype-positive suppressor factors that bind (2) to anti-idiotype T_H cells in the complex, where they are cleaved (3) to release nonspecific suppressor factors that suppress (4) other cells in the complex.

conceivable that the antigen-specific inhibition of immune responses passively transferred with IgG antibodies (Concept 10-2) and that the antigen-specific augmentation of immune responses passively transferred with IgM antibodies is mediated (at least in part) by $T_{Fc\gamma}$ and $T_{Fc\mu}$ cells, respectively.

10-5 Tolerance for self-antigens requires an active response from the immune system

Relationship to the immune response pathway

Elimination of foreign antigens and tolerance to self-antigens are both active and continuing responses by the immune system. These two responses presumably involve the same network of potential responses and yet lead to opposite consequences for self- and nonself-antigens. Although a vertebrate has the genetic information necessary to synthesize antibodies against self-antigens, it normally blocks expression of this information in effector cells. The mechanism of tolerance induction is unclear, but its consequence is that lymphocytes carrying cell-surface receptors specific for self-determinants are either irreversibly inactivated (clonal amnesia), eliminated (clonal abortion), or suppressed.

The pathway for the immune response can be viewed as having two branches (Figure 10-10). In one branch of the pathway, an antigen induces synthesis of a reactive anti-image carried on antibodies and T_C cells that triggers elimination reactions upon binding antigen. In the other branch, the antigen induces synthesis of an antigen-identical image carried on suppressors, which, upon binding to specific lymphocyte receptors, inhibits their function. During an immune response, both branches of the pathway are activated—one to eliminate the offending antigen and the other to regulate the response and to suppress it once the antigen has been removed.

The same pathway is useful in describing the phenomenon of tolerance, which is characterized by the absence of ability to respond to antigen with synthesis of reactive antibody. Antibody synthesis could be blocked by inactivation or elimination of B cells or T cells, which must cooperate in the branch of the pathway leading to antibody synthesis. Alternatively, antibody synthesis could be blocked because B cells or T cells are suppressed due to an enhancement of the branch of the pathway leading to synthesis of effector T_S cells. It is not yet clear which, if either, of these possibilities is quantitatively the more important.

Tolerance due to clonal amnesia or abortion and tolerance due to clonal suppression can be distinguished by mixing lymphocytes from a tolerant host with lymphocytes from a normal host. Tolerance mediated by suppressors will prevent normal lymphocytes from reacting to the tolerogenic antigen, whereas tolerance due to clonal amnesia or abortion cannot be transferred to normal lymphocytes (Figure 10-12). Both types of tolerance have been demonstrated by this test. It should be borne in mind, however, that these measurements do not necessarily indicate that the detected deficiency is the primary one. For example, the primary lack of a particular B-cell clone might predispose to the development of the detected T_S cells. Alternatively, the primary action of some T_S cells might be to eliminate or inactivate certain clones of B cells.

Induction of tolerance in immature lymphocytes

B cells and T cells appear to be particularly sensitive to antigen at an early stage in their differentiation from precursor lymphocytes. At this stage, contact with even low concentrations of antigens paralyzes or eliminates immature B cells and T cells with cognate receptors. Because lymphocytes continue to differentiate in the bone marrow

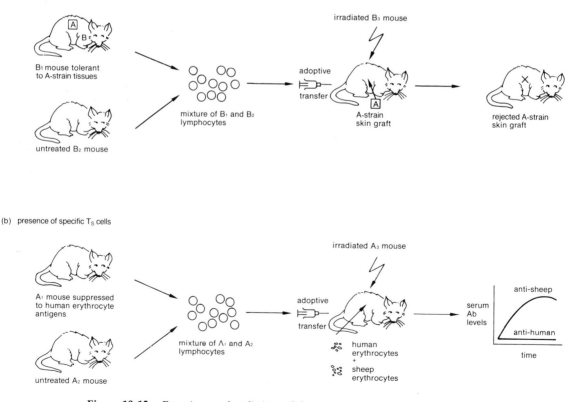

Figure 10-12   Experiments that distinguish between suppression and deletion of self-reactive clones as mechanisms for tolerance.

and thymus throughout an individual's lifetime, paralysis or elimination of self-directed clones must be an active and continuous check against production of anti-self-immunity. Maintenance of tolerance requires the continued presence of the tolerance-inducing (tolerogenic) antigen, presumably to activate continually the process for removal of newly developing self-directed B and T lymphocytes.

One plausible mechanism for paralysis of self-directed B cells derives from the properties of their surface immunoglobulins. Newly developing virgin B_μ cells have a limited capacity to resynthesize their receptor immunoglobulins. Exposure to multivalent antigens or to anti-immunoglobulin antibodies leads to capping and shedding of their receptor immunoglobulins. Over an experimental observation period of 1–3 days, their receptor immunoglobulins are not resynthesized. The cells remain viable but, upon adoptive transfer to an immune-deficient host, are unable to restore immune responsiveness. By contrast, mature $B_{\mu+\delta}$ cells respond to receptor capping by resynthesizing their surface immunoglobulins within 1 day. Arrays of self-antigens on host cells could plausibly accomplish the continual inactivation of self-directed B cells. Comparable studies of T-cell receptor turnover will soon be feasible.

Induction of tolerance in mature lymphocytes

Some insight into tolerance has come from experiments on its induction in mature animals, with the reservation that the mechanisms of tolerance induction in mature and immature lymphocytes may differ. Certain antigens administered under certain conditions can induce tolerance by paralyzing or eliminating mature lymphocytes. Mature lymphocytes are far more difficult to inactivate with a tolerogenic antigen than are immature lymphocytes. B cells and T cells respond differently to the induction of tolerance. Very low (subimmunogenic) doses of an appropriate antigen generally inactivate only T cells. However, some evidence suggests that this *low zone tolerance* also can be induced in B_μ cells but not in other B cells. Very high doses of antigen induce a *high zone tolerance* in both B cells and T cells, but it is more rapid and long lasting in T cells. Tolerance in either cell type can block synthesis of specific antibodies because B cells and T cells must cooperate to produce a complete humoral immune response (Figure 10-2).

The route of antigen administration and the form of the antigen can determine whether it elicits immunity or tolerance. Administration of antigens via the bloodstream or, in some cases, orally favors the induction of tolerance, whereas their administration intracutaneously (in the skin), subcutaneously (just under the skin), or intramuscularly favors the induction of immunity. Protein antigens, when administered in the form of an aggregate, are always immunogenic, whereas soluble monomeric forms of the same determinants may be immunogenic or tolerogenic depending on the dose. In general, high doses of monomeric antigen favor tolerance. However, even monomeric antigens are always immunogenic if administered with adjuvants, which are particulate-containing oily substances that promote protein aggregation. (An adjuvant, when mixed and injected with antigen, serves as a tissue depot that slowly releases the antigen and also as a lymphoid system activator that nonspecifically enhances the immune response.)

One type of experimentally induced tolerance is somewhat better understood and may have important clinical applications. Very high doses of polysaccharide antigens cause paralysis of most of the antigen-specific B cells by binding to all their surface receptors. This binding is reversible, but if the antigen is present at high enough levels, it can nevertheless prevent B-cell activation by a process termed *receptor blockade*, whose molecular basis is still unclear. A small amount of humoral antibody is produced but is then bound by the excess antigen. In a similar way, unnatural D isomers of polypeptide antigens also induce tolerance by blockade of B-cell receptors. This blockade is essentially irreversible, presumably because mammals lack proteases that can degrade polypeptides of D amino acids. Although the normal turnover of receptor immunoglobulin is measured in hours to days, B cells bearing D-isomer antigens persist for weeks. Thus receptor blockade also affects the metabolism of receptor immunoglobulin.

Breakdown of tolerance Tolerance induction by some of the described mechanisms predicts that self-reactive lymphocytes are actually present in an activatable form but are held in check. This prediction is supported by a variety of studies indicating that vertebrates commonly carry normal B cells bearing immunoglobulin receptors directed at self components. In autoimmune diseases, the normal regulatory checks and balances are breached, leading to a breakdown in tolerance and expression of self-directed antibodies (Concept 12-7).

Selected Bibliography

Natural immunological tolerance

Owen, R. D., "Immunogenetic consequences of vascular anastomoses between bovine twins," *Science* **201**, 400(1945).

The preceding seminal paper started it all; cattle that normally reject immunogenetically different blood cells will specifically *tolerate* them if exposed by fetal vascular anastomoses.

Induced immunological tolerance

Billingham, R. E., Brent, L., and Medawar, P. B., "Actively acquired tolerance of foreign cells," *Nature* **172**, 603(1953).

The preceding classic paper demonstrates that Owen's phenomenon could be experimentally induced and that it represents a specific *immune* tolerance as predicted by Burnet's self-nonself models of immune recognition.

Tolerance at the level of T and B cells

Chiller, J. M., Habicht, G. S., and Weigle, W. O., "Cellular sites of immunologic unresponsiveness," *Proc. Natl. Acad. Sci. USA* **65**, 551(1970).

Nossal, G. J. V., "Cellular mechanisms of immunologic tolerance," *Annu. Rev. Immunol.* **1**, 33(1983).

The preceding studies distinguish the relative susceptibility of T and B cells to tolerance induction.

Actively induced immune regulation

Gershon, R. K., and Kondo, K., "Infectious immunological tolerance," *Immunology* **21**, 903(1971).

Green, D. R., Flood, P. M., and Gershon, R. K., "Immunoregulatory T-cell pathways," *Ann. Rev. Immunol.* **1**, 439(1983).

Weissman, I., and Lustgraaf, E. C., "Antibody formation and repressor systems," *Transplantation Bulletin* **28**, 134(1961).

The first and third papers outline the speculations and experiments that challenged the idea that tolerance was simply due to a lack of reacting cells, but that tolerance might be due to an active, suppressive, and specific arm of the immune system. The second paper is the most recent of a long line of developments in the field by Gershon, who is responsible not only for identifying the cell types responsible for immunoregulation but also for the demonstration that misregulation by these cells has profound medical consequences.

Immune regulatory circuits and networks that are based on antigens and on idiotypes

Herzenberg, L. A., Tokuhisa, T., and Hayakawa, K., "Epitope-specific regulation," *Ann. Rev. Immunol.* **1**, 609(1983).

Jerne, N. K., "The immune system," *Sci. Am.* **229**, 52(1973).

Jerne, N. K., "Towards a network theory of the immune system," *Ann. Immunol.* (Inst. Pasteur) **125 C**, 373(1974).

Rajewsky, K., and Takemori, T., "Genetics, expression, and function of idiotypes," *Ann. Rev. Immunol.* **1**, 569(1983).

The preceding papers provide the ideas and experiments that regulatory cells in the immune network may involve recognition systems centered on antigenic epitopes or on idiotopes of the antibodies recognizing such epitopes.

Additional concepts introduced in the problems

1. Antibody inhibition of the immune response. Problem 10-4.
2. Antigenic competition. Problem 10-5.
3. Transplantation tolerance. Problems 10-9 and 10-10.

Problems

10-1 Indicate whether each of the following statements is true or false. Explain the error in each statement you consider to be false.

(a) Tolerance is an active process that exhibits a high degree of specificity.

(b) Antibodies that react with self-molecules are generally not produced because genes that code for self-antibodies are not inherited.

(c) Anti-self-immunity does not develop because we do not possess MHC-linked high immune response genes to self-antigens.

(d) Identical twins do not reject blood transfusion because the twins share all genetically encoded blood group antigens and therefore accept them as self.

(e) An immunoglobulin idiotope is unique to a particular V_H-V_L pair.

(f) An immunoglobulin idiotype is unique to a particular V_H-V_L pair.

(g) We do not respond to norepinephrine as an antigen because it is present at sufficient concentrations to induce tolerance in *both* B and T cells.

10-2 Supply the missing word or words in each of the following statements.

(a) Immunological _____ is the process that normally prevents lymphocytes from reacting with self-antigens.

(b) Administration of DNP-d (glu, lys) to mice will lead to DNP tolerance caused by B lymphocyte _____ .

(c) The network theory states that immunoglobulins can be considered both as _____ and as _____ .

(d) Single immunoglobulin variable-region antigenic determinants are called _____ .

(e) Freemartin cattle are nonidentical twins that tolerate each other's blood-cell antigens because they had a common _____ during _____ development.

10-3 An interesting experiment was done to investigate the question of whether tolerance, or immunological unresponsiveness, is an active or a passive state. Normal adult mice were thymectomized, irradiated, and then reconstituted with syngeneic bone-marrow cells so that they lacked T cells. Thirty days later, all the mice were given 3×10^7 normal thymocytes intravenously and then divided into three groups. Group 1 received 8×10^7 spleen cells from mice immunized with sheep red blood cells (SRBC), while Group 3 received spleen cells from mice tolerant to SRBC. Group 2 mice received only the thymocytes. All the mice were then challenged with SRBC and, at an appropriate time thereafter, their anti-SRBC antibody titers were measured by hemagglutination (Concept 3-4). Figure 10-13a indicates total antibody titers; Figure 10-13b shows the titers of mercaptoethanol-resistant antibody. (IgM activity is destroyed by reducing agents such as mercaptoethanol, hence the level of resistant antibody corresponds roughly to that of antibody of the IgG class.) With reference to the figure, answer the following questions.

(a) Compare the responses of groups 1 and 2. Does the difference seem reasonable?

(b) Now compare groups 2 and 3. What response would you expect if normal thymocytes alone were injected? If the tolerant spleen cells alone were injected? What do you conclude about the interaction between the two cell populations? Can you propose a mechanism to explain this effect? Suggest an experiment to test your proposed mechanism.

10-4 The preceding problem underscores the interdependence of the interaction between cellular components of the immune system. A facet of this interaction is the ability of antibody itself to influence the humoral response. One research group passively immunized AKR mice with anti-SRBC IgG just prior to, or shortly after, a single injection of SRBC. Figure 10-14 gives the numbers of plaque-forming spleen cells at various times after immunization with SRBC, determined by the Jerne plaque assay. With reference to this figure, answer questions (a) and (b).

Figure 10-13

The anti-SRBC response of thymus-deprived mice given normal thymocytes and spleen cells from three different donors (Problem 10-3). Groups 1, 2, and 3 are described in the text. (a) Total antibody. (b) Mercaptoethanol-resistant antibody. [From R. Gershon and K. Kondo, *Immunology* **21**, 903(1971).]

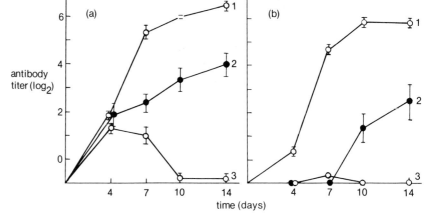

(a) What do you conclude from the data shown?

(b) What simple explanation can you suggest for this effect?

(c) A second research group extended these experiments to an *in vitro* system in which they cultured spleen cells with SRBC and anti-SRBC IgG. In addition, these researchers fractionated the anti-SRBC IgG into IgG_1 and IgG_2 subclasses and added anti-SRBC antibody of each subclass separately to spleen cell cultures. The observed production of plaque-forming cells is plotted against antibody concentration in Figure 10-15. How do you interpret these results?

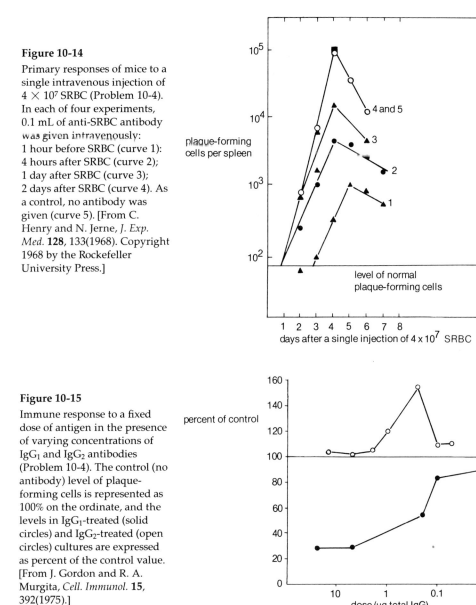

Figure 10-14

Primary responses of mice to a single intravenous injection of 4×10^7 SRBC (Problem 10-4). In each of four experiments, 0.1 mL of anti-SRBC antibody was given intravenously: 1 hour before SRBC (curve 1); 4 hours after SRBC (curve 2); 1 day after SRBC (curve 3); 2 days after SRBC (curve 4). As a control, no antibody was given (curve 5). [From C. Henry and N. Jerne, *J. Exp. Med.* **128**, 133(1968). Copyright 1968 by the Rockefeller University Press.]

Figure 10-15

Immune response to a fixed dose of antigen in the presence of varying concentrations of IgG_1 and IgG_2 antibodies (Problem 10-4). The control (no antibody) level of plaque-forming cells is represented as 100% on the ordinate, and the levels in IgG_1-treated (solid circles) and IgG_2-treated (open circles) cultures are expressed as percent of the control value. [From J. Gordon and R. A. Murgita, *Cell. Immunol.* **15**, 392(1975).]

(d) The researchers then added anti-SRBC antibodies to some cultures containing chicken red blood cells (CRBC) instead of SRBC. Figure 10-16 shows the anti-CRBC responses they obtained. What is the significance of this experiment?

(e) Are the results in part (c) consistent with your answer to part (b)? If not, how would you modify your answer to part (b)?

(f) Gordon and Murgita also tested F(ab')$_2$ fragments of the IgG antibodies from each subclass, but these fragments had no significant effect, either positive or negative. Remember that F(ab')$_2$ fragments lack most of the heavy-chain constant regions, but they still contain both antigen-binding sites, and they specifically bind antigen almost as well as complete immunoglobulin molecules. How does this observation bear on your explanation of the results in Figure 10-16?

10-5 The control mechanisms demonstrated in the preceding problems all share the characteristic of immunological specificity. The phenomenon of antigenic competition provides an interesting counterpoint. How do animals respond when challenged with two different antigens, one after another? In one such experiment, mice were immunized with either sheep red blood cells (SRBC) or horse red blood cells (HRBC) and then, several days later, were challenged with the other antigen. Table 10-1 shows the resulting splenic responses as production of plaque-forming cells (PFC) 5 days after the last injection.

(a) What is the apparent effect of these temporal sequences of immunizations?

(b) When the mice in group I were immunized with bovine serum albumin, HeLa cells (a human cell line), or *Brucella abortus* (a gram-negative bacterium) instead of SRBC on day 0, the results were essentially the same. What does this observation indicate about the immunologic specificity of the effect?

(c) Several hypotheses have been advanced to explain this effect. One possibility is that lymphocytes specific for the two antigens compete *in vivo* for space, for some limiting nutrient, or for some helper-cell population (T cells or accessory cells such as macrophages). Prior exposure to one antigen gives the corresponding lymphocytes a competitive advantage and hence reduces the response to the second antigen. Alternatively, this phenomenon could reflect a positive control mechanism. Specifically stimulated lymphocytes could inhibit the initi-

Figure 10-16

The plaque-forming cell response to sheep red blood cells (SRBC) or chicken red blood cells (CRBC) in the presence of IgG$_1$ or IgG$_2$ anti-SRBC antibodies (Problem 10-4). C indicates a control in which no antibodies were added. [From J. Gordon and R. A. Murgita, *Cell. Immunol.* **15**, 392(1975).]

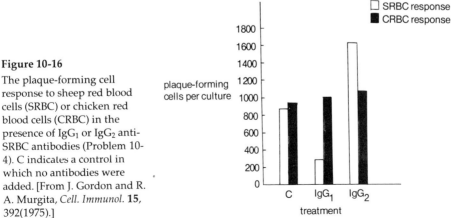

Table 10-1 Antigen Competition Between Sheep Red Blood Cells (SRBC) and Horse Red Blood Cells (HRBC) (Problem 10-5)

Group	Immunizing Antigen and Time of Administration		Assay (Day 8) Test Antigen	PFC/10^6 Spleen Cells
	Antigen 1 (day 0)	Antigen 2 (day 3)		
I	—	HRBC	HRBC	205 ± 45
	SRBC	HRBC	HRBC	13 ± 5
II	—	SRBC	SRBC	626 ± 58
	HRBC	SRBC	SRBC	78 ± 15

[From G. Moller and O. Sjoberg, *Cell. Immunol.* **1**, 110(1970).]

ation of new responses via nonspecific soluble factors or other means. Discuss the critical variables that must be considered in the design of experiments that discriminate between these two alternatives.

10-6 The preceding problems present several unusual situations in which an organism fails to respond to a set of antigenic determinants. How does the immune system normally become tolerant to its own self-antigens while retaining the ability to respond to nonself-antigens? An Australian scientist and his colleagues investigated this process. They began by looking at the surface immunoglobulin (sIg) on bone-marrow (BM) and peripheral lymphocytes of mice. To mouse lymphocyte suspensions they added increasing concentrations of ^{125}I-antiglobulin (^{125}I-labeled rabbit antibodies specific for mouse immunoglobulin), and they recorded the percentages of radiolabeled cells (sIg$^+$) in each population as shown in Figure 10-17. In this assay, there is an inverse linear relationship between the amount (or density) of sIg on a cell and the minimum concentration of ^{125}I-antiglobulin that labels the cell: the greater the amount of sIg on a cell, the lower the concentration of ^{125}I-antiglobulin required to label it. With regard to the data on lymph-node and spleen cells in Figure 10-17, answer the following questions.

(a) Is there a variation in the amount of sIg per cell among sIg$^+$ spleen and lymph-node cells?

(b) Can you deduce the approximate percentage of B cells in each population?

(c) Compare these populations with bone-marrow cells. Do these data provide a reliable estimate of the number of BM sIg$^+$cells?

(d) Is the variation in the amount of sIg per sIg$^+$ cell comparable for bone-marrow cells and the other two cell populations? (*Note:* At antiserum concentrations greater than 10μg/mL, nonspecific binding becomes significant and consequently limits the assay.)

(e) What do these data suggest to you about the maturation of lymphocytes in the bone marrow?

10-7 (a) The Australian researchers cited in Problem 10-6 next studied the maturation of bone-marrow cells by *in vivo* labeling with ^{3}H-thymidine. They found that 1

Figure 10-17

The incidence of labeled small lymphocytes in suspensions of cells from lymphoid tissues of CBA mice following exposure to rabbit ^{125}I-antimouse globulin at various concentrations (Problem 10-6). [From D. G. Osmond and G. J. V. Nossal, *Cell. Immunol.* **13**, 117(1974).]

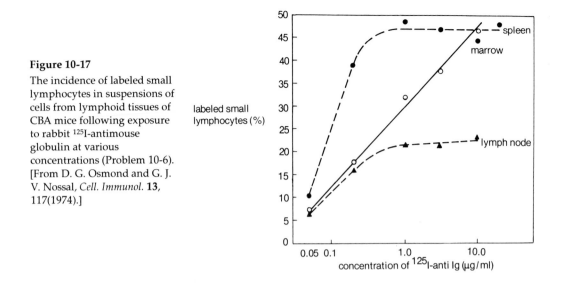

labeled small lymphocytes (%)

concentration of ^{125}I-anti Ig (μg/ml)

hour after intraperitoneal injection of ³H-thymidine, large bone-marrow lymphocytes (diameter $> 8\,\mu$) had been labeled but small lymphocytes (diameter $< 8\,\mu$) had not. When these same cells were treated with ¹³¹I-antiglobulin, only the small lymphocytes were labeled. Rarely was a doubly labeled cell detected. What can you infer about the biochemical events that occurred in the large and small lymphocytes?

(b) Some mice were given ³H-thymidine at 8-hour intervals over a 4-day period. Analyses of their bone-marrow cells gave the following results: first, the proportion (and absolute number) of small lymphocytes labeled with a 1 μg/mL concentration of ¹³¹I-antiglobulin remained approximately constant; second, the percentage of small lymphocytes labeled with ³H-thymidine increased monotonically, 83% of the cells having been labeled after 84 hours; third, the proportion of doubly labeled cells also increased monotonically, but only after a considerable time lag as shown in Table 10-2. What does the increase in the number of small lymphocytes labeled by ³H-thymidine suggest?

(c) What does the time lag before the appearance of doubly labeled cells suggest?

(d) New cells are apparently being produced, yet the proportion and absolute number of bone-marrow sIg⁺ cells remain roughly constant. How might this constant pool size be maintained?

(e) After 84 hours of continuous labeling, only 5% of the small lymphocytes in the periphery (blood, lymph nodes, and spleen) were labeled. What additional facts do you need to compare the number of labeled cells that migrate to the periphery with the number of new cells generated in this period?

10-8 The investigators mentioned in the preceding two problems carried out several experiments to test the immunologic capabilities of bone-marrow cells. They injected marrow or spleen cells into irradiated syngeneic hosts after culture *in vitro* for up to 3 days before adoptive transfer. Then they challenged the recipient animals with 5 μg of DNP conjugated to polymerized *Salmonella* flagellin (DNP-POL). Nine days later they determined the numbers of anti-DNP plaque-forming cells in the host spleens.

Table 10-2 Percentages of Bone-Marrow Small Lymphocytes Labeled After Administration of ^{3}H-Thymidine *in Vivo* and Exposure to ^{131}I-Antiglobulin *in Vitro* (Problem 10-7)

Duration of ^{3}H-Thymidine Labeling (hr)	Double-Label Experiments,[a] Using ^{131}I-Antiglobulin Concentrations of:					
	1.0 μg/mL			0.2 μg/mL		
	^{3}H	^{131}I	^{131}I + ^{3}H	^{3}H	^{131}I	^{131}I + ^{3}H
12	17.5	31.8	0			
26	41.7	24.0	0.5	44.2	17.2	0
33	51.7	35.1	1.2	51.8	20.8	0
50	64.8	27.9	6.6	63.5	16.6	1.8
57	71.8	20.3	11.5	68.5	17.5	3.7
74	77.6	15.9	17.8	70.4	11.3	5.0
83	82.6	10.3	16.4			

[a]Numbers indicate percentages of cells singly labeled with ^{3}H, singly labeled with ^{131}I, and doubly labeled with ^{131}I and ^{3}H as indicated by column headings.
[From D. G. Osmond and G. J. V. Nossal, *Cell. Immunol.* **13**, 132(1974).]

Table 10-3 summarizes the results of several experiments with this system. Notice that, in experiment III, varying concentrations of DNP conjugated to horse γ globulin (DNP-HGG) were added during the *in vitro* incubation period. With reference to the table, answer the following questions.

(a) What effect does *in vitro* incubation have on the spleen cell response? How might this result be explained?

(b) How do the marrow cells respond to culture? How might this result be explained? What do the kinetics of this effect suggest?

(c) Now consider experiment III in Table 10-3. What might be the relevance of the data?

(d) What do you think might have happened to the 800 potential plaque-forming cells whose development was inhibited by 0.4 μg DNP-HGG in experiment III? Do your answers to Problems 10-6 or 10-7 provide a possible explanation?

(e) How could you determine whether the nonresponsiveness is due to a suppressor cell population? Assuming that there is no suppressor cell population, what experimental results would you expect?

10-9   There are two general mechanisms by which tolerance might be established in the developing organism. Potentially reactive cells could be killed or irreversibly paralyzed, or they could be reversibly suppressed. The latter mechanism would require the constant presence of a suppressive factor, either humoral or cellular. A group of Israeli researchers interested in this problem incubated thymocytes from a Lewis rat with the thymic reticulum (thymic epithelial tissue) from the same rat *in vitro*. They then measured the ability of these lymphocytes to mount a graft-versus-host response (GVHR) in syngeneic animals after varying intervals in culture. They in-

Table 10-3   Adoptive Transfer Experiments with Bone-Marrow and Spleen Cells (Problem 10-8)

Cell Source	Number of Cells	Hours Incubated *in vitro*	Antigen Concentration Added *in vitro*	Anti-DNP Plaque-Forming Cells on Day 9
I Spleen	10^7	0	—	1600
		3	—	1400
		24	—	900
		72	—	400
II Bone marrow	2×10^7	0	—	400
		3	—	400
		24	—	400
		48	—	700
		72	—	1200
III Bone marrow	2×10^7	72	—	1200
		72	0.004 µg/mL DNP-HGG	900
		72	0.04 µg/mL DNP-HGG	650
		72	0.4 µg/mL DNP-HGG	400
		72	4.0 µg/mL DNP-HGG	250

[Data adapted from G. J. V. Nossal and B. Pike, *J. Exp. Med.* **141**, 904(1975). Copyright 1975 by the Rockefeller University Press.]

jected treated lymphocytes into a rat's right footpad and untreated control lymphocytes into the left footpad. After several days, they compared the number of cells in the lymph node that drains the right foot with the number of cells in the corresponding left lymph node to determine the magnitude of the GVHR. They also measured the cytotoxic potential of the lymphocytes in the right lymph node against syngeneic or allogeneic fibroblasts, with the results as shown in Table 10-4. With reference to the table, answer the following questions.

(a) Should thymocytes generate a GVHR in syngeneic recipients or specifically lyse syngeneic target cells? What do these data show?

(b) Outline the sequence of events that must occur to develop a GVHR. Which of these events occur *in vitro* and which occur *in vivo* in this experiment? What do these results suggest about one mechanism of tolerance?

(c) What is the minimum incubation time *in vitro* necessary to develop a strong response? How does this interval compare with the average generation time of lymphocytes, which is 10–16 hours? Could you attribute the appearance of anti-self-reactive cells to the differentiation of precursor cells *in vitro*? If not, how else could you explain this phenomenon?

(d) Combine your answers in parts (a)–(c) to formulate a model for the development of natural tolerance.

10-10   To distinguish between active suppression and clonal abortion as the mechanism for transplantation tolerance induced in neonatal mice, the following experiments were conducted. Neonatal CBA mice were inoculated intravenously with 2×10^7

Table 10-4 Kinetics of Autosensitization of Lewis Thymus Lymphocyte Cells Against Lewis Fibroblasts (Problem 10-9)

Sensitization Time *in Vitro* (hr)	Popliteal Lymph-Node Assay Average Cells per Right Lymph Node[a]	Lysis of Target Fibroblasts[b] Lewis	Lysis of Target Fibroblasts[b] BALB/c
0	3×10^6	11.9 ± 1.2	10.9 ± 0.4
2	3×10^6	9.1 ± 0.7	10.8 ± 0.6
6	8×10^6	17.0 ± 1.5	8.8 ± 1.7
24	12×10^6	21.6 ± 0.6	10.5 ± 2.0

[a]The control left lymph nodes contained an average of 2×10^6 cells per node.
[b]5×10^6 lymphocytes from the right lymph nodes of each group were incubated with BALB/c or syngeneic Lewis mouse target cells for 65 hours. The lysis of Lewis fibroblasts was significantly greater than that of the BALB/c controls at 6 and 24 hours ($p < 0.01$).
[From I. R. Cohen and H. Wekerle, *J. Exp. Med* **137**, 224(1973). Copyright 1973 by the Rockefeller University Press.]

Table 10-5 Effects of Allogeneic Lymphocyte Injections on Transplantation Tolerance in Neonatal Mice (Problem 10-10)

Mice	Original Graft* A(H-2a)	Second Graft† A(H-2a)	Second Graft† C3H(H-2k)	Second Graft† B10.A(4R) (H-2h4)
Thymectomized	10.2	>100	15.4	12.3
Sham thymectomized	9.8	11.0	11.0	12.9

*Mean survival time of skin graft in days after the injection of C3H cells.
†Mean survival time of skin graft in days after the second grafting.

spleen and lymph-node cells from (CBA $\times$ A)F$_1$ mice. These putatively tolerant CBA mice were either thymectomized or sham thymectomized within 4–5 weeks of birth, and they were challenged with an A-strain skin graft when they were 7–9 weeks old. After each animal had maintained its A-graft in excellent condition for at least 100 days, it was inoculated intraperitoneally with 15×10^7 spleen and lymph-node cells from C3H mice that had been sensitized against A-strain cells. Fifty days later the mice received a second skin graft from a donor of a different strain. The results are shown in Table 10-5. CBA and C3H mice are H-2k, whereas A mice are H-2a(KkIk/dDd). With reference to the table, answer the following questions.
(a) Explain why injection of C3H anti-A lymphoid cells would induce rejection of the original A-graft.

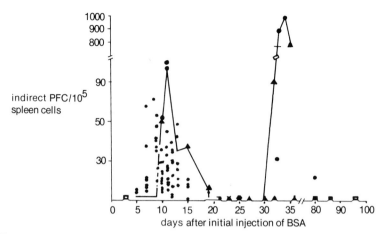

Figure 10-18

Quantitation of indirect plaque-forming cells (PFC) following injection of bovine serum albumin (BSA) (Problem 10-11). Rabbits were given daily subcutaneous injections of 1 g of BSA for six weeks. Each solid circle represents the number of PFC directed against BSA from spleen cells of an individual rabbit so treated. The solid line represents the response of a rabbit given a single intravenous injection of 20 mg of soluble BSA on day 0 and again on day 30. [From J. M. Chiller, C. G. Romball, and W. O. Weigle, *Cell. Immunol.* **8**, 29(1973).]

(b)   Why is the C3H skin graft rejected even though it has the same H-2 haplotype as CBA? Are you seeing a primary or a secondary response?

(c)   Explain the acceptance of the second A-graft in thymectomized mice and rejection in sham thymectomized mice. Does this result favor active suppression or clonal abortion? Explain.

10-11   Simply injecting large amounts of antigen into an animal does not always insure a strong immune response. Normal adult rabbits were injected subcutaneously with 1 g of BSA 6 times a week for 6 weeks. At various times, individual rabbits were sacrificed, their spleens removed, and the number of indirect plaque-forming cells (cells that secreted either IgM or IgG specific for BSA) was measured. With reference to the results shown in Figure 10-18, answer the following questions.

(a)   Compare the primary and secondary responses to 20 mg of BSA with the response to 1 g of BSA given 6 days per week for 6 weeks. What seems to have happened?

(b)   Some of the rabbits unresponsive to BSA were immunized with 5 mg of human γ globulin (HGG) on day 30, and they responded normally to the HGG. Why is this an important control and what does it prove?

(c)   Some newborn rabbits were injected subcutaneously with 150 mg and 250 mg of soluble BSA on the first and third days of life, respectively. No plaque-forming cells were detected for more than a month after the last injection. What do you conclude about neonatal animals? (Immunization with 0.5 mg BSA normally elicits a vigorous immune response in adult rabbits.)

10-12   BALB/c mice were immunized with a set of closely related BALB/c phosphorylcholine binding myeloma proteins (T15, M167, M511, and M603), all of

Table 10-6 Response of BALB/c Mice to Immunization with Phosphorylcholine-Binding (PC) Myeloma Proteins (Problem 10-12)

Immunogen	Proportion of Mice Responding[a]
T15	0/8
M167	18/18
M603	18/24
M511	4/9

[a]Response measured with the ^{125}I-labeled myeloma protein used as immunogen. Sera from immunized mice were incubated with 100 ng of labeled protein, and then goat antiserum to mouse Ig was added. The resulting immune precipitate was assayed for radioactivity. The goat antiserum to mouse Ig was absorbed with the myeloma protein used as labeled antigen in the assay. If the precipitate had three times the counts contained in the control precipitate using normal BALB/c serum, the response was considered positive. In practice, greater than 10% of the cpm precipitated was usually a positive response. [The data in Tables 10-6, 7, and 8 are adapted from experiments by C. A. Janeway, N. Sakata, and H. N. Eisen.]

Table 10-7 Specificity of the Antisera Made in BALB/c Mice (Problem 10-12)

	^{125}I-Labeled Proteins—Percent Bound				
Immunogen	M167	M603	M511	T15	Serum IgA (κ) (Nonphosphorylcholine-Binding)
M167	<u>54</u>	12	10	6	2
M603	0	<u>30</u>	0	0	1
M511	4	8	<u>19</u>	5	1

Values are the percent of added ^{125}I-labeled myeloma precipitated. Assays were conducted as described in Table 10-6. Values underlined are the percent precipitated when the immunogen and the labeled test protein were the same.

which consist of α heavy chains and κ light chains. The response data are given in Tables 10-6 and 10-7. With reference to these data, answer questions (a)–(c).

(a) Discuss the specificity of the three antisera in terms of idiotopes and idiotypes. How would you test whether binding in the 4–12% range is specific?

(b) The myeloma proteins are all originally from BALB/c mice. The ability to make these sera would seem to contradict our common sense notions about self-tolerance. Why do BALB/c mice make antibodies to these myeloma proteins?

(c) Can you give a reason why the T15 protein appears to be an exception? In a related experiment, an adoptive transfer system was used to study the response of BALB/c mice to the myeloma proteins as diagrammed in Figure 10-19. The results are shown in Table 10-8. With reference to the table, answer the following questions.

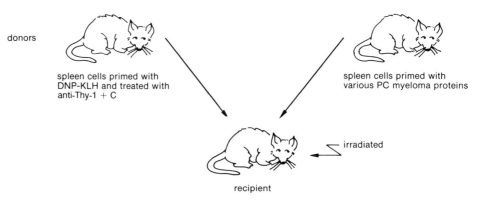

donors

spleen cells primed with
DNP-KLH and treated with
anti-Thy-1 + C

spleen cells primed with
various PC myeloma proteins

irradiated

recipient

Figure 10-19   Strategy for adoptive transfer experiments to study the response of BALB/c mice to various myeloma proteins (Problem 10-12).

(d) What carriers are the T cells from donor 2 recognizing in the recipient mice?

(e) In a general qualitative sense, do the T cells in Table 10-8 appear to be as discriminating as the B cells in Tables 10-6 and 10-7? What does this result suggest about the comparative sizes of the B-cell and T-cell repertoires of antigen-binding receptors?

Answers

10-1   (a) True

(b) False. Genes that code for anti-self-antibodies are inherited. Tolerance probably results from the elimination or paralysis of lymphocyte clones that produce anti-self-antibodies.

(c) False. We possess Ir genes that enable recognition of self-MHC components and use them to recognize foreign antigens in the context of self. Either we lack T cells that see self as a sufficient stimulus or else these T cells are eliminated or suppressed.

(d) True

(e) False. An idiotope could be a public or a private variable-region determinant and is not necessarily generated by the association of V_L and V_H regions.

(f) True

(g) False. We do not respond to norepinephrine as an antigen because the molecule is too small; it is equivalent to a hapten unattached to a carrier, and it is therefore nonimmunogenic.

10-2   (a) tolerance

(b) receptor blockade

(c) antibodies; antigens

(d) idiotopes

(e) blood vasculature; embryonic

10-3   (a) That specifically SRBC immune spleen cells would augment the response to SRBC seems reasonable.

(b) The results of group 2 illustrate the response of mice injected with thymocytes

Table 10-8 Results of Adoptive Transfer Experiments (Problem 10-12)

	Donor 1		Donor 2			
Group	Spleen Cells Primed with	Spleen Cells Treated with	Spleen Cells Primed with	Spleen Cells Treated with	Recipients Boosted with	Anti-DNP Response
1	DNP-KLH	anti-Thy-1 + C	M167	NMS + C	DNP-M167	30.9
2	DNP-KLH	anti-Thy-1 + C	M167	anti-Thy-1 + C	DNP-M167	0.6
3	DNP-KLH	anti-Thy-1 + C	M603	NMS + C	DNP-M167	4.5
4	DNP-KLH	anti-Thy-1 + C	M603	NMS + C	DNP-M603	35.4
5	DNP-KLH	anti-Thy-1 + C	M603	anti-Thy-1 + C	DNP-M603	1.2
6	DNP-KLH	anti-Thy-1 + C	M167	NMS + C	DNP-M603	7.4

Irradiated recipient mice received spleen cells from two separate syngeneic donors. One donor provided DNP-KLH primed spleen cells treated with anti-Thy-1 antibody. The other donor gave spleen cells primed with the myeloma proteins shown. Recipients were boosted with DNP covalently coupled to one of the myeloma proteins. The numbers shown measure the binding capacity of the resulting anti-DNP sera; higher numbers mean a larger response. NMS: normal mouse serum; C: complement.

alone. A very poor response would be expected if only the tolerant spleen cells had been injected. From the results observed with group 3, it appears that the tolerant spleen lymphocytes also actively suppress the response of the normal thymocytes. The active suppression affects IgG production more severely than IgM production. This result might have been expected because T cells are not absolutely required for a primary IgM response. One might hypothesize that the suppressor T cells kill or inhibit cells responsible for the generation of IgG specific for SRBC. The proposed specificity of this effect could be tested by simultaneously administering SRBC and a second, unrelated antigen. In fact, there does seem to be a generalized, nonspecific depression of the immune system in such experiments. These observations emphasize the important regulatory role that T cells may play in the immune response, but they also emphasize the need for specificity controls in these types of experiments.

10-4 (a) Injection of anti-SRBC antibody 1 hour before or 4 hours after SRBC diminishes the number of plaque-forming cells, reflecting a decreased number of specifically stimulated B cells. Therefore, injected IgG reduces the primary humoral (IgM) response to a cognate antigen.

(b) The simplest explanation is that the specific IgG interferes with the afferent arm of the response to antigen. The IgG could bind to free or accessory cell-processed SRBC antigens and prevent recognition by other specific B cells or helper T cells. Alternatively, the IgG may act by promoting the phagocytosis and digestion of the SRBC before they can elicit an immune response.

(c) Specific IgG_1 antibodies inhibit the response, but specific IgG_2 antibodies actually stimulate the response significantly.

(d) The anti-SRBC antibodies had negligible effects on the anti-CRBC response, thereby demonstrating that the inhibitory effect of added antibody is specific.

(e) The inhibition by IgG agrees with the previous results, but the stimulation by specific IgG_2 antibodies indicates that a more complex explanation is required. If the only differences between specific IgG_1 and IgG_2 antibodies are subtle variations in the heavy-chain structure, then the simple "recognition-interference" hypothesis seems invalid.

(f) The finding that specific F(ab')$_2$ fragments of either subclass are neither stimulatory nor inhibitory underscores the importance of the heavy-chain constant regions in this control mechanism and strengthens the argument against the simple recognition-interference explanation in part (b). Perhaps some additional element—for example, T cells or macrophages with Fc receptors—is required for antibody inhibition of immune responses.

10-5 (a) The response to the second (competing) antigen is sharply reduced, regardless of which antigen is administered first and which second.

(b) This effect does not depend on relatedness of the antigens. The mechanisms underlying this so-called antigenic competition must be nonspecific.

(c) The central problem is to distinguish between an active suppression and a failure to compete successfully for some limiting factor. Unfortunately, there is considerable experimental evidence on both sides of the question. Clearly, suppressor cells do exist, and some groups have reported the adoptive transfer of antigenic competition by T cells. Other groups report that addition of normal T cells relieves antigenic competition, which suggests that T cells are the limiting factor. Still other experiments strongly suggest that limitation of binding sites for T-cell receptors on accessory cells is the cause. Important variables seem to be the exact timing and the dose of antigen, the physical state of the antigens, whether the competing antigenic determinants are on the same or different molecules, whether the experiment is done *in vivo* or *in vitro* (the microarchitecture of the lymph nodes may influence this phenomenon critically), and finally whether accessory cells such as macrophages are present.

10-6 (a) There is some variation in the sIg per cell, but both populations show a plateau at about 1 μg/mL antiserum.

(b) The percentages of lymphocytes labeled at the plateau is a good measure of the total number of sIg$^+$ cells or B cells. Hence about 45% of the splenic lymphocytes and about 20% of the lymph-node lymphocytes are B cells.

(c) These data do not allow an estimate of the number of B cells because no plateau is evident. The assay would have to be carried out to higher antiserum concentrations to determine whether the marrow curve would reach a plateau. However, at antiserum concentrations greater than 10 μg/mL, nonspecific labeling becomes significant and invalidates the assay.

(d) The lack of a plateau up to 10 μg/mL antiserum demonstrates a greater variation in the amount of sIg per cell among sIg$^+$ marrow cells. An even greater variation is implied, in that there may be cells with still smaller amounts of sIg that are not labeled by even 10 μg/mL antiserum.

(e) If there is a continuous variation in the surface density of sIg, from cells with no sIg to cells with large amounts of sIg, then perhaps the density of sIg is a measure of the cells' maturity. The acquisition of sIg may be a critical step in lymphocyte maturation.

10-7 (a) The large lymphocytes synthesized DNA, which implies that they are rapidly dividing cells, whereas the small lymphocytes are not.

(b) Bone-marrow small lymphocytes are derived from dividing precursors; if there is no migration of cells into bone marrow, these small lymphocytes must be descendants of the rapidly dividing large marrow lymphocytes. Furthermore, the pool of small lymphocytes must be turning over rapidly; within 4 days, the majority of the unlabeled small lymphocytes were replaced by labeled small lymphocytes recently generated from the large blast cells.

(c) This lag indicates that newly formed small lymphocytes have little, if any, sIg. Apparently, it takes 30–40 hours before the sIg density is sufficient for the cell to be labeled by 1 μg/mL antiglobulin. This observation further supports the idea that lymphocytes mature and acquire increasing amounts of sIg during 3–4 days in the bone marrow.

(d) Mature cells could migrate from the marrow and enter the bloodstream or peripheral lymphoid organs. Alternatively, some lymphoid cells could differentiate into other cell types, or they could simply die.

(e) You would need to know the size of the peripheral lymphoid pool (which includes the nodes, spleen, peripheral blood, interstitial fluids, lymph vessels, thymus, and gut-associated lymphoid tissue) and the percent of those cells that are labeled. [Notice that recently migrating cells may preferentially home to one organ (e.g., the spleen) so that measurement of only one organ may give erroneous results.] Then you would have to calculate the number of small lymphocytes generated in all of the bone marrow and estimate the number of labeled cells that should have migrated in 3½ days. If this number greatly exceeded the number of labeled cells in the periphery, then you should look for evidence of cell death.

10-8 (a) *In vitro* incubation significantly decreases the spleen cell response. Cell death *in vitro* may explain this result.

(b) *In vitro* incubation significantly increases the bone-marrow cell response, particularly during the last 24–72 hours. This period is the same as the time during which ^{3}H-thymidine-labeled BM cells acquire detectable amounts of sIg (recall Problem 10-7). These kinetics suggest that new B cells matured during the culture interval.

(c) The molar concentrations of the added DNP-HGG range down to 10^{-10} M. Many serum proteins are present at these or much greater concentrations, even early in ontogeny. This result, which shows that developing B cells are inhibited by minute amounts of their specific antigens *in vitro*, may reflect the process by which tolerance to self-antigens is induced *in vivo*.

(d) The potential anti-DNP B cells may have been irreversibly inactivated or forced out of the bone marrow into the periphery. Alternatively, binding to antigen early in development may cause cell death.

(e) A mixture of one culture incubated with antigen and one incubated without should give results equivalent to the average of those obtained with the two cultures separately.

10-9 (a) Thymocytes should not react in any way against syngeneic cells, yet the data show a strong graft-versus-host response (GVHR) and specific cytotoxicity.

(b) In a GVHR, the T_A and T_C precursors must first be triggered by binding to their specific antigens. Then the cells undergo blast transformation and several rounds of division. (During this stage, other white blood cells are attracted to the site, probably by chemotactic lymphokines.) Finally, effector cells (e.g., cytotoxic lymphocytes) appear. In this experiment, only the triggering occurs *in vitro*; the proliferation and the generation of effector cells occur *in vivo*. This result could imply that tolerance is normally maintained by interfering with the triggering of self-specific lymphocytes.

(c) Two to six hours is the minimum incubation time required—much less than the average generation time for lymphocytes. Therefore, it is unlikely that this effect can be explained by the *in vitro* differentiation of precursor cells. It seems more likely that naturally occurring anti-self-reactive clones are reversibly suppressed *in vivo*, and that this suppression is lost *in vitro*, or that these autoreactive T cells will never be permitted to leave the thymus and undergo this reaction in the periphery.

(d) Any model should incorporate reversible suppression of self-reactive cells mediated at the level of recognition or triggering and not at the levels of proliferation or effector function. Other mechanisms are probably used concomitantly, thereby giving the organism several control mechanisms to prevent autoimmune reactions.

10-10 (a) Anti-A T_C lymphocytes kill A cells.

(b) Though C3H and CBA have the same H-2 haplotype, there are most likely to be differences in the *minor* transplantation antigens, which will elicit *weak* immune responses. Injection of C3H cells was the initial challenge, so rejecting the C3H skin graft is a secondary response which is equal in magnitude to the primary response toward the *major* transplantation antigen (B10.A(4R)).

(c) The original A-graft is rejected by C3H anti-A cells, which in turn are cleared by the CBA host. The rejection of the second A-graft has nothing to do with C3H cells. The breakdown of tolerance in sham thymectomized mice can be explained by clonal abortion. The original A-graft was accepted as self. All lymphocyte clones that can respond to A-graft are aborted. When the A-graft is removed, A-responding lymphocyte clones are regenerated through the thymus. They are not aborted because A is not around during their maturation. In the thymectomized mice, these clones are not regenerated, hence the tolerance. Active suppression would predict that the existing T_S cells would suppress the activity of newly regenerated A-responding lymphocytes so that the sham thymectomized mice should be tolerant. Therefore, this mechanism is not supported by the data.

10-11 (a) The massive doses of BSA inhibit the development of a normal immune response. The rabbits have become unresponsive (tolerant) to the antigen. This result is a typical example of high zone tolerance.

(b) The control result proves that the BSA has not suppressed the whole immune system. Rather, the unresponsiveness, or tolerance, is specific for the tolerance-inducing antigen. The animals can still react normally to other antigens.

(c) Neonatal animals are more sensitive to the induction of tolerance than are adults. Their immune system has not yet matured and is apparently paralyzed easily by moderate amounts of antigens.

10-12 (a) Antiserum to M603 appears to be specific for M603 private idiotopes, whereas the antisera to M167 and M511 show considerable, but not absolute, specificity. It would be fair to propose that the anti-M167 detects private idiotopes on M167 and public idiotopes in common with M603 and M511; the cross-reactivity with T15 is suspect. Similarly, the anti-M511 antiserum probably contains a low titer of anti-M511 private idiotopes and possibly some antibodies restricted to public idiotopes on phosphorylcholine-binding IgA(k) antibodies. All three antisera are anti-idiotypic in that they define their cognate immunoglobulin molecule. To clarify the specificity of these sera, each binding test against a particular labeled protein should be carried out in the presence of 5–10-fold excess unlabeled proteins of another type. For example, let us assume that the anti-M167 serum gives 54% binding to M167 in the presence of unlabeled T15 or IgA(k) antibodies, 44% in the presence of unlabeled M603, 40% in the presence of unlabeled M511, and 42% in the presence of all four unlabeled antibodies. One could conclude that anti-M167 did not detect idiotopes on M167 shared with T15 or IgA(κ), but it did contain antibodies directed against public idiotopes shared by both M603 and M511.

(b) The best guess is that M167, M511, and M603 antibodies are not commonly expressed in BALB/c mice and, therefore, were not present at sufficient concentrations to either induce tolerance in or to immunize the BALB/c mice used to make the anti-idiotypic antibodies used in this study. In fact, there is only one V_H germline gene that gives rise to all four myelomas, and three of the four V_H genes expressed in the myelomas have undergone extensive somatic mutations in their coding sequences. Similarly, M167 and M511 derive from a single germline V_κ gene, and both have undergone several coding sequence mutations. Thus somatic mutation has altered both V_H and V_κ genes, and these alterations apparently render these antibodies immunogenic in the host of origin.

(c) Perhaps T15 is expressed as such throughout the life of the host in sufficient concentrations to induce tolerance in (or to suppress) the host specifically. In fact, V_H T15 and V_κ T15 are unaltered from the germline, and they are expressed at high levels throughout neonatal and adult life in BALB/c mice.

(d) Lines 1, 2, and 6 show that these T_H cells collectively recognize the M167 idiotype, some of them recognizing cross-reactive idiotopes on M603. Lines 3–5 show that those T_H cells are mainly M603 idiotype specific.

(e) Although one would be tempted to conclude that M603 anti-idiotypic antibodies are more specific than M603-specific T_H cells, one could not do so without a clearer idea of signal-to-noise ratios in Table 10-7. No conclusion can be made about the comparative specificity of the anti-M167 T_H and B cells. Thus these experiments do *not* discriminate between T- and B-cell repertoires of antigen-binding receptors.

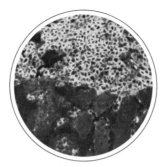

CHAPTER 11

Tissue Transplantation

Chapter Outline

The replacement of severely injured tissues and organs has been a clinical objective for as long as medicine has been practiced. Up to the early 20th century, the failure of transplanted grafts between individuals was ascribed variously to supernatural, technical, or physiological barriers. With the discovery that blood transfusions and tissue grafts were targets of immune reactions, the discipline of immunogenetics was founded, ushering in a modern immunology. This chapter considers the immunogenetics of transplantation antigens, the effector functions mediating transplant rejection, and the current status of clinical transplantation.

Concepts

11-1   Transplanted tissues are accepted or rejected on the basis of their histocompatibility antigens

Grafts from an individual to himself (*autografts*) almost invariably succeed and are especially important in treatment of burn patients. Likewise, grafts between two genetically identical individuals (*syngeneic* grafts) almost invariably succeed. However, grafts between two genetically dissimilar individuals of the same species (*allogeneic* grafts) or between individuals of different species (*xenogeneic* grafts) do not normally succeed. The major reason for transplant rejection is an immune response to the cell-surface antigens that distinguish donor from host. The tissue antigens that induce an immune response in other individuals are called *histocompatibility antigens*, and the genes that specify their structure and synthesis are called *histocompatibility genes*.

Major histocompatibility antigens

In all species tested, there appear to be two categories of histocompatibility genes. Genes of the major histocompatibility complex (MHC; Chapter 6) specify antigens that induce rapid rejection of grafts, whereas minor histocompatibility genes specify antigens that cause a slower graft rejection. The MHC is a chromosomal region encompassing a number of closely linked genes that are highly polymorphic within a species, and they are all involved in immune response and cellular recognition functions. A comparison of the MHC regions of humans and mice is shown in Figure 11-1.

The analysis of histocompatibility genetics in mice required the development of inbred strains produced by repeated brother–sister mating through 20 or more generations. Except for sex, all mice in an inbred strain are virtually identical genetically. Therefore, there is MHC identity within an inbred strain. However, due to the high degree of MHC polymorphism, there is MHC nonidentity between most such strains. In mice, the MHC was the second histocompatibil-

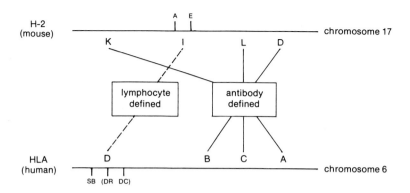

Figure 11-1 Arrangement of subloci in the MHC complexes of mice and humans. In both species, antigens specified by the MHC were first identified as serologically defined antigens (K, L, D and Ia antigens in mice, Ia [DR, DC, SB], B, C, and A antigens in humans) or as lymphocyte defined antigens (I-A and I-E in mice; D in humans). Serologically defined class I antigens are found on almost all cells, whereas the lymphocyte defined class II antigens are present only on cells in some tissues.

ity locus named and, therefore, it is called H-2. Each combination of particular alleles within the MHC is called an H-2 *haplotype* and is named by a letter, for example, H-2^a or H-2^b. Accordingly, the genetic designation of inbred strains, which are homozygous at the MHC, is H-2$^{a/a}$, H-2$^{b/b}$, and so on. If two inbred strains of mice that differ only in the H-2 region—for example, H-2$^{a/a}$ and H-2$^{b/b}$—are crossed, the F$_1$ progeny will have the genotype H-2$^{a/b}$. F$_1$ progeny will accept grafts from either parental strain, but neither parental strain will accept grafts from the F$_1$ progeny (Figure 11-2). These observations indicate that MHC genes are expressed codominantly. If F$_1$ progeny are crossed to obtain an F$_2$ generation, three-fourths of the offspring will accept grafts from either one of the original parent strains, and half will accept grafts from both (Figure 11-2). In general, the probability of graft acceptance from parent to F$_2$ in crosses between inbred strains of mice is ($\frac{3}{4}$)^n, where n equals the number of distinct histocompatibility differences between the two strains. In the simplified example just given, the H-2 locus was the only histocompatibility difference. In reality, for two inbred strains chosen at random, $n \geq 30$, indicating that there are at least 29 distinct minor histocompatibility loci (Figure 11-3).

Human MHC antigens, which are called HLA antigens, also show extensive polymorphism (Figure 11-1; Chapter 6). Because humans are an outbred species, almost all individuals are heterozygous for HLA genes. This fact is critical in the choice of a donor for organ or tissue transplants. Mild immunosuppression (Concept 11-4), which

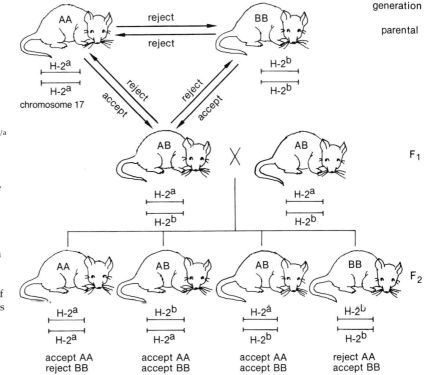

Figure 11-2
The genetics of histocompatibility antigens in inbred mice. Each inbred mouse strain is homozygous for the H-2 complex (e.g., $H-2^{a/a}$ or $H-2^{b/b}$). Both sets of products are expressed in the heterozygous F_1 hybrids. The F_1 progeny, therefore, produce H-2 antigens that stimulate an immune response in either parental strain, whereas neither parental strain expresses H-2 antigens foreign to the F_1 hybrid. In the F_2 generation there is a classical Mendelian 1:2:1 distribution of homozygous and heterozygous genotypes.

allows long-term retention of grafts between individuals differing only at minor histocompatibility loci, is insufficient when an MHC difference is involved. Figure 11-4 illustrates the usual situation in a human family. Because the parents normally possess four distinct MHC haplotypes, all grafts between parents, from parents to children, or from children to parents will involve at least one MHC incompatibility. However, sibling grafts have a 25% chance of MHC compatibility.

Minor histocompatibility antigens and H-Y antigen

Minor histocompatibility antigens represent any of a number of limited polymorphisms of cell-surface determinants and may be tissue specific or sex specific. Because HLA matching is widespread in clinical transplantation, minor histocompatibility antigens become important targets for rejection of tissue and organ grafts. Immune responses to minor histocompatibility antigens that are polymorphic within a particular species can also provide immunological tools for the study of these cell-surface antigens as important markers of cell lineage and function. For example, most of the mouse T-cell and B-cell differentiation markers (Tables 7-1 and 7-3) were discovered through immunizations to reveal minor histocompatibility antigens.

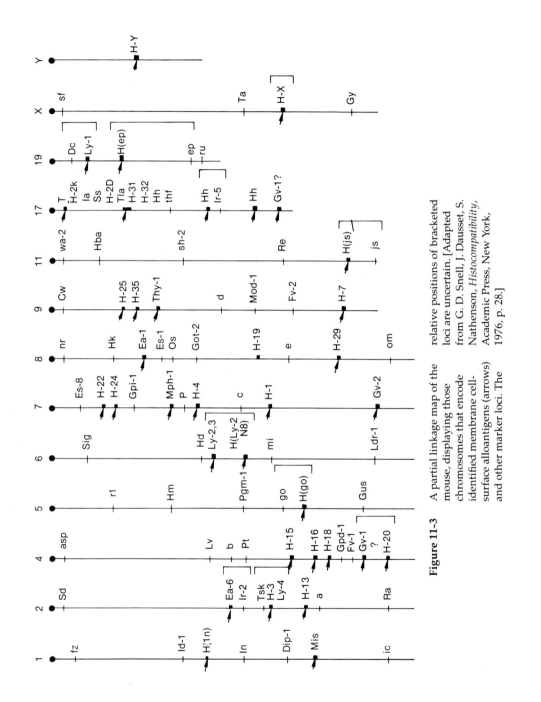

Figure 11-3 A partial linkage map of the mouse, displaying those chromosomes that encode identified membrane cell-surface alloantigens (arrows) and other marker loci. The relative positions of bracketed loci are uncertain. [Adapted from G. D. Snell, J. Dausset, S. Nathenson, *Histocompatibility*, Academic Press, New York, 1976, p. 28.]

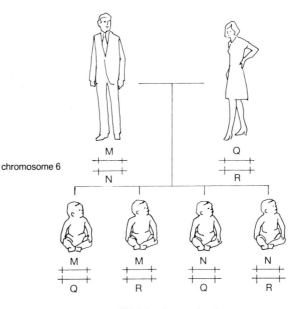

Figure 11-4 The genetics of human histocompatibility antigens. Because humans are outbred and the HLA system is highly polymorphic, it is likely that any two parents will possess four distinct MHC haplotypes (e.g., M/N, Q/R). The children of these parents will express one of four distinct haplotype groups: M/Q, M/R, N/Q, and N/R. Each parent will express one HLA haplotype foreign to each child, and thus parental grafts are rejected by the children. Each child will express one HLA haplotype foreign to each parent, and thus grafts from the child are rejected by parents. On the average, a graft from one child to another will have a one-in-four chance of histocompatibility at the HLA locus.

A particularly interesting minor histocompatibility antigen was identified following the discovery that female mice of certain inbred strains regularly rejected skin grafts from syngeneic males. This immune response was attributed to antigen(s) coded for or regulated by the Y chromosome, and the male-specific antigen has become known as H-Y. Whereas the T-cell-mediated immune response to this antigen may be quite intense, especially in second and subsequent grafts, the antibody response is weak. Because each inbred mouse strain is naturally congenic with respect to H-Y, immunity to H-Y has become an important system for the study of immunity to an individual minor histocompatibility antigen and for the analysis of the specificity of T_C cells.

Surprisingly, serological and cell-mediated immunity analyses of H-Y antigen show little or no antigenic polymorphism between mouse strains, and they show no known antigenic divergence during evolution with species as widely separated as mice and humans! This very unusual degree of evolutionary conservation of the only known gene expressed (or controlled) by the vertebrate Y chromosome has led several investigators to propose that H-Y antigen must serve an essential function that cannot survive variation. There is some evidence that molecules bearing H-Y determinants play a primary role in the embryological organization and development of the testis, and anti-H-Y sera have proved invaluable in unraveling some clinical puzzles involving patients with disordered sexual phenotypes.

11-2 Effector T cells are primarily responsible for rejection of tissue and organ transplants

Mixed lymphocyte responses and the importance of accessory cells

When lymphocytes from two genetically different individuals of a species are mixed in cell culture medium, the T cells of each individual respond to the MHC antigens of the other by differentiating and proliferating. Presumably this process, which is called the *mixed lymphocyte response*, involves an activation sequence analogous to that observed in response to viral antigens—for example, Concept 8-7. Allogeneic antigens (alloantigens) presented on accessory cells stimulate precursor T_A, T_D, and T_C cells, and then effector T_A cells secrete interleukin 2 and other lymphokines to cause maturation of effector T_C cells (Figure 11-5).

Most members of the population of T_A cells respond to Ia alloantigens, called HLA-D alloantigens in humans (Chapter 6), whereas an infrequent fraction respond to K or D alloantigens (HLA-A, B, or C alloantigens in humans). Most precursor T_C cells respond to K or D alloantigen, whereas an infrequent fraction respond to Ia alloantigens. This preferential stimulation of T_A and T_C cells by different classes of alloantigens follows their normal pattern of MHC restriction in cellular interactions (Concept 8-7), but the reason for this correspondence is not clear. As in the response to a foreign antigen, the continued proliferation of T_A cells is dependent on the presence of alloantigen, but T_C cells, once stimulated, can proliferate in the absence of alloantigen as long as interleukin 2 is supplied. As a result, T_C cells predominate late in a mixed lymphocyte response.

Because T_A cells recognize Ia antigens and because Ia antigens (at least I-A and I-E encoded antigens) are heterodimers composed of α and β chains, an F_1 hybrid between two parental strains will possess Ia antigens lacking in either parent (see Figure 8-21). In fact, when T_A cells from one parent (M) responsive to Ia antigens on F_1 hybrid (M $\times$ N) accessory cells are analyzed at a clonal level, a high proportion of clones react with F_1 cells but not with the cells of the other parental

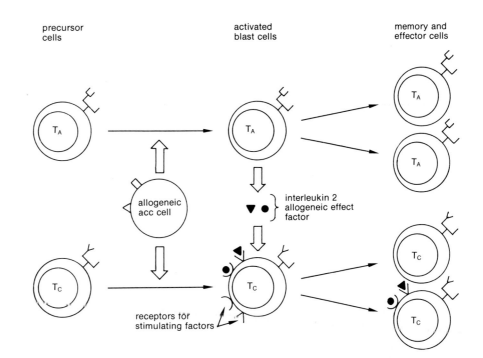

precursor
cells

activated
blast cells

memory and
effector cells

Figure 11-5 Activation events in a mouse allogeneic mixed lymphocyte response. Small T_A cells recognize I region-encoded alloantigens, enlarge, and release interleukin 2 and other factors such as allogeneic effect factors. Small precursors of T_C cells almost simultaneously recognize K/D-encoded alloantigens, enlarge, and express receptors for interleukin 2 and allogeneic effect factors. (Even in long-term maintained antigen-specific T_C clones, reexposure to alloantigens is necessary for continual expression of interleukin 2 receptors.) The continued division of T_A cells requires reexposure to the I region-encoded alloantigens. It is believed that both specific effector cells (e.g., the T_C blast at bottom) and increased clones of specific memory cells of both T_A and T_C subclasses are generated.

(N) type. Thus MM hosts rendered tolerant to fully *allogeneic* NN cells may not be tolerant to tissues from their (MN) F_1 progeny.

The importance of accessory cells in graft rejection is illustrated by the following example. For years, infrequent (and sometimes notorious) reports have appeared that organ grafts "conditioned" by long-term maintenance *in vitro* are not rejected by MHC different hosts. It was recently found that such forms of conditioning lead to the loss of immune accessory cells. Such a loss could render the activation of T_A cells deficient because the stimulatory Ia antigens are not expressed on the parenchymal cells of most organs. When as few as 5000 allogeneic macrophages are injected intravenously, such allotransplants are

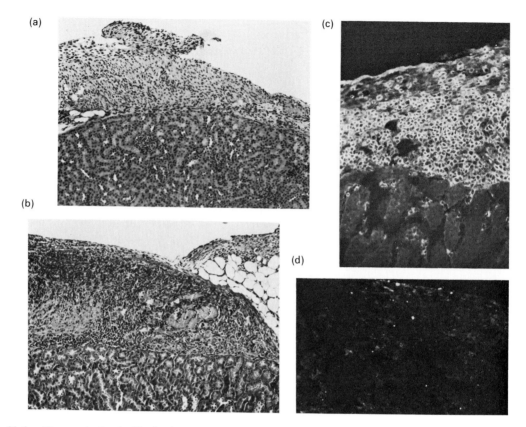

Figure 11-6 Tissue rejection by T cells. A slice of heart tissue from a strain-C mouse was transplanted under the kidney capsule of another strain-C mouse (a), or a strain-B mouse (b), 6 days before these sections of tissue were removed for analysis. In (a) the pale tissue on top is heart muscle, and the dark spots are cardiac muscle nuclei. The darker tissue below is normal kidney tissue. In (b) the pale appearance of heart muscle is obscured by the infiltration of many small, dark spots that are lymphocytes and macrophages. An anti-T-cell stain of another section from (b), which is shown in panel (c), demonstrates that a high proportion of the infiltrating cells are T lymphocytes. An anti-B-cell stain of the same tissue, which is shown in (d), demonstrates that B cells are rare or nonexistent in the lymphoid infiltrate. By 12 days after grafting, all allogeneic grafts were rejected and all syngeneic grafts were retained. [Photographs by M. Billingham, R. Warnke, and I. Weissman.]

rejected promptly even if they have been in place for months. Presumably these allogeneic macrophages function as accessory cells for presentation of their own MHC Ia as well as K/D antigens to the host's precursor T-cell population, thereby facilitating their development into effector T cells.

T_D and T_C cell recognition of allografts

Although effector T_D and T_C cells are responsible for graft rejection (Figure 11-6), the precise mechanism by which they accomplish it is not yet clear. As described in Chapter 8, effector T_A, T_D, and T_C cells normally recognize foreign antigenic determinants in the context of

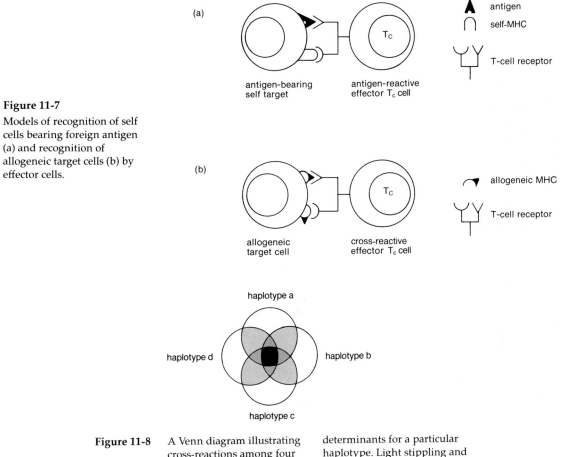

Figure 11-7
Models of recognition of self cells bearing foreign antigen (a) and recognition of allogeneic target cells (b) by effector cells.

Figure 11-8 A Venn diagram illustrating cross-reactions among four different hypothetical haplotypes. The set of determinants for each haplotype is represented by a circle. Clear spaces within a circle represent private determinants for a particular haplotype. Light stippling and dark stippling represent public determinants shared by two or three haplotypes, respectively, and blackened regions represent determinants common to all four haplotypes.

self-MHC molecules on their target cells (Figure 11-7). The puzzle in allograft rejection is that the target cells display *nonself*-MHC molecules. Although allograft rejection could involve recognition by some new mechanism, it seems likely that recognition will involve a version of the more familiar one. In this regard, it is important to remember the great structural similarity of all MHC molecules of the same class (Concept 6-4). Although each of the 30 or more distinct haplotypes must include unique MHC determinants (*private determinants*), they are also likely to include many other MHC determinants (*public determinants*) that are common to several haplotypes (Figure 11-8). Thus a T cell that responds to allogeneic cells could do so by

Figure 11-9

Diagrammatic representation of an experiment illustrating that a fraction of the T-cell population responds to each major histocompatibility haplotype. Thoracic duct lymphocytes from rat X contain T cells specifically reactive to strain-Y MHC antigens (●), and T cells reactive to other antigens (o). Injection of these cells into the tail vein of a strain-Y rat whose thoracic duct is cannulated allows circulating lymphocytes to traverse the rat's lymphoid tissues over a 24-hour interval and then enter the cannula. T cells reactive to strain-Y's MHC antigens are retained in lymphoid tissues, whereas the others enter the thoracic duct. In this hypothetical example based on experiments by W. L. Ford and colleagues, nearly 15% of the cells were retained.

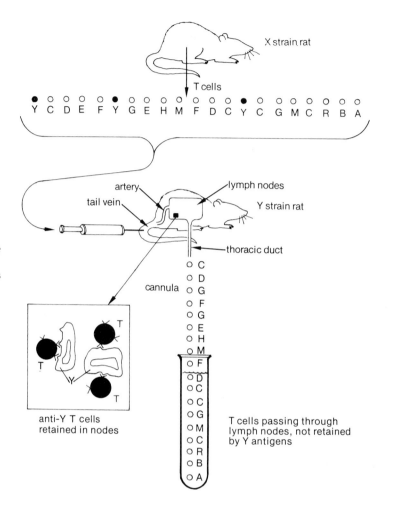

recognizing a nonself-MHC determinant with the same receptor that recognizes a foreign antigen in the context of a common, self-MHC determinant (Figure 11-7b). Whatever the mechanism for recognition, it must account for the high proportion of T cells that recognize and respond to the MHC molecules from different individuals of the same species. In mice and rats, as many as 1–12% of T cells can respond to an MHC haplotype difference (Figure 11-9). Several experiments indicate that these MHC alloreactive cells are probably progeny of those clones of cross-reactive T cells that responded initially to environmental antigens in the context of self-MHC determinants.

Graft rejection due to minor histocompatibility antigens

Graft rejection due to minor histocompatibility differences in MHC-matched transplants involves associated recognition of the foreign minor histocompatibility antigen and self-MHC determinants in the usual way (Figure 11-7a). Some mixed lymphocyte experiments have

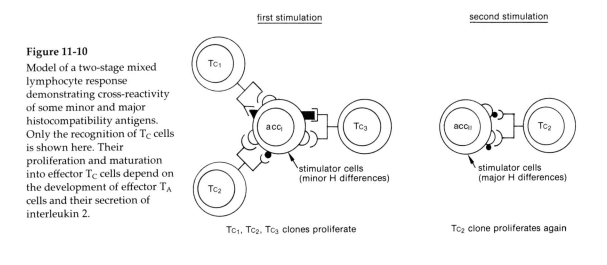

Figure 11-10

Model of a two-stage mixed lymphocyte response demonstrating cross-reactivity of some minor and major histocompatibility antigens. Only the recognition of T_C cells is shown here. Their proliferation and maturation into effector T_C cells depend on the development of effector T_A cells and their secretion of interleukin 2.

demonstrated that, within the population stimulated by minor histocompatibility differences, there is a subclass of T cells that also recognizes and responds to an independent allogeneic MHC antigen (Figure 11-10). Presumably this cross-reactivity results from a similarity between certain determinants of the minor histocompatibility antigen and those of the allogeneic MHC antigen.

11-3 Antibodies to histocompatibility antigens can cause rejection or protection of transplants

Rejection of transplants involving blood cells or vascular tissue

Modern clinical transplantation includes the transplantation of whole organs with their own blood vessels sutured to those of the host; the transplantation of tissues such as skin; the local implantation of avascular cells or aggregates of cells (e.g., insulin-producing pancreatic islets of Langerhans); and the intravenous injection of bone-marrow cells to replace bone-marrow stem cells in patients with deficient hematopoiesis. The primacy of cellular immunity in graft rejection was first established with skin and tumor grafts. Skin and tumor cells are susceptible to cell-mediated damage but are relatively resistant to antibody-mediated damage. Thus the passive transfer of reactive antibodies does not usually lead to rejection of skin and tumor grafts. However, blood cells and vascular endothelial cells, which are exposed to the complement system, are quite susceptible to antibody-dependent complement-mediated destruction. Thus, whenever transplants involve donor blood cells or vascular endothelial cells, humoral antibodies can contribute significantly to their rejection.

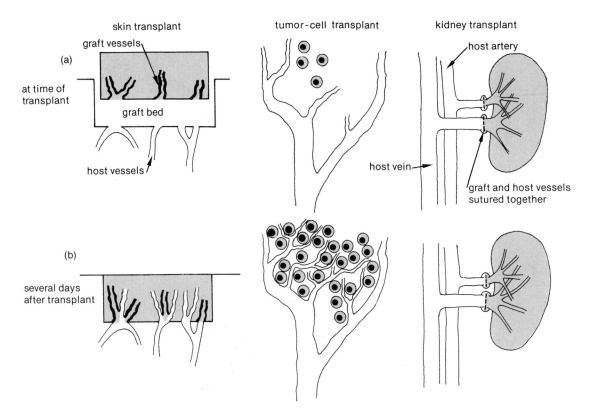

Figure 11-11 The vascular supply of various transplants. (a) At the time of transplantation, only organ grafts (e.g., kidneys) have the blood vessels surgically joined and, because they have an immediate blood supply, they do not release stimuli for host vessel proliferation. By contrast, both skin grafts and tumor cells release angiogenic (blood-vessel inducing) factors. (b) Host vessel proliferation may result in the establishment of new channels or in the natural anastomosis (joining) of host and donor vessels.

Hyperacute graft rejection

Whereas skin and tumor grafts are vascularized by new host blood vessels whose growth is induced by angiogenic factors released by the donor cells, the vessels in an organ graft are entirely donor in origin (Figure 11-11). Therefore, in organ grafts, humoral antibodies encounter donor antigens on endothelial cells of vessel linings. These cells are susceptible to antibody-mediated damage in which complement components become activated and localized to vascular endothelial cells of the graft. The resulting combined cytotoxic and acute inflammatory reactions shut off the blood supply to the organ graft, causing its death. If alloreactive antibodies preexist in the host, they may act on the new graft even as it is being sutured into place, resulting in a *hyperacute rejection*. The grafted organ turns gray due to anoxia, and histological examination of the graft vessels demonstrates blood clotting and massive accumulation of polymorphonuclear leukocytes. In addition, immunofluorescence analysis demonstrates immunoglobulin and complement bound to vessels.

One way that alloreactive antibodies can be induced in the host is by prior blood transfusions. Although histocompatibility antigens are virtually absent from red blood cells, they are expressed profusely on the surfaces of blood leukocytes. Repeated transfusions of blood that contains significant numbers of leukocytes induce antibodies directed at major and minor histocompatibility antigens. Not only can such antibodies induce hyperacute rejections of subsequent organ transplants, but also they can interfere with bone-marrow transplants by eliminating blood cells and their hematopoietic precursors. Thus great care must be taken to avoid leukocyte-contaminated blood transfusions in patients that may eventually require organ or bone-marrow transplants.

Transplant protection mediated by antibodies

Although antibodies to major and minor histocompatibility determinants may cause hyperacute rejection of organ allografts and interfere with bone-marrow transplants, such antibodies may act in different circumstances to interfere with T-cell immunity and prolong graft survival. This phenomenon, called *immunological enhancement,* is described more fully in Chapter 13. Briefly, alloreactive antibodies may interfere with the development or function of effector T_D and T_C cells by competing with T cells for antigenic determinants on antigen-presenting or target cells, or by augmenting the development of suppressor cells or suppressor factors. In MHC nonidentical grafts, antibodies to Ia molecules block the development of effector T_A and T_D cells, whereas antibodies to H-2 K/D determinants block the development of effector T_C cells or interfere with target cell lysis. Either class of antibodies is sufficient to prolong graft survival, providing additional evidence for cellular cooperation in rejection of organ grafts *in vivo.*

If the few cases of hyperacute rejection of kidney allografts are excluded from consideration, patients receiving kidney transplants that are mismatched at the HLA-D locus generally have a significantly longer survival of their transplants if they have received multiple prior blood transfusions. Thus prior blood transfusions can increase the survival of some renal transplant patients.

11-4 Nonspecific immunosuppression is currently used for human transplantation

Nonspecific immunosuppressive agents

Nonspecific immunosuppression of the host with antimitotic agents, adrenal steroids, and antilymphocyte sera permits long-term survival of most MHC-matched allografts and of about 40% of allografts that differ in MHC determinants. Recent studies with a new fungal agent,

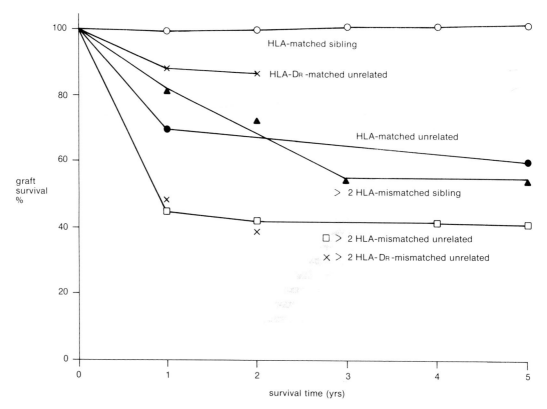

Figure 11-12   Human kidney transplants between HLA-typed donors and hosts. Matching transplants for serologically defined HLA-A, B, and C specificities increases the probability of survival significantly, and early data indicate that matching for HLA-DR (or HLA-D by mixed lymphocyte reactions) gives a better correlation with survival. The increased survival of sibling grafts compared to grafts between unrelated individuals probably reflects the likelihood of mismatches at several minor histocompatibility loci and could also be due to the likelihood that matched HLA gene products are in fact identical.

cyclosporin A, offer promise for dramatic increases in allograft survival. However, all such immunosuppressed patients are immunodeficient (Concept 12-5), and a significant proportion of them suffer life-threatening infections. Even anti-T-cell sera are relatively nonspecific, in that all T cells are susceptible to even the most highly purified serum. Because most sera are not highly purified, other cell and tissue systems are at risk as well.

Monoclonal antibodies against specific human T-cell subclasses might prove very useful immunosuppressive reagents for organ transplantation. There is a good correlation between successful immunosuppression of a graft rejection episode and low levels of certain T-cell subclasses. Therefore, specific alteration in the ratio of T-cell subclasses using monoclonal antibodies might permit increased allograft acceptance.

Factors contributing to transplant success

The current range of success rates for heart and kidney transplants is 55% to 95%. Three factors have allowed increases in the success rates to these levels. First, donor grafts with a minimum number of histocompatibility differences are selected after MHC matching by antibody typing (which detects HLA-A, B, C, and DR differences) and by mixed lymphocyte reactions (which detect HLA-D differences). MHC-matched transplants fare much better than donor–host combinations with one or more HLA differences (Figure 11-12). Second, several kinds of analysis for impending rejection allow the physician to maintain the appropriate level of immunosuppressive therapy. These analyses include monitoring anti-donor antibodies and anti-donor T_C cells; measuring complement levels to detect rapid complement consumption; and analyzing tiny biopsy specimens of graft tissue for viability of graft cells, extent of inflammatory cell infiltration, and immunohistochemical identification of the type of infiltrating lymphocytes. Third, careful monitoring for infectious diseases is crucial in preventing morbidity and mortality of patients with healthy grafts. Monitoring for lymphoid system cancers is also important because they are increased about 35-fold in immunosuppressed transplant patients. The more specific immunosuppressive drug cyclosporin A has relatively low toxicity for nonlymphoid cells, but it may induce an even higher incidence of subsequent lymphoid malignancies than other immunosuppressive drugs.

11-5 Bone-marrow transplantation can promote survival of subsequent organ allografts

Whole-body irradiation and total hematolymphoid replacement

Whole-body irradiation is a significant immunosuppressant that acts by killing B cells, T cells, and their hematopoietic precursors directly. The dose required for such suppression is lethal to the host because pluripotent hematopoietic stem cells are eliminated (Concept 7-2). Irradiated hosts often die from blood-clotting anomalies because they have no platelets, or from overwhelming infections because they have no phagocytes. In the 1950s, several scientists found that total hematolymphoid replacement of lethally irradiated hosts could be accomplished by the transplantation of bone-marrow cells. Because the transplanted cells are of donor origin, they reconstitute a donor hematolymphoid system. Two major problems have restricted this form of therapy: a physician's understandable hesitancy to administer a potentially lethal dose of whole-body irradiation and the potential for a graft response against the host.

Graft-versus-host responses

Bone-marrow cell suspensions inevitably contain a few percent of mature T cells, presumably from the blood. Some of these grafted T cells recognize and respond to host major and minor histocompatibility antigens. The result of such recognition is a T-cell graft response directed at the host. The first sites of such a reaction are the lymphoid organs to which T cells home. These organs are rich in host MHC antigens, and a phase of massive proliferation of donor T-cell clones is followed by host inflammatory and repair processes that are usually ineffective. The resulting coexistence of donor immune components and host responses leads to a massive enlargement of these lymphoid organs. Meanwhile, the spread of cytotoxic and inflammatory cells to all other organs bearing MHC antigens leads to their destruction and, ultimately, to the death of the host. (In animals, the combined weight loss due to anti-gastrointestinal tract reactions and the increased lymphoid organ size has led to a quantitative and sensitive assay of T-cell immunity, an assay which has proved valuable to the understanding of T-cell subclasses and cellular immunity.)

In humans, graft-versus-host responses have proved to be the major stumbling block for bone-marrow transplantation. However, successful transplants of hematolymphoid cells have been achieved in recent animal experiments by eliminating donor T cells with anti-T-cell antibodies. MHC matching of donor and host is still important because the donor-derived T cells must still mature in a thymus bearing *host* MHC antigens. If developing T cells acquire their MHC restriction during passage through the thymus (Concept 7-5), then if donor and host are not matched, the maturing T cells would "learn" to recognize and protect the host-cell but not the donor-cell population. In a subsequent viral infection, the elimination of infected donor cells would presumably require that the foreign viral antigens be recognized in the context of *donor* MHC antigens. Despite these considerations, infected donor cells are successfully eliminated on some experiments even in the absence of MHC matching. In these cases, perhaps a subset of host MHC-restricted T cells shows cross-reactivity to infected donor cells as discussed in Concept 11-2 and Figure 11-10.

Bone-marrow transplants

Replacement of the irradiation-eliminated hematolymphoid system of the host by donor bone-marrow cells permits subsequent successful allogenic transplantation of donor grafts. This tolerance presumably arises because immature T and B cells directed at donor antigens are eliminated or paralyzed by their continual exposure to the donor bone-marrow cells that have become part of the host. As illustrated in Figure 11-13, a strain-A mouse that has had its own hematolymphoid system replaced by a bone-marrow transplant from an (A × B)F$_1$ hybrid mouse will accept organ grafts from the F$_1$ hybrids and from

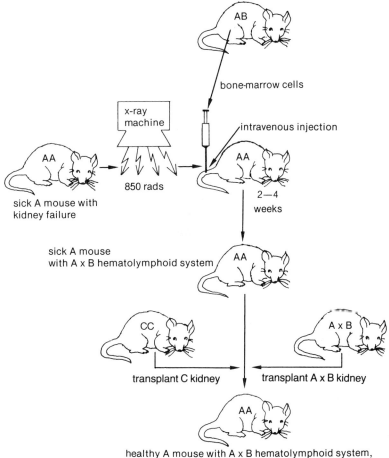

Figure 11-13

A strategy for replacement of the host hematolymphoid system and subsequent successful allogeneic graft transplantation.

strain-B mice, but it will reject grafts from strain-C mice. If strain-C bone-marrow cells had been injected following irradiation, subsequent strain-C kidney grafts might also have been accepted. It should be noted that this kind of tolerance would not extend to donor organs bearing polymorphic organ-specific antigens.

A similar kind of transplantation tolerance can be created in unirradiated rodents by transfusion of spleen or bone-marrow cells from an (A × B)F$_1$ hybrid, for example, into immunologically immature fetal or neonatal strain-A hosts. These animals are also tolerant to subsequent donor grafts because anti-donor T and B cells are continually eliminated or paralyzed by exposure to donor cells that are part of the host. This procedure works only in animals that are accessible for transfusion before the full onset of immune competence. Humans have probably passed that stage by the end of the second trimester of gestation, long before organ failure and the need for transplantation have become apparent.

Total lymphoid irradiation	The successful radiotherapy of Hodgkin's disease has provided a relatively safe immunosuppressive method for delivering high dose irradiation to all lymphoid sites, but at the same time avoiding most bones so that patients do not require a bone-marrow transplant. Somewhat surprisingly, such patients are depressed in certain T-cell functions for the rest of their lives. Animals and some patients have received total lymphoid irradiation and subsequently have accepted transplants of MHC nonidentical bone marrow without either a host or a graft reaction. Such subjects contain donor and host hematolymphoid systems in peaceful coexistence. Although it is believed that the specific irradiation protocol somehow inhibits the generation and survival of effector T_A and T_C cells, the exact basis for the lack of mutual immune responses is not yet known. Total lymphoid-irradiated hosts do contain high levels of suppressor cells and suppressor activity. A specific irradiation procedure that permits successful bone-marrow transplants would be quite useful for replacement of hematolymphoid functions or as a preparative step for a subsequent organ transplant from the bone-marrow donor.
Goals of modern transplantation research	Despite the problems, modern immunological research may eventually find a safe method of allotransplantation. The goal of this research is to remove or inactivate selectively those clones of host T cells that recognize donor MHC antigens, leaving the rest of the T-cell repertoire intact. Among the most promising areas of endeavor are current research with monoclonal antibodies, with external removal of specific alloreactive T cells on absorbent columns, and with isolation and cloning of specific T_S cells and suppressor factors.

Selected Bibliography

General

Billingham, R., and Silvers, W., *The Immunobiology of Transplantation*, Prentice-Hall, Englewood Cliffs, N.J., 1971. A short, lucid presentation of the biological basis of tissue and organ transplantation.

T-cell response to transplants

Butcher, G. W., and Howard, J. C., "Genetic control of transplant rejection," *Transplantation* **34**, 161(1982).

Loveland, B. E., and McKenzie, I. F. C., "Which T cells cause graft rejection?" *Transplantation* **33**, 217(1982).

The two preceding papers present sometimes contrasting views as to the type of effector T cell (T_D versus T_C) that is responsible for graft rejection, the class (I versus II) of graft MHC antigens recognized, and the genetic control of their activation.

Approaches to clinical transplantation

Lafferty, K. J., Prowse, S. J., Simeonovic, C. J., and Warren, H. J., "Immunobiology of tissue transplantation: a return to the passenger leukocyte concept," *Ann. Rev. Immunol.* **1**, 143(1983).

Najarian, J. S., "Immunological aspects of organ transplantation," *Hospital Practice* **61**, October (1982).

Strober, S., and Weissman, I. L., "Immunosuppressive and tolerogenic effects of whole body, total lymphoid, and regional irradiation," in *The Current Status of Modern Therapy*, J. R. Salaman (Ed.), Lancaster, England, MTP Press, **7**, 19(1981).

Additional concepts introduced in the problems

1. The fetus as an allograft. Problem 11-11.

2. Organ-specific polymorphic transplantation antigens. Problem 11-13.

Problems

11-1 Indicate whether each of the following statements is true or false. Explain the error in each statement you consider to be false.

    (a) When a female from one inbred mouse strain is crossed to a male of another strain, skin grafts from the mother to her F_1 male offspring will always be accepted.

    (b) Following the cross in part (a), skin grafts from the father to his F_1 female offspring will always be accepted.

    (c) Skin grafts from a human mother to her son are always accepted.

    (d) Kidney graft rejection in humans is always caused exclusively by cell-mediated immunity.

    (e) Bone-marrow grafts from an $(A \times B)F_1$ mouse offspring to one of its lethally irradiated parents are usually accepted and save the parent's life.

    (f) Bone-marrow grafts from an inbred parent to a lethally irradiated $(A \times B)F_1$ offspring are usually accepted and save the offspring's life.

11-2 Supply the missing word or words in each of the following statements.

    (a) A skin graft from a Lewis rat to a C57BL mouse is called a(n) _____, whereas a BALB/c mouse graft to the same host is called a(n) _____.

    (b) The major limitation to standard treatment for graft rejection in humans is _____ due to _____.

    (c) T lymphocytes from a strain-A mouse tolerant of strain-B tissues proliferate in response to $(A \times B)F_1$ stimulator cells due to formation of novel _____ in the stimulator cells.

    (d) Hyperacute rejection of organ allografts involves infiltration of _____.

    (e) In grafts from strain-A mice to F_2 offspring of an $(A \times B)F_1$ reciprocal cross, an acceptance rate of 9/16 indicates that A and B strains have _____ distinct histocompatibility differences.

11-3 Consider the following series of experiments on graft transplantation among mice from four inbred strains (A/J, BALB/c, C57BL, and SJL). Skin was grafted from A/J female mice onto A/J, BALB/c, and C57BL females, and the results are shown in Table 11-1a. Six weeks later, some of the original mice received another skin graft, and the results are shown in Table 11-1b. The remainder of the mice that had received the first skin grafts from A/J donors were sacrificed. The serum from the BALB/c mice was pooled, as were the cells. The effect of immune cells was studied by giving new BALB/c mice skin grafts with or without immune BALB/c cells injected intravenously 3 days before grafting (Table 11-1c). The effect of immune serum injected intravenously was also studied (Table 11-1d). With reference to the data in Table 11-1, answer the following questions.

Table 11-1   Skin-Graft Experiments (Problem 11-3)

(a) The Survival of Skin Grafts from Donor A/J Females to Other Inbred mice

Recipient	Number of Grafts	Number of Rejections	Mean Survival Time of Graft
A/J	20	0	–
BALB/c	40	40	14 days
C57BL	40	40	11 days

(b) The Survival of Second Grafts in Inbred Mice

Skin-Graft Donor	Skin-Graft Recipient	Number of Grafts	Number of Rejections	Mean Survival Time of Graft
A/J	A/J	10	0	–
A/J	BALB/c	10	10	8 days
A/J	C57BL	10	10	8 days
SJL	A/J	10	10	11 days
SJL	BALB/c	10	10	11 days
SJL	C57BL	10	10	11 days

(c) The Effect of Injected Immune Cells upon Graft Rejection

Skin-Graft Donor	Skin-Graft Recipient	Cells	Number of Grafts	Number of Rejections	Mean Survival Time of Graft
BALB/c	BALB/c	–	5	0	–
A/J	BALB/c	–	5	5	14 days
A/J	BALB/c	+	5	5	8 days
SJL	BALB/c	+	5	5	11 days

(d) The Effect of Injected Immune Serum upon Graft Rejection

Skin-Graft Donor	Skin-Graft Recipient	Serum Injected	Number of Grafts	Number of Rejections	Mean Survival Time of Graft
A/J	BALB/c	–	10	10	14 days
A/J	BALB/c	+	10	10	17 days
SJL	BALB/c	+	10	10	11 days

(a) Is graft rejection an immune phenomenon? What would be the evidence for such an assertion?

(b) Is graft rejection mediated by the cellular system or the humoral system? What is the evidence for your choice?

(c) Briefly outline an experiment that would support your answer to part (b) independently.

(d) Does serum from immune mice strengthen or weaken the immune response? Suggest an explanation for the serum transfer results in Table 11-1d.

(e) How does the host's immune system distinguish foreign grafts from syngeneic grafts?

11-4 Organ transplantation among humans has required the use of immunosuppressants to block the graft-rejection process. Some immunosuppressants act primarily as inhibitors of cell division (e.g., anti-metabolites that are analogues of the nucleotide bases); others act primarily by destroying lymphocytes (lymphocytolytic agents such as the adrenal steroids); and others are both lymphocytolytic and anti-proliferative (e.g., X rays and DNA alkylating agents). Immunosuppression can also be achieved with antilymphocyte serum (ALS). Each of these immunosuppressants lacks one critical feature that the ideal immunosuppressant should have. What is this feature?

11-5 A colleague of yours has a 45-year-old patient who requires a kidney transplant. Your colleague proposes to treat him by whole-body irradiation, replacement of his hematolymphoid system cells with marrow cells from the patient's 22-year-old son, and then transplantation of a kidney to the patient from his son, who has agreed to the operation. Your colleague reasons that the operation should succeed for his human patient because it has been shown to succeed in inbred mice that receive transplants from an F_1 offspring (Figure 11-13). Would you advise him to proceed with the operation or not? Give your argument.

11-6 (a) Suppose that you are a young transplant surgeon repaying your medical school loans by 2 years of medical service in an isolated community hospital that lacks a doctor as well as money and transportation facilities. You soon find that, due to inbreeding, the community has a high incidence of congenital renal failure, and that the resulting childhood mortality rate approaches 10% of individuals up to age 21. To counteract the high mortality rate, the average family has 12 children; thus most mothers are highly multiparous (have had multiple pregnancies). You decide to treat the disease by transplanting kidneys from normal children to their defective siblings. You know that the major human transplantation (HLA) antigens can be defined by agglutination of human leukocytes using serum from multiparous women who have become immune to paternal HLA antigens. This test can be adapted to determine identity or nonidentity of the paternally inherited HLA haplotype among sibling children. Mixed lymphocyte reactions (MLR) between siblings can be used as a further test of HLA identity. How would you apply these tests and interpret the results to identify most efficiently the best donor sibling for a diseased child?

(b) Having defined the best match, you now seek an immunosuppressant. Lacking money and transportation facilities, you remove the thymus from a young patient who has just died, disaggregate the tissue, and inject it into a horse to make anti-T-cell serum (ALS). Two weeks later, the horse serum will agglutinate thymocytes at serum dilutions of up to 1:10,000. You transplant a kidney into your first recipient and inject 5 mL of the ALS. Within 6 hours, the patient's red blood cell (RBC) count falls from 5×10^6 RBC/mm^3 of blood to 1.5×10^6 RBC/mm^3. What has happened, and what should you do?

(c) Following a blood transfusion, the patient develops an infection of *Staphylococcus albus* at the surgical incision site. Knowing that *S. albus* is usually nonpathogenic, you check the differential white blood count and find that the patient's total leukocyte count has fallen from 10,000 cells/mm³ to < 100 cells/mm³. What has happened now?

(d) Following appropriate therapy, the patient heals at the incision site, but by 2 days post transplant it is clear that the transplanted kidney is failing. You do a kidney biopsy and see an infiltration of the glomeruli by polymorphonuclear leukocytes (PMNs). What would be the most likely cause of PMN infiltration? How could you make the correct diagnosis?

(e) Treatment of the kidney biopsy as suggested in the answer to part (d) reveals unbroken green lines outlining the glomerular tufts. Why is the kidney failing? Assuming that another matched sibling is available for a second transplant, what could you do to improve the chances of success?

(f) After you have finally made successful transplants in a few children, a smallpox infection threatens the community, and you find that no one has been vaccinated. Should you vaccinate everyone in the town?

11-7 (a) When white blood cells from person X are mixed with white blood cells of person Y, the X lymphocytes will proliferate and some of them will become T_C cells, able to lyse lymphocytes from person Y. The generation of these specific killer T cells will be most enhanced if the histocompatibility genes of X and Y differ (1) at the I locus, (2) at the D and K loci, (3) at both I and D/K loci, or (4) at neither locus. Which of these four choices is the best answer?

(b) Describe which kinds of cells from person X specifically recognize person Y's MHC antigens and trigger the production of specific T_C cells.

(c) Describe lineage relationships, cellular interactions, MHC products recognized, and effector cell functions in all of person X's reactions to person Y's cells.

11-8 (a) Histologists use the term *blast* to denote large, rapidly dividing cells whose descendants are usually further differentiated. Such cells are often seen in lymph nodes that are responding to an antigenic challenge. Specific antigens provoke the appearance of blast cells in cultures derived from specifically immunized individuals but not in cultures from unimmunized individuals. The degree of blast transformation can be quantified by adding ³H-thymidine to these cultures. Only the actively replicating blast cells take up ³H-thymidine. These radiolabeled cells can be counted by radioautography or by other methods. In one study, researchers cultured mixtures of lymphocytes from pairs of individuals. In each pair, the lymphocyte donors were either monozygotic twins, dizygotic twins, or unrelated individuals. After 5 days, ³H-thymidine was added to each culture for a short period. The number of labeled cells in each culture was found to be as shown in Figure 11-14. Compare the results obtained with monozygotic twins to those obtained with unrelated individuals. What does this pattern of reactivity suggest about the nature of this immune reaction?

(b) The major histocompatibility complex in humans (HLA) is polymorphic; that is, there are many allelic variants of the genes in this complex among the population. Given this property of the HLA complex, how can you explain the variability in the dizygotic twin results shown in Figure 11-14?

(c) Suppose that a person had suffered acute kidney damage and needed a transplant to survive. In addition, suppose that this person had several siblings, all willing to donate a kidney. How could you decide which sibling to use as a donor?

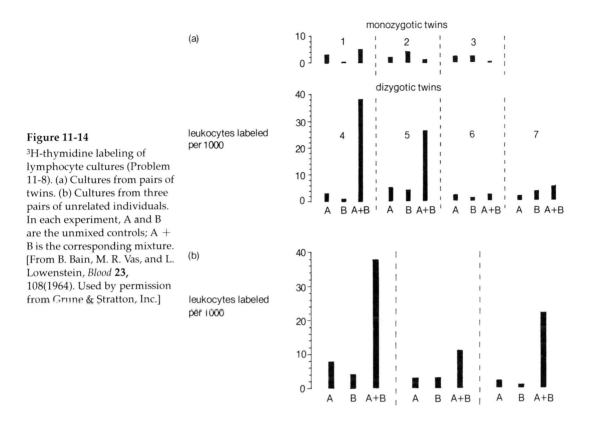

Figure 11-14

^{3}H-thymidine labeling of lymphocyte cultures (Problem 11-8). (a) Cultures from pairs of twins. (b) Cultures from three pairs of unrelated individuals. In each experiment, A and B are the unmixed controls; A + B is the corresponding mixture. [From B. Bain, M. R. Vas, and L. Lowenstein, *Blood* **23,** 108(1964). Used by permission from Grune & Stratton, Inc.]

(d) Assume that the mixed lymphocyte reaction is determined by identity or non-identity at a single locus and that the products of this locus are expressed in a codominant fashion on the surfaces of cells in a heterozygote. What sort of reaction would you expect if you mixed lymphocytes from a child with lymphocytes from one of its parents? Why?

11-9 The large lymphocytes generated in a mixed lymphocyte response begin mitosis after 2 days in culture. If the lymphocytes in a mixed culture come from donors of different sexes, the response of each donor's lymphocytes can be assayed independently by determining the karyotypes of the mitotic cells. This technique was used to examine mixed lymphocyte reactions between parental and F_1 lymphocytes. Using inbred rats of four strains—L, DA, BN, and F—various male-female, parental-F_1 combinations were tested with the results shown in Table 11-2. Remembering that inbred animals are essentially homozygous at all loci, answer the following questions.

(a) Describe the pattern of reactivity. What do you infer from the results with regard to the rats' histocompatibility genes?

(b) Suppose the reactions between parental and F_1 lymphocytes were examined using outbred humans as donors. How and why would the results differ from those obtained with inbred rats?

(c) Suppose that the parental human cells were inactivated by X irradiation or treatment with mitomycin C, a fungal antibiotic, to prevent DNA synthesis

Table 11-2 Mixed Lymphocyte Reactions Between Cells from Inbred Parental (Homozygous) Rats and Their F_1 (Heterozygous) Offspring (Problem 11-9)

Culture Mixture	Sex	Number of Mitoses on Day: 5	6	7	11	Totals
L/L ($\female$) + DA/L ($\male$)	$\female$	1	19	38	0	58
	$\male$	0	1	7	0	8
L/BN ($\female$) + L/L ($\male$)	$\female$	0	0	0	0	0
	$\male$	1	9	49	1	61
F/BN ($\female$) + F/F ($\male$)	$\female$	0	0	0	0	0
	$\male$	3	24	23	4	54
L/BN ($\female$) + DA/L ($\male$)	$\female$	4	19	23	0	46
	$\male$	8	15	14	0	37

[From D. B. Wilson, W. Silvers, and P. Nowell, *J. Exp. Med.* **126,** 655(1967). Copyright 1967 by The Rockefeller University Press.]

and mitosis. What result would you expect in a mixed lymphocyte reaction between inactivated parental cells and untreated cells from an F_1 individual? What results would you expect if the F_1 lymphocytes were inactivated and the parental lymphocytes were untreated?

(d) Can you think of a situation in which measuring the response of each donor's lymphocytes independently would be important?

11-10 One technically simple way to assess the number of mature T cells in a population of lymphocytes is to test for their ability to mount a graft-versus-host response (GVHR). Mature T cells injected into an allogeneic, immunologically incompetent host (e.g., an immature newborn or a suitably irradiated adult) will react against the host. The GVHR is directed against all tissues, and within 7 days it can cause marked loss of body weight due to liver and gastrointestinal tract damage. In this same period of time, there is a great enlargement of the spleen, termed *splenomegaly*, due initially to proliferation of the injected T cells that migrate to the spleen. Later, damage to host spleen cells results in inflammation, repair, and regeneration. The increase in spleen weight is commonly used to indicate the magnitude of the GVHR, which in turn provides an estimate of the proportion of mature reactive T cells among the injected lymphocytes.

One research group, investigating the way T-cell precursors mature in the thymus, isolated from calf thymus a mixture of factors collectively named *thymosin*. The group incubated CBA mouse bone-marrow cells with this factor and then injected the cells into adult, irradiated (C57BL $\times$ CBA)F_1 hosts. The magnitudes of the ensuing GVHRs are given in Table 11-3. With reference to the table, answer the following questions.

(a) Why is the ratio of spleen weight to body weight, rather than simply the absolute spleen weight, used in measuring the GVHR?

Table 11-3 Stimulation of GVHR of Allogeneic Bone-Marrow Cells by Thymosin *in Vitro* (Problem 11-10)

Injected Cells Experimental Groups	Number of Host Animals	Spleen Weight (mg)/Body Weight (g)	p Values[a]	Spleen Index[b]
(C57BL × CBA)F$_1$ bone-marrow cells (syngeneic)	60	2.08 ± 0.10	–	–
CBA bone-marrow cells preincubated with:				
saline	62	2.65 ± 0.10	–	1.27
100 μg thymosin	28	3.74 + 0.36	<0.01	1.80
10 μg thymosin	21	3.99 + 0.30	<0.01	1.92
1 μg thymosin	9	3.78 + 0.37	<0.01	1.82
100 μg spleen extract	8	3.23 + 0.40	0.05	1.55
10 μg spleen extract	12	2.97 + 0.17	>0.2	1.43
1 μg spleen extract	8	2.45 + 0.23	>0.5	1.18

[a]p value is a statistical measure of the probability that the observed difference between experimental and control values could be due to statistical fluctuations rather than to a real difference in the mean values. A p value of 0.05 means that the results could have happened by chance 5% of the time; this difference is considered significant. A p value of 0.01 or less is considered highly significant.

[b]Spleen index $= \dfrac{\text{allogeneic (spleen weight/body weight)}}{\text{syngeneic (spleen weight/body weight)}}$

[From A. L. Goldstein, A. Guha, M. L. Howe, and A. White, *J. Immunol.* **106**, 777(1971).]

(b) What does line 1 in Table 11-3 indicate?

(c) What seems to be the effect of thymosin? Give two hypotheses for thymosin action.

11-11 Pregnancy presents the immune system with a special challenge. The immune system normally recognizes and reacts against foreign antigens, yet during pregnancy the mother's immune system must *not* react against the foreign paternal antigens expressed on fetal cells. The following experiments illustrate one immunologic control mechanism that may help to protect the fetus. Lymphocytes were taken during the third trimester of pregnancy and then again 2 months *post partem* (after delivery) from five pregnant women who had already borne several children. Each batch of cells was incubated with a sample of the father's lymphocytes, which had been inactivated by mitomycin C. After 24–48 hours, the release of macrophage migration inhibition factor (MIF) was measured. MIF release after only 24–48 hours in culture is an indication that the maternal lymphocytes had previously been sensitized to the paternal antigens. Either 15% autologous plasma (from the same mother) or 15% homologous plasma (from another pregnant but unrelated woman) was included in each mixed lymphocyte culture. The results are shown in Figure 11-15. With reference to the figure, answer the following questions.

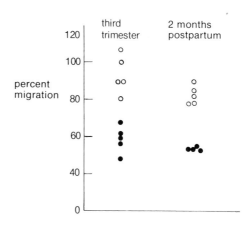

Figure 11-15 Migration of macrophages in supernatant fluid from mixed lymphocyte cultures (Problem 11-11). Percentages were determined by comparison to migration in control supernatant fluid derived from cultures of maternal lymphocyte alone. Open circles (o) indicate values obtained with mother; father cultures in autologous plasma. Solid circles (●) indicate values obtained with the same cultures in homologous plasma. [From H. Pence, W. Petty, and R. Rocklin, *J. Immunol.* **114,** 525(1975).]

(a) Consider the cultures incubated with homologous plasma (solid circles). How do you interpret these results? Were the maternal cells sensitized to paternal antigens? If so, how might they have become sensitized?

(b) Which paternal cell-surface antigens are most probably being recognized by the maternal lymphocytes?

(c) Consider the cultures to which autologous plasma was added (open circles). Was MIF released by the maternal cells in these cultures? Suggest an explanation for the results.

(d) When the autologous plasma was fractionated on a Sephadex G-200 column, the active fraction was found to elute with IgG. How may further proof that the active factor is an immunoglobulin be obtained?

(e) The results in Figure 11-15 demonstrate that maternal lymphocytes can recognize and respond *in vitro* to paternal antigens, and yet the fetal "allograft," which expresses these antigens, is not rejected. Using all the information presented, propose as complete a model as you can for the control mechanism involved. What is the active factor that suppresses the normal response? Where did it come from? Is it immunologically specific? Does it exert its effect on afferent (antigen-processing and presentation), central (T- and B-lymphocyte recognition and response), or efferent (effector-cell or product interaction with antigen) arms of the immune response? Is the mother "tolerant" to paternal antigens?

11-12 (a) A little girl comes to your clinic with aplastic anemia, a disease in which the body fails to produce blood cells. One successful treatment of this disease is bone-marrow transplantation. All her family members are willing to donate marrow, but you need to choose one as a histocompatible donor. Your patient

has had no previous transplants. She has two parents, and (luckily) three siblings. The results of HLA typing follow. Remember that in these heterozygous
individuals, all the MHC products are expressed as cell-surface proteins on the
appropriate cells.

	A locus	B locus	D locus
Mother (M)	A1/A2	B1/B2	D1/D2
Father (F)	A3/A4	B3/B4	D3/D4
Brother 1 (B1)	A1/A3	B1/B3	D1/D3
Brother 2 (B2)	A2/A3	B2/B3	D2/D3
Sister 1 (S1)	A2/A4	B2/B4	D2/D4
Patient	A1/A3	B1/B3	D1/D3

You decide to test the lymphocytes of these family members with those of your
patient by doing a one-way mixed lymphocyte reaction. You irradiate the test
cells, incubate them with the patient's cells for 5 days, and assay proliferation
by measuring the uptake of ^{3}H-TdR into high molecular weight DNA at the
end of 5 days. Fill in the following table with the results you would predict.
Indicate a vigorous response (high levels of ^{3}H-TdR incorporation) with ($++$),
a moderate one with ($+$), and no response with ($-$).

Stimulator cells
(All irradiated before the test)

	M	F	B1	B2	S1
Patient's cells					

(b) The whole family gets the flu, a viral disease (and a very serious problem for
the patient). In the course of treatment, you take a blood sample from each
family member. You purify the peripheral blood lymphocytes and do a cell-
mediated lympholysis reaction. You mix the cells from the patient with ^{51}Cr-
labeled targets taken from the flu-ridden family members, leave them for 4
hours, and measure the amount of ^{51}Cr released into the medium. Fill in the
following table with your predicted results, using ($++$) to indicate high levels
of killing, ($+$) to indicate moderate levels of killing, and ($-$) to indicate no
killing above control levels.

	M	F	B1	B2	S1
Patient					

(c) Which family member would you choose as the bone-marrow donor for your
patient?

(d) The results of the two kinds of assays are different. Why do the test cells react
vigorously to allogeneic cells in the mixed lymphocyte reaction but not in the
cell-mediated lympholysis reaction?

11-13 CBA and C57BL/6 are two different inbred strains of mice that carry H-2^k and H-2^b
haplotypes, respectively. Strain-CBA mice were injected neonatally with (CBA $\times$
C57BL/6)F$_1$ hematopoietic cells. To your surprise, these mice later reject C57BL/6
and (CBA $\times$ C57BL/6)F$_1$ skin grafts. You check for chimerism by typing lymphocytes from these mice for H-2 haplotype and find that some carry H-2^k-coded molecules and some also carry H-2^b-coded molecules. Serum obtained after these
chimeric animals had rejected the C57BL/6 skin graft is tested for its ability to lyse
various tissues in the presence of complement with the results shown in Table 11-4.
With reference to this table, answer the following questions.

Table 11-4   Complement-Mediated Lysis of Cells from Various
Tissues by Serum from Chimeric Mice (Problem 11-13)[a]

	Tissue			
Strain	Bone Marrow	Spleen	Lymph-Node Lymphocyte	Epidermal Cell
CBA			−	−
C57BL/6		−		+
(CBA × C57BL/6)F$_1$			−	

[a]Cell lysis is scored "+" if >20% target cells are lysed.

(a) Explain the rejection of C57BL/6 and (CBA × C57BL/6)F$_1$ skin grafts.
(b) Fill in the blank spaces with predicted results.
(c) (CBA × C57BL/6)F$_1$ spleen and lymph node lymphocytes were injected intravenously into chimeric mice like those in this problem 3 days before the skin graft. Will the C57BL/6 skin graft be rejected if active suppression is the *operating* mechanism of tolerance? If clonal abortion is the mechanism? Briefly explain each answer.

Answers

11-1   (a) True
(b) False. The female offspring recognizes and rejects the paternal tissue through an immune response to H-Y antigens.
(c) False. The son inherits only one of the maternal HLA haplotypes and, because of the extensive HLA polymorphism, the other haplotype-encoded transplantation antigens will induce graft rejection.
(d) False. Hyperacute rejection occurs if the host has preformed antibodies to donor HLA determinants.
(e) True
(f) False. Although the graft will be accepted, the few T cells of parental type will recognize the H-2 antigens of the other parent in the offspring and mount a lethal graft-versus-host response.

11-2   (a) a xenograft; an allograft
(b) infection; immunosuppression
(c) hybrid Ia antigens
(d) polymorphonuclear leukocytes
(e) two

11-3   (a) Graft rejection is an immune phenomenon. This phenomenon shows an accelerated second response: the BALB/c and C57BL mice reject the second A/J skin graft faster than they did the first graft. In addition, the second response shows specificity: a previous A/J skin graft does not accelerate rejection of an SJL graft. Finally, this phenomenon involves a distinction between self and nonself: A/J mice never reject an A/J skin graft.

(b) Graft rejection is mediated by the cellular system. Mice that received immune cells showed an accelerated response when grafted for the first time with A/J skin. They rejected their first grafts in 8 days, whereas mice that did not receive immune cells took 14 days to reject their first grafts (Table 11-1c, d). The ability to reject grafts can be transferred by cells but not by serum.

(c) If the cellular system is primarily responsible for graft rejection, then animals deficient in T cells should show an impaired ability to reject grafts. Therefore, you could test neonatally thymectomized mice or nude mice (which congenitally lack a thymus) for their ability to reject grafts from a different mouse strain.

(d) Injection of immune serum lengthens the mean survival time of the graft (Table 11-1d); that is, it weakens the immune response to the graft. Destruction of grafted tissue presumably requires intimate contact between host lymphocytes and the grafted cells. Humoral antibodies that are specific for antigenic determinants on the surface of the grafted tissue cells may bind tightly to the surface of grafted cells and prevent host lymphocytes from recognizing or binding to the grafted cells. Any of the other mechanisms operative in antibody inhibition of the immune response could also be involved. Such humoral antibodies are termed *blocking* antibodies because they block the cellular immune response. They provide an example of how the humoral immune system can interfere with the functioning of the cellular immune system. Blocking antibodies may play an important role in the impairment of cellular immunity against cancer cells (Chapter 13).

(e) Graft rejection is caused by the presence of histocompatibility antigens on the surface of cells that are different in the donor graft from those found on the host cells. This process is easily studied in inbred strains of mice because of the genetic identity of individuals within the strain. In mice, the H-2 locus codes for the cell-surface antigens that play the most important role in the graft rejection process. Mice that differ at this locus will reject transplants from one another rapidly.

11-4   None of these immunosuppressants exhibits specificity. Each kills rapidly dividing cells or lymphocytes indiscriminately. Theoretically, the ideal immunosuppressant would remove just those lymphocytes that could react with the foreign cell-surface antigens of the transplant. To find a method for imposing such specific tolerance is one of the major goals of transplantation biology.

11-5   Inbred mice are homozygous for MHC determinants. Consequently, when mice of two inbred strains are crossed, their F_1 progeny express all the MHC antigens that are expressed in either parent. Thus, if T cells of any F_1 individual are transferred to either parent in a marrow transplant, they will not recognize or react to any parental antigens as nonself determinants. By contrast, because humans are invariably heterozygous for MHC antigens, a given F_1 individual will receive only half the MHC determinants of either parent. In a bone-marrow transplant, the remainder of the parental determinants will be recognized as nonself by any F_1 T cells that are injected, and a multisystem graft-versus-host immune response will ensue. Because such a response is usually fatal to the recipient, your colleague would be well advised not to proceed with the operation as planned.

11-6   (a) In a family with many children, the multiparous mother is highly likely to have antibodies to the products of both paternal HLA haplotypes because, assuming no crossing-over within the MHC, each child has an equal probability of expressing either one of the two paternal haplotypes. Therefore, blood leukocytes from all children will agglutinate in maternal serum. Siblings can be matched for paternal haplotype by using leukocytes from the diseased child to absorb the maternal serum exhaustively at its agglutination end point. The absorbed serum may then be tested for the ability to agglutinate leukocytes from other siblings. Those whose cells are still agglutinated must express the other paternal haplotype, whereas those whose cells are not agglutinated express the same paternal haplotype as the diseased child.

A transplant donor, however, must also be matched for maternally inherited HLA antigens, again because each child has an equal probability of inheriting either maternal haplotype. Identity of maternal HLA antigens can be determined using a mixed lymphocyte reaction in which blood lymphocytes from the intended recipient are incubated separately with lymphocytes from each of the siblings that were found to express the same paternal haplotype in the preceding test. After 5 days, the number of lymphocytes that are undergoing blast transformation are counted in each of the cultures. Lack of any blast transformation indicates HLA identity.

(b) The horse presumably made antibodies to surface antigens that are shared by RBCs and thymocytes. While you give the patient a blood transfusion, you could prove this assumption by showing that absorption of the ALS with an equal volume of RBCs removes its RBC agglutinating activity without lowering the thymocyte agglutinating power.

(c) The horse also made antibodies against antigens that are shared by all leukocytes but are not present on RBCs. The acute bacterial infection is almost certainly due to a lack of polymorphonuclear leukocytes (PMN). To treat this condition, you could "plasmaphorese" the patient (remove the plasma from blood samples, returning the packed cells) to reduce the blood level of antibody, transfuse him with a PMN concentrate, and give back RBC, PMN, and a preparation of ALS that had been absorbed with these cells and B cells.

(d) The PMN could infiltrate because of local infection or local complement activation by anti-kidney antibodies. The former would be unlikely to affect only glomeruli. To test for the latter, you could use fluorescein-tagged antihorse-immunoglobulin or anti-human-C3 on the kidney biopsy.

(e) The tests show local deposition of antibody and C3 on the glomerular basement membrane (Figure 12-4b). This result indicates that your ALS contains anti-basement-membrane antibodies, which were presumably induced by basement membranes contained in the thymus mash and which are now causing an acute inflammatory reaction that is leading to failure of the transplant. You should remove the transplant, absorb the ALS with the failing kidney, and put in another HLA-matched donor kidney along with the absorbed ALS.

(f) You should vaccinate everyone in town *except* the transplant recipients. Although the live vaccinia virus used for smallpox vaccinations is normally nonpathogenic, it will cause a severe generalized infection and, probably, death of these recipients due to their T-cell deficit caused by your immunosuppressive treatment. Consequently these individuals must be kept in isolation and *not* vaccinated.

11-7 (a) 3

(b) T_A and T_C precursor cells specifically recognize MHC antigens. Accessory cells may also be involved, but not in the specific recognition and response to antigens. B cells are not involved.

(c) T_A cells from person X recognize HLA-D antigens from person Y and proliferate. These T_A cells stimulate person X's T_C-cell precursors that recognize HLA-A,B,C antigens of person Y, thereby causing formation of specific T_C cells from these precursors. T_D cells of person X respond to HLA-D antigens of person Y and become poised to effect delayed hypersensitivity. T_H cells of person X recognize HLA-D antigens of person Y and help the B cells of person X respond to the HLA-A,B,C antigens of person Y by proliferating, differentiation to plasma cells, and secreting antibody.

11-8   (a) Cells from genetically identical monozygotic twins hardly respond to one another, whereas cells from unrelated donors undergo active lymphocyte proliferation when mixed. This observation implies that lymphocytes react only to genetically disparate cells in a manner reminiscent of transplant rejection *in vivo.*

(b) At any particular genetic locus, dizygotic twins will be either identical or quite different. Thus some pairs will be identical at their HLA loci and hence will not react with each other, whereas other pairs will differ and hence will react.

(c) A sibling who is identical to the prospective recipient at the HLA locus should be chosen. Identity can be assayed by culturing the recipient's lymphocytes with the cells from each sibling. The mixture that gives the lowest reactivity will identify the sibling whose HLA locus is most similar to that of the recipient. The kidney should be transplanted from the most similar donor to minimize the possibility of rejection.

(d) Because histocompatibility genes are codominant, F_1 lymphocytes will express both maternal and paternal histocompatibility antigens. Therefore, unless the parents had closely similar histocompatibility genotypes, the F_1 lymphocytes will differ from either parent's cells, and a vigorous mixed lymphocyte reaction should ensue.

11-9   (a) Parental lymphocytes account for 173 of the 181 mitotic figures observed. Clearly, F_1 lymphocytes are not stimulated to undergo blast transformation by parental cells, whereas parental cells respond strongly to F_1 cells. This result shows that lymphocytes are stimulated only by foreign histocompatibility antigens. Quantitative differences in the antigens expressed do not trigger a response.

(b) Unlike inbred rats, humans are likely to be heterozygous, particularly at the highly polymorphic histocompatibility loci. Thus F_1 lymphocytes will probably carry some, but not all, of each parent's histocompatibility antigens. Hence, F_1 cells should respond actively against parental cells. In fact, the results should be similar to those in line 4, Table 11-2.

(c) Inactivation of human parental lymphocytes would allow direct demonstration of the result predicted in part (b), that F_1 cells will generally react to parental cells. If the F_1 cells were inactivated, the response of the parental cells could be determined. In general, this technique allows independent determination of the two responses in a mixed lymphocyte reaction under conditions where karyotype analysis cannot distinguish the two cell populations.

(d) For organ transplants, it is necessary to know whether the donor's kidney cells will trigger an immunologic response in the recipient. Whether recipient cells can trigger the donor's lymphocytes is irrelevant because no donor lymphocytes are knowingly transferred. If the donor lymphocytes are inactivated as in part (c), then a mixed lymphocyte reaction between these cells and lymphocytes of the recipient will furnish the required information.

11-10   (a) Use of the spleen/body weight ratio is intended to correct for variations in the normal body weights and spleen weights of individual mice. It also magnifies the observed response because the GVHR causes an increase in spleen weight and a decrease in body weight.

(b) Line 1 in Table 11-3 provides a control value for recipient mice in which no

GVHR should have occurred because these mice received syngeneic cells.

(c) Thymosin somehow increases the magnitude of the GVHR. One possible explanation is that it induces maturation of at least some bone-marrow cells into functional T cells. If so, thymus-cell differentiation antigens (e.g., Lyt-1, 2, 3; TL) and other T-cell characteristics should also be expressed. Another possibility is that thymosin acts on the few immunocompetent cells in bone marrow to increase their activity or their number. The difference in the effects of thymosin and spleen extract are quantitative but not qualitative, suggesting that thymosin activity may not be confined to the thymus or that similar factors are produced in the spleen. Unfortunately, the experiments shown here do not verify that the thymosin effect is acting only through specific graft-versus-host reactions because no experimental group of syngeneic bone-marrow donors treated with thymosin or spleen extracts is used. The appropriate control for each group in the calculation of spleen indices would be a syngeneic injection from donors treated with the same dose of the same extract. (This control series was included in subsequent experiments, verifying the hypothesis that thymosin acted to augment specifically the graft-versus-host activity of CBA donor bone-marrow cells.)

11-11 (a) Supernatant fluid from cultures containing homologous plasma significantly inhibited macrophage migration. This result indicates the presence of MIF and thus demonstrates that the maternal lymphocytes were sensitized to paternal antigens. This sensitization probably occurred during one or more previous pregnancies. Homologous plasma does not interfere with this response, and it provides needed nutrients.

(b) Because the major histocompatibility antigens are usually immunologically dominant, the mother is probably responding primarily to paternal HLA antigens.

(c) Supernatant fluid from these cultures had essentially no effect on macrophage migration. Hence autologous plasma somehow inhibited the sensitized maternal lymphocytes from reacting to the paternal cells. This finding may be interpreted to demonstrate the existence of a mechanism to protect the fetus from reactive maternal lymphocytes. Moreover, the observation that only autologous plasma inhibits this mixed lymphocyte reaction indicates that this mechanism may be immunologically specific. Conceivably the autologous plasma could have contained anti-MIF factors or antibodies, or macrophage chemotactic factors that enhance their migration. The control with homologous plasma would be insufficient unless the control plasma were shown to have similar specific inhibiting activities when cells from the plasma donor were placed in a similar reaction with her spouse's cells. Thus it is critical to do the appropriate controls and to identify in autologous plasma the factor that prevents MIF formation or activity.

(d) If the inhibitory factor is an immunoglobulin, then removal of immunoglobulins with appropriate anti-Ig antisera should abolish the inhibition of MIF release by autologous plasma. Alternatively, purified immunoglobulin from autologous plasma should inhibit release of MIF.

(e) The active factor is probably IgG, and the effect is immunologically specific. Thus autologous IgG molecules appear to prevent MIF release and, by inference, the total immunological response. Both these humoral factors and the sensitized maternal lymphocytes arise in response to paternal antigens on fetal cells, which have presumably somehow entered the maternal circulation. Thus both could be specific for paternal antigens. If so, specific IgG could bind to paternal antigens and block recognition by maternal lymphocytes. To prove this hypothesis, one could absorb autologous plasma with paternal or unrelated cells. The specific IgG should bind specifically to the paternal cells, and the plasma, which would still contain all other IgG molecules, should have no protective effect. With regard to the question of tolerance, the mother's system may not recognize small doses of paternal antigens, but her lymphocytes can respond to those antigens and could probably reject a skin transplant. Consequently, the mother is, to a limited extent, unresponsive, but she is not truly tolerant. Thus neither these experiments nor any others reported to date adequately explain why the fetus is not rejected by the mother.

11-12 (a)

M	F	B1	B2	S1
+	+	−	+	++

(b) Patient

M	F	B1	B2	S1
+	+	++	+	−

(c) Brother 1.

(d) The mixed lymphocyte reaction is a 5-day test. You measure the development of reactivity (blast transformation) during that period. Thus the capacity of the patient to develop an allogeneic response is measured. Because she is totally different from S1 and shares some, but not all, antigens with all other family members, the (+) or (++) response is seen. In the cell-mediated lympholysis test, you are assaying reactivity that is already there because the assay is short term. The patient's T cells have already been sensitized to flu virus in the context of her own MHC antigens, and thus they respond by killing cells of that haplotype. Because she shares some HLA-A and B antigens with M, F, and B2, there is killing of their cells. She shares all antigens tested with B1, so his cells are killed as efficiently as her own. She shares no HLA-A or B with S1, so her T cells do not have the capacity (in this short-term assay) to kill S1's cells.

11-13 (a) The C57BL/6 genome encodes a tissue-specific antigen (Sk) that is expressed on epidermal cells but not on cells of the hemopoietic lineage. This antigen is not present in CBA mice. Although their lymphoid tissue becomes chimeric, the CBA mice were not tolerized against the Sk antigen and, therefore, they would be expected to reject both C57BL/6 and (CBA × C57BL/6)F_1 skin grafts, assuming dominant or codominant expression of Sk.

(b) The completed table of results should appear as follows:

	Bone marrow	Spleen	Lymph node	Epidermal cell
CBA	−	−	−	−
C57BL/6	−	−	−	+
F_1	−	−	−	+

(c) (CBA × C57BL/6)F_1 mice are tolerant to the Sk antigen (self). If active suppression is the mechanism of self-tolerance, the F_1 lymphocytes should contain specific T_S cells that will transfer tolerance upon injection, so that C57BL/6 skin grafts will be tolerated. If clonal abortion is operating, the F_1 cells will have no effect on the host, and the skin grafts will be rejected as before.

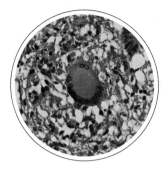

CHAPTER 12

Immunopathology

Chapter Outline

Diseases involving the immune system can be grouped into two general classes. *Deficiency* diseases result when a component of the system fails to function. These diseases manifest themselves clinically by low resistance to infection and loss of immunologic surveillance functions. *Hypersensitivity* diseases result when the system reacts under inappropriate conditions. Some diseases of both classes are congenital, whereas others are acquired. Medical practice and research have provided detailed phenomenological descriptions of these diseases, with the hope that suffering from them can be alleviated through knowledgeable intervention. These immunopathologies also provide important clues to still poorly understood immunological principles. This chapter considers the cellular and molecular bases of deficiency diseases, the inappropriate responses of T cells and B cells in hypersensitivity diseases, and the relationship between specific major histocompatibility genes and specific diseases.

Concepts

12-1   Failure of a host's nonlymphoid defenses to stop invading microorganisms can lead to infection

Resistance to infection depends on a combination of nonspecific innate functions and specific adaptive immune responses of T cells and B cells. The nonspecific functions prevent invasion by the vast majority of microorganisms. Some of the most important of these functions are: maintenance of epithelial surface integrity; action of antibacterial substances such as lysozyme (in secretions, an enzyme that attacks bacterial cell walls) and C-reactive protein (an inducible serum factor that binds to bacterial cell-wall phosphorylcholine residues and activates complement-mediated opsonization and lysis); maintenance of local pH conditions (e.g., acidity in the stomach and vagina); and mechanical expulsion of microorganisms by various mechanisms such as the sneeze reflex and ciliary movement on respiratory tract epithelia. Failure of any of these innate defenses may lead to infection, even in the absence of an immunologic deficiency.

For example, some microorganisms, including the bacteria *Vibrio cholerae*, *Shigella dysenteriae*, and a diarrhea-causing strain of *E. coli*, attach to intestinal epithelial cells via receptors specific for cell-surface components. If attachment is not prevented, the organisms proliferate and release toxins that can be fatal. The cholera toxin, which is a protein consisting of two subunits, A and B, linked by disulfide bonds, binds the cell-surface glycolipid GM_1 by subunit B and releases subunit A, which triggers the cell to excrete Cl^- ions at a high rate. The concomitant transudation of Na^+ ions and H_2O from the tissue fluids to the intestinal lumen can give rise to an explosive and often lethal diarrhea.

Attached *Shigella* bacteria are taken up by endocytosis and then proliferate intracellularly with release of toxins that block ribosomal function. Intestinal cells die, releasing *Shigella* endotoxins into the bloodstream where they can activate the alternative complement pathway (Concept 9-2) to produce a vicious systemic shock. In some cases, the endotoxin activates both the complement and coagulation systems, causing erythrocyte lysis, platelet consumption, and microclots in the kidney blood vessels. This associated disease is called the *hemolytic-uremic syndrome*.

IgA antibodies normally supplement the body's innate defenses against infection by microorganisms at mucosal epithelial surfaces (Concept 9-1). However, some bacteria evade this protection by producing enzymes that cleave IgA. Certain strains of *Streptococcus* and *Neisseria*, a subtype that causes gonorrhea following pilus and outer membrane protein attachment to cells in the mucosal surfaces of the genital tract, produce specific IgA proteases. Protozoal parasites, such as trypanosomes and schistosomes, also produce specific immunoglobulin proteases.

If microorganisms successfully invade epithelial barriers, most of them are removed by the phagocytic system, which also stimulates the specific functions of T-cell and B-cell immunity. Because most immunologic reactions also end with phagocytosis and degradation of the antigenic microorganisms, malfunction of phagocytic cells is an appropriate topic with which to begin the discussion of lymphoid system deficiencies.

12-2 Deficiencies in phagocytic functions often result in lethal bacterial infections

Phagocyte functions

The elimination of invading microorganisms by phagocytic cells is a multistep process (Concept 9-5). It includes chemotactic attraction of phagocytes to the site of infection, adherence of the phagocyte to the blood-vessel wall near the site of infection, movement of the phagocyte through the vessel wall by diapedesis, chemotactic attraction to the microorganisms, phagocytosis of invading microorganisms, intracellular union of phagosomes and lysosomes, and enzymatic halogenation of microbial cell walls, leading to their breakdown by various acidic hydrolases. In normal hosts, most microorganisms are eliminated by this process, and consequently they are nonpathogenic; a few types of microorganisms regularly escape the phagocytic system and hence are pathogenic. However, in patients with malfunctioning phagocytic cells, normally nonpathogenic organisms, called *opportunistic pathogens,* become pathogenic and cause recurrent infections. Such phagocytic malfunction diseases are relatively rare and are usually inherited. Practical diagnosis of these disorders involves isolation and testing of blood phagocytes for (a) motile responses to chemotactic factors, (b) ability to phagocytize a range of microorganisms, (c) ability to kill phagocytosed microorganisms, and (d) ability to generate hydrogen peroxide (H_2O_2), which is required in the lysosomal halogenation of microorganisms and can be measured *in vitro* using the redox-sensitive dye nitroblue tetrazolium.

Human phagocytic-cell diseases

Several forms of phagocytic-cell disease have been described in humans. One group of rare diseases involves defective leukocyte chemotactic responses to N-formylmethionyl peptides that are characteristic of the N termini of proteins formed during bacterial but not eucaryotic protein synthesis. Patients with these diseases are exceedingly susceptible to the formation of bacterial (usually staphylococcal) abcesses, often in the skin (boils). Some of these patients have very high serum levels of IgE, but the connection between these findings is unexplained.

Chediak–Higashi syndrome involves a lysosomal defect in phagocytes and other cells (Figure 12-1a). These cells have abnormally large lysosomes that lyse bacteria ineffectively and fuse sluggishly with phagosomes although phagocytosis is normal. Polymorphonuclear leukocytes normally have two types of cytoplasmic granules: (a) *azurophilic* granules containing myeloperoxidase (involved in the respiratory burst of these cells when activated), acid hydrolases, lysozyme and proteases and (b) *specific* granules, which contain lactoferrin. In the leukocytes from patients with Chediak-Higashi syndrome, the azurophilic and specific granules are fused. These patients are extremely sensitive to light (photophobic) and are partial albinos due to a related defect of intracellular vesicles in the pigmented cells of the retina and skin. The disease is hereditary, caused by an autosomal recessive gene, and it is usually fatal in childhood. Related disorders have been found in mink (Aleutian mink disease), cattle, and mice (beige mice). Beige mice also show profound defects, not yet understood, in natural killer cells.

Several rare phagocytic dysfunctions result from defects of lysosomal enzymes involved in the respiratory burst required in the halogenation of microorganisms following phagocyte activation. These diseases include severe glucose-6-phosphate dehydrogenase deficiency, myeloperoxidase deficiency, and glutathione reductase deficiency. Cells from patients with some of these diseases phagocytize but do not kill most bacteria, which continue to grow inside the phagocytes and induce a prolonged local inflammatory reaction. The combination of activated phagocytes and surrounding cells growing in a nodule is identifiable histologically as a *granuloma*. Such *chronic granulomatous diseases*, which are usually fatal in childhood, can exhibit either an X-linked recessive or an autosomal recessive form of inheritance (Figure 12-1a).

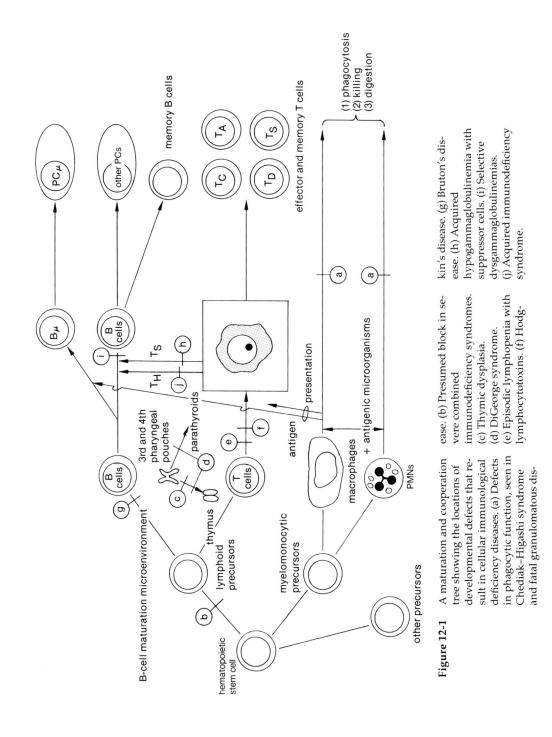

Figure 12-1 A maturation and cooperation tree showing the locations of developmental defects that result in cellular immunological deficiency diseases. (a) Defects in phagocytic function, seen in Chediak–Higashi syndrome and fatal granulomatous disease. (b) Presumed block in severe combined immunodeficiency syndromes. (c) Thymic dysplasia. (d) DiGeorge syndrome. (e) Episodic lymphopenia with lymphocytotoxins. (f) Hodgkin's disease. (g) Bruton's disease. (h) Acquired hypogammaglobulinemia with suppressor cells. (i) Selective dysgammaglobulinemias. (j) Acquired immunodeficiency syndrome.

Table 12-1 Complement Deficiency and Associated Diseases in Humans

Deficient Component	Associated Diseases
C1r	Hypersensitivity diseases, infections
C1s	Hypersensitivity diseases
C2	Hypersensitivity diseases, infections
C3	Infections
C3b inhibitor	Infections
C4	Hypersensitivity diseases
C5	Infections (mainly Neisseria)
C6, C7, C8	Infections (mainly Neisseria)

12-3 Deficiencies in complement components can lower resistance to infection or be associated with hypersensitivity diseases

Hereditary deficiencies in several of the complement components involved in acute inflammation (Concept 9-2) are usually associated with a decreased resistance to bacterial infections, an increased incidence of hypersensitivity diseases, or both (Table 12-1). Deficiency of C1-esterase inhibitor, which is a control element in complement activation, leads to a condition known as *hereditary angioneurotic edema*. Normally, activation and deactivation of the complement system is under strict control. In patients with this deficiency, the reactions of the activated system go unchecked, causing recurrent episodes of local acute inflammation at sites of activation. The results are vessel dilation and transudation of fluid into the tissue spaces in the upper respiratory tract, gastrointestinal tract, and skin. If activation occurs in the throat at or near the larynx, it can cause death by suffocation.

12-4 Deficiencies in T cells, B cells, or both lead to generalized immune diseases

Patients with defects in T cells are especially susceptible to intracellular viral and bacterial infections, whereas patients with defects in B cells are especially susceptible to extracellular infections, mainly those caused by bacteria. Patients with defects in both T-cell and B-cell sys-

Table 12-2 Properties of Human Blood Lymphocyte Classes That Can Be Assayed in Diagnostic Tests

Properties	T Cells	B Cells	Monocytes
Percentage representation among nucleated blood mononuclear cells (excludes granulocytes)	60–70%	10–15%	10–20%
Presence of cell-surface:			
κ chains or λ chains	–	+	–
μ chains + δ chains	–	+	–
γ chains	–	2–5%[a]	–
α chains	–	2–5%	–
Fc receptors[b]	–	>80%	+
C3 receptors[c]	–	50–80%	+
native sheep erythrocyte receptors	+	–	–
human T-cell surface antigens (see Table 7-2)	+	–	–
Mitogenic response to:			
concanavalin A	+	–	
phytohemagglutinin	+	–	
pokeweed mitogen	+	+	

[a]Percentages indicate the fraction of B cells that possesses the marker.
[b]Under conditions where T cells with Fc receptors are not detected.
[c]Including cells that possess receptors for the split products of C3 (C3b and C3d). Different assays can distinguish among B cells with C3b receptors, B cells with C3d receptors, and monocytes with C3b receptors.

tems are extraordinarily susceptible to intracellular and extracellular infections. Vaccination of T-cell deficient individuals with live, attenuated (nonpathogenic) viruses is usually fatal.

T-cell deficiencies

Several congenital defects can lead to a specific lack of T cells. The diagnosis of T-cell deficiency requires evidence that T cells are absent from the blood and lymphoid tissues. Patients with T-cell deficiencies lack testable T-cell functions such as graft rejection and activation of blood lymphocytes in response to the T-cell mitogenic lectins concanavalin A and phytohemagglutinin (Table 12-2). One such defect, known as *thymic dysplasia,* is characterized by disorganized tissue in the thymus (Figure 12-1c), but it is otherwise poorly understood. A second defect, known as the *DiGeorge syndrome,* is characterized by lack of the thymic (and parathyroid) inductive microenvironment, presumably as a result of improper formation of the third and fourth pharyngeal pouches during embryogenesis (Figure 12-1d). This abnormality is congenital but not heritable. Children with the syndrome can be recognized clinically because they also lack parathyroid hormones and therefore cannot maintain appropriate calcium levels in the blood. Consequently, they suffer muscle spasms (hypocalcemic tetany) soon after birth. The T-cell deficiency in DiGeorge syndrome patients is extensive but not absolute.

A defect in the formation of the thymic inductive microenvironment is also found in mice; however, this abnormality is heritable. The epithelial cells of the affected animals have several defects, including the absence of hair follicles. Consequently, these mice are hairless, and the autosomal recessive gene responsible for their multiple defects is called *nude* (*nu*). As in DiGeorge's syndrome, the T-cell deficiency in *nu/nu* mice is striking but not absolute.

Some congenital T-cell deficiency patients lack a purine metabolic enzyme, purine nucleoside phosphorylase, which catalyzes conversion of the purine nucleosides inosine and guanosine to hypoxanthine and guanine, respectively. These patients accumulate high levels of deoxyguanosine and deoxyguanosine triphosphate. The latter metabolite, dGTP, is a potent inhibitor of ribonucleotide reductase, which is necessary for conversion of ribonucleotides to deoxyribonucleotides. Deoxyguanosine and dGTP are selectively toxic for dividing T cells, their proliferating thymic precursors, and some T-cell lymphomas, but not for resting T cells, apparently, or for B cells. T-cell division is required for expression of cell-mediated immunity but, at least in experimental models, T_H-cell division is not required for B-cell help. How dividing plasma cell precursors are spared dGTP toxicity is still unclear. Nevertheless, in this case an apparently specific cell maturation defect is, in fact, an enzyme defect that leads to selective cell killing by an accumulated metabolite.

An epidemic, adult-onset, selective T-cell deficiency called *acquired immunodeficiency syndrome* has recently surfaced in the United States. Most patients suffer severe infections by opportunistic pathogens, with the pneumonia-causing protozoan, *Pneumocystis carinii*, heading the list, closely followed by a herpes-type virus, *cytomegalovirus*. Most of these patients die of their opportunistic pathogen or of an unusual cancer, called *Kaposi's sarcoma*. Most of the patients are male homosexuals who are very active sexually; about 10% are users of intravenous drugs; 6% are Haitian immigrants. Most informative are a group of acquired immunodeficiency syndrome patients who were well until they received as little as a single blood transfusion or blood products transfusion from donors who were subsequently found to have the acquired immunodeficiency syndrome. Hemophiliacs are particularly at risk for this mode of "infectious" transmission. The epidemiology of the syndrome strongly suggests a transmissable immunosuppressive infectious agent as the cause. In man a retrovirus, HTLV 3 (or LAV), is implicated. A similar epidemic outbreak in monkey colonies has been documented, and the plasma of these monkeys contains filterable agents, probably viruses, which transmit the disease. The level of circulating lymphocytes is low in humans with the acquired immunodeficiency syndrome, with the defect occurring mainly in the T4 (generally containing the helper) T-cell subset. Thus the ratio of helper to suppressor/cytotoxic subclasses of T lymphocytes is reversed. Patients with the syndrome suffer defects in all aspects of cell-mediated immunity, including contact sensitivity, delayed-type hypersensitivity, and natural killer and natural cytotoxic cell activity. In spite of the low ratio of T4-identified "T_H" cells, humoral immunity and the levels of all antibody classes appear to be normal. A significant proportion of the patients are HLA-DR5, suggesting that this determinant may represent a low responder allele of an immune response gene to the immunosuppressive agent, perhaps via the *preclusion phenomenon* (Concept 8-9). Because a significant proportion of these patients (about 33%) develops a highly malignant form of Kaposi's sarcoma, a role for T-cell immunity in the immunosurveillance of this cancer (Chapter 13), or of agents causing this cancer, is likely.

B-cell deficiencies

A total congenital lack of B cells, their progeny, and their products, which results from an X-linked recessive gene defect, is known as *infantile sex-linked agammaglobulinemia (Bruton's disease)*. Patients with this syndrome (Figure 12-1g) are especially susceptible to pyogenic (pus-causing) bacterial infections of the skin and respiratory tracts, beginning at about 6 months of age, when placentally transferred maternal immunoglobulin has disappeared. The lives of these patients can be saved by inoculation with gamma globulins pooled from several different donors.

Patients with *selective dysgammaglobulinemias* are characterized by lack of particular immunoglobulin classes in the blood (Figure 12-1i). Several selective dysgammaglobulinemias have been reported, including deficiencies in IgM, IgA, IgM and IgA, IgA and IgG, or IgM and IgG. Deficiencies in IgM and IgG are usually accompanied by susceptibility to pyogenic infections. Deficiencies of IgA, or IgA and IgG, are often associated with gastrointestinal tract disorders, such as diarrhea, and with poor intestinal absorption of fats and fat-soluble vitamins. However, the connection between these symptoms is not understood. Most IgA-deficient patients are healthy with disease manifestations largely limited to patients with combined IgG_2/IgG_4 and IgA deficiencies. As noted in Concept 9-1, selective IgA deficiency may be ameliorated by transepithelial secretion of Sc-J-IgM complexes.

Several acquired B-cell defects are also known. These diseases, all poorly understood, include both complete and partial deficiencies of B cells and their immunoglobulin products. Patients with one type of *acquired agammaglobulinemia* have normal levels of B cells but no plasma cells (Figure 12-1h). *In vitro* analysis shows that some of these patients possess a class of T_S cells that prevents stimulation of antibody formation; others possess T_S cells but lack helper cells, and one patient was recently found with normal levels of T_H and T_S cells, but his precursor T_H cells were insensitive to antigenic stimulation. Thus, this disease may be classified more properly as a T-cell abnormality.

Combined T-cell and B-cell deficiencies

The congenital lack of T cells and B cells is known as *severe combined immunodeficiency* (Figure 12-1b). These patients have no serum immunoglobulins, they lack a lymphoid thymus, and their blood, spleen, lymph nodes, Peyer's patches, tonsils, and appendix also lack lymphocytes. In some patients, bone-marrow cell transplants may completely repopulate both T-cell and B-cell systems. Three distinct genetic bases for these diseases have been described: an X-linked recessive and two autosomal recessive defects. In one of the autosomal recessive diseases, the primary defect is known to be a lack of the metabolic enzyme adenosine deaminase, which catalyzes the conversion of adenosine to inosine. In the absence of this enzyme, deoxyadenosine and deoxyadenosine triphosphate (dATP) can accumulate intracellularly with depletion of intracellular ATP pools. dATP is highly and perhaps selectively toxic to both dividing T and B lymphocytes, perhaps because of its inhibition of ribonucleotide reductase. The enzyme deficiency is also toxic to resting T and B lymphocytes because of ATP depletion. Therefore, the resulting immunodeficiency is not a specific maturational defect of lymphocytes, but it is secondary to a generalized enzyme defect. Transfusion with leukocyte-free fresh blood sometimes restores the ability of these patients to metabolize adenosine, with a concomitant return of immune function.

12-5 Some immunodeficiencies are secondary to other diseases or their treatments

Immunodeficiencies resulting from disease

Immunological deficiency may be secondary to diseases that result in the accumulation of immunosuppressive products. For example, defective function of the kidney or liver leads to an accumulation of toxic substances that can depress immune responses, and patients with virus infections often release immunosuppressive products into the blood, as do many patients with advanced cancers. For example, patients with *Hodgkin's disease*, which is a cancer of lymph-node cells in the macrophage lineage, acquire an immune deficiency because the surface receptors of their T cells appear to be blocked by serum factors that are elevated markedly (Figure 12-1f). Some evidence also suggests that these patients have elevated levels of T_S cells that control the release of immunosuppressive prostaglandins. Consequently, although the malignant cells may be limited to a single lymph node, these patients exhibit a whole-body deficiency of T-cell functions and immunity to viral infections (especially Herpes viruses), even though they have normal numbers of peripheral T cells as measured by T-cell antisera.

Patients with *Cushing's disease* develop an immunodeficiency because cortisone and cortisol, two hormones of the adrenal cortex, are secreted in excess. At increased concentrations, these hormones act as potent anti-inflammatory agents, lyse most resting T cells and B cells directly, and decrease the levels of blood monocytes. Patients with Cushing's disease become extremely susceptible to infection, particularly to those agents usually controlled by the T-cell system. The increased secretion of the two hormones may sometimes be episodic, related to periods of emotional or physical stress.

Patients with *ataxia telangiectasia*, a rare disease inherited as an autosomal recessive disorder, have a general defect in DNA synthesis with a particular defect in their ability to repair X-ray-induced damage to DNA. The first clinical symptoms of this disease appear as effects on the cerebellum, resulting in disorders of balance and movement (ataxia). As patients grow older, they develop pathological alterations in their small veins with the formation of *telangiectases* (*tel*, end; *angio*, vessel; *ectases*, stretching out), which are highly dilated, tortuous venous networks visible in the skin and the whites of the eyes. In early life, their immune system appears normal. Beginning in about the fifth year of life, these patients develop a progressive immune deficiency that is characterized by defective cellular immunity and, often, by a total lack of IgA, IgE, IgG$_2$, and perhaps IgG$_4$. The thymus is alymphoid in these patients by the time the immunological defects appear. The progressive loss of serum IgG$_2$, IgG$_4$, IgA, and IgE, but not IgM or IgG$_1$, suggests that this disease may involve an acquired dysfunction of some critical cell class or process involved in B-cell maturation or the immunoglobulin class switch or both. These patients suffer from recurrent bacterial and viral upper respiratory tract infections, presumably due to the IgA deficiency in fluid secretions and the IgG$_2$ and IgG$_4$ deficiency. (IgG$_2$ and IgG$_4$ are the main human IgG subclasses involved in formation of antibodies to polymeric bacterial surface antigens.) No clear relationship between the X-ray sensitivity of the cells from these patients and their subsequent pathology has yet been established, although a preponderance of their chromosome breaks are on the heavy-chain chromosome (14). Surprisingly, many of these patients have a form of diabetes in which insulin receptors on cells are blocked, quite possibly by immunoglobulins.

Another unexplained, multisystem, progressive disease that results in loss of T cells is called *immunodeficiency with thrombocytopenia and eczema* (*Wiskott–Aldrich syndrome*). Thrombocytopenia means lack of platelets, and eczema is a skin disorder characterized by an inappropriate response of the IgE system to antigens. Patients with this disease are born normal, but at an early age they have problems with bleeding due to lack of platelets, which are important in the blood-clotting process. They develop eczematous skin rashes and show a progressive loss of T-cell functions. The underlying pathological process that causes this distinctive combination of immunodeficiency, thrombocytopenia, and eczema is unknown, but the triad of symptoms disappears following successful bone-marrow transplantation. T-cell replacement selectively cures the eczema.

Immunodeficiencies resulting from medical therapy

Many therapeutic treatments suppress the immune system, either intentionally or inadvertently. These treatments are inherently dangerous because the resulting immunodeficiency lowers resistance to disease. (Diseases *caused* by medical therapy are called *iatrogenic diseases*.) Immunosuppressive therapies are commonly used in control of inflammation, treatment of cancer, and transplantation of organs.

The potent anti-inflammatory effect of the adrenocortical hormones, cortisone and cortisol, and their inducer, adrenocorticotropic hormone, has led to widespread use of these agents in the control of diseases that have a major inflammatory component. Prolonged use of these hormones has the same effects as Cushing's disease and may make infections fatal.

Chemotherapy and X-ray therapy of most cancers involve the use of agents that inactivate dividing cells, and they can cause interphase death of small lymphocytes (Concept 8-2). Because cell division is necessary to generate most effector cells of the immune system, the prolonged use of anticancer agents depletes cells important for host immunity.

Transplantation operations to replace defective organs often introduce foreign antigenic tissue into the recipient. Adrenocortical hormones and anticancer drugs, as well as antisera against lymphocytes of the T-cell series and total lymphoid irradiation are used to suppress the host's rejection reactions (Chapter 11). All these agents cause non-specific immunosuppression that leads to immunodeficiency.

12-6 Some immunopathologies are secondary to normal immune responses

Active immune responses may also cause disease. Collectively, these immunopathological disorders are known as *hypersensitivity diseases*, although it is not always the case that the immune response is "hyper." Classically, clinical immunologists have divided these diseases into four main categories based on their predominant effector components: (a) cytotoxic T cells; (b) direct antibody plus complement reactions; (c) immune complexes of antigen, antibody, and complement; and (d) IgE plus mast-cell reactions (Table 12-3). Although these

Table 12-3 Pathological Classifications of Immune-Mediated Tissue Damage (Hypersensitivity Diseases)

Classification	Name	Predominant Effector Components
Type I	Anaphylactic	IgE + mast cells or basophiles
Type II	Cytotoxic	IgM or IgG (anti-self) + complement
Type III	Immune complex	IgM or IgG in immune complexes with antigen and complement
Type IV	Cell mediated	T cells

categories are useful, it has become increasingly apparent that hypersensitivity diseases often involve multiple components of the immune system, whether directed against self- or foreign antigens.

Damage by T cells: Lymphocytic choriomeningitis, tuberculosis, and contact sensitivity

In some instances, activated T cells initiate or promote disease by immune responses to microorganisms. For example, *lymphocytic choriomeningitis virus* infects the choroid membrane of the third and fourth lateral ventricles of the brain and the membranous meninges that cover the brain. Lethal neurological damage results, not from the virus itself, but from the cellular immune response to the infected cells. In the absence of an immune response (e.g., in a thymectomized host), the viral infection is not lethal.

T-cell immunity can also contribute to a disease condition if the immune response does not eliminate the microorganism. The tubercle bacillus that causes *tuberculosis* infects primarily host macrophages in the lungs (Figure 12-2). Most of these bacilli are killed within the activated macrophages, but a few survive, perhaps by releasing a substance that prevents fusion of phagosomes and lysosomes. Resistant bacilli can proliferate inside macrophages in the face of an active cellular and humoral immune response. This continued infection produces a chronic inflammation with the formation of granulomas (much as in the granulomatous diseases, Concept 12-1) at the expense of valuable lung tissue. Macrophages infected with the tubercle bacillus may swell to look like epithelial cells (epithelioid), and they may fuse to form giant multinucleate syncytial cells (Figure 12-2b). The resulting histopathological appearance is characteristic of tuberculosis granulomas. The signals for repair that normally accompany chronic inflammation cause proliferation of fibroblasts at the outer edges of the growing granuloma, resulting in formation of a fibrous tissue covering. Cells in the central core of the granuloma begin to die due to the lack of oxygen, the action of nonspecific cytotoxins characteristic of chronic inflammation (Concept 9-4), and the continued proliferation of tubercle bacilli. When the dead and dying cells in the core

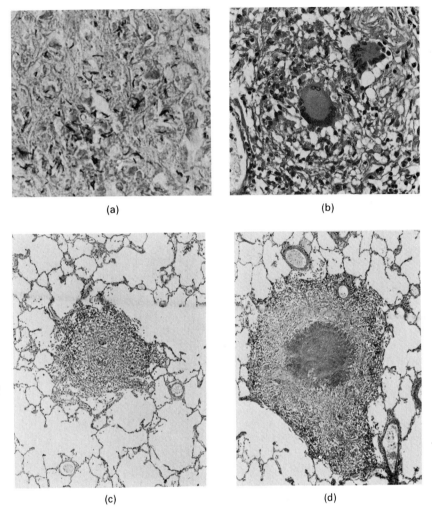

(a)

(b)

(c)

(d)

Figure 12-2
The histological appearance of tuberculosis in the lung. (a) A high-power view of tubercle bacilli inside macrophages. A dye that stains the rodlike bacilli is used. (b) A high-power view of cells in an early granuloma. The large multinucleate cells are characteristic of this process. Most of the dark nuclei are lymphocytic; other cells include macrophages and cells involved in repair and regeneration. (c) A low-power view of a central granuloma surrounded by relatively normal lung tissue (large air sacs separated by lacy-thin alveolar walls). The granuloma contains a central zone of giant cells and fibrous tissue, with a shell of lymphocytic infiltrate. (d) A higher-power view of a granuloma containing a core of dead tissue and surrounding fibrous tissue, giant cells, and a shell of lymphocytic infiltrate. [Photographs by R. Rouse and I. Weissman.]

rupture through the fibrous wall of the granuloma, they spread live tubercle bacilli to neighboring sites, eventually destroying sufficient lung tissue to kill an untreated host. The bacillus that causes *leprosy* is closely related to the tubercle bacillus, and it produces a similar destructive host response following preferential infection of macrophages in the skin and around nerves.

T-cell immunity to environmental haptens can cause a local, destructive immune response called *contact sensitivity*. Environmental haptens can bind to proteins or cell membranes in the skin and induce a local T-cell immune reaction to the hapten-conjugated proteins on cells. These haptens can be natural products (e.g., the active small molecules in poison ivy and poison oak leaves) or industrial reagents such as picryl (trinitrophenyl) chloride, which can form conjugates with cell-surface proteins through the ϵ-amino groups of lysine side chains. Sufficient concentrations of these contact-sensitizing agents

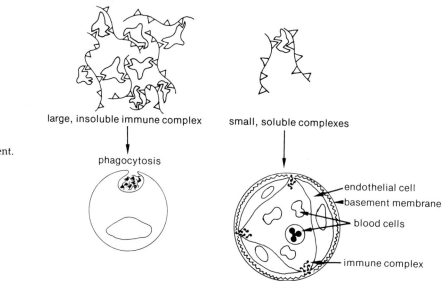

Figure 12-3

Fates of large and small complexes of antigen, antibody, and complement.

large, insoluble immune complex

small, soluble complexes

phagocytosis

endothelial cell
basement membrane
blood cells
immune complex

may induce a T-cell immune response that results in a chronic inflammatory focus as well as direct lysis of hapten-conjugated target cells.

Immune-complex diseases

Immune complexes of antigen, antibody, and complement can cause local, destructive, inflammatory lesions. Immune complexes may form in an immune response to a multideterminant antigen if antibody and antigen concentrations are appropriate (Concept 3-6). Large complexes are phagocytized, but smaller complexes may escape phagocytosis and pass between vessel endothelial cells to deposit on subendothelial basement membranes (Figure 12-3). If these complexes activate complement, they may induce an acute local inflammation at the site of deposition. This effect is usually transient, as antigen and complexes are cleared and antibody levels rise. However, if the inducing antigens are reintroduced or are produced endogenously or by organisms that cannot be eliminated, recurrent or continuous immune-complex diseases occur, leading to serious inflammatory problems. Immunofluorescence microscopy is often helpful in diagnosing immune-complex diseases because of the characteristic granular deposition of immunoglobulin, complement, and antigen on basement membranes underlying the cells that line blood vessels (Figure 12-4a).

The local inflammatory response initiated by immune-complex deposition and complement activation may cause release of vaso-active peptides that induce vasodilation, thereby revealing larger areas of vascular basement membrane. This process is especially notable in the small capillary tufts of the kidney glomeruli where blood filtration takes place (Figure 12-5). Normally, the kidney glomeruli allow

Figure 12-4

Immunofluorescence of renal immunoglobulin deposits in glomerulonephritis. (a) Immune-complex nephritis with granular deposits of IgG. (b) Goodpasture's syndrome with linear deposition of IgG on glomerular basement membranes. [Photographs by D. Rice and R. Kempson.]

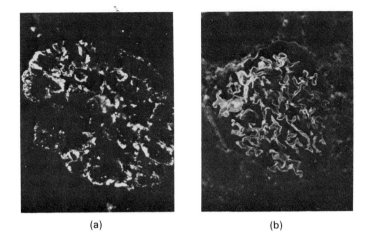

(a)   (b)

passage of small molecules, such as urea, but prevent passage of most serum proteins from the vascular lumen into the space that constitutes the beginning of the urinary tubules (Bowman's space).

As immune complexes settle on the epithelial side of the glomerular basement membrane, they continue to activate complement, thereby increasing vasodilation and deposition of more immune complexes. Larger complexes may be trapped primarily in the phagocytic mesangial cells lining the vascular stalk of the glomerulus, whereas smaller complexes continue to settle on either side of the basement membrane. In both cases, these complexes induce release of chemotactic factors that attract polymorphonuclear leukocytes, which tend to disrupt the attachment of epithelial-cell foot processes to the glomerular basement membrane. The polymorphonuclear leukocytes degranulate to release pyrogens (factors that stimulate brain centers to raise body temperature) and hydrolytic lysosomal enzymes that destroy large areas of the basement membrane. At this stage, serum proteins leak into Bowman's space and the kidney's function of clearing small molecules decreases dramatically. As phagocytic cells remove bound immune complexes, cells, and tissue debris, the glomerular endothelial and epithelial cells are replaced by cell division. The acute inflammation of the glomeruli is called *acute glomerulonephritis.* One type is commonly induced by the immune response to a particular protein (M protein) in streptococci. An acute glomerulonephritis that does *not* involve antibody can occur in blood infections by gram-negative organisms that activate the alternative complement pathway (Concept 9-2).

In addition to the acute glomerulonephritis just described, immune complexes may deposit in skin blood vessels to cause local rash and tissue damage (*Arthus phenomenon*); they may deposit in systemic blood vessels to cause *necrotising vasculitis* (*necro:* dead or dying); they may deposit in lymph nodes to cause swollen glands (*lymphadenitis*);

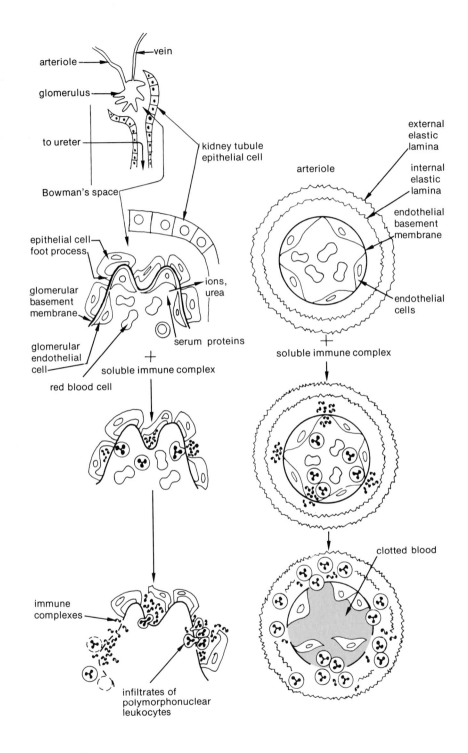

Figure 12-5
Immune-complex deposition injury to a kidney glomerulus (left) or to an arteriole (right). See text for details.

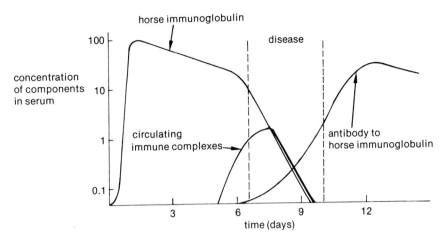

Figure 12-6

The time course of major events in serum sickness.

they may deposit in the small arteries in nodal foci throughout the body to cause *periarteritis nodosa* (in 10–20% of these patients the immune complexes contain hepatitis B viral antigens); and immune complexes may also deposit in joints to cause *arthritis*.

Serum sickness is an example of an immune-complex disease in which the initial antigen load is large. This disease was most common in the era before antibiotics, when serum from immunized animals was injected into humans to provide passive immunity to a particular pathogen or its toxins. Figure 12-6 illustrates the course of events in serum sickness following injection of horse immunoglobulins. The levels of horse immunoglobulins at first fall slowly, reflecting the intrinsic degradation rate of these proteins. Beginning at about day 8, the levels begin to fall more rapidly as the foreign protein begins to be eliminated by immune-complex formation. Concomitant with immune elimination of free horse immunoglobulins is an increase in antigen–antibody complexes and the appearance of the typical disease pattern: fever, rash, joint lesions, appearance of serum proteins in the urine (proteinuria), and retention in the serum of substances, such as urea, that are normally cleared by the kidneys. These indications of inflammatory disease subside as immune complexes disappear from the serum and free antibodies to horse immunoglobulins appear.

Systemic lupus erythematosis is a multisystem autoimmune disease in which immune complexes involving a variety of endogenous cellular components (especially nucleic acids) deposit in skin, joints, arteries, muscle, pericardium, and glomeruli. The antibodies directed against nucleic acids can be specific for RNA, single-stranded DNA, or double-stranded DNA. The life-threatening pathology of this disease is usually either kidney failure due to glomerular involvement or the side effects of immunosuppressive and anti-inflammatory drugs. The associated joint disease apparently lacks a T-cell component and is

Figure 12-7

Two LE cells (lupus erythematosis) from the blood of a patient with active disease. These LE cells are polymorphonuclear granulocytes which phagocytosed the nuclei of cells bearing antinuclear antibodies and are considered to be diagnostic for the disease systemic lupus erythematosis.

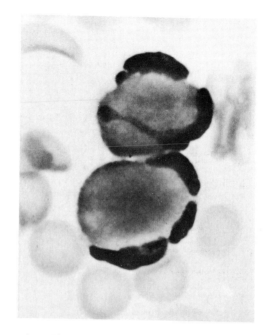

primarily an immune-complex disorder. Perhaps treatment of lupus patients with anti-inflammatory agents reverses the arthritis for this reason, whereas similar treatment of rheumatoid arthritis patients only temporarily abates the progress of their joint disease.

The etiology of systemic lupus erythematosis is not understood, but lupus patients have many types of antibodies specific for normal cellular components. Target cells of unknown type are presumably lysed in an initial, perhaps autoimmune, event to release cytoplasmic components and nuclei, which in turn elicit characteristic autoimmune responses. A hallmark of this disease is the presence in the blood of polymorphonuclear leukocytes that have phagocytosed IgG-coated cell nuclei (Figure 12-7). Of biological interest is the recent finding that lupus patients often have high concentrations of antibodies to small nuclear RNAs and/or to classes of proteins associated with them. Some of these RNAs have sequences that are complementary to the intron-exon boundaries in natural genes, suggesting that they may participate in the splicing step in messenger-RNA processing.

12-7 A breakdown in immunological tolerance can cause autoimmune diseases

Mechanisms of tolerance breakdown

Immune responses to self components represent a failure of immunological tolerance. As a result, forbidden clones of T cells and B cells emerge bearing receptors for self-antigens, which can lead to the production of self-directed antibodies, cytotoxic T cells, and inflammatory T cells. Such a breakdown in tolerance produces an autoimmune response that can cause disease. Autoimmune responses usually arise because certain helper T cells are induced or critical suppressor T cells are inhibited. For example, an immune response to nonself-antigens can activate lymphocytes that bear anti-self receptors which had been maintained in a state of nonreactivity. A set of functional B-cell clones often remains inactive only because the appropriate helper T cells are inactive. Sometimes the introduction of a foreign antigen attached to a self-antigen can break tolerance by inducing a helper T cell that can stimulate self-reactive B cells to produce autoantibodies. For example, dinitrophenol (DNP) modified autologous thyroglobulin can induce thyroglobulin-specific antibodies because the modification presents a foreign antigenic determinant in the context of self-determinants (Figure 12-8). The new antigenic determinant may result from the dinitrophenol hapten itself or from a secondary conformational change. A similar situation arises when thyroglobulin from another species is injected because it also presents unique foreign determinants in the context of self-antigens (Figure 12-8). Once induced, the antibodies to self-determinants on thyroglobulin can eliminate all circulating thyroglobulin, theoretically permitting the emergence of other T-cell and B-cell clones that are reactive to self thyroglobulin.

The example with heterologous thyroglobulin is especially relevant to patients who receive animal-hormone replacement therapy—for example, with bovine insulin or bovine adrenocorticotropic hormone. This same general process may also underlie the brain and nerve damage that can follow a rabies vaccination if the vaccine is prepared in heterologous tissue. A similar situation may be responsible for heart damage during *rheumatic fever*, which involves certain streptococci that carry antigenic determinants that cross-react with heart muscle. In general, whenever self- and foreign antigenic determinants are linked together, they have the potential for inducing self-reactive antibodies.

The failure of antigen-specific suppression by suppressor T cells may also allow clones of anti-self-lymphocytes to be activated. Loss of specific T_S cells or nonspecific loss of this class of cells could result in the spontaneous appearance of autoantibodies. This notion is supported by the finding that animals postnatally deprived of their thymus have a higher incidence of autoantibodies, and that animals with a genetic predilection for autoimmune diseases show an accelerated course of these diseases when thymectomized. In addition, several mouse strains with genetically determined autoimmune disorders all have abnormally high B-cell activity, and they apparently have defects in suppressor T-cell function. Analysis with monoclonal antibodies directed against T-cell-surface differentiation markers and MHC markers may help to identify the precise defects in these strains.

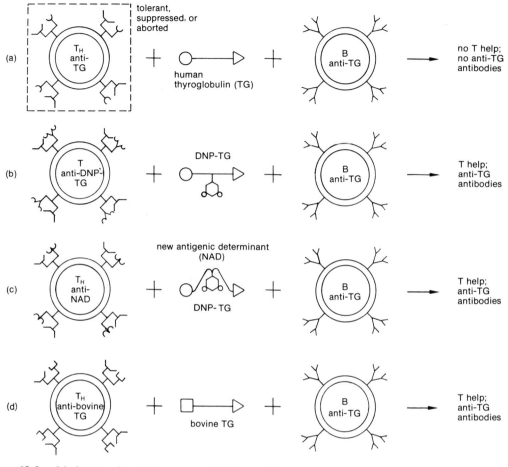

Figure 12-8 Mechanisms by which tolerance to an autologous thyroglobulin (TG) may be broken. (a) Normal tolerance; lack of active antithyroglobulin T_H cells prevents triggering of antithyroglobulin B cells. Hapten modification of thyroglobulin by DNP, for example, can result in stimulation of T_H cells that react to either (b) DNP-thyroglobulin or (c) new antigenic determinants revealed on the hapten-modified thyroglobulin. (d) Injection of thyroglobulin from another species (e.g., bovine thyroglobulin) may stimulate T_H cells reactive to specific antigenic determinants on bovine thyroglobulin.

Perhaps a similar analysis of human cell-surface markers will be useful in the diagnosis and therapy of some human autoimmune disorders.

Self-directed humoral immunity

Antibodies to self-antigens can cause disease in several ways. Antibodies to cell-surface antigens can cause cell death by direct complement-mediated cell lysis, by antibody-dependent cell-mediated cytotoxicity, and by opsonization. Antibodies against cell-surface receptors can interfere with cell functions. Finally, antibodies against supporting basement membranes can interfere with tissue function.

The most common cell types affected are blood cells—lymphocytes, platelets, polymorphonuclear leukocytes, and erythrocytes. In the rare disease known as *episodic lymphopenia with lymphocytotoxins*, patients periodically produce a serum autoantibody that lyses T cells in the presence of complement (Figure 12-1e). These episodic decreases in T-cell numbers are accompanied by the typical immunodeficiencies associated with T-cell absence (Concept 12-4). Autoantibodies to platelets (thrombocytes) can induce *thrombocytopenic purpura*—a general name for platelet-loss diseases. Autoantibodies to platelets may arise after some infections, after some drug therapies, or spontaneously. The resulting decrease in blood-clotting functions leads to multiple hemorrhages that are most visible in the skin and gums as purple spots (purpura). *Agranulocytosis* is a disease caused by autoantibodies to polymorphonuclear leukocytes; it renders patients highly susceptible to bacterial infections. This condition can be induced by drug treatment—for example, by amidopyrine and sulfa drugs, such as sulfapyridine and sulfathiazole. In *autoimmune hemolytic anemias,* autoantibodies directed at antigens on erythrocyte surfaces produce hemolysis (cell lysis that releases free hemoglobin into the serum) and anemia (decreased numbers of circulating erythrocytes). This disease is often initiated by antibodies against drugs like penicillin, quinidine, and α-methyl dopa, which adsorb to red cells.

One special case of an autoimmunelike disease directed at red blood cells is the occasional immunological attack of mother on fetus. During birth, a mother usually receives a small infusion of fetal blood. If an antigen known as Rh is present on fetal blood cells but lacking in the mother, then the mother may produce anti-Rh IgG antibodies. This response to a foreign blood-cell determinant is the same as that occurring after transfusion of mismatched blood, which is followed by massive immune hemolysis (*transfusion reaction*). However, the danger in the case of Rh incompatibility is that the anti-Rh IgG can cross the placental barrier in a *subsequent* pregnancy to cause massive antibody destruction of Rh-positive red blood cells in the fetus (*erythroblastosis fetalis*). This disease does not occur when there is a maternal-fetal incompatibility for the A-B-O blood groups because the mother's IgM antibodies, which do not cross the placenta, bind to and remove fetal blood cells, thereby preventing the induction of an IgG response.

Antibodies to cell-surface receptors can cause disease by interfering with receptor function. For example, antibodies to acetylcholine receptors at nerve–muscle junctions are found in patients with *myasthenia gravis,* a progressive (and usually fatal) disease beginning with muscle weakness and fatigue and ending with loss of breathing control by the diaphragm and trunk muscles. These antibodies impede neuromuscular transmission by coating the receptors and also by increasing their rate of breakdown by antigenic modulation, by lysis, and by opsonization for phagocytes, which remove or digest them.

Another disease caused by receptor blockade is *insulin-resistant diabetes.*

Anti-receptor antibodies against receptors also can stimulate receptors, thereby mimicking the effect of an endogenous specific ligand. The best-known example of this phenomenon is *Graves' disease* or hyperthyroidism. Patients with this disease almost always have antibodies directed against the thyroid-cell receptor for thyroid-stimulating hormone, which is produced by the pituitary. When administered to suitable hosts, these antibodies bind to the hormone receptors and stimulate thyroid gland cells to produce and excrete increased levels of thyroid hormones. Such antibodies are known clinically as long-acting thyroid stimulators (LATS).

Autoantibodies to vascular basement membranes can cause disease by initiating an acute inflammatory response that interferes with tissue function. In a particularly striking form of this condition, called *Goodpasture's syndrome*, autoantibodies are produced against determinants common to kidney glomerular and lung alveolar basement membranes. In the glomerulus, the result is an even, linear deposition of immunoglobulin and complement on the endothelial side of the basement membrane, which may induce glomerulonephritis with infiltration of polymorphonuclear leukocytes, much as in immune-complex diseases (Concept 12-6). However, these two conditions can be distinguished readily by the appearance of the immunoglobulin deposits in immunofluorescence microscopy (Figure 12-4b). Immunopathogenic levels of antibodies to glomerular basement membranes have been observed in kidney transplant patients after kidney rejection and as a consequence of immunosuppressive treatment with impure anti-lymphocyte serum.

Self-directed cellular immunity

A breakdown in tolerance resulting in cellular immunity to endogenous antigens can lead to an immunopathologic destruction of vital tissues. Depending on the distribution of the inducing self-antigen, the effector phase of T-cell immunity may be organ-specific or widespread. In certain human diseases, organ-specific, T-cell destruction is a prominent component, but, as with most autoimmune responses, it is not clear what triggered the self-directed immunity. Experimentally, organ-specific autoimmunity can be readily induced by injection of heterologous organ homogenates.

Patients with *Hashimoto's thyroiditis* all exhibit a chronic inflammatory reaction in the thyroid, and T cells from some of these patients are reactive to human thyroid antigens (Figure 12-9). In some cases of adrenal insufficiency (*Addison's disease*), cellular immunity is directed at adrenal cell antigens.

In encephalomyelitic diseases, such as *multiple sclerosis*, in which demyelination of central and peripheral nerves is prominent, it is likely that cellular and humoral immunity contribute to the characteristic inflammation (neuritis) and destruction (neuropathy) of nerve

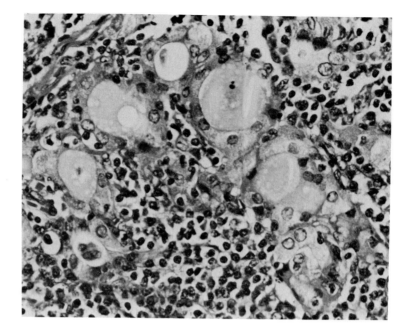

Figure 12-9

Thyroid from a patient with Hashimoto's thyroiditis. The predominant cell types that infiltrate the thyroid are lymphocytes and macrophages. [Photograph by R. Rouse.]

fibers. Peripheral neuritis without central nervous system lesions also may occur; for example, patients with relapsing polyneuritis produce monoclonal IgM antibodies directed against myelin proteins in peripheral nerves only. Immune demyelination may not be due simply to a breakdown in tolerance. Systemic injection of autologous brain tissue with an adjuvant leads to an *experimental autoimmune encephalomyelitis*. It appears that brain antigens are not normally presented to lymphoid organs (the brain has no lymphatics) and, therefore, that sensitization to brain antigens does not occur. However, once brain-specific cellular and humoral immunity have developed, the effector mechanisms can penetrate the blood–brain barrier to bring about the autoimmune disorder.

Diseases with complex, multisystem manifestations that result from loss of an important class of cells may have a T-cell autoimmune origin. A likely example is *juvenile-onset diabetes mellitus*, which is caused by lack of β cells in the islet-of-Langerhans of the pancreas. Patients with this disease show ample evidence of immune responses to their self-antigens, including T-cell and B-cell immunity to β-cell membrane and cytoplasmic antigens, as well as to insulin. Immune responses to insulin receptors on other cells are not found in juvenile-onset diabetes mellitus, and they are only a rare cause of insulin-resistant diabetes mellitus.

Animal studies support the view that cellular autoimmunity is involved in the pathogenesis of juvenile diabetes mellitus. For example, diabetes can be induced in rats and mice by the drug streptozocin, which probably induces specific damage to islet cells, and by several viruses—including encephalomyocarditis virus, coxsackievirus B4, and two strains of reovirus—all of which infect pancreatic islet-of-Langerhans cells. In all cases, the islet-cell damage produces a cellular autoimmunity to these cells and causes diabetes. On the basis of such evidence, it is thought that cellular immunity to virally infected cells may play a central role in the genesis of juvenile diabetes mellitus. Such a mechanism could be reconciled with the known genetic predilection for this disease, for example, by an increased sensitivity to viral infection conferred by specific MHC genes as described in Concept 12-9.

Inappropriate cellular as well as humoral immunity may contribute to several diseases. For example, some patients with *pernicious anemia* are unable to absorb vitamin B_{12}, which is necessary for erythroid and myeloid differentiation in the bone marrow. These individuals are usually deficient in intrinsic factor, a polypeptide that binds vitamin B_{12} and allows its absorption across the intestinal epithelium. In some of these patients, the stomach parietal cells, which normally produce intrinsic factor, are deficient, presumably as a result of parietal-cell-specific cellular autoimmunity. In others, the parietal cells produce and excrete intrinsic factor normally, but the factor is neutralized by specific humoral autoantibodies.

Rheumatoid arthritis is another example of a chronic autoimmune disorder in which the characteristic joint lesions involve both cellular and humoral immune responses. A prominent feature of this disease is the deposition in the joints of IgM-IgG-complement complexes. The IgM antibodies are directed against IgG antigenic determinants; these IgM antibodies in the serum are called *rheumatoid factor*. Continuing inflammation eventually leads to the destruction of both cartilage and bone in the joint. Helper T cells have been implicated in several aspects of the disease: they are prominent in the cellular infiltrate in the joints; they stimulate resident macrophages to release proteases, inflammatory mediators, and a factor that stimulates the synovial cells lining the joint cavities to release collagenase, an enzyme that destroys the collagen matrix cartilage; they activate osteoclasts, bone cells whose normal function is to digest bone matrix during bone growth repair; and they probably contribute to the local production of autoantibodies, some of which activate the complement system to cause acute inflammation.

12-8 Clinical allergy is caused by an exaggerated IgE response

Allergic responses

Some individuals develop exaggerated IgE responses to environmental, drug, or microbial antigens. Reexposure to even minute amounts of these antigens can then trigger release of mast-cell products, either locally or systemically. The specific IgE mast-cell complexes are so persistent that such a response may occur long after the synthesis of IgE directed against the original immunogen has ceased. Individuals who exhibit such responses are said to be allergic to the inducing antigens. Such reactions are often called *atopic* or *anaphylactic.* (The IgE antibodies also are called *reaginic* antibodies, and antigens that induce these reactions are called *allergens.*)

The pathological manifestations of IgE-antigen interaction are due to mast-cell degranulation that results in the release of histamine, heparin, a chemotactic factor for eosinophilic leukocytes, and the leukotrienes (C4, D4, and E4) that cause prolonged constriction of bronchial smooth muscle cells (Concept 9-3). Pathological allergic reactions differ from other antibody reactions by their independence of complement, by their induction in response to minute doses of antigen, by their production of vascular and smooth muscle effects that appear in minutes, rather than hours, and by their susceptibility to prevention with antihistamines and to treatment with epinephrine. Epinephrine prevents mast-cell degranulation by raising cellular cAMP levels, and it also antagonizes the action on smooth muscles of histamine and leukotrienes.

Allergic diseases may have systemic or local manifestations, depending on the route of entry of the antigen and the pattern of deposition of IgE and mast cells. Most local manifestations occur on epithelial surfaces at the site of entry of the allergen. Allergic individuals characteristically give rapid responses in skin testing, have high serum IgE levels, and often have increased blood and tissue concentrations of eosinophilic leukocytes.

Systemic anaphylaxis (anaphylactic shock) results from an IgE-basophil (the equivalent in the blood of a mast cell) response to intravascular antigen. The release of mast-cell mediators produces a biphasic response of vasoconstriction followed by peripheral vessel dilation. The result is a pooling of blood in the periphery and a concomitant drop in blood pressure (*shock*). Individuals who are sensitized to the venom toxins of biting and stinging insects may suffer fatal anaphylactic shock as the result of a simple bee sting.

Food allergies involve intestinal IgE mast-cell responses to ingested antigens. These responses may affect the upper gastrointestinal tract, causing vomiting, or the lower gastrointestinal tract, causing cramps and diarrhea. If sufficient antigen is ingested, systemic anaphylaxis and skin reactions may occur.

Skin reactions of the IgE mast-cell system may be acute or chronic. If acute, they may be a cause of *hives* (urticaria); if chronic, they may result in atopic dermatitis, a type of eczema, whose cause is unclear.

Allergic reactions of the upper respiratory tract are usually grouped together and called hayfever (*allergic rhinitis*). Some patients affected by this condition develop large nasal polyps that presumably result from chronic atopic reactions to nasal allergens. Reactions of the lower respiratory tract usually center in the bronchi and bronchioles, causing constriction and airway obstruction, and they are a major cause of *asthma*. The acute effects are probably due to histamine release, and the long-term effects are probably due to leukotrienes C4, D4, and E4.

Desensitization

IgE-mediated diseases are usually treated by *desensitization* procedures that involve the periodic injection of just suballergic doses of the allergen. Desensitization treatments may induce an IgG response that competes with IgE for the allergen, or they may induce specific suppressor T cells that block the synthesis of IgE directed against the allergen. Receptor blockade with monovalent, nonmetabolizable antigens may prove to be another approach to desensitization; it would prevent expression of an existing allergy by inactivating IgE mast-cell complexes, and it would prevent further production of IgE antibodies by blockading B_ϵ cells. It is also conceivable that chemically synthesized or genetically engineered IgE-specific Fc peptides could compete effectively for mast-cell and basophil Fc_ϵ receptors, thereby blocking access to IgE antibodies.

12-9 The predilection for some immunologic diseases is linked genetically to the major histocompatibility complex

The finding that human leukocyte antigens (HLA) are important in tissue transplantation (Concept 11-1) stimulated widespread investigation into the numbers and genetic relationships of these antigens. Although the major histocompatibility complex, which codes for these antigens, is highly polymorphic, particular MHC determinants occur with higher than expected frequencies in patients with certain diseases. Table 12-4 lists diseases that show significant associations with particular MHC determinants. Although this list is undoubtedly still incomplete, it suggests that immunopathology plays an important role in many diseases.

The cellular and molecular bases for the relationship between particular MHC determinants and diseases is not known, but they could involve any of several phenomena. Diseases associated with D-region determinants, which are the counterparts of I-region immune response genes in mice (Concept 8-9), could involve an inadequate or augmented response to a particular antigen. Diseases associated with A, B, or C MHC determinants could arise for several reasons. A particular MHC determinant could be the target of an autoimmune response. T_H- or T_S-*associated recognition* of a particular MHC determinant could be unusual, resulting in an inappropriately high or low response to cells that bear associated antigens. It is even conceiv-

Table 12-4   Examples of Associations Between Particular Diseases and the MHC in Humans

Disease	Linked HLA Region Determinant	Disease Risk of Persons Who Bear Determinant (Relative to Disease Risk in the Population at Large = 1)	Description of Disease
Inflammatory diseases:			
ankylosing spondylitis	B(27)	100–200	Inflammation of the spine, leading to stiffening of vertebral joints
Reiter's syndrome	B(27)	40	Inflammation of the spine, prostate, and parts of the eye (the uvea, which is the iris, the ciliary body, and the choroid)
acute anterior uveitis	B(27)	30	Inflammation of the iris and ciliary body
juvenile rheumatoid arthritis (Type II)	B(27)	10–12	A multisystem inflammatory disease of children characterized by rapid onset of joint lesions and fever
psoriasis	B(13)	4–5	An acute, recurrent, localized inflammatory disease of the skin (usually scalp, elbows, and knees), often associated with arthritis
celiac disease	B(8) D(Dw3)	9–10	A chronic inflammatory disease of the small intestine; probably a food allergy to a protein in grains
multiple sclerosis	D(DR2)	5	A progressive chronic inflammatory disease of brain and spinal cord that causes hardening (sclerosis) and loss of function in affected foci
rheumatic fever	DR(antibody 833)	4–5	An autoimmune disease wherein antibodies raised during β-hemolytic streptococcal pharyngitis cross-react with heart tissue to give rise to a damaging myocarditis and valvulitis

(table continues on next page)

Disease	Linked HLA Region Determinant	Disease Risk of Persons Who Bear Determinant (Relative to Disease Risk in the Population at Large = 1)	Description of Disease
Allergies:			
ragweed hayfever	many loci, direct linkage shown in family studies	difficult to calculate	An IgE-mediated allergic response to ragweed extracts
Endocrine diseases:			
Addison's disease	D(DR3)	4–10	A deficiency in production of adrenal gland cortical hormones
diabetes mellitus	D(DR3, DR4)	2–5	A deficiency of insulin production; pancreatic islet cells usually absent or damaged
Graves' disease	D	10–12	A hyperactivity of the thyroid; patients often produce an IgG antibody that stimulates thyroid function
Malignant diseases:			
acute lymphocytic leukemia	A(2)	1.2–1.4	A cancer of lymphocytes, usually in children
Hodgkin's disease	A(A1)	1.5–1.8	A cancer of lymph-node cells; local inflammation is prominent, as well as selective deficiency in cellular immunity and T-cell functions

able that MHC structures could serve as sites for attachment and entry of potentially pathogenic viruses. If the MHC is important for nonimmunologic cell interactions during development, then some MHC determinants might cause inappropriate development. Some of the extensive polymorphism of MHC determinants could conceivably be the result of their associations with diseases, which would constitute a powerful selective force in evolution.

Selected Bibliography

Textbooks for detailed reading

Stites, D. P., Stobo, J. D., Fudenberg, H. H., and Wells, J. V., *Basic and Clinical Immunology*, 4th ed., Lange Medical Publications, Los Altos, Cal., 1982.

Twomey, J. J., Ed., *The Pathophysiology of Human Immunologic Disorders*, Urban and Schwarzenberg, Baltimore, Md., 1982.

Clinical immunology and immunopathology are rapidly becoming independent disciplines. Each of the preceding texts covers these expanding fields in extensive clinical and histopathologic detail. These texts are useful as well-written, current reference books, and they are probably most valuable for students of clinical medicine and practicing physicians.

Immunological deficiency diseases

Good, R. A., Varco, R. L., Aust, J. B., and Zak, J., "Transplantation studies in patients with agammaglobulinemia," *Ann. N.Y. Acad. Sci.* **64**, 882(1957).

Porter, H. M., "The demonstration of delayed-type reactivity in congenital agammaglobulinemia," *Ibid.* **64**, 932(1957).

The preceding articles give two early views of the immune defect in agammaglobulinemia.

Carson, D. A., Lakow, E., Wasson, D. B., and Kamatami, N., "Lymphocyte dysfunction caused by deficiencies in purine metabolism," *Imm. Today* **2**, 234(1982).

Johnston, R. B., "Defects of neutrophil function," *New Eng. J. Med.* **307**, 434(1982).

Schroff, R. W., Gottlieb, M. S., Prince, H. E., Chai, L. L., and Fahey, J. L., "Immunological studies of homosexual men with immunodeficiency and Kaposi's sarcoma," *Clin. Immunol. and Immunopath.* **27**, 300–314(1983).

Autoimmunity, immune-complex disease, and antibody-mediated injury

Burnet, F. M., *Autoimmunity and Autoimmune Disease*, F. A. Davis, Philadelphia, Pa., 1972.

The preceding book is a scholarly and speculative approach to the problem of autoimmunity.

Cohen, I. R., Ben-Nun, A., Holoshitz, J., Maron, J., and Zerubavel, R., "Vaccination against autoimmune disease with lines of autoimmune T lymphocytes," *Immunol. Today* **4**, 227(1983).

Dixon, F. J., "Murine SLE models and autoimmune disease," *Hosp. Practice* **3** (March), 63(1982).

McFarlin, D., and Waksman, B., "Altered immune function in demyelinative disease," *Immunol. Today* **3**, 321(1982).

Smith, H. R., and Steinberg, A. D., "Autoimmunity—a perspective," *Annu. Rev. Immunol.* **1**, 1975(1983).

Theofilopoulos, A. N., and Dixon, F. J., "Autoimmune diseases: immunopathology and etiopathogenesis," *Am. J. Pathol.* **108**, 321(1982).

IgE-mediated clinical allergy

Austen, K. F., "Tissue mast cells in immediate hypersensitivity," *Hosp. Practice* **11** (Nov.), 98(1982).

Marsh, D. G., Meyers, D. A., and Bus, W. B., "The epidemiology and genetics of atopic allergy," *New Eng. J. Med.* **305**, 1551(1981).

Weissmann, G., "The eicasanoids of asthma," *New Eng. J. Med.* **308**, 454(1983).

Additional diseases and concepts introduced in the problems

1. Adult onset dysgammaglobulinemia. Problem 12-3

2. Myasthenia gravis. Problem 12-4

3. DiGeorge syndrome. Problem 12-5

4. Partial lipodystrophy glomerulonephritis. Problem 12-6

5. Mouse X-linked immunodeficiency. Problem 12-10

6. Autoimmune hemolytic anemia. Problem 12-11

7. Hereditary angioedema. Problem 12-12

8. Scrapie and Kuru. Problem 12-13

Problems

12-1   Indicate whether each of the following statements is true or false. Explain the error in each statement you consider to be false.

(a) Chronic granulomatous disease is a phagocytic cell dysfunction caused by defective membrane receptors for IgG and IgM Fc regions.

(b) Recurrent pneumonia in patients with cystic fibrosis (a disease in which thickened mucous secretions prevent normal mucous flow) is a good example of failure of innate immunity mechanisms.

(c) The blood of children with Bruton's disease (X-linked agammaglobulinemia) usually lacks mature B cells.

(d) Antagonists of mast-cell degranulation can inhibit the development of kidney disease in systemic lupus erythematosis (SLE).

(e) Acquired immunodeficiency syndrome (AIDS) is an epidemic immunodeficiency caused by autoantibodies to immature stages of B-cell development.

(f) Contact sensitivity is a skin reaction that can be transferred passively with reaginic (IgE) antibody.

(g) Evidence that structural genes for immunoglobulin H chains are on the X chromosome was first demonstrated by the genetic analysis of Bruton's disease.

(h) Lymphocytic choriomeningitis virus is nonlethal in thymus-deprived hosts.

(i) The immunopathological injury formerly associated with rabies virus vaccination involved the activation of an autoimmune process.

(j) The activating agent in part (i) was a passenger virus present in the primary host cells.

(k) The effector cells in part (i) were in the T-cell series.

(l) Clinically, patients treated with antilymphocyte serum (ALS) would be expected to show a rapid decrease in circulating long-lived antibodies (e.g., antibodies to polio virus).

(m) Patients who lack the enzyme adenosine deaminase have a selective deficit in development of plasma cells (plasmacytopoiesis).

(n) The most common cause of immunological deficiency in man is medical care.

(o) The predisposition for ankylosing spondylitis is genetically linked to the major blood-group antigen locus, ABO.

12-2   Supply the missing word or words in each of the following statements.

(a) The lack of an appropriate immune response to infection in the case of severe combined immunodeficiency is due to the failure in development or function of _____ and _____ cells.

(b) Rheumatoid arthritis is associated with serum antibodies, usually of the _____ class, which react against _____ .

(c) Patients with hayfever have abnormal concentrations of _____ antibodies, which, upon combination with their cognate antigen, activate _____ .

(d) Linear deposition of antigen–antibody complexes on the glomerular basement membrane is detected by fluorescent anti-IgG antibody in _____ .

(e) Patients with the disease described in part (d) may also have such patterns in basement membranes of _____ .

(f) As a pharmacologist, you wish to prepare a cytotoxic agent to be used as a preventative for people with bee sting sensitivity. The purpose of your agent will be to eliminate _____ cells.

(g) Hyperacute rejection of organ allografts involves infiltration of _____.

(h) _____ is a disease of complement regulation. The disease involves recurrent, local episodes of acute inflammation that may be fatal when they affect the larynx.

(i) Patients with _____ have disorders of balance and movement as well as immune deficiency.

(j) Rheumatic fever is an example of an autoimmune disease induced by _____ .

(k) Skin lesions caused by poison oak involve an immune hypersensitivity of the _____ system.

(l) Patients who develop progressive vaccinia viral infections following vaccination for smallpox most likely suffer from a disease that affects _____ lymphocytes.

(m) C3 deficiency results in a decreased resistance to _____ infections.

(n) Systemic lupus erythematosis results in immunological injury to several organs because of the production of _____ .

(o) Systemic anaphylaxis is a life-threatening consequence of immune hypersensitivity, and it should be treated with _____ and _____ .

(p) _____ are generally oily substances that serve as tissue depots and otherwise nonspecifically stimulate the immune response when injected with immunizing antigens.

12-3 A clinical investigator and colleagues at the National Institutes of Health studied several patients with common variable hypogammaglobulinemia. These patients presented an intriguing contrast to autoimmune patients. They had greatly reduced levels of serum immunoglobulins (less than 2 mg/mL IgG compared to about 12 mg/mL normally and less than 0.1 mg/mL IgM plus IgA compared to 4–5 mg/mL normally), but they had variable numbers of Ig^+ B cells, ranging from normal to significantly reduced. The patients ranged in age from 16 to 54 years. The clinical investigation team isolated peripheral blood lymphocytes from each patient and cultured them *in vitro* for 7 days in the presence of pokeweed mitogen, which is active on human B cells. The amount of immunoglobulin secreted was measured by sensitive radioimmunoassays. Table 12-5 summarizes data from normal control individuals and from the patients. Table 12-6 shows the results when lymphocytes from one patient were cultured together with lymphocytes from three different normal individuals. With reference to these tables, answer the following questions.

(a) What do you conclude from these data?

(b) The clinical investigation team then treated some lymphocytes from patient 2 with an anti-immunoglobulin antiserum plus complement and cultured the remaining cells with normal lymphocytes. The results were equivalent to those shown in Table 12-5. What do you conclude from this observation?

(c) Cells from five patients inhibited more than 85% of the immunoglobulin production in mixed cultures. However, cells from three other patients with common variable hypogammaglobulinemia had no inhibitory effects whatsoever. For those patients with an inherent B-cell defect only, indicate each major point at which development might be blocked in the life history of B cells from stem cells.

12-4 Muscles are stimulated to contract when the nerve endings at neuromuscular junctions release acetylcholine (ACh). This transmitter binds to acetylcholine-receptor

Table 12-5 Effects of Pokeweed Mitogen (PWM) on
Immunoglobulin Biosynthesis by Peripheral Blood Lymphocytes
from Normal and Hypogammaglobulinemic Individuals
(Problem 12-3)

	IgG[a]	IgA[a]	IgM[a]
Control individuals:			
without PWM	212	303	537
with PWM	1641	1698	3715
Hypogammaglobulinemia patients:			
with or without PWM	100	100	100

[a]Expressed as geometric mean immunoglobulin synthesis in nanograms for 7-day
culture of 2×10^6 lymphocytes. [Adapted from T. Waldmann, et al., *Lancet* **2**,
609(1974).]

Table 12-6 Immunoglobulin Synthesis by Normal Lymphocytes Co-Cultured with
Lymphocytes from Patient 2 with Common Variable Hypogammaglobulinemia (Problem 12-3)

	IgG		IgA		IgM	
	Amount[a]	Percent Inhibition	Amount[a]	Percent Inhibition	Amount[a]	Percent Inhibition
Normal A alone	1640		640		2860	
Patient 2 alone	0		0		26	
Co-culture 2 + A	0	100	14	98	400	86
Normal B alone	1920		2120		11200	
Patient 2 alone	0		12		0	
Co-culture 2 + B	60	97	80	96	0	100
Normal C alone	1120		760		4600	
Patient 2 alone	0		12		0	
Co-culture 2 + C	70	94	130	83	448	90

[a]Expressed as nanograms synthesized per culture in the presence of pokeweed mitogen during a 7-day period. [From T.
Waldmann, et al., *Lancet* **2**, 609(1974).]

(AChR) proteins in muscle-cell membranes to depolarize the membrane and initiate
muscular contractions. A group of clinical researchers injected rats with from 1.1 to
350 picomoles of purified electric eel AChR protein suspended in complete Freund's
adjuvant. This immunization elicited a set of physical symptoms that included
weight loss, generalized muscular weakness, a characteristic hunched posture with
chin and elbows on the floor, and jerky movements of the head and forelimbs when
attempting ambulation. The animals were graded, as shown in Table 12-7, on the
following simple scale: 0, no definite weakness; +, weak grip with fatigability;

Table 12-7 A Syndrome in Rats After a Single Challenge with Eel AChR (Problem 12-4)

Dose (pico-moles)	Number of Animals with the Syndrome			Maximum Severity[c]		
	Total[a]	Early[b]	Late[b]	$+$	$++$	$+++$
350	21/23	21	15	2	2	17
110	10/10	9	9	0	2	8
55	2/2	2	2	0	1	1
35	8/9	6	6	1	1	6
11	6/11	5	4	3	2	1
3.5	7/9	6	4	2	5	0
1.1	0/10	0	0	0	0	0
0	0/10	0	0	0	0	0

[a]Number with syndrome/number injected.
[b]Rats were observed for up to 80 days. Early: before day 16; late: generally after day 20.
[c]See text.
[From V. A. Lennon, J. M. Lindstrom, and M. E. Seybold, *J. Exp. Med.*, **141**, 1365(1975). Copyright 1975 by the Rockefeller University Press.]

$++$, hunched posture with head down, movements uncoordinated; $+++$, severe generalized weakness, no grip, tremulous, moribund. Figure 12-10 shows a rabbit injected with AChR before (left) and after (right) reversal of neuromuscular blockade by a drug that markedly increases ACh levels. With reference to the table, answer the following questions.

(a) Can you explain all the symptoms (including weight loss) by a single underlying cause?

(b) What further studies could you do on the sera of these rats to test your explanation?

(c) The adjuvant was absolutely required to induce the clinical syndrome. Can you suggest a reasonable explanation for this requirement?

(d) Thymectomized rats do not develop this syndrome. In view of this finding, what models would you propose to explain the results of AChR immunization?

(e) A human disease called *myasthenia gravis* is characterized by weakness and fatigability of voluntary skeletal muscles, particularly of the head, neck, upper limbs, and respiratory apparatus. The number of acetylcholine binding sites is reduced in biopsied nerve–muscle junctions in these patients.

Furthermore, immunosuppressive therapy is often beneficial to these patients. What do you infer from these data? Might this disease have an autoimmune etiology? What further studies would you carry out to test this possibility?

(f) Serum or purified immunoglobulins from myasthenia gravis patients and controls were added to purified AChR, and ^{125}I-labeled α-bungarotoxin (a molecule that binds specifically to AChR) was added to assay availability of binding sites.

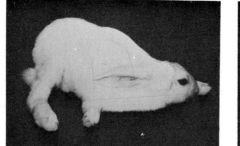 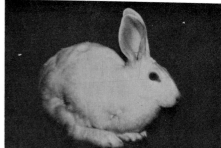

Figure 12-10   The effect of acetylcholinesterase inhibitors on paralysis (Problem 12-4). The left photograph shows a rabbit 5 days after the third injection of acetylcholine receptor. The right photograph shows the same animal 1 minute after receiving 0.3 mg of edrophonium intravenously. [From J. Patrick and J. Lindstrom, *Science* **180**, 871(1973). Copyright 1973 by the American Association for the Advancement of Science.]

The results are shown in Table 12-8. What conclusions can you draw from these data?

(g) Blood lymphocytes from myasthenia gravis patients and controls were incubated with purified AChR (or with medium alone) for 5 days and then tested for AChR-stimulated DNA synthesis by measuring the incorporation of ^{3}H-thymidine into cellular DNA. The ratio of

$$\frac{\text{cpm (AChR)}}{\text{cpm (medium)}}$$

is termed the *stimulation index* for a population of lymphocytes, and usually a stimulation index of >2 is significant. It is assumed that only T cells from immune hosts respond. The data are presented in Figures 12-11 and 12-12. What conclusions can be drawn from these data? Give three hypotheses to explain why these patients may have a decreased frequency of ^{125}I-α-bungarotoxin muscle receptors.

(h) Suppose that one could induce myasthenia gravis-like symptoms in mice by the injection of anti-AChR antibodies and that the syndrome, although controllable with drugs, lasted at least several months. Could the syndrome be due to receptor blockade by injected antibodies?

(i) Suppose that the mice in part (h) gave data such as those described for humans in parts (f) and (g). Propose several lines of *in vivo* and *in vitro* analysis by which you could elucidate the immunopathological mechanisms of this disease.

12-5 (a) Your patient is a newborn child with multiple minor congenital anomalies involving the lips and ears. There is no history of congenital defects in two siblings. You incubate a cord blood sample with phytohemagglutinin for cytogenetic analysis, but you obtain insufficient mitoses for analysis. The child begins to have tetanic seizures, although there is no evidence of intrauterine or postnatal infection. Blood analysis is unremarkable except for a lower serum calcium, low white blood count, and an increased ratio of polymorphonuclear leukocytes to lymphocytes. Intravenous fluid and calcium relieve the tetany.

Table 12-8   Serum and IgG from Myasthenia Gravis Patients and Controls Assayed for Ability to Inhibit Binding of ^{125}I-Labeled Bungarotoxin to Extracted Muscle AChR (Problem 12-4)

Patient	Tensilon Test[a]	Binding of ^{125}I-Bungarotoxin to AChR Preincubated with:	
		Serum[b]	IgG[b]
J. F.	+	0.56 ± 0.06	0.56 ± 0.06
C. S.	+	0.97 ± 0.006	1.01 ± 0.06
D. S.	+	0.57 ± 0.06	0.58 ± 0.03
B. J.	+	1.03 ± 0.01	1.02 ± 0.11
R. Y.	−	0.75 ± 0.04	0.88
Controls		1.00 ± 0.03	1.00 ± 0.03

[a]Indicates transient disappearance of muscle weakness following injection of Tensilon, a drug that increases ACh levels.
[b]Mean ± standard deviation (when more than one determination is made), normalized to mean of control values.
[From R. Almon, C. Andrew, and S. Appel, *Science* **186,** 55(1975). Copyright 1975 by the American Association for the Advancement of Science.]

Figure 12-11

Stimulation indexes in response to acetylcholine receptor in 21 controls and 21 patients with myasthenia gravis (MG) (Problem 12-4). The triangles represent controls with an unrelated muscular disorder (amyotrophic lateral sclerosis). The mean and standard error of the mean are indicated for the two populations. Stimulation index values greater than 2.0 are considered positive responses. [From D. P. Richman, J. Patrick, and B. G. W. Arnason, *N. Eng. J. Med.* **294,** 694(1976). Reprinted by permission from the *New England Journal of Medicine* **294,** 694(1976).]

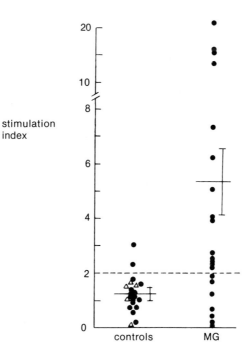

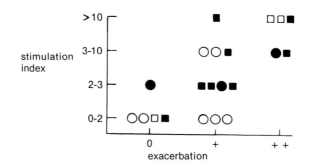

Figure 12-12 The cellular immune response to acetylcholine receptor in myasthenia gravis as a function of the activity of the disease (Problem 12-4). O indicates stable disease in an exacerbation serious enough to lead to hospitalization, and + + indicates severe exacerbation requiring respiratory assistance. Squares denote males and circles females; open symbols represent patients younger than 50 years of age, and closed symbols represent patients older than 50 years of age. [From D. P. Richman, J. Patrick, and B. G. W. Arnason, *N. Eng. J. Med.* **294**, 694(1976). Reprinted by permission from the *New England Journal of Medicine* **294**, 694(1976).]

Do you expect to find any abnormalities in level of function of serum-IgA secretory component? If so, why?

(b) A mild cold virus infection is endemic in the pediatric neonatology staff. Your patient develops a severe tracheobronchitis. You begin to suspect that fluid and calcium did not cure everything. You order a repeat cytogenetic analysis to confirm your suspicions. How should you order the analysis to be carried out?

(c) You are required to do an emergency tracheostomy to save the infant's life. The tracheostomy is successful and you are about to suture the incision when it occurs to you to remove a paratracheal lymph node for biopsy. What might you expect to see in histological sections of this tissue?

(d) What are your diagnosis and suggestion for therapy?

(e) As a physician with a modern training in human genetics, what advice will you give to the parents regarding future pregnancies?

12-6 (a) A high proportion of patients with *partial lipodystrophy* (symmetric loss of fat from the face, arms, and trunk in a dermatomal distribution) suffer from a form of glomerulonephritis. A group of investigators from Hammersmith Hospital in London reported [*N. Eng. J. Med.* **294**, 461, 495(1976)] that these patients have normal serum levels of complement components 1 and 4 but abnormally low serum levels of C3; furthermore, C3 disappears rapidly on injection into these patients. The relationship between the lipodystrophy and the glomerulonephritis is obscure. Biopsies of the kidney in these patients reveal granular deposits of C3 with no detectable immunoglobulin in the glomeruli. What do you think is involved in activating and mediating the glomerulonephritis? Think in terms of causative processes, factors, and cells.

(b) Can you think of a laboratory test that will confirm your activation hypothesis?

(c) Would you classify this disease as an autoimmune disorder? As an immune hypersensitivity disease? As an allergic disorder?

12-7   (a)   Chronic arthritis may occur as a complication of intestinal bypass surgery for morbid obesity. For example, one report [*N. Eng. J. Med.* **294**, 121(1976)] records an analysis of five arthritic postoperative patients. Their serum levels of complement components C3 and C4 were abnormally low, but they had no rheumatoid factor (IgM anti-IgG). Components of the alternative complement pathway were present in their serum in activated forms. In addition, they had circulating serum complexes containing IgM, IgG, C3, C4, and C5. The IgG antibody in these complexes was directed against bacteria that usually inhabit the gastrointestinal tract. The complexes were found in the serum preceding episodes of arthritis, but they were absent after remission. Propose a model for the pathogenesis of this disorder.

           (b)   How would you propose to treat this disorder?

12-8   The patient is a 15-year-old boy with a lifelong history of diarrhea and gastrointestinal-tract infections with the fungus *Candida albicans*. *Candida albicans* is usually nonpathogenic, but in cases of immune deficiency, it becomes an opportunistic pathogen. This patient was sent to a clinical investigation team. Suspecting an immunologic deficiency disease, these investigators tested his levels of serum immunoglobulins, blood lymphocytes, and salivary IgA, with the results shown in Table 12-9. With reference to this table, answer the following questions.

           (a)   What do you conclude from these data?

           (b)   Propose a model for his disease and a test to confirm or rule out your model.

           (c)   From the results of the test shown in Table 12-10, what do you conclude is the basic defect in this patient? Propose a therapy.

           (d)   The investigative team prescribed oral bovine colostrum, and the patient responded well and recovered. How does this therapy work?

12-9   This problem deals with a hypothetical clinical syndrome.

         A sick mouse arrives in your veterinary clinic for consultation. He (Michael) has a fever of 2 weeks duration and a cough productive of 20 μl per day of purulent material. You culture his sputum and the major bacterium present is the usually nonpathogenic rough (nonencapsulated) form of *Diplococcus pneumoniae*. His antibody levels to this organism are low (compared to the level of antibodies in the serum of his mate, Minifred; both Michael and Minifred are shown to have equivalent antibody responses to the mousepox virus, *Ectromelia*). You isolate the various components of the *Diplococcus* cell wall and assay for the corresponding cognate antibodies by two-stage radioimmunoassay (Table 12-11). You also undertake a genetic analysis of this disease and obtain the results shown in Table 12-12 with the two mice and their offspring. With reference to these tables, answer questions (a) through (c).

           (a)   On which chromosome does the susceptibility gene map? Devise a brother–sister mating cross that would test your hypothesis and give the expected results, citing only the relevant gene locus or loci.

           (b)   Can you rule out the hypothesis that this disease is carried by a sex-linked gene? Why or why not?

           (c)   Do you think that the defect in this disease will be revealed by typing blood cells with the following panel of antibodies: anti-Ia^b; anti-Lyt-1; anti-Lyt-2; anti-κ; anti-λ?

           (d)   Several weeks after the illness has swept the Mouse family, you note on retesting that Minifred no longer has serum anti-*D. pneumoniae* antibodies. You test her serum (in the central well) in an Ouchterlony test against the acute-phase sera (in the outer wells) you drew the first week and get the result shown in Figure 12-13. How do you explain this result? (Be very specific in the terms you

Table 12-9 Levels of Serum Immunoglobulin, Immunoglobulin-Bearing Lymphocytes, and Salivary IgA in Normal Adults and a 15-year-old Patient (Problem 12-18)

	Serum Immunoglobulin (mg/mL)			Immunoglobulin-Bearing Blood Lymphocytes (Percent[b])				Salivary (mg/mL)
	IgG	IgM	IgA	IgG	IgA	IgM	IgD	IgA
Normal adults:								
mean	12.7	1.3	2.7	8.7	4.2	6.0	7.5	7.2
range[a]	(10–15)	(0.8–2.0)	(1.3–3.8)	(5.8–12.6)	(2.0–6.2)	(2.3–10.0)	(4.0–10.8)	(3.8–10.0)
Patient:								
Test 1[c]	11.3	1.2	1.2	8.0	13.0	8.0	14.0	0.2
Test 2[c]				11.0	10.8	13.0		
IgA-deficient patients:								
mean	—	—	—	—	—	—	—	0.3
range[a]	—	—	—	—	—	—	—	(0.1–0.4)

[a]Figures in parentheses represent mean ± standard deviation.
[b]Expressed as percent of total peripheral blood lymphocytes.
[c]Tests 1 and 2 represent two independent determinations on the patient.
[Data from W. Strober, R. Krakauer, H. L. Klaeveman, H. Y. Reynolds, and D. L. Nelson, *N. Eng. J. Med.* **294,** 351(1976). Used by permission from the *New England Journal of Medicine* **294,** 351(1976).]

Table 12-10 Salivary Concentrations of Free Secretory Component in Normal Controls, IgA-Deficient Patients, and the Patient Under Study (Problem 12-8)

Individuals Tested	Secretory Component (μg/mL)
Normal controls:	
mean	220
± standard deviation	(40–400)
Patient	$<$10
IgA-deficient patients	170–$>$1000[a]

[a]Range observed among ten patients tested. Six of these patients showed $>$1000 μg/mL. [Data from W. Strober, R. Krakauer, H. L. Klaeveman, H. Y. Reynolds, and D. L. Nelson, *N. Eng. J. Med.* **294,** 351(1976). Used by permission from the *New England Journal of Medicine* **294,** 351(1976).]

Table 12-11 Levels of Antibodies to *Diplococcus* Cell-Wall Components in the Sera of Two Mice (Problem 12-9)

	Antibody Level (μg/mL)	
Cell-Wall Component	Michael	Minifred
Carbohydrate (CH)	220	200
Phosphorylcholine (PC)	5	870
Proteoglycan (PG)	27	85
Lipopolysaccharide (LPS)	5	5

Table 12-12 Data from Genetic Analysis of Two Mice and Their Offspring (Problem 12-9)

Marker Tested	Chromo-some	Parents		Offspring					
		Michael	Minifred	Larry	Avram	Arthur	Fran	Ken	Count
Hemoglobin (electrophoresis)	7	Diffuse(D/D)	Sharp(S/S)	D/S	D/S	D/S	D/S	D/S	S/S
H-2	17	a/c	b/c	a/b	a/b	c/c	b/c	a/c	c/d
Ig-H chain	12	a/d	b/d	b/d	a/d	a/b	a/b	a/d	d/f
Ig-κ chain	6	b/b	b/b	b/b	b/b	b/b	b/b	b/b	b/b
Ig-γ chain	16	a/c	b/d	a/b	a/b	b/c	b/c	c/d	d/?
Anti-CH ($>$100 μg/mL)		+	+	+	+	+	+	+	+
Anti-PC ($>$100 μg/mL)		−	+	+	−	+	+	−	+
Anti-PG ($>$50 μg/mL)		−	+	−	+	−	+	+	+
Anti-LPS ($>$50 μg/mL)		−	−	−	−	−	−	−	+
Susceptibility to *D. pneumoniae*		yes	no	no	yes	no	no	yes	no
Percent B cells in blood		20	25	22	31	27	54	22	10

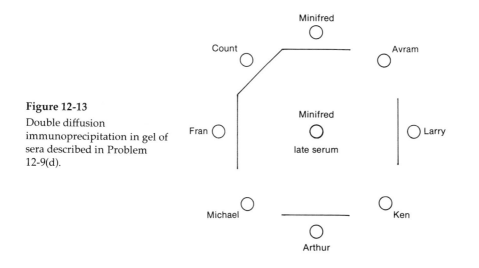

Figure 12-13

Double diffusion immunoprecipitation in gel of sera described in Problem 12-9(d).

use to describe the type of determinants seen by Minifred's late serum on the acute-phase serum immunoglobulins.) What steps would you take to confirm your explanation?

(e) You decide to prepare hybridomas by fusing Minifred's B cells from the frozen samples of acute-phase and late-phase blood cells The late-phase B lymphocytes give rise to 4 out of 500 hybridoma clones that produce antibodies that bind to acute-phase IgM isolates from Minifred, Larry, Arthur, Fran, and Count only. This binding assay is blocked by preincubating the acute phase IgM with *D. pneumoniae*. Diagram what is happening in the blockade test.

(f) These four clones detect the immunoglobulin products of 6 out of 77 clones from Minifred's *acute-phase* B-cell hybridomas. Five of these acute-phase-derived hybridomas produce and release IgM or IgG immunoglobulins: the sixth one makes only an intracellular μ chain, and the intracellular μ chain reacts with the late-phase hybridoma antibodies.

You isolate the mRNAs from the sixth (intracellular μ) hybridoma and, using reverse transcriptase, prepare exact cDNA copies for insertion into λ bacteriophage. You screen phage plaques with a C_μ-labeled DNA probe and select three λ phage clones (from 5000 plated) that hybridize with the probe and therefore represent DNA copies of the entire μ chain mRNA. They prove to be identical to each other by restriction endonuclease mapping as shown in Figure 12-14. The region hybridizing with the C_μ probe contains all C_μ domains. Diagram the region from C to D using immunoglobulin gene terminology.

(g) You find an enzyme (X) that cuts just 50 bases 5' to the C_μ hybridizing region of the clone, and you subclone the fragment that extends from C to the X restriction site (C → X fragment). You use a labeled C → X probe to examine fragments following endonuclease digestion, size separation by gel electrophoresis, transfer to nitrocellulose, and hybridization according to the Southern procedure, and you obtain the results shown in Figure 12-15. Explain each of the intense bands. Identify the chromosome to which each band is linked, and label each band accordingly (See Table 12-11).

(h) Try to explain the molecular basis of Michael's disease. (*Hint:* You should explain bands present as well as bands absent.) Why do Minifred and Arthur lack the disease?

Figure 12-14

Restriction endonuclease map of the μ-chain cDNA insert described in Problem 12-9(f).

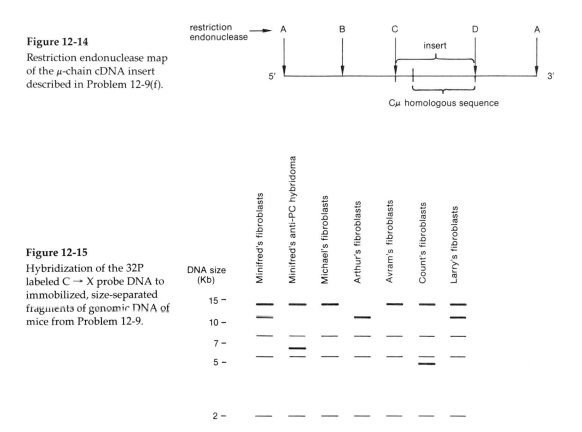

Figure 12-15

Hybridization of the 32P labeled C → X probe DNA to immobilized, size-separated fragments of genomic DNA of mice from Problem 12-9.

12-10 The CBA/N mouse strain has an X-linked immune defect that affects the response of B cells to certain antigens, including phosphorylcholine (PC). Male mice from a CBA/N × BALB/c cross are hemizygous for the X-linked immune defect and cannot respond to PC. Female mice are phenotypically normal and can respond to PC. The response of female mice is extremely homogenous, and virtually all of the antibody produced expresses the T15 idiotype. Adoptive transfer experiments were performed to test the T-cell helper capability of male mice. Keyhole limpet hemocyanin (KLH)-primed T cells from either male or female mice were mixed with PC-primed B cells from female mice and transferred along with an antigenic boost of PC-KLH into lethally irradiated female mice. The response was measured as before but, in addition, the number of anti-PC antibody plaque-forming cells (PFC) that expressed the T15 idiotype was determined. With reference to the results shown in Table 12-13, answer the following questions.

    (a) In terms of the anti-PC–PFC response, what conclusions can you draw about the ability of male T cells to participate in an anti-PC response?

    (b) What is the significance of the mixture experiment in line 3?

    (c) What do the data indicate about the reactivity of T-helper-cell subpopulations present in the male and female mice?

12-11 (a) Under normal circumstances, humans do not make antibodies to self-components, e.g., red blood cell (RBC) antigens. What are three possible explanations for this type of self-tolerance?

Table 12-13   Responses of Immune-Defective Male and Female Mice to Phosphorylcholine (PC) (Problem 12-10)

T-Cell Donor KLH-Primed	Total PC-PFC	Geometric Mean PFC/Spleen	
		T15$^+$ PFC	(Percent T15$^+$)
1. Female	5,200	4,600	88
2. Male	6,120	1,680	27
3. Female + male	12,000	6,700	56

(b)   Certain human autoimmune disease states are characterized by an abnormal immune response to self-antigens. One example of autoimmunity is the hemolytic anemia associated with the use of the anti-hypertensive drug, alpha-methyldopa. Approximately 15% of patients taking alpha-methyldopa have circulating antibodies directed against red-cell antigens. Suggest three possible mechanisms for alpha-methyldopa induced autoimmunity. Be specific about the types of antigens detected by the autoimmune antibodies.

(c)   To investigate further the mechanism of methyldopa-induced autoimmunity, immunoglobulin was isolated from patients with hemolytic anemia, labeled with ^{125}I, and tested in a radioimmunoassay for binding to RBC from various sources, with the results shown in Table 12-14. What do these data suggest about the origin of alpha-methyldopa induced anemia? Does this narrow your choices in part (b)?

12-12   (a)   A chronic, noninflammatory edema called *hereditary angioedema* (HAE) is an autosomal dominant genetic defect caused by the malfunction of a complement or complement-associated component. Complement components were isolated from the serum of a patient with HAE, treated with EDTA (a chelating agent for divalent cations), and chromatographed on DEAE cellulose (an ion-exchange resin that separates polypeptides on the basis of charge). One of the HAE complement components so treated gave three peaks the sizes of which were 11S, 7S, and 4S. The material from the 11S peak was found to bind IgM-coated sheep red blood cells (SRBC) by recognizing a site on the CH$_2$ domain of the IgM molecule. (IgM-coated SRBC were made by raising IgM antibodies to SRBC, isolating these antibodies, and allowing them to bind SRBC *in vitro*.) Material from the 7S peak and from the 4S peak could not bind IgM-coated SRBC. Which complement component was treated with EDTA and chromatographed to give three subunits?

(b)   What is the identity of the material in the 11S peak?

(c)   In a second experiment, the native complement component described in part (a) was allowed to bind IgM-coated SRBC before EDTA treatment. The cells were then treated briefly with EDTA and the supernatant collected. When the supernatant was chromatographed on DEAE cellulose, a prominent peak, whose size was 4S, resulted. The material from this peak could cleave both *p*-toluenesulfonyl-L-arginine-methyl ester (TAME) and N-acetyl-L-tryosine-ethyl ester (ATEe), whereas the 4S material from the first experiment could not

Table 12-14 Binding to Red Blood Cells (RBC) of Radiolabeled Immunoglobulin from Patients with Methyldopa-Induced Autoimmune Hemolytic Anemia (Problem 12-12)

Test Cells	cpm-Bound Radioactivity/10^6 RBC
Normal RBC	15,800
Normal RBC + methyldopa	14,600
RBC from patients with alpha-methyldopa induced hemolytic anemia	16,500
Blank tube	<200

do so. What is the 4S peak and why can it cleave TAME and ATEe in the second experiment and not in the first?

(d) What is the 7S peak in the first experiment?

(e) When the whole serum from a normal person was added to the 4S material obtained in the second experiment, it was found that the 4S material could no longer cleave TAME or ATEe. When the whole serum from the person with HAE was added to the 4S material obtained in the second experiment, the cleavage of TAME or ATEe was unaffected. Give two possible explanations for the genetic defect associated with HAE.

(f) How could you distinguish between your hypotheses?

12-13 (a) Scrapie, in sheep, and kuru, in man, are transmissible lethal degenerative diseases of the central nervous system; their etiologies are still a mystery. Kuru is apparently transmitted in New Guinea Fore cannibals by their eating the brains of diseased foes. Although scrapie transmission is less clear, parenteral or intracerebral injection of brain extracts from scrapie-positive sheep will transmit the disease to other sheep, and it will transmit a similar disease in a mouse model. Brain extracts from scrapie-negative sheep will not transmit the disease. Although most neurologists and microbiologists initially believed these diseases to be transmitted by viral agents, two experiments on the scrapie agent do not support a classical viral etiology. In the first experiment, scrapie-agent-containing extracts were bombarded with increasing doses of ionizing or ultraviolet irradiation [T. Alper et al., *Nature* **214**, 764(1967)]. According to radiation target theory, the smaller the target (in this case the scrapie agent), the greater the radiation dose required to inactivate the target. In this experiment, the calibrated target mass of the scrapie-agent activity was no more than 150,000 daltons. What would be the coding capacity of a virus of this mass?

(b) In the second series of experiments, a variety of enzymes, chemicals, and pharmacological inhibitors were tested against the scrapie agent, and, in all cases, the transmissible biological activity appeared to reside in lipophilic polypeptides and not in polynucleotides [S. B. Prusiner, *Science* **216**, 136(1982)]. Using all of the preceding information and your insights into immunopathology, develop an immunological model for the transmission and pathogenesis of scrapie (and kuru).

Answers

12-1   (a)   False. In chronic granulomatous disease, Fc receptors are intact; lysosomal enzyme functions are defective.

         (b)   True

         (c)   True

         (d)   False. SLE kidney disease is caused by complement-fixing immune complexes, not by the IgE system.

         (e)   False. AIDS is marked by a selective deficit of $T4^+$ cells and deficient cell-mediated immunity.

         (f)   False. Contact sensitivity is a manifestation of cellular immunity.

         (g)   False. H-chain structural genes are not X linked. Bruton's disease is an X-linked defect in the development of B cells.

         (h)   True

         (i)   True

         (j)   False. The activating agent was brain protein that bore cross-reacting antigens similar to those of human nervous tissue.

         (k)   True

         (l)   False. ALS affects circulating T cells predominantly, although it may affect circulating B cells if the serum is not completely specific due to improper absorption. ALS treatment does not remove long-lived antibodies.

         (m)   False. These patients have a combined T-cell and B-cell immune system defect.

         (n)   True

         (o)   False. It is linked to the human MHC, the HLA locus.

12-2   (a)   T, B

         (b)   IgM, IgG immunoglobulins

         (c)   IgE, mast cells

         (d)   Goodpasture's syndrome

         (e)   pulmonary (lung) alveoli

         (f)   mast (or B)

         (g)   polymorphonuclear leukocytes

         (h)   Hereditary angioneurotic edema

         (i)   ataxia-telangiectasia

         (j)   cross-reacting antigen

         (k)   T-cell (or cellular-immunity)

         (l)   T

         (m)   bacterial

         (n)   immune complexes

         (o)   epinephrine, antihistamines

         (p)   Adjuvants

12-3   (a)   In the presence of the mitogens, normal cells synthesize considerable amounts of immunoglobulin. Even without mitogen, they secrete some immunoglobulin. However, even with mitogen, the hypogammaglobulinemia patients' cells secrete virtually no immunoglobulin. Furthermore, the patients' cells suppress immunoglobulin secretion by normal cells. Therefore, these patients seem to suffer from hyperactive suppressor cells.

         (b)   The suppressor cells either do not carry surface immunoglobulin or are not sensitive to lysis by anti-immunoglobulin and complement for some other reason. (The authors concluded that the suppressor cells were T cells, but they provided no direct evidence for that conclusion.)

(c) The generation of small pre-B lymphocytes from large pre-B precursor lymphocytes could be blocked, or the small pre-B lymphocytes could fail to mature further. Either eventuality would cause complete absence of sIg$^+$ cells, as well as agammaglobulinemia. Immature B lymphocytes could have an internal biochemical defect that would result in failure of V-gene formation on either H- or L-chain genes. Other defects could prevent B-cell stimulation subsequent to antigen binding, including blocks at any point along the pathway of blast transformation and immunoglobulin synthesis: for example, in mRNA processing or transport from the nucleus, or in the addition of carbohydrate, or in the secretory process. Alternatively, inhibition by other cells could prevent immunoglobulin synthesis or secretion.

12-4 (a) The immunization protocol elicits antibodies specific for the acetylcholine receptor that is likely to carry cross-reacting antigens in electric eel and rat. These antibodies probably bind at neuromuscular junctions and impair voluntary muscle stimulation. The muscular weakness, hunched posture, and jerky movements could all be traced to impairment of head and forelimb muscles. Weight loss would follow from failure to eat due to impairment of head and neck muscles and inability to move to the food supply.

(b) You could confirm the presence of self-reactive antibodies and determine the precise effect of the antibodies on the neuromuscular system.

(c) Clearly, organisms normally do not make such antibodies. A strong adjuvant is needed to break the natural tolerance to the self-antigens of the AChR protein.

(d) The syndrome may represent a direct manifestation of T effector cells. Alternatively, if AChR were a thymus-dependent antigen in terms of B-cell triggering, humoral antibody could cause the syndrome.

(e) Myasthenia gravis could be due to autoantibodies against acetylcholine receptors. Again, you could test sera for antibodies specific to human neuromuscular junctions. You might also test these sera against purified AChR from electric eels.

(f) Some patients with myasthenia gravis have serum immunoglobulins that partially block subsequent binding of α-bungarotoxin to AChR. In additional tests of such patients, about half showed definite or possible inhibition. The immunoglobulin binding could cause neuromuscular blockade *in vivo*, thereby accounting for both the disease process and the finding that the concentration of muscle-binding sites is reduced in these patients.

(g) Patients with myasthenia gravis also show evidence of cellular immunity specific for AChR, and the degree of hypersensitivity correlates directly with the severity of the disease process. Thus T-cell immunity is implicated in this disease process, and the reduced frequency of muscle AChR in these patients may be due to (1) the cytotoxic and/or inflammatory effects of effector T cells, (2) competitive inhibition of receptor sites by T cells or cell-free T-cell factors, or (3) competitive inhibition of receptor sites by specific antibody.

(h) This syndrome could be due to receptor blockade only in its initial phases because the half-life of most antibodies in mice is hours to days, not months. AChR and/or complexes of anti-AChR with AChR in this instance probably induce a prolonged immune response to the AChR.

(i) The mice show evidence of both T- and B-cell immunity to AChR. To demonstrate that immunopathogenic effector function, you would have to test the effects of various subclasses of immunoglobulins and lymphocytes on *in vitro* receptor binding and on muscle stimulation by ACh. You could also fractionate immunoglobulins and cells for passive or adoptive transfer of the disease to normal, syngeneic hosts. Particularly useful for the cell-transfer studies would be fractionation procedures allowing enrichment or depletion of cells bearing surface Ig, C3 receptors, Fc receptors, Thy-1, L3T4, Lyt-1, Lyt-2, and Lyt-3. In each case, you would have to demonstrate that the putative effect of each transferred agent was a direct action of that agent rather than induction of a secondary process.

12-5   (a) There is no reason to suspect any abnormalities in levels of secretory component. If you wished to check these levels, you should assay saliva rather than serum.

      (b) Because you suspect that the patient has a T-cell deficit, you should order separate assays of blood lymphocytes with phyothemagglutinin (which stimulates T cells only) and pokeweed mitogen (which stimulates both T and B cells) to test your suspicion.

      (c) In the histologic sections, you should see intact primary follicles and medullary development of plasma cells, but you should see total lymphocyte depletion of the diffuse cortex.

      (d) Your diagnosis should be DiGeorge syndrome (thymic aplasia). You must either keep the child in a germ-free isolater for life or investigate the possibilities of thymus transplant. If you consider a transplant, you must take into account the problem of a graft-versus-host reaction. Also, you must supply calcium or parathyroid hormones for life.

      (e) The parents need not worry about future pregnancies because this syndrome results from a nongenetic congenital defect, perhaps due to intrauterine trauma, toxin, or infection.

12-6   (a) The glomerulonephritis involves activation of the alternate complement pathway, either by endogenous release of activators or by a subclinical infection with endotoxin-producing bacteria. The latter alternative seems unlikely in the absence of a specific antibody response. The activated C3 becomes deposited in the glomeruli, and it activates an acute inflammatory response involving vasoactive peptides and infiltration of polymorphonuclear leukocytes.

      (b) If the activating agents are in the blood, then serum from these patients should fix complement spontaneously, thereby lowering the complement titer of a standard serum.

      (c) There is no reason to believe that this inflammatory disorder involves any of the specific elements of the immune system.

12-7   (a) It is likely that recurrent release of gastrointestinal bacteria into the bloodstream is occurring due to an imperfection in the surgical procedure. These bacteria are inducing a specific immune response. The arthritis is probably due to immune-complex-activated, complement-dependent acute inflammation.

      (b) You should treat the symptoms with anti-inflammatory agents and attempt to find the locus of infection to eliminate recurrence. If you can find no locus of infection, you must entertain the possibility that the immune response is directed against cross-reacting endogenous antigens and try to identify them or plan immunosuppressive therapy.

12-8   (a) The boy's serum immunoglobulin levels are normal. Likewise his levels of B-cell subclasses are normal, with a possibly significant increase in B_α and B_δ cells (perhaps $B_{\alpha\delta}$ as there is no increase in $B_{\mu\delta}$ cells; double staining for α and δ was not carried out). There is no evidence here of immune deficiency.

      (b) The patient is deficient in salivary IgA. Either IgA or IgA-synthesizing cells do not reach the submucosal tissues, or there is a defect in production or function of secretory component. You might test the latter possibility by developing an

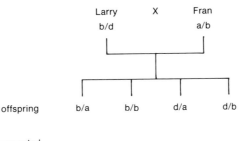

Larry   X   Fran
b/d   a/b

offspring   b/a   b/b   d/a   d/b

expected disease predilection   resistant   resistant   susceptible   resistant

Figure 12-16

Answer to Problem 12-9(a).

immunoassay that would measure secretory component (SC) specifically. The investigating team developed a radioimmunoassay for this purpose.

(c) The patient suffers from a defect in production of functional SC. The defect could be either failure of synthesis or production of an altered component that neither binds to IgA nor is secreted. Any therapy must either restore epithelial production of functional SC or replace gastrointestinal IgA. IgA is in highest concentrations in colostrum and milk.

(d) Presumably bovine colostrum contains IgA, some of which is anti-*Candida* or is directed against substances that promote *Candida* infection. How IgA protects epithelial surfaces other than by combining with antigenic microorganisms is still unknown.

12-9   (a) Chromosome 12. Michael, Avram, and Ken all share disease susceptibility to *D. pneumoniae*, lack of anti-PC antibody responses, and chromosome 12 haplotypes (a/d). Chromosome 6 is ruled out because all mice in this cross appeared to be the same at the Ig-κ-chain region. Chromosome 16 is ruled out because the deficiency does not co-map with either the Ig-λ a or c allele. Chromosome 17 is also an unlikely choice because Larry and Avram are identical at this haplotype, yet Avram has the immunodeficiency while Larry does not. (The results also indicate that Count is not the result of a Michael/Minifred cross.) The hypothetical defective haplotype on chromosome 12 is a/d. Because any brother $\times$ sister mating must include Fran, who is a/b at that locus, the most informative cross would be with Larry, who, like Fran, is not immunodeficient (Figure 12-16).

(b) Yes. Michael would have to carry the disease susceptibility gene that is passed on to Avram and Ken. If it were an X-linked trait, he could transmit it to his female offspring only. If it were a Y-linked trait (the first Y-chromosomal disease susceptibility trait), all male offspring should inherit it, yet Larry and Arthur did not.

(c) Anti-Ia^b, no; anti-Lyt-1, no; anti-Lyt-2, no; anti-μ, no; anti-δ, no; anti-κ, no; anti-λ, no. The only antibodies that might have helped would be anti-allotypic or anti-idiotypic.

(d) Minifred has antibodies against antigenic determinants present in her own acute-phase serum as well as in Count's, Fran's, Arthur's, and Larry's, but none are present in the three diseased members of the family. Because the determinants are on the acute-phase serum immunoglobulins and because they are raised against Minifred's own immunoglobulins, it is unlikely that these autoantibodies detect isotypic or allotypic specificities. It would be reasonable

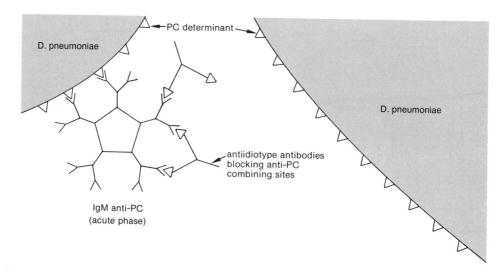

Figure 12-17   Answer to Problem 12-9(e). A   bacterial PC or anti-idiotypic
diagram of anti-PC antibodies   antibodies.
interacting either with the

to propose that these antibodies are directed against idiotypic determinants on these immunoglobulins.

You could test this model by isolating the immunoglobulins from Minifred's acute-phase serum and showing that the antigenic determinants seen by the late-phase antibodies are present on F(ab) but not Fc fractions of these immunoglobulins. This test could be accomplished by redoing the Ouchterlony test but including, in the central well with Minifred's late-phase serum, an excess of her acute-phase antibody F(ab) or Fc fractions. The F(ab) fragments containing the idiotypic determinants should combine with the anti-idiotypic antibodies, preventing the formation of precipitin lines (of identity) against Fran's, Count's, Minifred's, Larry's, and Arthur's immunoglobulins.

(e) See Figure 12-17.

(f) See Figure 12-18.

(g) All bands represent V_H subgenic elements from chromosome 12. The 14Kb band is a V_H-hybridizing segment from the IgH^d haplotype, and almost certainly it does not encode functional anti-PC (V_H) binding sites. The 11Kb band is from IgH^b haplotype, and, at least in Minifred's case, it almost certainly encodes a functional anti-PC V_H; it is rearranged to a 6Kb V_H-containing band in the anti-PC hybridoma. The 5Kb band is further evidence of Count's parentage.

(h) Avram and Michael each have only one anti-PC V_H homologous band, the 14Kb band that is apparently nonfunctional. In the IgH^a haplotype chromosome 12, no anti-PC V_H gene is present. Thus Avram and Michael cannot construct a gene-encoding, functional anti-PC heavy chain. Minnie and Arthur lack the disease because the anti-PC V_H^b gene is functional.

12-10   (a) Male cells give normal levels of anti-PC–PFC, but most of these antibodies lack the T15 idiotype.

(b) This experiment shows that the lack of T15 idiotype-positive PFCs in CBA/N males is *not* due to an idiotype-specific suppressor population present at the time of assay.

Figure 12-18
Answer to Problem 12-9(f).

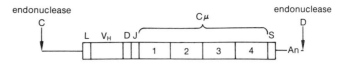

(c) Males have adequate T_H cells for most PC responses, but they cannot trigger $T15^+$ B cells from CBA/N females; such $T15^+$ B cells are adequately triggered by CBA/N female T_H cells.

12-11 (a) The three possible mechanisms for self-tolerance are: (1) tolerance at the B-cell level by clonal abortion or amnesia; (2) tolerance at the T_H-cell level but not at the B-cell level by clonal abortion or amnesia; and (3) tolerance at the T_H-cell or B-cell level or both by active suppression—for example, by T_S cells.

(b) Mechanism 1. Alpha-methyldopa binds to all red blood cells, thereby inducing an anti-alpha-methyldopa antibody response that directly removes all cells with the hapten alpha-methyldopa bound to them. Mechanism 2. Alpha-methyldopa binds to all red blood cells, thereby revealing a red blood cell neoantigen, which then acts as the inducer and target of an antibody response. Mechanism 3. Alpha-methyldopa binds to red blood cells and creates a determinant recognized by T_H cells, which then acts to trigger anti-self B cells to give rise to an autoantibody response to normal red blood cell determinants.

(c) The antibodies appear to bind to normal red blood cells to the same extent they bind to alpha-methyldopa derivatized cells *in vitro* or to red blood cells from patients with alpha-methyldopa-associated hemolytic anemia. Thus the antibodies detect normal red blood cell antigens, clearly favoring mechanism 3.

12-12 (a) Complement component 1.

(b) C1q.

(c) The 4S peak is C1s, the serine esterase. It has been activated by C1r following the binding of C1q to IgM in the second experiment, whereas, in the first, the C1s subunit was disassociated from C1r and q before being activated.

(d) The 7S peak is C1r.

(e) Serum from a normal person contains an inhibitor of the serine esterase, whereas serum from the HAE patient does not. The defect in the patient could result from (1) a point mutation in the gene for the inhibitor, making a nonfunctional product, or (2) an effective deletion of the inhibitor product resulting from either a deletion of the inhibitor gene or a mutation in a regulatory gene controlling the synthesis of the inhibitor.

(f) If you had antibodies against the inhibitor, you could probably distinguish between (1) and (2) by determining whether or not the serum from a patient with HAE could react with the antibodies.

12-13 (a) An animal virus with a mass of 150,000 daltons would be smaller than any yet identified. Even if the agent consisted entirely of DNA or RNA, double-stranded nucleic acid of molecular weight 150,000 could contain a maximum of 2500 nucleotide pairs, whereas a single strand could contain up to 5000 nucleotides. These nucleic acids could encode 1–4 average size proteins (molecular weight 50,000) using one reading frame. For comparison, functional retroviruses have a single-stranded RNA genome of 8200 nucleotides, whereas functional papova viruses have a double-stranded DNA genome of 5226 nucleotide pairs. These considerations suggest the possibility that the scrapie agent does not carry information in a nucleic acid sequence and that the transmission of its biological information might not occur by the classical nucleic acid replication model.

(b) To explain its behavior, the scrapie agent must possess at least three properties. It must have (1) *recognition sites* to target it to the parts of the central nervous system that are eventually destroyed, (2) *effector functions* to trigger the pathologic process, and (3) a means by which these two functions can be *replicated* faithfully in the affected host to produce the stable transmissible agent. Viruses usually encode this information in three or more distinct macromolecules. To support a hypothesis that the scrapie agent is exclusively polypeptide in nature (this hypothesis is certainly not yet proven), one must consider how polypeptides can mimic infectious agents and bring about their own replication.

The antigen-specific molecules secreted or displayed by lymphoid effector cells join *recognition sites* and *effector functions* into a single molecule (e.g., antibodies, T_S-cell receptors, T_H-cell receptors). Thus an antigen-specific molecule could contain information to recognize target determinants in the central nervous system, and it could also contain information to trigger localized cytopathic functions (e.g., complement-mediated inflammation and cell lysis by IgM and some IgGs). If the destruction of the target structure bearing the recognized determinant led to conversion of this determinant to a potent immunogen, then the resulting host immune response could generate more antigen-specific molecules of the same class, recognition function, and effector function.

In scrapie, the brain antigen alone must not have the capacity to induce such antigen-specific molecules; perhaps local modifying agents such as serine esterases (Answer 12-12c) could cleave a nonimmunogenic molecule to reveal an immunogen. All that is required is that the immunogen always induce effector molecules of defined class, receptor specificity, and function, much as bacterial cell-wall phosphorylcholine reproducibly induces antibodies of restricted isotype (IgM, IgG_3, IgA) and restricted idiotype (see Problem 12-10). In light of this argument, a polypeptide of molecular weight 150,000 becomes a conceivable infectious agent. If a similar antigen-specific molecule could withstand digestion and cross the gastrointestinal tract epithelium, then a similar explanation would be conceivable for kuru.

In theory, this model for an immune-based polypeptide capable of recognition, effector function, and induction of a like (or identical) molecule is conceivable for other polypeptide systems, including hormones (and their receptors), growth factors (and their receptors), and even endogenous viruses (and their receptors). The important point is that not all transmissible agents must be nucleic acid in nature or use nucleic acid replication for their multiplication in a suitable host.

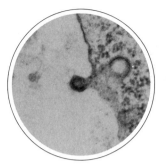

CHAPTER 13

Cancer Biology and Immunology

Chapter Outline

The immunosurveillance functions of the immune system provide the body's principal defense against cancer. Cancer cells have lost the growth control of normal cells and gained the ability to invade new tissue. The transformation of normal cells into cancer cells by chemical, physical, and viral agents is now beginning to be understood. Expression of new cell-surface antigens by cancer cells usually allows their recognition and elimination by the surveillance functions of the immune system. When cancer cells escape this surveillance, life-threatening tumors can result. This chapter begins by describing cancer cells and current knowledge of the mechanisms by which they arise from normal cells. Subsequent sections deal with immune-related aspects, including the future of immunological approaches to cancer prevention, diagnosis, and therapy.

Concepts

13-1   Cancer cells divide when they should not

Malignant and benign neoplasms

Normal growth is regulated so that the proportion of proliferating cells in an organ increases or decreases to balance the rate of cell loss, thereby maintaining constant organ size. Cancer cells do not respond normally to such regulation. Consequently, some or all of their descendants may proliferate inappropriately to produce tumors (Figure 13-1).

The localized swelling referred to as a tumor may be caused by cell proliferation, inflammation, or infection. A tumor caused by cell proliferation is called a *neoplasm* (new growth). Neoplasms that invade surrounding tissues and ultimately spread throughout the body are called *malignant* neoplasms or cancers. Neoplasms that form noninvasive tumors that do not spread to distant sites are called *benign* neoplasms. Tumors that arise from epithelial cells are called *carcinomas* (Figure 13-2), and those that arise from stromal or mesenchymal cells are called *sarcomas* (Figure 13-3).

Growth of solid tumors

All solid tumors exhibit two growth phases: a first phase in which cells gain nutrients by diffusion from the surrounding intercellular fluids, and a second phase in which the tumor appears to induce proliferation of host blood vessels that nourish the tumor mass. Most cancer cells possess more active membrane transport systems than those of normal cells for uptake of metabolites. Despite this competitive advantage, the maximum size to which a tumor can grow without a vascular supply appears to be a spheroid about 1 mm in diameter. Beyond this size, availability of nutrients to interior cells limits their proliferation and can eventually cause their death. However, most tumors greater than 1 mm in diameter appear to release (or cause the

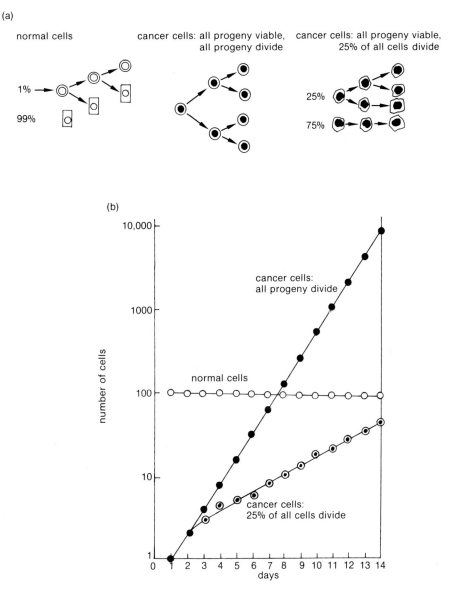

Figure 13-1 Growth kinetics of normal and neoplastic cells. The example shown considers 100 representative cells in a typical organ. Normally 99 of these cells will be differentiated and nondividing, and the remaining one will be a dividing stem cell. At each division, the stem cell gives rise to a daughter stem cell and a differentiated cell, as diagrammed in (a). The resulting rate of increase in cell number just compensates for the rate of cell loss from the tissue, so that the total number of viable cells remains constant [(b), open circles]. If one of the 100 cells becomes a cancer cell of which all progeny are dividing cells as diagrammed in (a), middle figure, then the number of cancer cells in the tissue will increase exponentially [(b), solid circles]. If one of the 100 cells becomes a cancer cell of which only 25% of the progeny give rise to two dividing daughters with each division as diagrammed in (a), right figure, then the number of cancer cells will increase more slowly [(b), open circles with solid centers].

Figure 13-2

Examples of carcinomas and their normal counterparts. (a) A section of skin with normal epidermis showing orderly maturation from a row of basal cells to layers of thin, dead surface cells that form a protective layer. (b) Invasive skin carcinoma composed of cells with frequent mitoses. Disorderly maturation is exhibited by the whorls of cells in the center of a mass of tumor cells, rather than on the surface as seen in normal epidermis. (c) Normal lining cells of the bladder (transitional epithelium) consisting of lower layers of cuboidal-shaped cells and a single top layer of flattened cells. (d) Malignant transitional cell carcinoma arising in the lining of the bladder. The cells are invading the underlying tissue as cohesive, but irregular, masses. [Photographs courtesy of R. Rouse.]

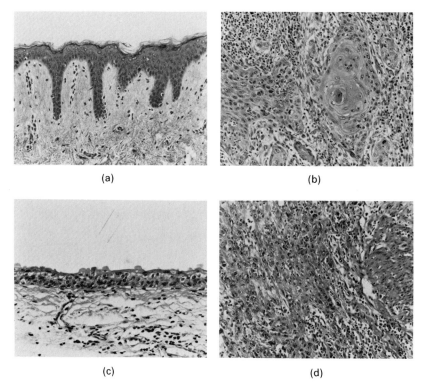

(a)

(b)

(c)

(d)

release of) *angiogenesis factors* that stimulate growth of host blood vessels. These new vessels penetrate the outer cell layers of the tumor. Subsequent tumor growth ensues by rapid proliferation of these outer layers, leaving behind an interior core of dead and dying cells (Figure 13-4). The actual growth rate of a tumor depends on the fraction of cells that are in the mitotic cycle, the average cell-cycle time, and the fraction of dying cells.

13-2 Cancer cells invade healthy tissues

Metastasis

The spread of cancer cells is termed *metastasis*. Ability to metastasize is a heritable property of malignant tumor cells. The first stage of metastasis is the spread of cancer cells into tissues surrounding the original tumor. The second stage begins with invasion of a vessel wall and entry of cancer cells into either the lymphatic or the blood vascular system (Figure 13-5).

Figure 13-3

Examples of sarcomas and their normal counterparts. (a) Normal bone, consisting of regular layers of calcified matrix. Very few cells are present; they include individual bone cells (osteocytes) within spaces and a row of bone-forming cells (osteoblasts) on the surface. (b) The histologic appearance of a malignant osteosarcoma, showing increased cellularity, with numerous large wild-looking cells. In some areas, the cells are laying down irregular, uncalcified bone matrix (upper left corner). (c) A low-power photograph of an osteosarcoma in a typical location at the end of the femur. The malignant neoplasm can be seen invading the medullary cavity, as well as eroding the cortex of the bone. Extensive bleeding and tissue death are common in these tumors. (d) Normal skeletal muscle with small, regular nuclei on the outer surfaces of the fibers. Cross striations are visible in most of the fibers. (e) The histologic appearance of a malignant rhabdomyosarcoma (sarcoma of rod-shaped [*rhabdo*] muscle [*myo*] cells), consisting of cells with centrally located, large, abnormally shaped nuclei. Some of the cells exhibit cross striations in their cytoplasm. (f) A higher-power view of a rhabdomyosarcoma showing a cell with prominent cross striations. [Photographs courtesy of R. Rouse and P. Horne.]

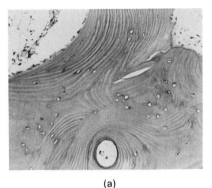

(a)

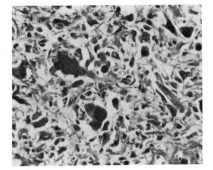

(b)

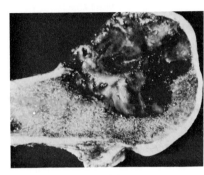

(c)

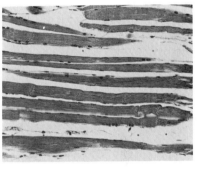

(d)

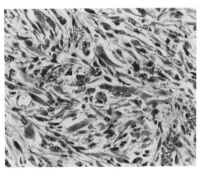

(e)

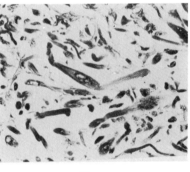

(f)

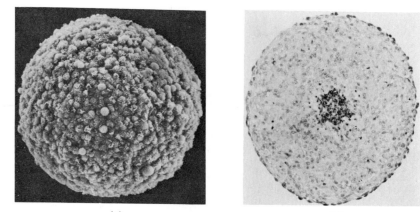

(a)

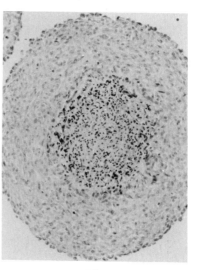

(b)

Figure 13-4

Multicellular tumor spheroids. (a) A scanning electron micrograph of a large spheroid of a breast cancer in mice. (b) A cross section of the spheroid in (a). The central core of dark cells represents a zone of cell death due to lack of nutrients. (c) A larger spheroid with a larger necrotic core. [Courtesy of R. M. Sutherland.]

(c)

Figure 13-5

A diagrammatic view of the routes of tumor cell invasion and the implications of these routes for the sites of distant metastases. Tumor cells that break off the original focus into the intercellular space enter afferent lymphatics and lodge in draining lymph nodes. Tumor cells that invade adjacent blood vessels enter the bloodstream and are distributed throughout the body.

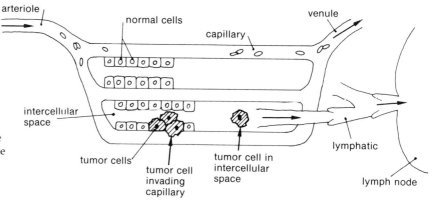

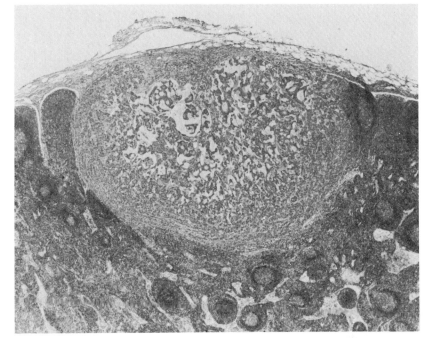

Figure 13-6
Lymph-node metastasis. The central light area is a metastatic breast cancer that has formed abnormal epithelial structures. The dark surrounding tissue is the lymph-node cortex with prominent secondary follicles. The light zones in the lower one-fifth of the photograph are medullary sinuses.
[Photographs courtesy of R. Warnke and P. Horne.]

Lymphatic metastases

Lymphatic vessels drain all intercellular fluid spaces in the body, conducting both particulate matter and fluid plasma into lymph nodes (Concept 7-1). Cancer cells that break free from a tissue or invade a lymphatic vessel almost always become trapped in the meshwork of a draining lymph node. If these cancer cells proliferate, the result is abnormal enlargement of the node (lymphadenopathy). Continued proliferation may result in release of cancer cells into the efferent lymphatic vessel leading from the lymph node to the next lymph node up the chain.

Some cancers have a predictable route of lymphatic metastasis. For example, breast cancers (Figure 13-6) that arise in the lateral portion of the breast spread via lymphatics to nodes in the armpit (axilla), whereas those arising in the medial portion of the breast usually spread to a chain of lymph nodes next to the breast bone (sternum) under the ribs (Figure 13-7).

Some metastatic cancers appear to spread almost exclusively via the lymphatics, whereas others also spread through the blood vascular system. Knowledge of these patterns of spread can be an important aid for therapeutic intervention in cases where the primary tumor can be diagnosed microscopically (e.g., Figure 13-6).

Hematogenous metastases

Cancer cells can enter the bloodstream in two ways. Proliferating metastatic cells in draining lymph nodes may enter a large collecting

Figure 13-7

A diagram of the lymphatic drainage of the breast. Lymph nodes in the axilla drain the lateral portion of the breast, while lymph nodes just under the ribs next to the sternum drain the medial portion of the breast.

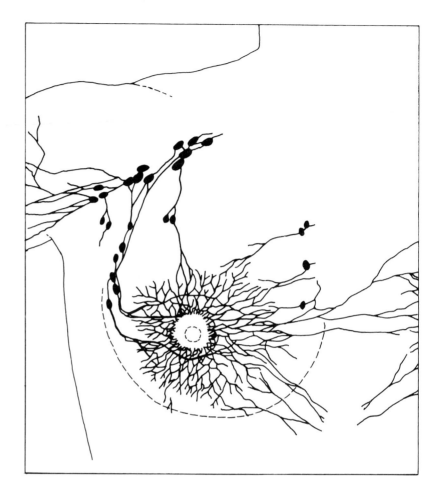

lymphatic such as the thoracic duct, which empties directly into the larger veins leading to the heart. Cancer cells may also enter the bloodstream by invading blood vessels directly (Figures 13-5 and 13-8). Cancer cells transported by the bloodstream are called *hematogenous* metastases. Metastatic cells that come to rest in small vessels begin a reverse invasion of the extravascular tissue spaces through the vessel wall, resulting in a new focus of the cancer that may be far from the original site.

Hematogenous metastases settle throughout the body, often in essential organs that cannot be removed without fatal results. Therefore, the consequences of hematogenous metastases are usually graver than those of lymphatic metastases. The frequency of metastases increases with the age of the cancer; the tendency to metastasize depends on tumor size and the inherent invasive potential of the cancer (Figure 13-9).

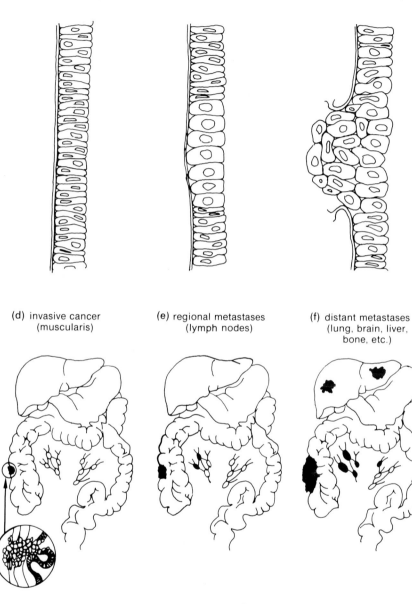

(a) normal

(b) cancer
in situ

(c) microinvasive cancer
(basement membrane)

(d) invasive cancer
(muscularis)

(e) regional metastases
(lymph nodes)

(f) distant metastases
(lung, brain, liver,
bone, etc.)

Figure 13-8 Successive stages in the development of a cancer of the colon (lower intestine). Going from left to right with time, an abnormal focus of cells invades the deeper muscular layer of the intestinal wall, spreads to local lymph nodes via the tissue lymphatics, and then spreads to the liver following entry into blood vessels. [Adapted from N. Berlin, *Hosp. Pract.* **10**(1), 83(1975).]

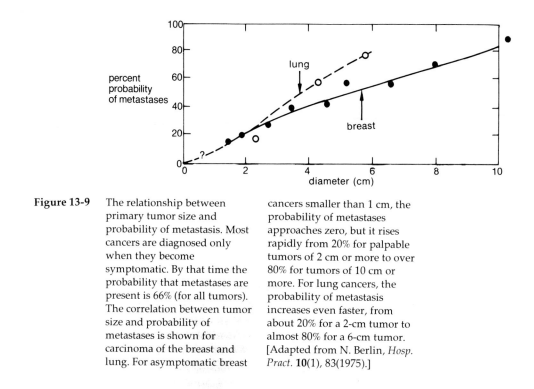

Figure 13-9 The relationship between primary tumor size and probability of metastasis. Most cancers are diagnosed only when they become symptomatic. By that time the probability that metastases are present is 66% (for all tumors). The correlation between tumor size and probability of metastases is shown for carcinoma of the breast and lung. For asymptomatic breast cancers smaller than 1 cm, the probability of metastases approaches zero, but it rises rapidly from 20% for palpable tumors of 2 cm or more to over 80% for tumors of 10 cm or more. For lung cancers, the probability of metastasis increases even faster, from about 20% for a 2-cm tumor to almost 80% for a 6-cm tumor. [Adapted from N. Berlin, *Hosp. Pract.* **10**(1), 83(1975).]

13-3   Cancers can be initiated by environmental factors and by viruses

Neoplastic transformation

Carcinogenesis, the process by which cancers arise, is only beginning to be understood. The conversion of a normal cell to a cancer cell is called *neoplastic transformation*. A transformed cell produces only transformed progeny, thereby giving rise to a clone of cancer cells. The preclinical development of a cancer, which occurs over a long period prior to diagnosis, probably involves a *progression* of transformations, giving rise to subclones of increasing malignancy. However, by the time they are clinically detectable, most cancers appear monoclonal—that is, as if they were derived from a single cell. Therefore, if a progression of transformations is involved, each must give a particular subclone such a competitive advantage that it can grow to dominate the tumor.

Carcinogens and promoters

Evidence that environmental factors could be responsible for carcinogenesis first came from epidemiological studies of cancer (Table 13-1). Tests in experimental animals confirmed that some common environmental substances—for example, cigarette smoke—are carcinogenic (Figure 13-10). Purification and fractionation of these substances

Table 13-1 The Progressive Increase of Bladder Tumors with Increasing Length of Exposure to Aromatic Amines[a] Among 78 Distillery Workers

Length of Latent Period (Years)	Length of Exposure in Years:					
	Up to 1	1	2	3	4	5 and over
	(Percentage of Workers with Tumors)					
Up to 5	0	0	0	0	0	0
10	0	0	0	0	0	11
15	0	17	22	0	10	45
20	4	17	22	40	30	69
25	9	17	22	70	70	88
30	9	17	48	70	80	94

[a]The statistics are given for bladder tumors among 78 men engaged under conditions of heavy exposure in the distillation of 2-naphthylamine and benzidine, two highly carcinogenic dyestuff intermediates. The group of workers who were exposed for only 4 years did not show a response for the first 10 years of observation, but after 20 years their bladder tumor incidence was up to 30%, and by 30 years it was as high as 80%. For the workers exposed for 5 years or more, the incidence observed in 30 years went up to 94%. [Courtesy of American Cancer Society.]

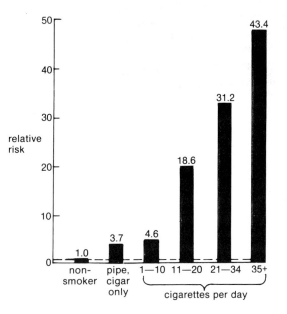

Figure 13-10

The relative risk of incurring lung cancer among nonsmokers and various groups of smokers. Those who smoke more than 35 cigarettes per day, for example, are more than 43 times as likely to develop cancer as those who do not smoke. [Courtesy of American Cancer Society.]

Table 13-2 Some Common Carcinogens and Promoters

Class of Compound	Carcinogens	Typical Source	Promoters	Typical Source
Polycyclic aromatic hydrocarbons	3,4-Benzpyrene (BP)	Coal tar; cigarette smoke; soot	Phorbolmyristate acetate (PMA)	Croton oil
	Methylcholan-threne (MC)	Coal tar; cigarette smoke; soot	Natural hormones	Ovary, adrenal, etc.
	Aflatoxin B_1	Aspergillus flavus (a fungus that grows on grains and peanuts)		
Aromatic amines	Dimethylamino-benzene (butter yellow; DAB)			
	2-Acetylamino-fluorene (AAF)			
Food preservatives	Nitrates convert secondary amines to nitrosamines	Preserved meats such as frankfurters		
Azo dyes		Dye industry		
Irradiation	X ray	Military; nuclear reactors; medical diagnosis		
	Ultraviolet	Sun		
Other chemicals	Asbestos	Insulating material		
	Bis (2-chlorethyl) sulfide (mustard gas)	Military		
	Vinyl chloride	Plastics industry		
Drugs	Diethylstilbesterol	Medical therapy		

sometimes led to loss of carcinogenic activity. Selective recombination of fractions, sometimes from separate sources (such as coal tar and cigarette smoke), restored activity. Such studies defined two classes of compounds active in chemical carcinogenesis: *carcinogens* and *promoters* (Table 13-2).

Carcinogens act acutely on target cells to cause an irreversible change in the cellular genome. This action is necessary but not sufficient for neoplastic transformation. Promoters stimulate cell division and cause neoplastic transformation of carcinogen-treated cells. At least two cell-division cycles in the presence of promoters are required

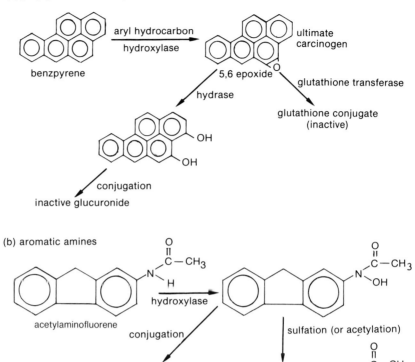

Figure 13-11

Metabolism of two classes of carcinogens in the liver by detoxifying enzymes that produce ultimate carcinogens as a byproduct.

for transformation. Promoter action is reversible, and it is not by itself carcinogenic. It must occur after carcinogen treatment to cause transformation.

Direct application of most environmental carcinogens to target cells *in vitro* does not lead to malignant transformation, even in the presence of appropriate promoters. Environmental carcinogens are modified metabolically *in vivo* to become *ultimate carcinogens.* The crucial modification usually takes place in the liver, where detoxifying enzymes catalyze conversion to highly reactive intermediates and then esterification of these intermediates with glucuronides (Figure 13-11). The inactive esters are excreted into the urine via the kidney tubule-cell transport system. The highly reactive intermediates are ultimate carcinogens. If their rate of production exceeds their rate of esterification, they may reach carcinogenic levels. For example, people with abnormally high levels of the detoxifying enzymes aryl hydrocarbon hydroxylases have greatly increased risk for some types of cancer.

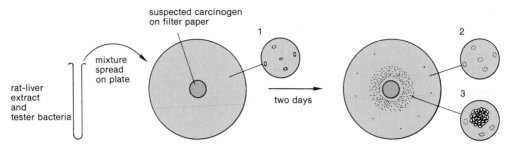

Figure 13-12 A diagrammatic representation of the Ames test for detection of mutagens. Mutagenesis is detected by mixing an extract of rat liver, which can convert carcinogens to ultimate carcinogens, with test bacteria that carry a mutant gene for histidine biosynthesis, so that they require histidine for growth. The mixture is then plated on a medium lacking histidine, and a dose of the substance to be tested is placed on a filter paper disc in the center of the plate. After two days, most of the bacteria have died for lack of histidine, but, in the vicinity of the disc, mutagenesis by the test substance has led to reversion of the defective *his* gene to a functional form in some of the bacteria, which have formed visible colonies. [Adapted from R. Devoret, *Scientific American* **241**, August 1979.]

Although the mode of action of ultimate carcinogens in transformation is not yet established, there is increasing evidence that most, if not all, of these compounds are potent mutagens. This generalization is the basis for analyses such as the *Ames test*, simple, inexpensive screening procedures that can detect low levels of environmental carcinogens, either as is or after conversion to ultimate carcinogens using a liver preparation, by their ability to increase the frequency of mutational events in bacteria and bacterial viruses (Figure 13-12). The physical agents that cause cancer, such as ultraviolet and γ irradiation, are also highly mutagenic, acting directly on nucleic acids to cause genetic changes. Therefore, carcinogens probably cause transformation by acting on DNA, but the primary effect of their action remains unclear.

Oncogenic DNA viruses

Certain DNA and RNA viruses, termed *oncogenic*, can transform the cells they infect and thereby induce tumor formation. There are several varieties of oncogenic DNA viruses, ranging from very simple to very complex. A classification of these viruses and the neoplasms they induce is given in Table 13-3. The simplest viruses, SV40 and polyoma, have been analyzed most completely. Both can undergo alternative routes of infection, depending on properties of the host cell that are not understood. In *permissive* cells, the virus appropriates the host

Table 13-3   Some DNA Oncogenic Viruses and Their Properties

Class	Virus	Genome Size (Molecular Weight)	Host Cell for Productive Infection	Host Cell for *in Vitro* Malignant Transformation
Papova	SV40 (Simian virus 40)	3×10^6	Monkey	Human, mouse, hamster
	Polyoma (*poly* = many, *oma* = tumors)	3×10^6	Mouse	Mouse, hamster, rat
	Papilloma (causes the benign skin tumors called warts)	5×10^6	?	Rabbit, human, cattle
Adenoviruses	Several types (e.g., adenovirus-12)	25×10^6	Human	Hamster, rat, human
Herpes	Herpes saimiri	100×10^6	?	Monkey
	Lucke carcinoma	100×10^6	?	Frog
	Marek's disease	100×10^6	?	Chicken
	Epstein–Barr virus (EBV)	100×10^6	Human (infectious mononucleosis)	Human (Burkitt's lymphoma)

synthetic machinery, produces 10^3 to 10^4 progeny virus particles per cell, and then causes cell lysis with release of the new virus. In *nonpermissive* cells, some viral genes are expressed, but the infection then aborts and the host cells survive. A small fraction of these cells undergo malignant transformation. The transformed cells retain one or a few viral genomes, integrated covalently into the host genome. DNA oncogenic viruses were first used to demonstrate that large primary RNA transcripts are processed (spliced) to form active smaller mRNAs. In SV40 virus infection (Figure 13-13), a set of messages derived from alternative splicing of early transcripts is directly involved in the neoplastic transformation of nonpermissive cells. The so-called large T antigen coded by one of these messages binds to the origin of transcription of the integrated SV40 genome and somehow causes transformation.

Whether DNA oncogenic viruses cause cancer in humans is not known. However, there is a striking correlation between primary liver cancers (hepatomas) and previous infection with hepatitis virus type B, both in woodchucks and in humans. Hepatitis virus infects (but does not transform) several cell types *in vitro*. Thus there is no direct evidence for a hepatitis B virus transforming gene. Infection with hepatitis B virus causes extensive and prolonged cell death and cell damage, with concomitant and prolonged liver cell proliferation,

Figure 13-13

Viral and integrated forms of the oncogenic DNA virus SV40. In a nonpermissive host, the viral DNA integrates into the cellular genome, and only early genes are transcribed. Alternative RNA processing pathways produce messages for two gene products, T and t, whose actions lead to transformation of the infected cell (see text).

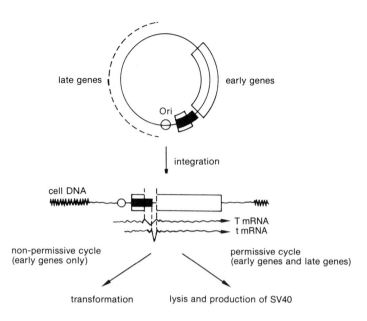

late genes

early genes

Ori

integration

cell DNA

T mRNA
t mRNA

non-permissive cycle
(early genes only)

permissive cycle
(early genes and late genes)

transformation

lysis and production of SV40

immune responses, and host repair processes. Perhaps one or more of these processes contributes to an increased incidence of neoplastic transformation.

Other candidates for human oncogenic DNA viruses are herpes viruses, complex enveloped viruses with large, segmented DNA genomes. A high incidence of Burkitt's lymphoma in restricted regions of Africa coincides with the geographic distribution of Epstein–Barr Virus (EBV); the lymphomas contain integrated EBV genomes and express EBV proteins. Nasopharyngeal carcinoma in East Asia is similarly linked to EBV. Less clear is the relationship of cervical cancer to herpes simplex type II virus (HSV II), but again epidemiological evidence indicates a link. Finally, the *acquired immunodeficiency syndrome* (Concept 12-4) leads to a highly malignant form of the cancer known as *Kaposi's sarcoma*. Patients with acquired immunodeficiency syndrome are often infected with a herpes virus, the opportunistic pathogen cytomegalovirus (CMV). While some early evidence indicated that the nuclei of tumor cells from a few of these patients harbor CMV genomes, it is most likely that CMV takes advantage of the patient's immunodeficiency and does not play a role in oncogenesis. The highly malignant variant of Kaposi's sarcoma also occurs with high incidence in patients immunosuppressed for transplantation and in parts of Africa in young children.

Oncogenic RNA viruses

Oncogenic RNA virus (*oncornavirus*) infections differ from DNA tumor virus infections in several respects. Oncornaviruses belong to a larger group called *retroviruses* because their replication involves a reversal of the normal transcription process. These viruses produce a polymerase called *reverse transcriptase* that uses the viral RNA as a template to transcribe a DNA copy initiated from a tRNA primer (Figure 13-14). The same enzyme converts the DNA copy to a double-stranded form, called the *provirus*, that can insert into the host-cell genome. The linear genomes of these viruses are small (about 8000 nucleotides in length) and simple, including only three or four genes and, in their DNA form, long-terminal-repeat (LTR) sequences at each end.

Oncornaviruses may be divided into two classes: rapidly transforming and slowly transforming viruses (Table 13-4). The rapidly transforming viruses can transform target cells directly *in vitro* by means of specific oncogenic genes (*onc* genes) that are discussed in the following section. Slowly transforming oncornaviruses lack known *onc* genes, and they cannot transform target cells *in vitro* although they eventually cause tumors in infected animals.

Oncornavirus-infected cells continually produce progeny virus by a budding process at the cell membrane. During budding, the viral core is in the shape of a C; hence these viruses are also called C-type viruses (Figure 13-15). The structural glycoproteins of the cell membrane budding site become the envelope glycoproteins of the virus, and they are coded by the viral genome. Budding occurs by evagination of the core-membrane complex, ending with a separation of viral and cellular membranes (Figure 13-16). Many retroviruses also produce *core* (*gag* gene product) polyprotein mRNAs that enter the endoplasmic reticulum and become expressed apparently erroneously as cell-surface glycosylated molecules that are not used in production of budded virions.

13-4   Transformation can involve changes in expression of normal cellular genes

Assay for oncogenes by DNA transfection

Recent experiments have demonstrated two important characteristics of neoplastic transformation. First, transformation involves changes in the cellular DNA, and second, these changes can cause transformation by affecting the activity of normal cellular genes. The evidence for these conclusions comes from so-called *transfection* experiments, in which DNA added to cultured cells under appropriate conditions is taken up and incorporated into the cell genome at low frequency. In general, intact DNA from neoplastic cells or cells infected with rapidly transforming virus will, in transfection experiments, lead to the neoplastic transformation of appropriate cultured target cells, whereas intact DNA from normal cells will not. Although freshly

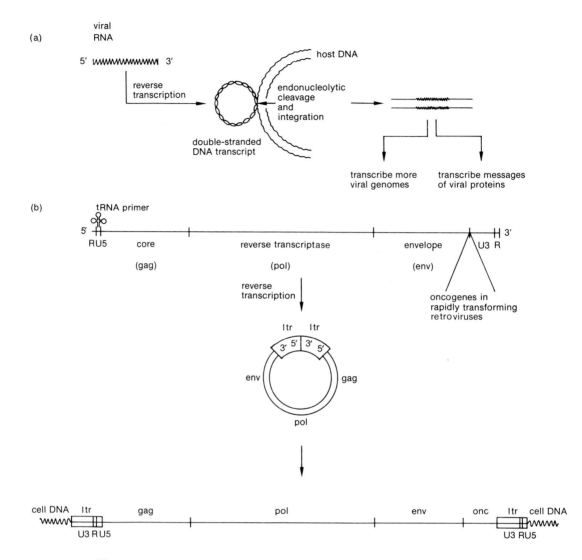

Figure 13-14   Events in the reverse transcription and integration of oncornavirus genes into host genomes. The enveloped virus penetrates into the target cell cytoplasm. Using an enzyme called *reverse transcriptase,* which it codes for and carries with it, the virus begins the transcription of its RNA nucleotide sequence template into a complementary DNA nucleotide sequence. The reaction requires as primer a host-cell transfer RNA (tRNA) that binds to a complementary sequence near the 5′ end of the viral RNA. A single-strand DNA is copied to the 5′ end of the viral RNA, and then synthesis continues at the 3′ end of the viral RNA but duplicating the long-terminal-repeat (LTR) region. During this process, the used viral RNA template is digested or removed, and a second-strand DNA copy is made using the reverse transcribed DNA as a template. The result is a double-stranded closed-circular proviral DNA copy of the viral RNA information with LTRs at both 5′ and 3′ ends. In cells susceptible to infection by this virus, the DNA provirus apparently integrates in host chromosomal DNA, where it may act as a site of transcription of new viral RNAs and individual gene messages. The LTR region contains a promoter as well as an enhancer sequence for DNA → RNA transcription and thus causes constitutive expression of both viral and nearby host genes.

Table 13-4   A List of Oncornaviruses and Their Effects

Name	Susceptible Species	Type of Tumor Induced	Transforming Gene
Rapidly transforming viruses:			
Rous sarcoma virus	Chickens; other aves	Sarcomas	$v\text{-}src$
Fujinami sarcoma virus	Chickens; other aves	Sarcomas	$v\text{-}fps$
Avian myeloblastosis virus	Chickens; other aves	Myeloid cells	$v\text{-}myb$
Avian erythroblastosis virus	Chickens; other aves	Erythroid cells	$v\text{-}erb$
Myelocytomatosis virus 29 (MC29)	Chickens	Myelomonocytic cells	$v\text{-}myc$
Harvey sarcoma virus	Rodents	Sarcoma	$v\text{-}ras^H$
Kirsten sarcoma virus	Rodents	Sarcoma	$v\text{-}ras^K$
Moloney sarcoma virus	Rodents	Sarcomas	$v\text{-}mos$
Abelson leukemia virus	Rodents	Hematopoietic tumors; pre B-cell tumors	$v\text{-}abl$
Simian sarcoma virus	Simians	Sarcomas	$v\text{-}sis$
Feline sarcoma virus (Gardner/Theilen)	Cats	Sarcoma	$v\text{-}fes$
Friend focus forming virus[a]	Rodents	Erythro and myelo-monocytic tumors	$v\text{-}sif$
Slowly transforming viruses:			
Avian leukosis virus	Chickens	B-cell leukemia	None identified
Gross leukemia virus	Rodents	T-cell leukemias	None identified
Radiation leukemia virus	Rodents	T-cell leukemias	None identified
Friend lymphatic leukemia virus	Rodents	T-cell leukemias	None identified
Moloney leukemia virus	Rodents	T-cell leukemias	None identified
Friend erythroleukemia virus	Rodents	Erythroblastic leukemias	gp52 envelope gene
Feline leukemia virus	Cats; baboons?	Leukemias	None identified
Bovine leukemia virus	Cattle	Leukemias	None identified
Mouse mammary tumor virus	Rodents	Mammary carcinomas	None identified

[a]Intermediate phenotype; rapidly transforming *in vivo* oncogenic retrovirus.

explanted normal cells do not usually serve as suitable targets for neoplastic transforming DNA, certain cultured lines of mouse fibroblast cells selected for their ability to proliferate and to survive beyond the ⌣50-generation senescence limit of most normal cells are suitable targets. Thus this assay measures the activity of certain cancer cell genes to *complete* the neoplastic progression of already immortalized mouse fibroblasts. There is not a strict concordance between cancer genes revealed by this assay and the malignant transformation potential of known retroviral *onc* genes; that is, many viral *onc* genes are not active in this assay. Nevertheless, the heritability of the transformed phenotype and its transmission by DNA transfection indicate that transformation involves heritable changes in the cell genome.

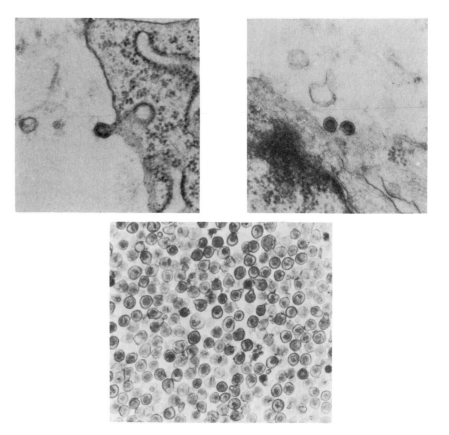

Figure 13-15
The budding of an oncornavirus. In (a) the virion bud is in the characteristic C configuration, whereas in (b) one completed virion is adjacent to a nearly completed particle. In (c) a concentrate of these viruses is shown. [Photographs courtesy of O. Witte and D. Rice.]

Relationship of oncogenes from viruses, normal cells, and tumor cells

The nature of several retroviral oncogenes (*v-onc* genes) is now known (Table 13-4). Several, including the oncogenes from *Rous sarcoma virus* (*v-src*) and *Abelson leukemia virus* (*v-abl*), code for cytoplasmic protein kinases that catalyze phosphorylation of tyrosine residues on specific sets of cellular proteins. Others, such as the oncogene from *avian myelocytomatosis virus* (*v-myc*), code for DNA-binding proteins found in the nucleus. Hybridization studies have shown that the *v-onc* genes are closely homologous to genes in normal mammalian cells. Most, if not all, of these cellular (*c-onc*) genes are potentially oncogenic in transfection assays. If a *c-onc* gene is combined artificially with an appropriate retroviral long-terminal-repeat sequence that apparently serves as a promoter of transcription, the recombinant *c-onc* DNA may, in many cases, transform cells in culture. These findings strongly support the view that DNA alterations may cause transformation by affecting the activity of normal cellular genes. The circle of evidence has been tightened with the demonstration that the active cloned oncogene from a spontaneous human bladder cancer is closely related to the *onc* genes *v-ras^H* and *c-ras^H*, previously characterized as a retroviral oncogene and its cellular homolog, respectively.

DNA transfection of freshly explanted fibroblasts with *v-* or *c-onc*

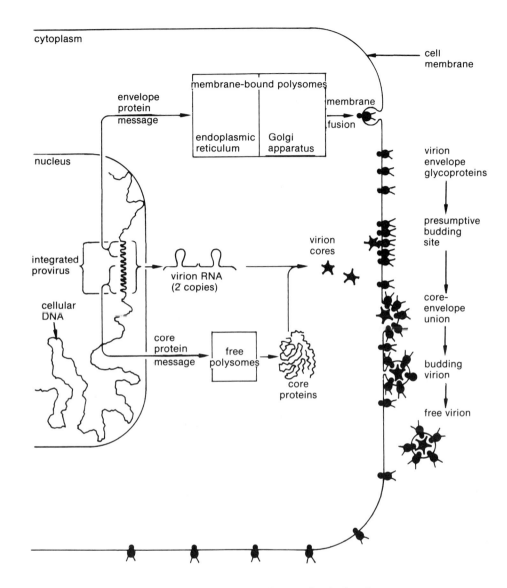

Figure 13-16 Cellular formation of oncornavirus budding sites. Virion mRNAs of two classes, core and envelope, are transcribed from integrated viral DNA copies. A core polyprotein is produced from core mRNA in the free polysome fraction, and then cleaved into several distinct proteins that combine with virion RNA to form the virion cores. Simultaneously, envelope mRNA is translated in polysomes bound to membranes of endoplasmic reticulum. This envelope precursor polyprotein is glycosylated, cleaved to its functional subunits, and inserted into the plasma membrane of the cell to form presumptive budding sites. Core assemblies bind to the inner surface of the presumptive budding sites and evaginate through them, with eventual separation of viral and cellular membranes.

genes has revealed synergistic actions of these genes in neoplastic transformation. One class of oncogenes apparently endows these cells with the ability to proliferate and survive beyond the usual sequence limit, whereas the other class of oncogenes complete the neoplastic progression of these (and other) immortalized cells. The first class of genes include the *myc gene*, the adenovirus *EIA gene*, and the SV40 *large T gene*, all encoding proteins that localize to the cell nucleus. The second class of genes include all of the *ras gene* family, and perhaps other oncogenes which encode proteins which localize to the cyto-plasmic face of the plasma membrane. These experiments have at least two important consequences: they implicate both cell membrane and nuclear sites as key elements in neoplastic proliferation, and they provide at least two independent events which are probably involved in tumor progression.

The way in which *slowly transforming* oncornaviruses cause lym-phocytic and mammary gland neoplasms *in vivo* remains unclear. One postulated mechanism, called the *promoter-insertion hypothesis*, is the chance integration of provirus next to a *c-onc* gene, whose ex-pression is thereby heightened by the promoter and/or enhancer ac-tivity of the viral 3' long-terminal-repeat sequence. A second model, called the *receptor-mediated leukemogenesis hypothesis*, proposes that T- and B-cell tumors proliferate in response to retroviral envelope "anti-gen" binding to lymphocyte cell-membrane antigen- or mitogen-spe-cific receptors. In addition to these models, transfection experiments using immortal mouse fibroblasts treated with DNA from tumors induced by slowly transforming oncornaviruses reveal the presence of an oncogenic element that is neither related to any retroviral se-quence, nor to any known *c-onc* gene, nor to any antigen receptor-encoding gene. Therefore, transformation by these viruses may be a multistep process involving several genomic changes.

Recent studies of the molecular genetic mechanisms of the chro-mosomal translocations that are characteristic of particular lymphoid cell neoplasms provide striking corroboration of the potential impor-tance of cellular oncogenes and/or antibody receptor genes in neo-plastic transformation (Figure 13-17). In human Burkitt's lymphoma, there is a reciprocal chromosomal translocation between the part of chromosome 8 bearing *c-myc* and one of the three chromosomes bear-ing immunoglobulin *V regions* (heavy chain, chromosome 14; κ chain, chromosome 2; λ chain, chromosome 22). In mouse plasmacytomas, there is a reciprocal chromosomal translocation between the part of chromosome 15 bearing *c-myc* and immunoglobulin heavy-chain chromosome 12 "switch" regions (Concept 4-6). The translocated, of-ten truncated, *c-myc* genes are transcriptionally active in these cells. Similar reciprocal chromosomal translocations involving other cellu-lar homologues of viral oncogenes have been reported in nonlymphoid neoplasms, including the well-known *Philadelphia chromosome* characteristic of human *chronic myelogenous leukemia*, in which the *c-abl* gene on chromosome 9 is translocated to chromosome

original chromosomes

translocated chromosomes

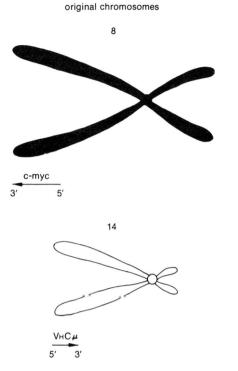

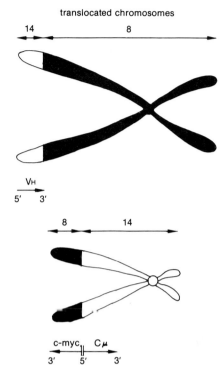

Figure 13-17   An example of a chromosomal translocation characteristic of Burkitt's lymphoma. The normal location of *c-myc* is at the tip (telomere) of the long arm of chromosome 8, with the *c-myc* gene reading in the centromere to telomere direction, as shown. The normal location of the $V_H...D...J_H$-C_μ region is near the telomere of the long arm of chromosome 14 with the $V_H \rightarrow$ C_μ reading (when rearranged) in the telomere to centromere direction. In Burkitt's lymphoma, the *c-myc* translocates to the S_μ switch site just 5′ from the C_μ (or rarely to another C_H switch sequence), while the telomeric region of chromosome 14 containing $V_H...D...J_H$ up to the S_μ site replaces *c-myc* on chromosome 8. A similar translocation in mouse plasmacytomas involves the movement of *c-myc* to the nonexpressed heavy-chain chromosome at the switch sequence upstream of the expressed C_H gene (e.g., S_α in a cell expressing IgA from its homologous chromosome). Such translocations of *c-myc* often result in the loss of the 5′ *c-myc* exon.

22, while the *c-sis* gene on chromosome 22 is reciprocally translocated to chromosome 9. The *sis* gene apparently encodes a polypeptide growth factor, the so-called *platelet-derived growth factor*. Thus an oncogene encodes a protein whose main normal function is the stimulation of proliferation by appropriate cells having cell-surface receptors for this protein.

In all of the preceding cases involving activation or change of particular cellular genes, no direct evidence is yet available that demonstrates whether the expression of such genes in neoplastic cells is the *cause* or the *consequence* of neoplastic transformation. However generated, the expression of these proteins provides ready targets for immunodiagnosis of cancer cells, and these targets might also prove to be antigenic targets for the host immune system.

13-5   Many cancers are antigenic in their host of origin

Demonstration of host immunity to tumors

In 1908, Paul Ehrlich postulated that cancer cells arise frequently, that they bear membrane changes recognizable as foreign antigens by the host, and that the immune system may be able to reject most of these cells. Fifty years later, Lewis Thomas proposed further that the evolution of cell-mediated immunity may have been driven by selection for *immunological surveillance* of newly arising neoplasms. If cancer cells are antigenic, they should induce a specific immune response in the host of origin. Tumor formation would then have to result from an immunoresistant cancer or an ineffective immune response. Demonstrating immunity of a host to its own tumor could therefore be difficult. Experimentalists in the early twentieth century attempted to circumvent this problem by transplanting tumor cells from the original host to a second animal of the same species. In every case, these tumors indeed began to grow and were then rejected. However, we now know that because these investigators did not use inbred strains, the immune responses observed were directed against donor transplantation antigens rather than against tumor-specific antigens. Only with the development of inbred strains of mice and rats did the demonstration of tumor-specific antigens become possible.

Tumor antigenicity and host immunity to tumors was first demonstrated by a three-stage experiment (Figure 13-18). A carcinogen-induced cancer was excised completely from its original host, and then varying numbers of tumor cells were transplanted to syngeneic hosts. The number of transplanted cells that reproducibly induced tumors in the recipient hosts was determined. Retransplantation of this number of tumor cells from the secondary hosts to the original host usually resulted in no tumor growth. This phenomenon was *specific* for the original tumor. Adoptive transfer of lymphocytes from the original host to genetically identical naive hosts conferred specific resistance to the original tumor. This transfer of immunity required the transfer of live lymphocytes, subsequently identified as T lymphocytes.

With the advent of sensitive techniques such as immunofluorescence and radioimmunoassay for assaying antibodies specific to tumor antigens, tumor-bearing hosts were shown to have both a cell-mediated and a humoral immune response to their own tumor antigens. The resulting humoral antibodies were used in cross-absorption studies to compare large numbers of tumors and normal cells. Thus it was possible to identify tumors with *cross-reacting antigens*, tumors with *tumor-unique* antigens, and tumors with antigens common to a subset of normal cells (*differentiation antigens*).

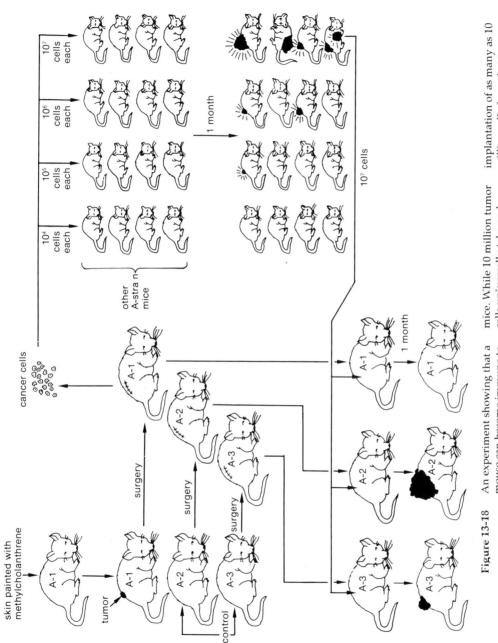

Figure 13-18

An experiment showing that a mouse can become immune to its own tumor. A mouse of strain A (A-1) has a carcinogen-induced skin tumor that is excised, and graded numbers of tumor cells are injected into other A-strain mice. While 10 million tumor cells universally take and eventually kill hosts, only 50% of A mice receiving one million cells have tumor takes. However, the original mouse (A-1) that had the tumor excised is now resistant to implantation of as many as 10 million cells from that tumor, while littermate controls (A-2 and A-3) are susceptible to as few as one million tumor cells. [Modified from experiments by R. Prehn.]

Figure 13-19

A clonal selection hypothesis to describe carcinogen-induced tumor-specific antigens. Several distinct cell types in a tissue adhere to each other by cell-specific surface properties. The carcinogen selectively transforms one of these types. The clonal progeny resulting from this transformation bear the same cell-specific determinants, but these cancer cells show a wide variety of morphological characteristics (pleomorphism). Because these malignant progeny no longer have complementary cells to adhere to, they tend to grow away from the original focus.

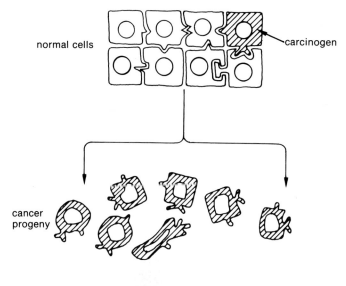

Tumor-specific antigens

In theory, apparent tumor-specific antigens could be new determinants or simply very rare normal determinants. Most tumors are populated predominantly by a single clone of cells, all of which share the cell membrane properties of the original transformed cell. Some of the surface determinants of each normal cell may be unique, or they may be shared by only a few other cells. If so, the concentration of these unique determinants will normally be far too low to trigger either an immunogenic or tolerogenic response. However, if such a cell gives rise to a transformed clone of identical cells, its surface molecules may provoke an immune response even if no new determinants are present. Thus a carcinogen-induced transformation may produce a change in the cell surface, or it may simply select for expansion of a rare subset of preexisting cells bearing unique cell-surface determinants (Figure 13-19).

In cancer research and therapy, four different classes of tumor antigens are distinguished. These are *oncofetal* antigens and three classes of tumor-specific antigens, induced by chemical carcinogens, oncogenic DNA viruses, and oncornaviruses, respectively.

Oncofetal antigens are found on the surfaces of cancer cells, but they are also expressed during a specific phase of embryonic differentiation. An important example is the carcinoembryonic antigens (CEA) of the colon. This set of antigens is found on the surfaces of all tumor cells derived from the gastrointestinal tract or derivatives of the fetal gastrointestinal tract, such as pancreas, liver, and gall bladder. These glycoprotein antigens are present on only a small subset of normal adult cells, so that the total body concentration of CEA is normally extremely small. Another important example is alpha-fetoprotein (αFP), normally secreted by yolk sac and fetal liver epithelial cells, and also produced by malignant yolk sac and liver cells. Although αFP is a secreted product, anti-αFP immune responses restrict growth of these neoplasms. Careful analysis has revealed that αFP is not solely a tumor antigen in adults, but it is normally expressed by the proliferating fraction of liver cells.

Members of the second class are tumor-specific antigens induced by chemical carcinogens. Each carcinogen-induced tumor expresses unique cell-surface antigens. When a single mouse is skin-painted with the carcinogen methylcholanthrene at several different sites, each of the resulting carcinomas will express cell-surface antigens that are identical on all cells within the tumor but different from the antigens expressed by the other methylcholanthrene-induced tumors. The following experiment suggests that in at least one case these antigens are unlikely to be normal cell-specific determinants. Mouse epithelial cells from the prostate were cloned *in vitro,* and several progeny cells from the same clone were independently transformed by carcinogen *in vitro.* The tumor-specific, cell-surface antigens were identical among the progeny of any given transformed cell, but the tumor-specific antigens of each transformed clone were unique. Other chemical carcinogens also show induction of diverse tumor-specific antigens.

These findings are important for at least two reasons. At the biological level, it is important to know whether chemical carcinogens somehow select for rare cells, each of which when cloned expresses a unique surface antigen present on the original cell just prior to transformation, or whether transformation invariably results in a genetic event that is expressed as a new cell-membrane antigen. If the second alternative is true, it will be important to establish whether neoplastic transformation is dependent on the membrane alteration. If so, transformation could be postulated to have its primary effect on cell-cell interactions or cell-membrane function, which as a secondary consequence promotes cell proliferation. For example, the new tumor antigen could be part of, or linked to, a cell-surface receptor-mitogen complex.

There is also an important clinical consequence of the finding that carcinogens induce unique tumor-specific antigens. If each new carcinogen-induced tumor bears only unique tumor-specific determinants, then it will be difficult if not impossible to prepare in advance a stockpile of specific immunologic reagents for tumor detection or treatment.

The third class of tumor-associated antigens comprises those induced by oncogenic DNA viruses. Each of these viruses induces unique nuclear and cell-surface antigens in cells that it transforms. For a particular virus, these antigens are always the same, regardless of differences in the tissue, the animal, or even the species in which the transformation occurs. Thus both the nuclear (T) antigens (Figure 13-20) and surface (S) antigens are diagnostic of the virus. However, both

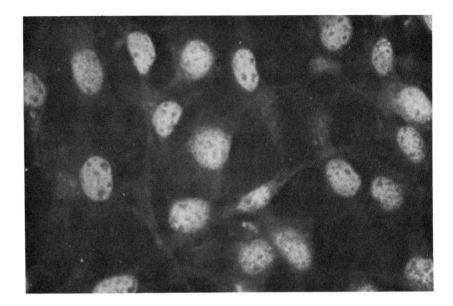

Figure 13-20
The detection of nuclear (T) antigens by immunofluorescence in cells infected with SV40. [Courtesy of C. Croce and K. Huebner.]

the T antigen and the cell-surface antigen are distinct from antigens of the viral protein coat, and the latter antigens are not detectable in transformed cells. Three of the major candidates for tumors induced by human DNA viruses (herpes viruses)—Burkitt's lymphoma, nasopharyngeal carcinoma, and uterine cervical cancer—do express tumor-associated cell-surface antigens that are the same on all tumors of a particular type.

The fourth class of tumor-associated antigens comprises those induced by oncornavirus transformation. Like the DNA tumor viruses, each RNA tumor virus induces specific antigens that are the same, regardless of differences in the host cell. By contrast, most, if not all, oncornavirus-specific tumor antigens are viral protein antigens. Some of these proteins represent *env* gene-encoded precursors of virus budding sites on the transformed cell membrane (Figure 13-16). Oncornavirus tumor antigens may have *group-specific* determinants in common with all viruses of a certain group (e.g., mouse leukemia viruses), *type-specific* determinants shared by only a few closely related viruses (e.g., Gross and radiation leukemia viruses), and unique virus-specific determinants. These determinants may be present on various virion polypeptides. At least one class of antigen, those carried on cell-surface glycosylated *gag* polyproteins, also are present on internal virion proteins.

Most of the leukemogenic oncornaviruses induce neoplasms that express normal differentiation antigens as well as viral antigens. In the mouse, one differentiation antigen, TL, may be anomalously expressed by thymic lymphomas from a mouse strain that does not normally express TL antigens on its thymocytes. Thus the control of

TL expression can somehow be interfered with by oncornavirus-induced transformation. In the special case of the murine oncornavirus-induced cell-surface antigens, the virion envelope protein may express virus-unique determinants, as well as determinants common to host differentiation antigens, in keeping with the homology between certain host genes and virion envelope genes.

13-6   Cancer cells are attacked by the cellular immune system

The immune response to cancers

The first experiment to define clearly the role of antibodies and cells in the immune response to cancers was carried out in the late 1940s. Cancer cells were placed into a cell-impermeable chamber with 0.2 μ diameter pores that allowed molecules, but not cells, to enter and exit. When the chambers were placed into hosts immune to the cancer cells, the cells survived and multiplied, although high concentrations of cancer-specific antibodies diffused into the chamber and bound to the cells. However, when the experiment was repeated with a chamber that contained pores large enough for cells to enter, the cancer cells were destroyed, and host lymphoid cells could be found infiltrating the tumor mass. Thus most tumors are not susceptible to attack by antibodies alone or by antibodies plus complement, but they are susceptible to attack by killer cells. Three kinds of killer cells may be involved in cell-mediated immunity to tumors: T_C cells, K cells (the cells responsible for antibody-dependent cell-mediated cytotoxicity), and the so-called natural killer and natural cytotoxic (NK/NC) cells. In most cancers, the T_C response is dominant. However, leukemias are quite sensitive to natural killer cells, to antibody and complement, and to antibody-dependent cell-mediated cytotoxicity. In general, cancers of the hematolymphoid system are sensitive to both humoral and cellular immunity, whereas all other cancers are susceptible to cellular immunity only.

Effects of immunodeficiency on tumor incidence

If the T-cell immune system is important for elimination of newly arising tumors, then animals and humans deficient in this system should be highly susceptible to induced tumors and should also have a high incidence of spontaneous tumors. Animals deprived of their thymus early in life are indeed extremely susceptible to various oncogenic viruses. For example, when neonatally thymectomized mice are exposed to Moloney sarcoma virus or polyoma virus, the animals suffer a high incidence of tumors that grow more rapidly than the tumors induced at low incidence in nonthymectomized littermate controls. Furthermore, the tumors from thymectomized animals are more highly antigenic on a per cell basis than the tumors in nonthymectomized littermates. These results, and those described in the preceding section, fulfill a postulate of the immunosurveillance hypothesis, that is, that the immune system responds to the antigens of endogenous neoplasms.

Another postulate of the hypothesis, that the cellular immune system has evolved to protect against a high rate of spontaneously arising neoplasms, is more controversial. As improvements in animal husbandry have allowed congenitally athymic animals to survive longer, it has been found that they do not have high incidence of death from cancer. Athymic mice, however, have strikingly increased levels of NK/NC cells, and these cells are highly active in tumor cell killing for several classes of cancer cells. For some types of carcinogen-induced cancers, the stage of transition between low malignancy and high malignancy is associated with a loss of susceptibility to elimination by natural killer cells. Nevertheless, further experiments are needed to determine whether athymic animals have a thymus-independent immune response that is sufficient for immunosurveillance, whether there is a nonimmune surveillance mechanism for removal of antigenic or newly arising tumor cells, or whether the assumption that tumors frequently arise by mutation simply is not true.

In apparent support of the hypothesis, humans with congenital immunodeficiency disease are strikingly susceptible to neoplasms. Nearly 10% of such immunodeficient children develop cancer. However, these cancers are principally derived from cells of the lymphoid system, and it is not certain whether the high rate of neoplasia is due to lack of immunosurveillance or to pathological consequences of the lymphoid system imbalance.

The best-documented examples of increased tumor incidence occur in adult-onset immunodeficiencies (Concept 12-4) and in patients treated with immunosuppressive drugs for allogeneic kidney transplants. The kidney transplant patients have an eighty-fold increased risk of developing cancer; about 60% of their cancers are of epithelial origin and about 40% of lymphoid origin. Again, it is unclear whether these cancers reflect the patient's immunodeficient state or whether they result from a pathological lymphoid disorder. The results are further complicated by the observation that the frequencies of the various epithelial neoplasms that develop in these patients do not correspond to the frequencies found in other groups of patients matched for age, sex, and geographic location. For example, immunosuppression causes little increase in the incidence of breast cancer or lung cancer, whereas it causes large increases in the incidence of some other epithelial neoplasms. Patients with *acquired immunodeficiency syndrome* (Concept 12-4) have a high incidence of Kaposi's sarcoma, but it is unclear whether the immunodeficiency predisposes to the emergence of antigenic tumor cells or to the emergence of antigenic agents that cause these tumors.

In summary, there is circumstantial evidence to support the immunosurveillance hypothesis, but the theory has not been conclusively tested. Still lacking is knowledge of all the immune mechanisms that could be involved and proof that cancers arise spontaneously at a high frequency.

13-7 Cancers may escape immunosurveillance by several mechanisms

Whatever the general validity of the immunosurveillance hypothesis, by the time a tumor is diagnosed most cancer patients demonstrate both cellular and humoral immunity directed specifically at cell-surface antigens of the tumor cells. How then do these tumor cells survive in what should be a hostile environment? Tumor growth under these conditions has been termed *immunological escape.* Transplantation experiments have shown that in some cases low doses of inoculated cancer cells "sneak through" to form tumors, whereas somewhat higher doses do not. Growth of small tumors is progressive despite evidence of an active host immune response. In other cases, termed *concomitant immunity*, a large primary tumor grows quite well, yet antigenic metastases are rejected by the host. In these cases, a small number of tumor cells are handled by the immune system, whereas a large number are not. Several different mechanisms of immunological escape have been found in research on experimental tumors; these studies form the basis for our current understanding of human tumor immunology.

Immunological tolerance

Animals injected before the development of full immunological competence with tumors or high concentrations of tumor-associated antigens maintain a specific unresponsiveness to these tumors if they are transplanted into the animals later in life. This phenomenon appears to be identical to that of immunological tolerance described in Chapter 10.

Immunoselection

Rare variant cells that have lost the original surface antigens occur in large tumor cell populations. In the face of an immune response against the antigenic tumor cells, the variants grow selectively to dominate the tumor. These cells may bear a different set of antigens and may in turn induce their own specific immune response. The immune response does not induce antigenic change; it merely selects for cells that have undergone antigenic change independently.

Antigenic modulation

The interesting phenomenon of antigenic modulation provides an example of how understanding the basic biology of microorganisms leads to an important clinical insight. In the 1940s, Beale and Sonneborn observed that treatment of paramecia with antibodies specific for their ciliary antigens leads to cessation of movement. However, if the paramecia are metabolically active, they soon begin to swim again, even in the continued presence of antibody. Further examination reveals that they have lost the antigens formerly present on their cilia and that they are expressing a new set of antigens. In the presence of antibody to the new antigens, modulation may occur again, with either reexpression of the first antigens or expression of another new set of antigens. These ciliary antigens are all encoded by nuclear genes of the paramecium.

Similar antigenic modulation has been demonstrated in two systems of mouse leukemic cells. Thymic leukemias induced in some mouse strains by murine leukemia viruses express TL antigens. Transfer of these thymic leukemia cells to hosts immune to TL antigens does not stop progressive growth of the tumor. Analysis of the leukemia cells growing in these hosts reveals no accessible cell-surface TL antigens. In tissue culture as well, when anti-TL antibody is added to TL-positive leukemia cells, the cells also lose accessible TL antigens within a few hours. In the absence of anti-TL antibodies, the TL antigens usually reappear. Immunoglobulin molecules on the surfaces of B cells and B-cell leukemias are also subject to antigenic modulation. In this case, it has been demonstrated directly that the original antigenic molecules are removed from the cell surface by capping in the presence of IgG followed by either endocytosis or shedding, or both.

Immunostimulation

A suggestion was first made in the 1950s that some aspect of the humoral immune response against a tumor may actually trigger cancer cells into more rapid or extensive proliferation. More recently, a cellular immune response was shown to promote increased outgrowth of antigenic tumor cells in a few tumor systems. Neither the class of humoral antibodies nor the type of immune cells (e.g., T_H or T_S) involved in immunostimulation is so far known. Immunostimulation could involve interactions among cell-surface determinants that are normally involved in control of cellular proliferation, such as mitogen-receptor complexes, but the mechanism of this phenomenon is still unclear.

Immunosuppression

There are several ways in which immunosuppression can occur in a cancer patient. The most common is iatrogenic immunosuppression—that is, immunosuppression caused by agents used to treat the cancer. Most anticancer agents, including ionizing radiation and cytotoxic drugs, have as side effects the destruction of lymphocytes and other cells important in the generation and maintenance of immunity. An unusual induction of immunosuppression occurs in the case of UV-light-induced skin neoplasms. In addition to the induction of neoplasms, UV induces a specific immunosuppression to antigens applied to or injected into the irradiated skin. Current evidence suggests that UV damages the antigen-presenting Langerhans cells in the skin, and that the damage is expressed by preferential induction of the suppressor T-cell circuits.

In some cancers, the tumors themselves seem to release immunosuppressive factors. The most striking example of this phenomenon is Hodgkin's disease, in which a small tumor in a single lymph node releases or induces the release of immunosuppressive factors that have a powerful effect on the entire cell-mediated immune system. Patients with Hodgkin's disease have a poor delayed hypersensitivity response and are abnormally sensitive to intracellular parasitic infections such as tuberculosis and herpes virus infections.

Finally, tumor cells may be infected with and actively produce immunosuppressive viruses. Two examples studied in the mouse are lactic dehydrogenase virus (LDV), which affects lymphocyte homing and function, and cytomegalovirus (CMV), which inhibits both cellular and humoral immunity by unknown mechanisms. The relationship of CMV infection to *acquired immunodeficiency syndrome* and *Kaposi's sarcoma* (Concepts 12-4 and 13-6) may therefore be complex.

Immunological enhancement

In some cases, animals that have been preimmunized with allogeneic grafts of disrupted cells from a certain tumor and then subsequently challenged with the same tumor will support its growth and eventually die. Nonimmunized animals challenged with the same tumor will allow it only brief growth and then reject it. Several experiments suggest a diversity of mechanisms to explain this paradoxical finding.

Immunological enhancement of tumor allograft growth may be accomplished by passive transfer of serum from an immunized host to a syngeneic nonimmune host. The serum antibodies could act by preventing immunization or by blocking effector functions. In support of the first possibility, enhancement is also observed if tumor cells precoated with enhancing antibodies are injected. However, enhancement results even if antiserum injection is delayed until as late as 7 days after tumor implantation. This result suggests that enhancement is due to blockade of the effector mechanisms that normally promote tumor rejection (Figure 13-21), although another possibility would be the type of antibody-induced antigenic modulation shown for TL antigens.

Experiments with an *in vitro* model system support the existence of serum-blocking factors that interfere with effector-cell mechanisms. Growth of tumor cells in tissue culture is often inhibited by lymphocytes from the tumor-bearing host (Figure 13-22). This lymphocyte effect can be blocked by addition of serum from the tumor-bearing host (Figure 13-23) but not by serum from hosts with another tumor type. This result could be due to a blockade of tumor target-cell

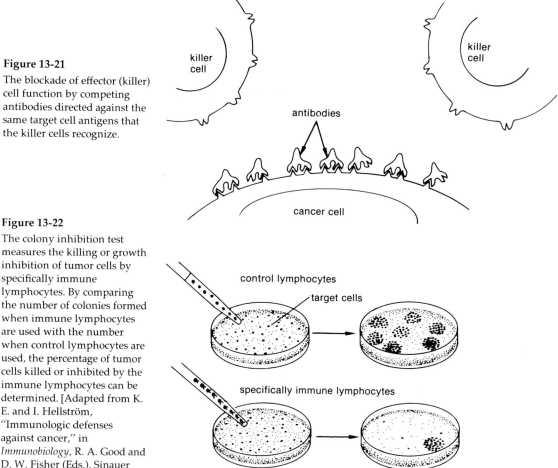

Figure 13-21

The blockade of effector (killer) cell function by competing antibodies directed against the same target cell antigens that the killer cells recognize.

Figure 13-22

The colony inhibition test measures the killing or growth inhibition of tumor cells by specifically immune lymphocytes. By comparing the number of colonies formed when immune lymphocytes are used with the number when control lymphocytes are used, the percentage of tumor cells killed or inhibited by the immune lymphocytes can be determined. [Adapted from K. E. and I. Hellström, "Immunologic defenses against cancer," in *Immunobiology*, R. A. Good and D. W. Fisher (Eds.), Sinauer Associates, Stamford, Conn., 1971, Chapter 21.]

antigenic determinants by anti-tumor antibodies, which would prevent attack by immune lymphocytes. If so, these experiments appear to indicate a basic antagonism between humoral and cell-mediated immunity to tumors. Alternatively, the serum-blocking factors could be solubilized tumor cell antigens that, either alone or complexed with anti-tumor antibodies, inhibit immune lymphocytes by blockade or elimination reactions (Figure 13-24).

In some cases of immunological tolerance as well as immunological enhancement, the dominant influence in specific inhibition of the immune response appears to be suppression—that is, suppressor T cells or products of suppressor T cells. In fact, serum-blocking factors could be suppressor factors. Thus it is possible that specific suppression also plays some role in the enhancement of tumor growth by inhibition of immune responses (Figure 13-25).

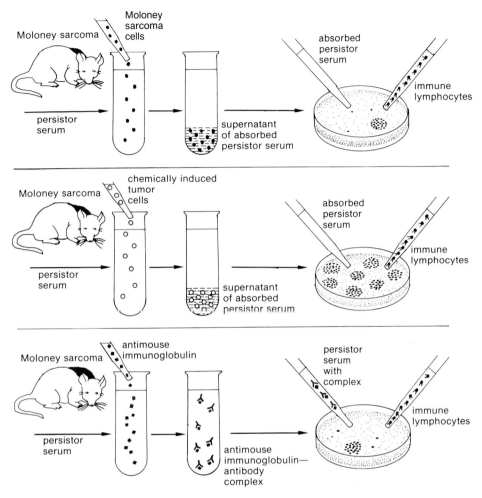

Figure 13-23 Two types of experiments provide evidence that the serum factors protecting persistent tumors contain specific antibodies. When persistor serum from an animal with a Moloney sarcoma is absorbed with Moloney sarcoma cells, the serum loses its ability to protect tumor cells (top). When cells from a different type of tumor (chemically induced) are used, the protective effect of the serum is unchanged (middle). The protective effect also is lost upon addition of goat anti-mouse immunoglobulin, which complexes and removes serum antibody (bottom). [Adapted from K. E. and I. Hellström; see Figure 13-22 legend.]

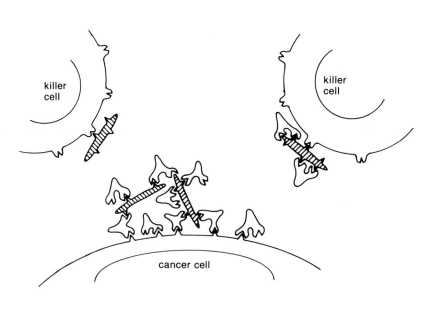

Figure 13-24

Two models of blocking-factor action. Antigen (shaded) or antigen–antibody complexes form lattices that may obscure target cell antigenic determinants or killer-cell receptors, or both.

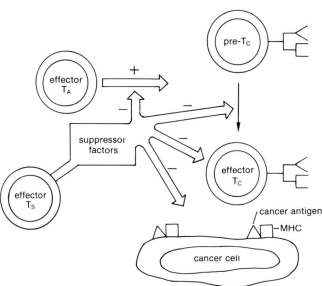

Figure 13-25

How suppressor T cells may block tumor immunity. T_S cells may affect T_C cells by having specificity for T cells, or for the combination of antigen with T_C, or for antigen alone. Alternatively, T_S cells may suppress by direct action on the tumor target cell and thus have receptor specificity for tumor antigens.

Defective associated recognition by T lymphocytes

Defective associated recognition of tumor antigens could derive from genetic defects and/or as congenital defects in the development of important interacting structures such as the thymus. The most likely defects of associated recognition are those already documented for several viral and minor antigen systems—the genetic preclusions of associated recognition of certain antigens in the context of particular I or K-D molecules (Concept 8-8). Preclusion could result in genetic predilections for cancer in some families. Thus it might be reasonable to study the HLA determinants in specific kinships with a high incidence of cancers. Because the phenomenon of preclusion does not define universally defective MHC gene products, the analysis of such families may require typing of all HLA determinants to allow the determination of precluded combinations. Such studies would also aid in the detection of Ir gene-mediated defects in tumor immunity.

13-8   Three kinds of methods are currently employed for cancer treatment in humans

Two of the commonly used therapeutic approaches to treatment of human cancers are localized, and one is systemic. The primary method of localized therapy is surgical removal of cancerous organs and tissues. This approach obviously requires a precise knowledge of the location and extent of the cancer, because only limited amounts of tissue can be excised.

The second method of localized therapy is the application of ionizing radiation (radiotherapy) to the site of known primary and suspected metastatic sites. The radiation results in irreparable damage to cellular DNA; those cells that enter the next cell cycle are unable to complete mitosis and die (mitotic death). A few cell types, such as lymphocytes, die without mitosis within hours after absorbing a lethal dose of irradiation (interphase death). Radiotherapy also requires precise knowledge of tumor location and extent. This treatment is most useful against tumors of lymphoid origin with known metastatic patterns, such as Hodgkin's disease, which can now be cured in up to 90% of all cases. Radiotherapy is also useful where an important structure must be cleared of cancer cells but can function subsequently without extensive cell division. For example, radiotherapy for laryngeal carcinoma leaves the patient with intact, functioning vocal cords, whereas the surgical approach usually does not.

The third method of cancer treatment is chemotherapy, the systemic administration of cytotoxic drugs. These drugs are designed to affect proliferating cells preferentially by interfering with pyrimidime and purine metabolism, DNA synthesis, or the process of mitosis (Figure 13-26, page 526). Because these drugs are accessible to all cells, malignant and normal, their major limitation is that they also kill normal cells.

With one or more of these therapeutic approaches, a number of cancers that were incurable 10 years ago can now be cured. However, these cures may be only partially effected by the therapeutic treatment. Many oncologists believe that all cancer therapies act to reduce the tumor cell load to a size that host defense mechansims can handle. In any case, curative cancer therapy must have as its goal the removal of all cancer cells because a single cancer cell left unimpeded will multiply to kill the patient.

13-9 Immunological methods may be important in the therapy, diagnosis, and prevention of cancer

Immunotherapy

Given the complexity of immune responses in patients with clinically detectable tumors, what are the prospects for development of cancer immunotherapy? Clearly humans often have both a humoral and a cell-mediated immune response to their own tumor antigens, but for some reason this response is not always effective.

Cell-mediated immunity provides the best defense against most cancers. However, attempts to increase the number of killer T cells, NK/NC cells, and antibody-dependent killer cells in a patient may result in expansion of inhibitory cell clones as well. Moreover, because the dimensions of the blocking-factor problem are not yet understood, it is not clear that increased clones of killer cells could compete with the blocking system. Even if T_C clones to tumor-specific antigens were introduced in large numbers, there is strong evidence that such *in vitro* cell lines do not express normal lymphoid cell homing receptors, and therefore the distribution of adoptively transferred T_C lines may lack the specificity of normally induced T_C effector cells.

Adoptive transfer of immunity to human cancer antigens from one patient to the next by transfer of uncloned live lymphocytes could be exceedingly dangerous because of the probable graft-versus-host response to the recipient's transplantation antigens. Such a response affects several of the body's important organ systems and is often fatal. In some cases of leukemia, transfer of lymphocytes from an HLA-matched donor leads to a milder form of graft-versus-host response, as well as some reduction of tumor load. Whether this results from a direct graft-anti-leukemia response or via some other mechanism (such as the release of potent lymphokines) is unknown.

An approach that has been tested is called *adjuvant immunotherapy*. In this method, the tumor is inoculated with BCG, an attenuated mycobacterium that is related to the tubercle bacillus and is an intracellular parasite of macrophages. The resulting immune response leads not only to the destruction of the intracellular forms of BCG but also to a massive increase in the number and activity of the phagocytic cells, as well as the production of interferon, an inducer of natural killer cells. BCG in combination with most immunogens heightens the immune response. In mice, it slightly but significantly increases the immune response to tumors. BCG may act as an immunological adjuvant by increasing the immunogenicity of the antigens it is mixed with or by increasing the activity of the macrophage system. This increased activity could be nonspecific, or it could involve an interferon-induced increase in either natural killer cells or antibody-dependent killer cells. Unfortunately, the effect of BCG on human tumors seems limited to those accessible to injection or infection with

BCG, and distant metastases and internal tumors are usually unaffected. BCG is potentially dangerous because increasing the immunogenicity of tumor cell antigens could increase the levels of blocking factors or suppressor cells as well as the cell-mediated immune response against a tumor.

Antibody therapy of tumors should also be approached with caution. Passive transfer of tumor-specific antibody into tumor-bearing hosts would be helpful mainly for leukemias and lymphomas, in which the cells are sensitive to antibody-triggered immunological destruction rather than to immunological enhancement. Recently, monoclonal antibodies to T-cell-specific differentiation antigens on human T-cell lymphocytic leukemias were infused into patients with these leukemias; in two cases, the leukemia cells underwent antigenic modulation. In contrast, monoclonal anti-idiotypic antibodies infused into a few patients with idiotype-positive B-cell lymphomas led to complete remissions. Triggering antibody-dependent, cell-mediated immunity would be another hypothetical approach, but this possibility will be impractical until more is known about the requirements for effective antibody in the triggering process. A most promising approach is to render noncytotoxic antibodies cytotoxic by attachment of radioactive nuclides or toxins such as ricin A chain.

Immunodiagnosis

The immunodiagnosis of cancer is likely to be an important addition to the clinician's armamentarium. Many tumors release specific cell-surface antigens into the bloodstream, and these antigens can be detected by radioimmunoassay (Chapter 3). There are three important limitations to this type of assay: first, antigen must be available in highly purified form so that the radioimmunoassay will be specific; second, the determinants must retain antigenicity when radiolabeled with iodine; and third, the antigen must be free to enter the circulation in tumor-bearing hosts.

Immunoassay also can be used to measure levels of serum antibody to a specific tumor antigen. Assays that detect antibody action on whole tumor cells *in vitro* may be used, so that it is unnecessary that purified antigen be available or that the tumor release antigen into the circulation. It is necessary only that antibody responses be related in some way to the presence or absence of tumor antigens in the host. High-titer tumor-specific antibodies (such as those obtained using hybridoma-monoclonal techniques) might be very useful in two other types of immunoassay: immunohistochemical identification of tumor cells in biopsy samples (Figure 13-27), and as markers for occult tumors whose antigens are accessible to circulating antibodies. In the latter technique, labeled tumor-specific antibodies are coinjected intravenously with nonbinding control antibodies, and the serum is sampled at various times to follow the specific disappearance from the bloodstream of the tumor-specific antibodies. If the antibodies are removed from the bloodstream by microfoci of tumor cells, it is theoretically possible that radioisotopic labeling of such antibodies

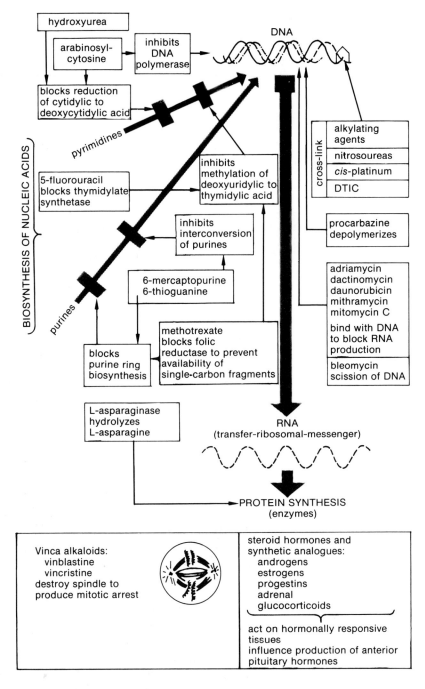

Figure 13-26
The actions of currently used anticancer chemotherapeutic agents. Three classes of agents are depicted: those that interfere with DNA synthesis or replication, those that affect the mitotic spindle and therefore arrest cells at metaphase, and those that act on tissues that require or are inhibited by steroid hormones. [Adapted from I. Krakoff, "Cancer Chemotherapy," in *CA—A Cancer Journal for Clinicians* **27**(3), 130(1977).]

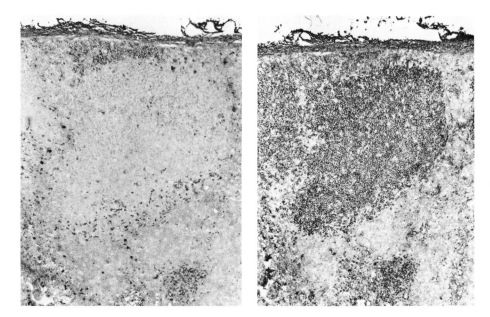

Figure 13-27　Immunohistochemical diagnosis of a lymph-node metastasis of a $\mu\kappa$ B-cell lymphoma. In (a) the lymph node is stained with an anti-λ chain antibody. Scattered $B_{\mu\lambda}$ cells surround a large unstained nodule in the region of a lymphoid follicle. In (b) a serial section is stained with an anti-κ chain antibody, demonstrating that the tumor nodule (a large cell lymphoma) is κ positive. [Courtesy of Dr. Roger Warnke.]

could be used to localize such micrometastases, and that toxic levels of radionuclides or protein toxins could be attached to these antibodies for therapeutic trials.

Immunological approaches to cancer prevention

Immunological techniques could also be useful in cancer prevention. If it ever becomes possible to identify infectious agents (such as oncornaviruses) that induce tumors bearing virus-specific antigens, then the possibility of vaccination with attenuated forms of these agents could be considered. However, as pointed out in Concept 13-7, induction of an immune response to a tumor-associated antigen may result in immunological enhancement rather than in protective immunity. Extensive animal testing would be required to determine the potential benefits and risks of such an approach before it could be applied to humans. Whereas immunodiagnosis and immunotherapy would be applied to patients with poor prognoses, vaccination would be carried out on a healthy population. Large-scale vaccination could not be justified unless the risk of inducing disease was proven to be virtually nonexistent.

Selected Bibliography

Where to begin

Cairns, J., "The origin of human cancers," *Nature* **289**, 353(1981).

Biology of cancer cells

Friedman, J. M., and Fialkow, P. J., "Cell marker studies of human tumorigenesis," *Transplant. Rev.* **28**, 17(1976).

Nowell, P. C., "The clonal evolution of tumor cell populations," *Science* **194**, 23(1976).

The preceding two articles are on the question of monoclonal versus multiclonal origins of cancers. They include a discussion of the factors involved in the progression of tumors of low malignancy into tumors of high malignancy.

Tannock, I. F., "Biology of tumor growth," *Hospital Practice* **18** (4), 81(1983). A highly readable and informative account of cancer growth and the basis for cancer chemotherapy.

Chemical and physical agents that cause cancer

Farber, E., "Chemical carcinogenesis," *N. Engl. J. Med.* **305**, 1379(1981).

Pitot, H. C., "Chemicals and cancer: initiation and promotion," *Hospital Practice* **18** (7), 101(1983).

The two preceding articles discuss the changes that occur in normal cells when carcinogens and promoters facilitate neoplastic transformation.

Mutations and cancer

Ames, B. N., "Carcinogenic potency," in "*Environmental Mutagens and Carcinogens,*" Sugimana, T., Kondo, S., and Takabe, H. (Eds.), Alan R. Liss, Inc., New York, 663–670 (1982).

McCann, J., "*In vitro* testing for cancer-causing chemicals," *Hospital Practice* **18** (9), 73(1983).

Are carcinogens mutagens, and if so, does their mutagenicity explain their mode of action in malignant transformation? The two preceding articles discuss these questions in depth.

Knudson, A. G., Hethcote, H. W., and Brown, B. W., "Mutation and childhood cancer: a probablistic model for the incidence of retinoblastoma," *Proc. Natl. Acad. Sci. USA* **72**, 5116(1975).

The preceding article is an epidemiological perspective on the interaction of heredity, environment, and mutation in the genesis of a cancer of the retina.

Oncogenic viruses and cellular oncogenes

Bishop, J. M., "Oncogenes," *Scientific American* **246** (3), 81(1982).

Weissman, I., and Bernhard, S., Eds., *Leukemia*, Dahlem Konferenzen, in press.

The two preceding treatises are on the transforming retroviruses and the cellular genes they acquire.

Cooper, G. M., "Cellular transforming genes," *Science* **218**, 801(1982).

Weinberg, R. A., "A molecular basis of cancer," *Scientific American* **249**, (5), 126(1983).

Land, H., Parada, L. F., and Weinberg, R. A., "Cellular oncogenes and multistep carcinogenesis," *Science* **222**, 771(1983).

The three preceding articles are on the identification of cancer genes by DNA transfection.

Rowley, J. D., "Human oncogene locations and chromosome aberrations," *Nature* **301**, 290(1983). Cellular oncogenes are often on "marker" translocated chromosomes in tumor cells.

Immunosurveillance of cancer: The beginnings of tumor immunology

Ehrlich, P., "Uber den jetzigen Stand der Karzinomforschung," in *The Collected Papers of Paul Ehrlich*, Vol. II, Pergamon Press, London, 1957, p. 550. Cited here is the famous 1908 speech by Ehrlich setting the stage for the study of tumor immunology.

Burnet, F. M., "The concept of immunological surveillance, *Prog. Exp. Tumor Res.* **13**, 1(1970).

Thomas, L., "Reactions to homologous tissue antigens in relationship to hypersensitivity," in *Cellular and Humoral Aspects of the Hypersensitive States*, Lawrence, H. S., (Ed.), Hoeber-Harber, New York, 1959, p. 529.

The preceding are two restatements of the Ehrlich hypothesis, with a more elaborate discussion of the possibility that development of immunosurveillance provided the selective pressure for evolution of cellular immunity.

Tumor antigenicity

Prehn, R. T., and Main, J. M., "Immunity to methylcholanthrene-induced sarcomas," *J. Natl. Cancer Inst.* **18**, 769(1957). In this landmark study it was demonstrated that hosts may show specific immunity to carcinogen-induced tumors, that such tumors express the same tumor antigens through hundreds of cell generations, and that each carcinogen-induced tumor possesses unique tumor antigens. A quarter of a century later, we know little more about these tumors.

Alexander, P., "Foetal 'antigens' in cancer," *Nature* **235**, 137(1972). A review of oncofetal antigens.

Gold, P., and Freedman, S. O., "Specific carcinoembryonic antigens of the human digestive system," *J. Exp. Med.* **122**, 467(1965). This paper (and a companion paper in the same journal issue) demonstrates that oncofetal antigens are expressed in humans.

Oettgen, H. F., "Immunological aspects of cancer," *Hospital Practice* **16** (7), 85(1981).

Weissman, I., "Tumor immunology, T-cell maturation, and cell neoplasia," *Progress in Experimental Tumor Research* **25**, 193(1980).

Relationship of immunosurveillance to killer-cell and immune-cell systems

Algire, G. H., Weaver, J. M., and Prehn, R. T., "Growth of cells *in vivo* in diffusion chambers. I. Survival of homografts in immunized mice," *J. Natl. Cancer Inst.* **15**, 493(1954). A classical paper that demonstrated the primacy of cell-mediated immunity over humoral immunity in the rejection of tumor transplants.

Haverkos, H. W., and Curran, J. W., "The current outbreak of Kaposi's sarcoma and opportunistic infections," *CA—A Cancer Journal for Clinicians* **321** (6), 330(1982).

Miller, J. F. A. P., Ting, R. C., and Law, L. W., "Influence of thymectomy on tumor induction by polyoma virus in C57B1 mice," *Proc. Soc. Exp. Biol. Med.* **116**, 323(1964). The T-cell system operates to regulate DNA virus-induced tumors.

Prehn, R. T., "The immune reaction as a stimulator of tumor growth," *Science* **176**, 170(1972). But immune cells also can augment tumor growth!

Immunological escape by tumor cells

Boyse, E. A., and Old, L. J., "Some aspects of normal and abnormal cell-surface genetics," *Ann. Rev. Genet.* **3**, 269(1969). Differentiation antigens, tumor antigens, and an extensive discussion of the TL antigen.

Hellstrom, K. E., and Hellstrom, I., "Lymphocyte-mediated cytotoxicity and blocking serum activity to tumor antigens," *Adv. Immunol.* **18**, 209(1974). Antigen–antibody complexes as blocking factors.

Kaliss, N., "The survival of homografts in mice pretreated with antisera to mouse tissues," *Ann. N.Y. Acad. Sci.* **64**, 977(1957). An important early paper on the phenomenon and mechanism of immunological enhancement.

Klein, G., "Immunological surveillance against neoplasia," *Harvey Lecture Series* **69**, 71(1975)

Immunotherapy

Miller, R. A., Maloney, D. G., Warnke, R., and Levy, R., "Treatment of B-cell lymphoma with monoclonal anti-idiotype antibody," *N. Eng. J. Med.* **306**, 517(1982).

Sears, H. F., Mattis, J., Herlyn, D., Hayry, P., Atkinson, B., Ernst, C., Steplewski, Z., and Koprowski, H., "Phase I clinical trial of monoclonal antibody in treatment of gastrointestinal tumors," *The Lancet* **1**, 762(1982).

Weissman, I., Nord, S., and Baird, S., "Immunotherapy and immunodiagnosis of metastatic neoplasms: prospects and progress," *Frontiers in Cancer Research*, Vaeth, J., (Ed.), Karger, Basel, 161(1972).

Additional concepts introduced in the problems

1. Principles of leukemia and tumor pharmacotherapy. Problem 13-6
2. Genetic control of antigens which may modulate. Problem 13-8
3. Effector cell specificity in tumor immunity. Problem 13-11
4. Anti-idiotype T cell regulation of plasmacytomas. Problem 13-13

Problems

13-1 Indicate whether each of the following statements is true or false. Explain the error in each statement you consider to be false.
(a) Cancer cells generally divide more rapidly than normal cells.
(b) The daughters of a cancer cell generally have identical morphological and metabolic characteristics.
(c) Most tumors appear to have one or more cell-surface tumor-associated antigens.
(d) Tumor-associated antigens that are expressed earlier in development as fetal membrane components cannot induce an immune response in the adult animal because of the lack of immunological responsiveness to self-components (tolerance).
(e) The spread of cancer viruses from one organ to another, causing *de novo* cancer induction in the second organ, is called *metastasis*.
(f) The site of metastatic spread via lymphatics is usually predictable, whereas the site of metastatic spread via the bloodstream is usually unpredictable.
(g) Rapidly transforming oncornaviruses contain a gene that codes for the malignant phenotype when expressed in host cells.
(h) Chemical carcinogens and X rays act by introducing new genetic information into the cell.
(i) At the time of clinical diagnosis, most cancers consist of several independent clones of malignant cells, presumably due to the multicentric origins of most cancers.
(j) Most oncogenic RNA viruses have an RNA-dependent DNA polymerase that permits the transfer of information from RNA to DNA.
(k) The fact that many cancers undergo several progressions in their malignant behavior is proof that somatic mutation plays a significant role in carcinogenesis.
(l) Each chemically induced tumor appears to express unique tumor-associated antigens.
(m) The lymphocytes from a patient dying of malignant melanoma can usually destroy his or her own tumor cells *in vitro*.
(n) Osteogenic sarcoma with a single diagnosed lung metastasis is most likely to be cured by surgery alone.

13-2 Supply the missing word or words in each of the following statements.
(a) Tumors with little cellular adhesiveness tend to _____ to distant sites rapidly.
(b) The three conventional forms of cancer therapy are _____, _____ , and _____ .
(c) Most anticancer drugs _____ the immune system.
(d) Following exposure to polyoma virus, _____ infections occur in permissive cells, whereas _____ infections occur in nonpermissive cells.

(e) _____ viruses appear to cause most spontaneous virus-induced cancers in animals.

(f) DNA copies of the RNA virus genome are made by the enzyme _____ .

(g) Cigarette smokers who have an exceptionally high risk of developing lung cancer may have abnormally _____ levels of the aryl hydrocarbon hydroxylase enzymes.

(h) The rapid loss of a cell-surface tumor antigen on contact with specific antibody is called _____ _____ .

(i) The cellular immune system may have evolved as a _____ system for cancer.

(j) Tumor-associated antigens that result in immune rejection are usually located in the cancer cell _____ _____ .

(k) _____ _____ appear to be composed of humoral antibodies and tumor-associated antigens.

(l) Ultimate carcinogens cause irreversible changes necessary for neoplastic transformation, but transformation also requires the subsequent action of another class of substances, termed _____ .

13-3 As an epidemiologist, how would you interpret the following data? In 1963, a study was initiated on 370 unionized asbestos insulation workers, all of whom had been working for at least 20 years. Previous analysis of members of the union between 1943 and 1963 had shown lung cancer deaths to be 6.8 times as frequent as expected from statistics on the general population. Among the 370 men, there were 87 who had no history of cigarette smoking. By April 1967, there had been no death from lung cancer in this group. By contrast, 24 of the 283 with a history of regular cigarette smoking had died of lung cancer, although less than 3 such deaths had been expected, given their smoking habits.

13-4 The entire SV40 genome is usually integrated into the host genome during transformation. The virus can be induced by fusion of the transformed cell with a permissive cell, leading to cell lysis and the release of mature infectious virions. Offer a possible explanation for this observation.

13-5 Polyoma virus infection occurs naturally in adult mice without apparent ill effect. However, when injected into newborn mice, the virus causes several different tumors. Can you offer an explanation for this surprising behavior?

13-6 Leukemia is a cancer of blood-forming cells, and it is usually restricted to one or another blood-cell type. The diagnosis and treatment of leukemia requires an understanding of leukemic cell growth kinetics. For most of the life history of a leukemia, the number of leukemic cells increases exponentially with time, usually doubling in number with each cell cycle. In leukemias that originate in or home to the bone marrow, a total body load of at least 10^{10} leukemic cells (~ 10 g of tumor cells) must be present before an experienced pathologist can diagnose leukemia by microscopic analysis of a sample of bone marrow. A total body load of 10^{11} leukemic cells must be present before diagnosis can be made by an examination of the blood, and 10^{12} cells must generally be present before a patient becomes aware that he is ill because of either bleeding or infection, caused by leukemic replacement of platelets or polymorphonuclear leukocytes, respectively. Nearly 10^{13} cells must be present before leukemic infiltration of vital organs causes death.

The elimination of leukemic cells by chemotherapeutic agents is usually an exponential function of dose; for example, if 10 mg of drug A eliminate 90% of the leukemic cells, then 20 mg will eliminate 99%, 30 mg will eliminate 99.9%, and so on. However, at a certain dose of any drug, the side effects become so severe that treatment with that drug must be stopped. Suppose that you are a clinical oncologist

Table 13-5 Properties of Six Drugs Used for Chemotherapy of Leukemia (Problem 13-6)

Drug	Dose to Eliminate 90% Leukemic Cells	Limiting Dose Because of Side Effects	Type of Side Effects
A	10 mg	30 mg	Gastrointestinal
B	5 mg	20 mg	Gastrointestinal
C	100 mg	200 mg	Bone-marrow depression
D	0.5 mg	1.0 mg	Gastrointestinal
E	50 mg	200 mg	Peripheral neuritis (tingling and pain)
F	10 mg	20 mg	Lymphocytopenia (infections)

treating a leukemia patient who has come to you with bleeding gums. You treat him initially with 30 mg of the drug A just described and, despite a few days of nausea and diarrhea (due to death of gastrointestinal tract cells), his gums clear up. However, he returns after 20 days, when his gums have again started to bleed. Assuming that the leukemic cells in this patient always double their number with each cell cycle, answer the following questions.

(a) What is the average cell-cycle time (interval between mitoses) for this patient's leukemia?

(b) How long before the first diagnosis did this patient's leukemia arise?

(c) In diagnostic chest X rays, you notice that a spot has appeared in the patient's lungs, and you correctly assume that it is a solid leukemic tumor. How long will it take for the tumor to increase in diameter from 10 mm to 40 mm?

(d) You have at your disposal the drugs listed in Table 13-5. Choose the optimal treatment for your patient, and explain the rationale for it.

(e) Assuming that all cells are accessible to the chemotherapeutic agents, how many leukemic cells will remain following your treatment? How long will the patient be in remission without symptoms?

(f) In a case similar to this one, the patient did not have a recurrence of bone-marrow-diagnosable leukemia for at least 5 years. Give two possible explanations for this striking remission.

13-7 How would you explain the following results?

(a) An antiserum raised against unfertilized mouse eggs in a xenogeneic host (of another species) is cytotoxic to SV40-transformed mouse cells but not to normal adult mouse cells.

(b) The serum from mice immunized with syngeneic SV40-transformed cells is not cytotoxic to mouse eggs, but it does contain antibodies directed against a tumor-specific surface antigen that appears in response to virus infection.

13-8 (a) In 1963, L. J. Old and his co-workers produced antisera in C57Bl/6 mice by immunization with spontaneous leukemias from (A $\times$ C57Bl/6)F$_1$ mice. These

Table 13-6 Tla Phenotypes and Genotypes (Problem 13-8)

Inbred Strain	Tla Phenotype of Normal Thymocytes	Phenotype of Leukemic Cells and Presumed Tla Genotype of Mouse
A	1,2,3,–	1,2,3,–
C57B1/6	–,–,–,–	,2,–,4
BALB/c	–,2,–,–	1,2,–,–
DBA/2	–,2,–,–	1,2,–,4

antisera were cytotoxic *in vitro* for cells of several C57B1/6 leukemias and for normal thymocytes from A and C58 strains. The cognate antigen was designated TL, and the locus coding for the antigen was called the Tla (*t*hymus *l*eukemia *a*ntigen) locus. TL was shown (at that time) to be a complex consisting of four antigens: Tla.1, Tla.2, Tla.3, and Tla.4 Normal inbred strains of mice fell into three groups based on the presence of these antigens, and leukemia cells fell into four groups (Table 13-6).

The three *normal* Tla phenotypes (haplotypes) behave as alleles at a single locus that maps about 1.5 centimorgans from the H-2D locus. However, the observations in Table 13-6 suggest that this locus includes more than simply structural genes for different subsets of the four antigens. What are these observations? Offer a genetic model to explain them.

(b) One striking observation has been made regarding mice immunized against Tla antigens and containing high titers of cytotoxic Tla antibodies. Such mice might be expected to resist syngeneic Tla-positive leukemias, but they do not; they are readily killed by such tumors. Moreover, the tumors recovered from such immunized hosts have lost their sensitivity to Tla antisera *in vitro* as well as their ability to absorb cytotoxic Tla antibodies. However, this loss is only temporary because a single passage of the tumors in nonimmunized syngeneic hosts allows the tumor to regain its ability to adsorb cytotoxic Tla antibodies. How would you explain these observations? The phenomenon they illustrate is formally similar to another cell-surface phenomenon described for receptor immunoglobulins. What is it? How would you test whether these two phenomena are mediated by similar mechanisms?

13-9 Suppose that you are a cancer immunologist studying the role of the immune response to two highly malignant fibrosarcomas from patients A and B. The cancer cells grow well in tissue culture, and the cultured cells are proven to be malignant by various tests. Serum, blood lymphocytes, and normal fibroblasts from patients A and B are readily obtainable. You conduct several tests in tissue culture with patient lymphocytes, serum, tumor cells, and normal target cells, adding serum to target cells at time zero and then adding lymphocytes 4 hours later, according to the experimental design indicated in Table 13-7. Several days later, you obtain the results shown. In all possible combinations, the growth of normal fibroblast colonies from patient A and patient B was unaffected by the addition of serum or lymphocytes, or both, from these patients. With reference to the table, answer the following questions.

Table 13-7 Immunologic Analyses of Tumor Cells from Two Fibrosarcoma Patients (Problem 13-9)

Experiment	Lymphocytes Added from Patient	Serum Added from Patient	Tumor Target Cells from Patient	Number of Tumor Colonies Growing
I	—	—	A	100
	—	A	A	97
	A	—	A	12
	A	A	A	98
II	—	—	B	101
	B	—	B	13
	A	—	B	98
III	B	—	A	15
	—	B	A	96
	B	A	A	99
	A	B	A	12

(a) By which of the following possibilities could one explain the continued growth of tumor in patient A: lack of an anti-tumor immune response, immunological tolerance, immunostimulation, immunoselection, immunological enhancement, or antigenic modulation? Discuss each possibility.

(b) What can you conclude concerning individual-specific and cross-reacting tumor-associated antigens on tumors from patients A and B, the ability of lymphocytes from each of these patients to recognize each of these antigens, and the specificity of serum factors from each of these patients?

13-10 As a young physician interested in immunology, you have a brilliant idea. One common type of leukemia is a cancer of the lymphocyte. Why not irradiate these leukemia patients with a dose of X rays sufficient to destroy all their lymphocytes (i.e., normal and leukemic cells) and then give them an adoptive transfer of spleen cells from another individual? The host's immune system is destroyed so there should be no graft rejection. All the leukemic cells are destroyed, hence the cancer should be cured. An older colleague finds your proposal highly amusing. Why?

13-11 (a) Some cancer cells express tumor-specific molecules that make the tumor antigenic to its host. One such tumor is a cancer called *Moloney sarcoma* (MS), which is induced by an RNA cancer virus, MSV (Moloney sarcoma virus). Transplantation of this tumor to syngeneic hosts leads to tumor growth and then regression. If the tumor is retransplanted to MS regressors, there is no tumor growth. Another tumor, EMT6, is a breast cancer that does not share tumor antigens with MS, and it is only weakly antigenic to its hosts. Serum from normal mice or from MS regressors was transfused into normal mice just prior to transplantation with an MS tumor on one side and an EMT6 tumor on the other. The transfusion did not affect the incidence or the growth rate of either tumor in these hosts. What conclusions can you draw from this result?

Table 13-8 Tumor Incidence of EMT6 and MS Transplanted into Normal or MS-Immune Syngeneic Hosts (Problem 13-11)

Group	Tumor[a]	Host[b]	Days after Inoculation:[c]		
			8	15	24
A. Growth of MS in normal and MS-immune hosts:					
1	MS	N	7/7	7/7	3/7
2	MS	MS-R	0/10	2/10	1/10
3	MS[d]	MS-R[d]	1/10	0/10	0/8
B. Growth of EMT6 alone or intermixed in normal and MS-immune hosts:					
1	EMT6	N	3/7	7/7	7/7
2	EMT6	MS-R	0/10	6/10	5/10
4	Mixture	MS-R	1/10	7/10	8/10
3	EMT6[d]	MS-R	0/10	6/10	6/8
3	Mixture[d]	MS-R	1/10	5/10	6/8

[a] 1.5×10^4 viable (6×10^4 total) EMT6 cells were inoculated into syngeneic hosts, alone or intermixed with 3×10^6 total (6×10^5 viable) MS cells. At other sites, 3×10^6 total (6×10^5 viable) MS cells were injected into these hosts.

[b] N = untreated BALB/c mice; MS-R = Moloney sarcoma regressor mice.

[c] Incidence of tumor-positive mice/total number mice given injections.

[d] In addition to EMT6 or MS flank injections, or both, a third site was injected with the same number of both tumor lines intermixed.

(b) The minimal number of viable EMT6 cells that will transplant a tumor to 100% of recipient hosts is 1.5×10^4 cells. Single-cell suspensions of EMT6 and MS were prepared and injected alone or intermixed into the skin of normal or MS-regressor (MS-R) hosts. The incidence of tumor growth is shown in Table 13-8. All hosts had tumors biopsied on day 24, and all tumors from group B were identified microscopically as EMT6. Consider Table 13-8, parts A and B, and compare the growth of EMT6 and MS in groups 1 and 2. What conclusions can be drawn and what hypotheses can you propose to explain the data?

(c) Consider Table 13-8, part B. Discuss the results in terms of effector-cell function and specificity. What can you say about the role in this reaction of T-cell lymphokines, such as lymphotoxin?

13-12 Immunity to Moloney tumor antigens can be tested *in vitro*, using ^{51}Cr-labeled Moloney lymphoma cells as targets. A research group compared the anti-Moloney immune responses, using lymphocytes and target cells from different strains of mice. They carried out these assays at a time following immunization, when T_C cells were the only killer cells that could recognize and eliminate Moloney target cells. The data from these experiments are shown in Tables 13-9, 13-10, and 13-11. [The tables are from E. Gomard, V. Duprex, Y. Henin, and J. P. Levy, *Nature* **260**, 706(1976).] With reference to these tables, answer the following questions.

(a) What conclusions can you draw from Tables 13-9 and 13-10?

(b) Discuss Table 13-11 in terms of T_C-cell receptor specificity.

Table 13-9 Specific ^{51}Cr Release from C57Bl and BALB/c Moloney Lymphoma Tumor Cells Attacked by Anti-MSV Lymphocytes from Different Strains (Problem 13-12)

Anti-MSV Spleen Cells from:	H-2 Genotype	Lymphoma Target Cells from: C57Bl	BALB/c
		(Percent Release)	
BALB/c	d/d	7	17
C57Bl	b/b	34	7
(BALB/c × C57Bl)F$_1$	b/d	39	16
BALB.B[a]	b/b	45	8
B10.D2[b]	d/d	7	24

[a]BALB mice with the H-2^b trait of C57Bl mice.
[b]C57Bl mice with the H-2^d trait.
[From E. Gomard, V. Duprez, Y. Henin, and J. P. Levy. *Nature* **260**, 706(1976).]

Table 13-10 Specific ^{51}Cr Release from C57Bl and BALB/c Moloney Lymphoma Tumor Cells Attacked by (BALB/c × C57Bl)F$_1$ Lymphocytes (Problem 13-12)

Immunization by:	Moloney Target Cells from: C57Bl	BALB/c
	(Percent Release)	
MSV inoculation	38	16
	13	8
	36	21
BALB/c Moloney lymphoma cells	6	34
	4	26
	0	12
C57Bl Moloney lymphoma cells	7	0
	13	0
	12	0

[From E. Gomard, V. Duprez, Y. Henin, and J. P. Levy, *Nature* **260**, 706(1976).]

Table 13-11 Blocking of Anti-MSV T-Cell-Induced Cytolysis by Preincubation of Target Cells with Various Sera (Problem 13-12)

Antiserum	Specific ^{51}Cr Release by BALB.B Moloney Lymphoma Target Cells (Percent Release)
BALB/c normal serum	18
BALB/c anti-C57Bl	0
BALB/c anti-C57Bl absorbed in BALB.B	17
BALB/c anti-C57Bl absorbed in B10.D2	4
BALB/c anti-BALB.B	0
C57Bl anti-BALB/c	19
AKR anti-Thy-1.2	19

[From E. Gomard, V. Duprez, Y. Henin, and J. P. Levy. *Nature* **260**, 706(1976).]

Table 13-12 The Action of M315-Immune T Cells on M315 Myeloma Cells

Effector: M315 Cell Ratio	Effector Cells	Viability	Percent of M315 Cells with Surface M315 IgA	Percent of M315 Cells that Secrete M315
M315 cells alone	None	94	89	45
50:1	Normal spleen	86	89	41
100:1	Normal spleen	85	84	40
200:1	Normal spleen	83	82	38
50:1	M315-immune spleen T cells	78	82	36
100:1	M315-immune spleen T cells	78	79	8
200:1	M315-immune spleen T cells	76	77	3

13-13   As a model system to study the role of idiotypes in the regulation of B cells, Lynch and his co-workers used two IgA BALB/c plasmacytomas, specific for DNP, that have different idiotypes, M315 and M460 [Lynch, R. et al., *J. Exp. Med.* **155**, 852(1982).] The results of their experiments turned out to have profound implications for tumor immunology, as well as for the mechanisms by which immunoglobulin genes are regulated in their expression. In the first experiment, mice were immunized with purified M315 or M460 IgA myeloma proteins and T cells were isolated from their spleens. The T cells were mixed back with the M315 cells in various ratios and the following observations made (Table 13-12).

(a)   What is the effect of M315-immune T cells on M315 plasmacytoma?
The immune spleen cells were then passed over anti-Lyt-1 or anti-Lyt-2 columns and the following observations made (Table 13-13).

Table 13-13   The Action of M315-Immune T Cell Subsets on M315 Myeloma

Effector: M315 Ratio	Treatment of Added M315 Immune Spleen Cells	Percent of M315 Cells That Secrete M315
M315 alone	—	55
50:1	No treatment	43
100:1	No treatment	8
50:1	Anti-Lyt-2 pass through	54
100:1	Anti-Lyt-2 pass through	50
50:1	Anti-Lyt-1 pass through	14
100:1	Anti-Lyt-1 pass through	6

Table 13-14   Selection of M315-Immune T Cells on Immunoglobulin Columns

Effector: M315 Ratio	Treatment of Spleen Cells	Percent M315 Cells Secreting
M315 cells alone	—	43
50:1	No treatment	12
100:1	No treatment	8
200:1	No treatment	3
50:1	IgM460 pass through	16
100:1	IgM460 pass through	10
200:1	IgM460 pass through	7
50:1	IgM315 pass through	35
100:1	IgM315 pass through	36
200:1	IgM315 pass through	34
12:1	Cells *eluted* from IgM315 columns	11
25:1	Cells *eluted* from IgM315 columns	4
50:1	Cells *eluted* from IgM315 columns	1

(b) What kind of cell is responsible for this suppression?
   The immune spleen cells were also passed over M315 or M460 immunoglobulin-coupled columns with the following effects (Table 13-14).
(c) What does this show about the specificity of the suppression?
(d) Why do the cells eluted from the M315 column show suppression at lower effector-to-target ratios?
(e) What kind of receptors are these effector cells likely to have?
(f) It was found that this suppression would occur even when the effectors and targets were separated by a 0.22-μ filter. What does this imply?

Table 13-15 Protein Synthesis in M315 Cells Coincubated with M315-Immune T Cells[a]

M315 Cells Treated with:	³H-Leucine Incorporated into:	
	M315 Ig	Total Cell Protein
Media	125,000	237,000
200:1 normal spleen	107,000	210,000
200:1 M315-immune spleen cells	9,000	112,000

[a]The numbers indicate the radioactive isotope levels incorporated into the designated proteins in counts per minute.

Studies were then done analyzing the amount of ³H leucine incorporated into M315 immunoglobulin and into the total cell protein of the M315 cells (Table 13-15).

(g) What does this say about this suppression?

Answers

13-1 (a) False. Many normal cells (e.g., cells of the gastrointestinal tract and bone marrow) divide more rapidly than most cancer cells. Tumor growth occurs primarily because cancer cell division is not regulated.

(b) True

(c) True

(d) False. If fetal components disappear before the maturation of the immune response (in most animals at or near birth), these components will be recognized as foreign in later life. Indeed, to maintain a state of tolerance or lack of immunologic reactivity, components must generally be exposed to the immune system throughout the individual's life.

(e) False. Metastasis is the property of cancer *cells* to move from one site to another, resulting in tumor cell colonization of the second site.

(f) True

(g) True

(h) False. They modify the existing genetic information or operate in an epigenetic manner. The only carcinogens known to introduce new genetic information into cells are viruses.

(i) False. For most types of cancer, most cancer cells in one patient are members of a single clone at the time of diagnosis. Although this observation has been taken as evidence for the unicentric origin of most cancers, it in fact only provides evidence that a single clone is dominant.

(j) True

(k) False. Although hypotheses of carcinogenesis by somatic mutation *predict* tumor progression, models of selective gene activation and inactivation are also consistent with the phenomenon of tumor progression.

(l) True

(m) True

(n) False. The finding of a blood-borne metastasis rules out the possibility of cure by surgery alone, as other micrometastases are surely present at unpredictable sites. Systemic chemotherapy and surgical or radiotherapeutic removal of the primary tumor are currently the only treatments of this disease pattern.

13-2   (a) metastasize
        (b) surgery, radiation, and chemotherapy
        (c) suppress
        (d) lytic, temperate (transforming)
        (e) RNA tumor (retro-)
        (f) reverse transcriptase (RNA-dependent DNA polymerase)
        (g) high
        (h) antigenic modulation
        (i) surveillance
        (j) plasma membrane
        (k) Blocking factors
        (l) promoters

13-3   This study appears to provide an example of the multiple factor etiology of lung cancer. Smoking alone should have caused 3 deaths, not 24. None of the 87 asbestos workers with no history of smoking died, hence it was not the asbestos alone. However, smoking and asbestos exposure in combination had an apparent multiplicative effect. The journal article goes on to conclude that asbestos workers who smoked had a risk of dying from lung cancer 8 times larger than that of smokers of the same age who had had no asbestos exposure, and 92 times larger than the risk of an individual who neither worked with asbestos nor smoked. A similar multiple factor effect has been demonstrated for smoking and uranium exposure.

13-4   One possible explanation may be that the transformed cell lacks a factor that permits the expression of later viral genes. The permissive cell supplies this factor and initiates the lytic pathway.

13-5   Adult mice are immune to polyoma. Under normal laboratory conditions, mice are presumably exposed to polyoma after the immune system has matured to the point of being able to generate an adequate response. In contrast, newborn mice with an immature immune system cannot generate an effective immune response rapidly enough to prevent malignant tumor growth.

13-6   (a) Because the patient arrived with bleeding gums, it is reasonable to assume a tumor load of $\sim 10^{12}$ cells. Drug A should eliminate 99.9% of them, leaving $\sim 10^9$ cells. These cells multiply to give 10^{12} cells again in 20 days. If each cell gives rise to two dividing progeny, and n is the number of doublings, then $(10^9)(2^n) = 10^{12}$, and $n = 10$. Thus ten cell cycles take place in 20 days, and the cell-cycle time is 2 days.

        (b) At first diagnosis, the patient had $\sim 10^{12}$ cells. If the leukemia began as a single cell (10^0), then $(10^0)(2^n) = 10^{12}$, and $n = 40$. Forty cell cycles would take 80 days, assuming that the cell-cycle time of 2 days is constant, that the cells multiplied exponentially throughout, and that there were no cells lost.

        (c) Because solid tumors grow roughly as spheroids, a 4-fold increase in diameter corresponds to a 64-fold increase in volume, and thus a 64-fold increase in cell number. Thus $2^n = 64$; $n = 6$ cell cycles, and 12 days should be required for the specified increase in tumor diameter.

        (d) Three principles should be followed in chemotherapy. (1) Simultaneous treatment with different drugs is preferential to sequential treatment, which allows clonal expansion of tumor cells between doses. More important, tumor resistance results from selection of drug-resistant variants, and the frequency of multiple-resistant variants will be the product of the frequencies of singly resistant variants. For example, if the frequency of a singly resistant variant is 10^{-5}, then the probability of a variant that is resistant to two drugs simultaneously is 10^{-10}. (2) Drugs used in combination should be those that do not lead to similar side effects. Thus, in this case, one cannot use any combinations of drugs A, B, and D, because they all damage gastrointestinal cells. (3) The preferred drugs are those with the highest therapeutic index—the ratio of toxic drug dose to effective drug dose. One should choose the drug that offers the best therapeutic index, regardless of its potency on a per milligram basis. Therefore, the best choice among A, B, and D is B, and the optimal treatment is concurrent administration of B, C, E, and F at their highest tolerance doses (20 mg for B, 200 mg for C, 200 mg for E, and 20 mg for F).

(e) If each drug acts independently and additively on the leukemic cell population, then the treatment recommended in part (d) should reduce the leukemic cell load from 10^{12} to 10^0 cells—that is, to a single cell. Assuming that recurrence of symptoms requires a 10^{12} cell tumor load, symptoms would recur after 80 days (see part (b)).

(f) This remission could be explained if some of the drugs acted synergistically rather than in an additive fashion, or if the total tumor cell load was reduced to a level at which host defense mechanisms, such as immunity, could eliminate the remaining leukemic cells.

13-7 The simplest interpretation is that SV40 transformation leads to the appearance in the cell membrane of both a fetal antigen to which adult mice are tolerant and a new tumor-specific surface antigen. Thus multiple membrane components may be induced during neoplastic transformation.

13-8 (a) No Tla antigens are expressed on normal thymocytes in C57B1/6 mice, but three of the Tla antigens are expressed on their leukemia cells. Similarly, only Tla.2 is expressed on normal thymocytes in BALB/c and DBA/2 mice, but additional Tla specificities are expressed on their leukemic cells. This observation suggests that each of the four strains carries at least two of the four Tla structural genes, that the Tla complex includes elements that control the expression of these genes, and that the structural genes are induced during leukemogenesis. Alternatively, these structural genes could be expressed in only a small subset of normal cells (e.g., up to 5% of C57B1/6 thymocytes could be Tla.1,2,4 and not be detectable using Old's assay), and these cells could be preferentially inducible by leukemogenic oncornaviruses.

(b) This observation is an example of antibody-induced removal of surface antigens, called *antigenic modulation*. It is similar to the loss of B-cell surface immunoglobulins in the presence of anti-immunoglobulin antibodies, the phenomenon called *capping*. Most capped immunoglobulins are lost from the cell surface, some by shedding (exocytosis) and some by internalization (endocytosis). The capping of cell-surface immunoglobulins has a well-defined series of steps (ring $\rightarrow$ patch $\rightarrow$ cap) and is prevented by metabolic inhibitors and microtubular inhibitors, implying an active energy-dependent process involving the intracellular cytoskeletal system. One could test the sensitivity of TL antigenic modulation to metabolic and microtubular inhibitors. One apparent difference is that antigenic modulation of TL antigens is supposed to be induced by monovalent Fab fragments, whereas the capping of immunoglobulins is not.

13-9 (a) Experiment I demonstrates that patient A's lymphocytes will prevent outgrowth of A tumor cell colonies, whereas his serum has no direct effect on A tumor cell growth. However, addition of A's serum to A tumor target cells before addition of lymphocytes blocks the immune effect of the lymphocytes on the tumor cells. Therefore, the patient has developed an anti-tumor immune response, ruling out the lack of immune responsivity, immunological tolerance to tumor antigens, and immunoselection of nonantigenic variants as explanations for continued tumor growth. Since neither arm of the immune response stimulates the growth of more A tumor colonies *in vitro*, it seems unlikely that immunostimulation is occurring *in vivo*. The specific inhibitory action of patient serum on cell-mediated tumor immunity could be the result of antibody-induced antigenic modulation. If so, one could predict that tumor cells taken directly from patient A would be nonantigenic and would reexpress tumor antigens only after tissue culture in the absence of patient serum or lymphocytes. Another likely possibility is the phenomenon of immunological enhancement, wherein tumor antigens are continually expressed, but serum-blocking and/or suppressor factors impede specific cell-mediated immunity.

(b)   It is likely that tumors from patients A and B share some surface antigens and that tumor A has some unique antigens as well. For example, lymphocytes from patient B recognize and react against both A and B tumor cells, but not against A and B normal cells. The most reasonable explanation is that these lymphocytes become sensitized to the cross-reacting antigens in B's tumor. Further evidence for this reaction comes from the ability of A serum to block the reaction of B's lymphocytes on A's tumor cells. A's lymphocytes, however, appear to react only to noncross-reacting tumor antigens in tumor A; they do not react against B's tumor cells, and B's serum will not block the reaction of A lymphocytes on A tumor cells. Two points are not clear: (1) it is possible that A's lymphocytes, if they are T cells, fail to react to B's tumor cells because of a possible lack of HLA-linked associated recognition, and (2) we know nothing about B's humoral response to his tumor.

13-10   Your colleague is amused for several reasons. First, to irradiate to eliminate *all* leukemia cells one would have to irradiate the patient's *whole body* with a tumoricidal dose of irradiation. Even if all leukemic cells were sensitive to X-ray-induced interphase death, a whole-body dose of ~ 2000 rads would have to be given to eliminate 10^{11-12} leukemic cells; if the cells died only by mitotic death, a dose of nearly 4000 rads would be required. At 600–800 rads for the whole body, sufficient numbers of hematopoietic stem cells are eliminated, so that death due to infection (allowed by insufficient numbers of phagocytes) or due to bleeding (caused by insufficient numbers of platelets) generally occurs in 10–20 days. At 1000–1200 rads for the whole body, sufficient numbers of intestinal epithelial stem cells are eliminated, so that death due to loss of body fluids through the denuded intestines occurs within 5–10 days. Although one may be able to transfuse hematopoietic stem cells, one cannot replace intestinal cells.

Even if the patient survived the irradiation, the lymphocytes from the donor would recognize the host antigens as foreign and initiate a GVHR, which generally leads to the death of the host.

13-11   (a)   Immunity to MS is not effected by the humoral immune system.

(b)   EMT6 cells grow less well in MS-R hosts. Perhaps there is a low-level antigenic cross-reactivity between these tumors, or perhaps MS activation of the immune system results in a more active host response to EMT6—for example, by nonspecific macrophage activation. MS grows and regresses in normal mice but does not grow in MS-R hosts (although EMT6 does). Specific cell-mediated immunity to MS tumors is established.

(c) Killer cells in this system recognize and destroy MS cells. Even though each EMT6 cell is entrapped in a 50-fold excess of MS tumor cells, the killer cell reaction to MS spares EMT6 cells. Thus both recognition and elimination in this reaction are highly specific *in vivo*. If T-cell lymphokines play any role in this reaction, they must act at extremely short range, and they cannot act effectively as diffusable nonspecific toxins.

13-12 (a) Table 13-9 shows that anti-MSV BALB/c lymphocytes recognize and react only to BALB/c Moloney lymphomas, that C57B1 strain lymphocytes react only to C57B1 strain Moloney lymphomas, that (BALB/c $\times$ C57B1)F_1 lymphocytes react to both C57B1 and BALB/c lymphomas, and that the required identity between killer and target is determined by the H-2 locus. Thus associated recognition of H-2 determinants is necessary for interaction of killer cells with target cells in this system. Table 13-10 demonstrates that (BALB/c $\times$ C57B1)F_1 lymphocytes may also demonstrate this restriction if the Moloney tumor antigens that stimulate the appearance of killer cells are presented in the context of one of the parental H-2 types. This result demonstrates the important point that the context of stimulation determines the range of recognition by killer cells and that not all (BALB/c $\times$ C57B1)F_1 anti-Moloney killer cells recognize Moloney target cells in the same way. One could propose that the repertoire of (BALB/c $\times$ C57B1)F_1 anti-Moloney prekiller cells is relatively extensive and that only those subsets recognizing Moloney antigens in the context of a particular H-2 type are stimulated by the cognate immunogen.

(b) Table 13-11 demonstrates that preincubation of target cells with anti-H-2 serum directed against the H-2 type of the target cells prevents killer-cell reactions to that cell, whereas antiserum to another antigen on that cell (Thy-1.2) does not prevent cytotoxicity. Furthermore, the table shows that the inhibitory activity of the H-2 antisera appears to be removed only by absorption with hosts expressing the correct H-2 type. One could propose that H-2 determinants on the target cells are in or close to the sites recognized by T_C-cell receptors and that masking them with antibodies prevents appropriate T_C-cell recognition of the target cells.

13-13 (a) The M315-immune T cells apparently do not kill more than 25% of the M315 targets, but they do eliminate detectable secretion (but not surface display) of M315 immunoglobulins.

(b) The inhibitory cells are most likely Lyt-1$^-$2$^+$. Most effector T_C and T_S cells express this phenotype.

(c) M315-immune T cells are retained on M315 immunoglobulin columns specifically. Thus the cells recognize the M315 immunoglobulins and/or molecules that copurify with them.

(d) The anti-M315 T cells represent a subset of the T-cell set. Those binding to M315 immunoglobulin columns are selectively enriched for M315 cell inhibition of M315 immunoglobulin secretion.

(e) The most appealing possibility is that the receptor on anti-M315 T cells is an anti-idiotypic receptor; however, binding to and reaction against a copurified antigen is still possible.

(f) The T cells release a suppressive factor that can traverse a 0.22-μ pore.

(g) Suppression in this case would appear to be specific inhibition of M315 immunoglobulin synthesis. Recent evidence indicates that the block is at the level of depressed levels of κ light-chain mRNA. [Parslow, T., Milburn, G. L., Lynch, R. G., and Granner, D. K., *Science* **220**, 1389–1391(1983).]

Index

The Natural Wedding

Ideas and Inspirations for a
Stylish and Green Celebration

Louise Moon

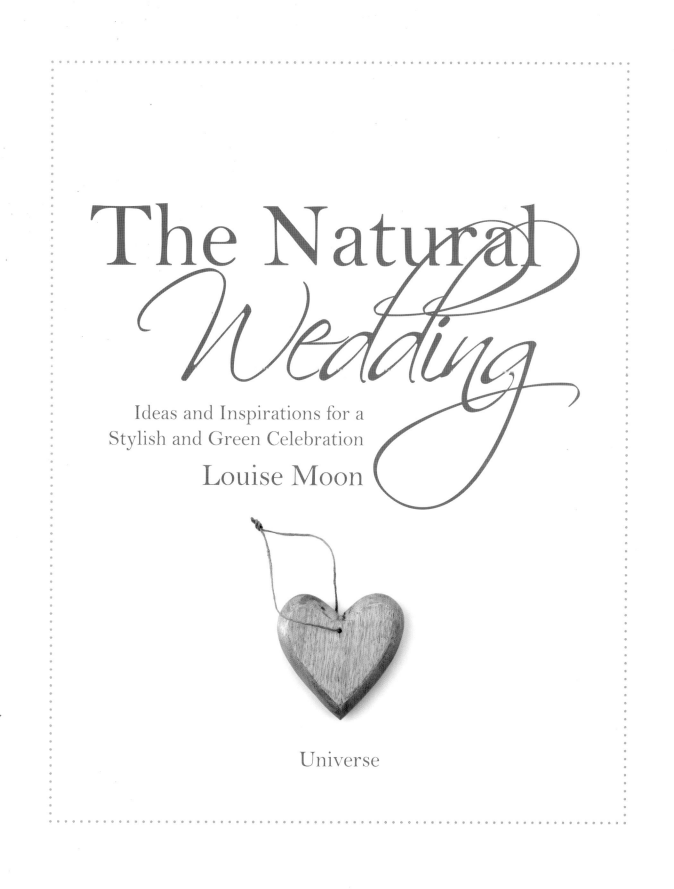

Universe

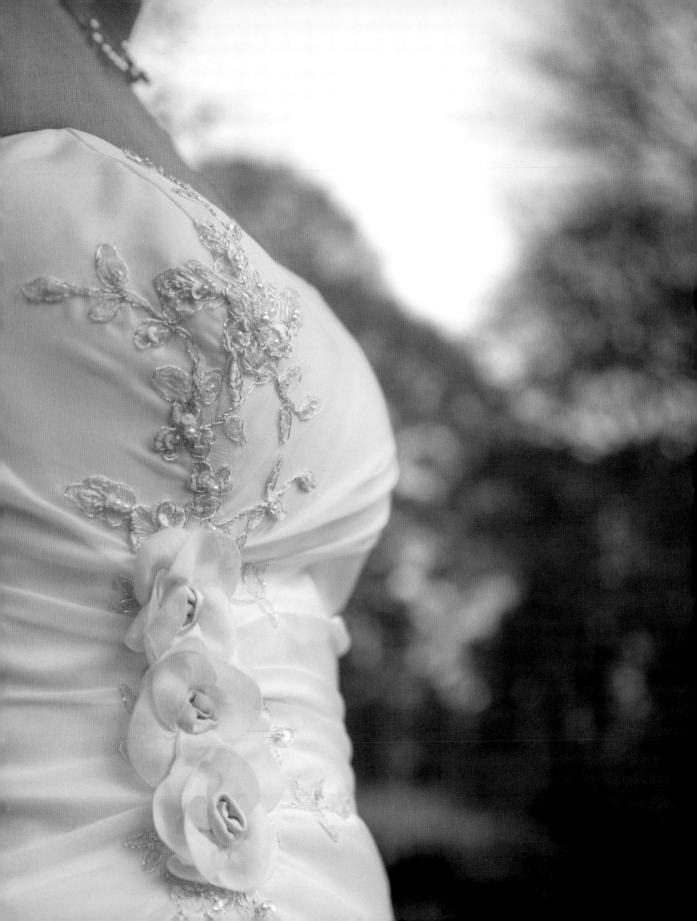

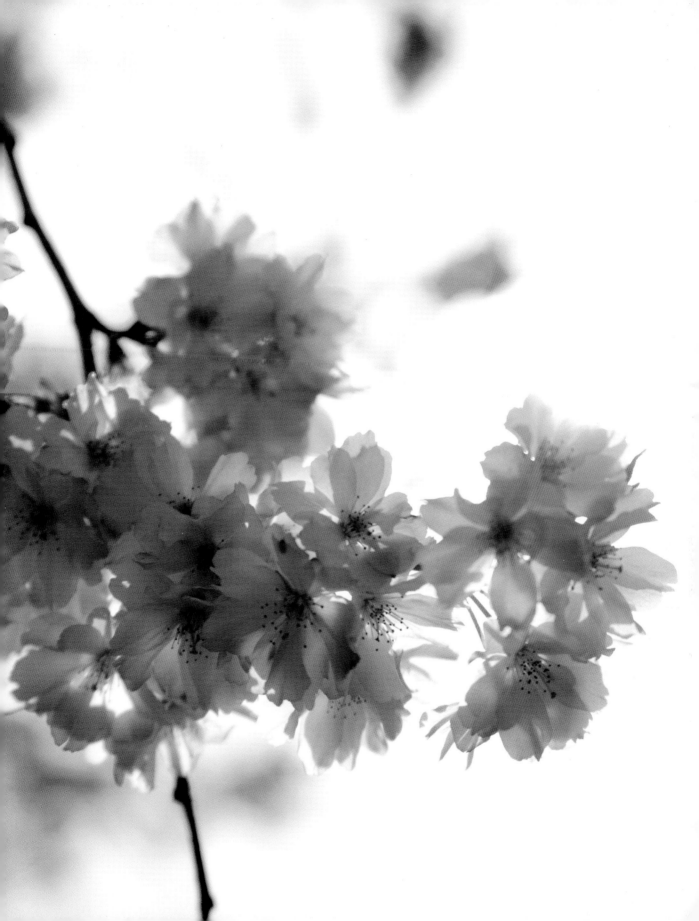

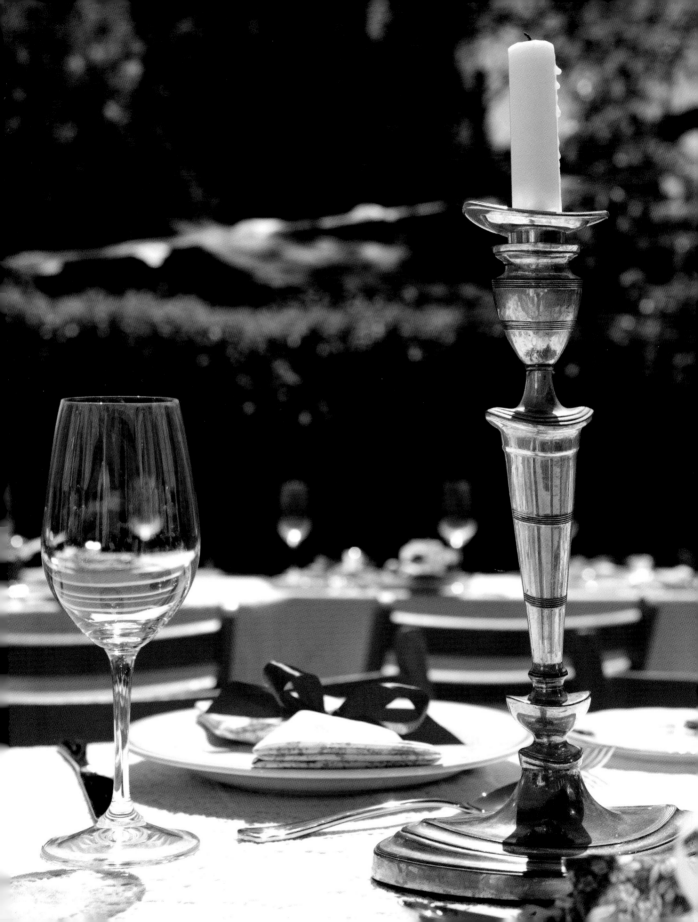

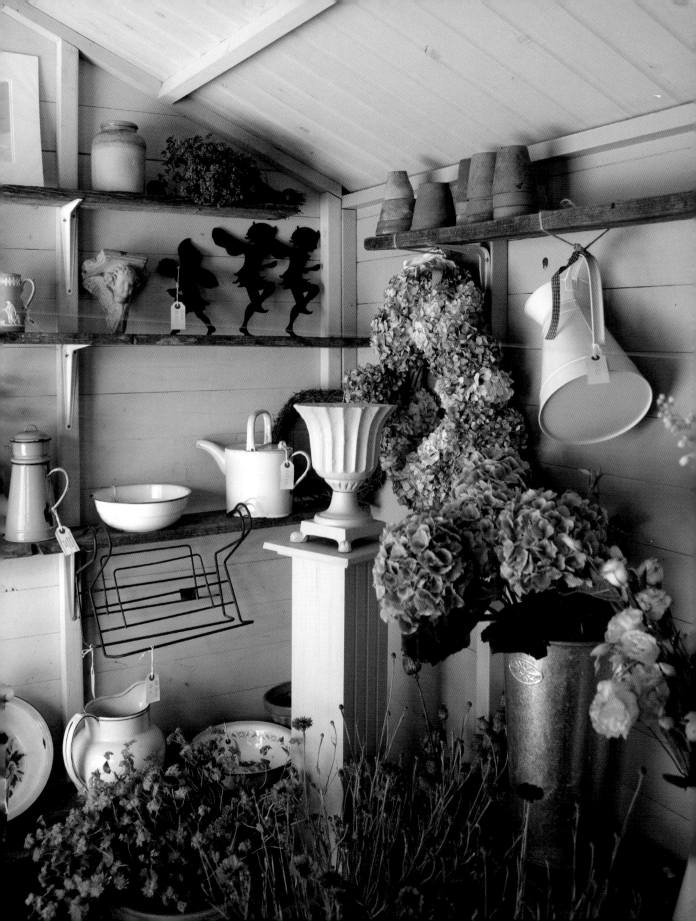

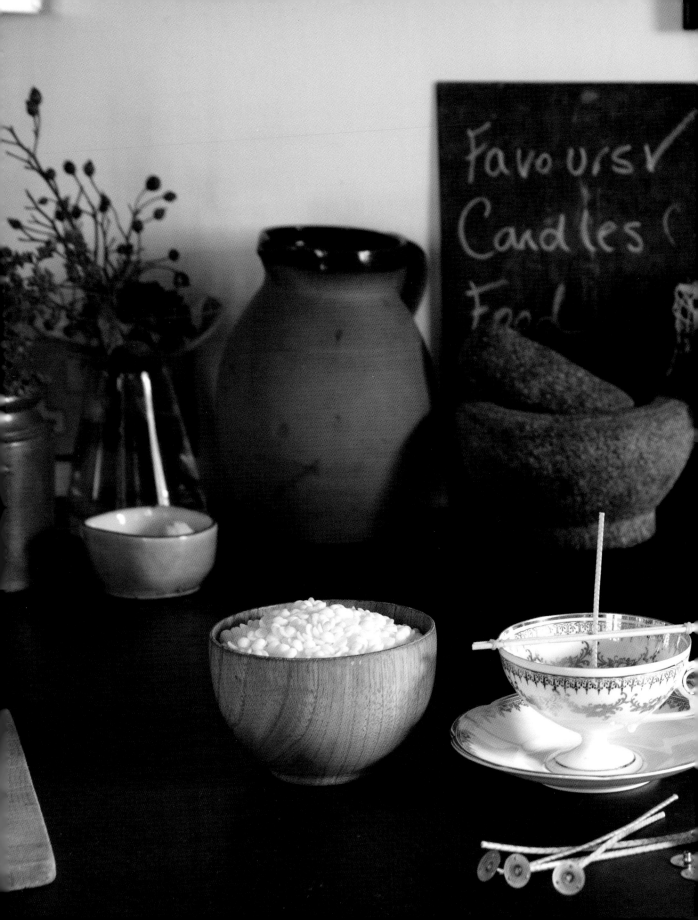

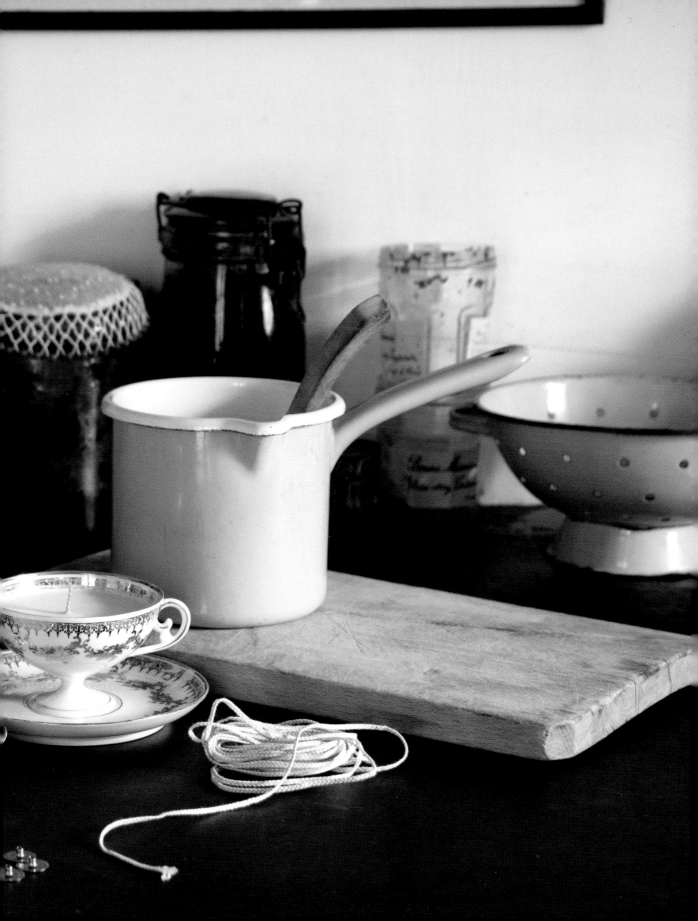

Contents

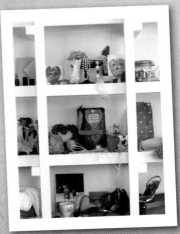

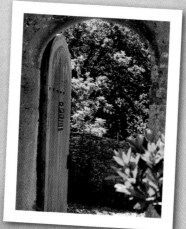

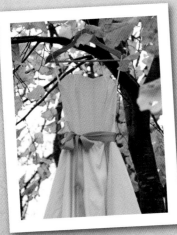

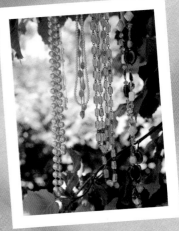

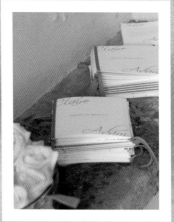

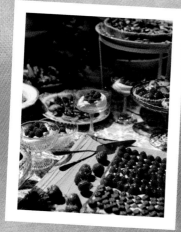

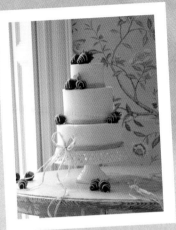

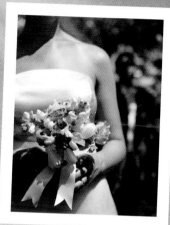

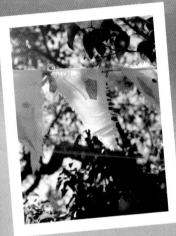

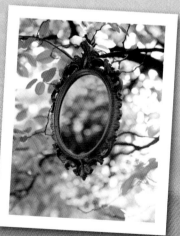

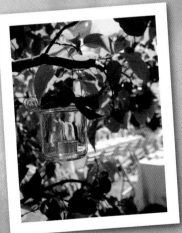

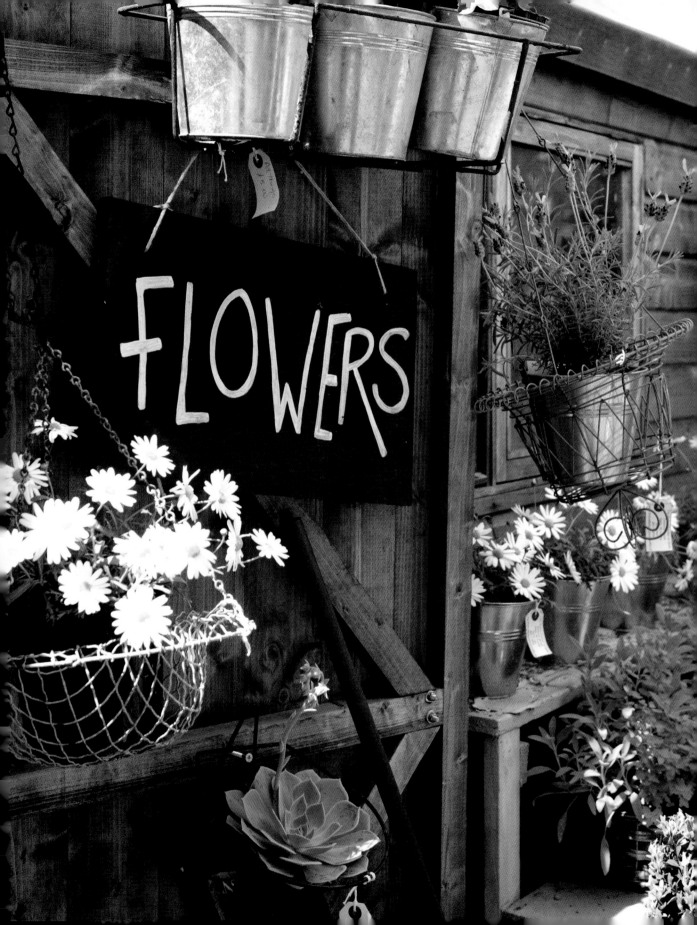

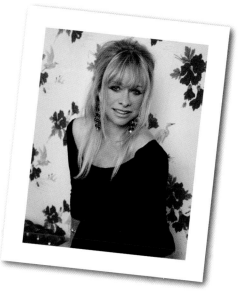

Foreword by Jo Wood

You want your wedding day to be the best day of your life, so why not plan it with an organic, eco-, and ethical conscience, ensuring your values and personality shine through. From sourcing a unique, one-off vintage dress to designing a locally sourced and seasonal menu, finding beautiful vintage crockery, or using a biodegradable tent, there really is an ecochoice out there for everyone.

The eco-option can also be kinder on the purse strings and offer you ways to make your day even more memorable, as I found when my daughter Leah got married in 2008. We used flowers from the garden and collected jam jars to use as water glasses instead of renting them. We even got a certificate from the council for all our recycling efforts.

If you don't have the time to research local vendors and grow your own, then why not approach a sustainable catering company to help get you started? I set up Mrs. Paisley's Lashings, with leading ecochef Arthur Potts Dawson, with this in mind. A percentage of our profits go toward funding gardens in schools, so we can encourage the next generation toward healthy, organic eating.

I'm delighted that Louise Moon is sharing her expertise in green weddings; we all need to be taking small steps toward a united, global environmental change, and where better to begin than your wedding. Why not start married life as you mean to go on?

I wish you all the very best with planning your big day; love your planet, go organic.

Jo Wood, founder of Jo Wood Organics
London, 2010

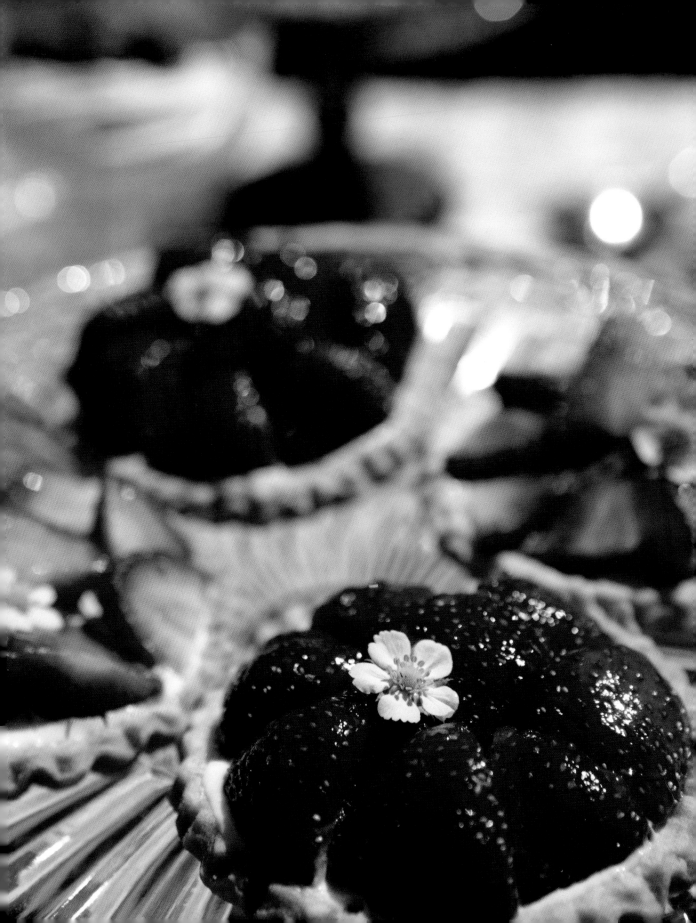

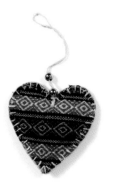
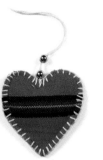
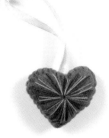
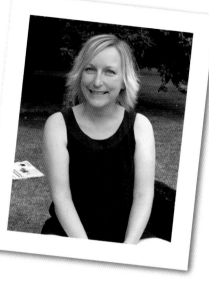

Introduction

My love of all things green and gorgeous started at an organic bed-and-breakfast in Dorset, many years ago. My fiancé and I ate delicious organic breakfasts, enjoyed 100 percent–natural toiletries, browsed in the town's ethical shops, buying ecowares and natural shampoos and soaps, and left with changed priorities.

Not long after, I launched EcoMoon, my wedding-planning business with a difference, designed to offer people a stylish alternative to the carbon-heavy and usually very expensive standard wedding. Current figures show that the average wedding can send 14.5 tons of carbon dioxide into the atmosphere—roughly double an individual human's carbon footprint for a year! This results in an expensive day, both for a couple's pockets and for Earth. So what is the alternative? Well, that is where my book comes in.

I wanted to write *The Natural Wedding* to provide couples with inspiration and advice on every aspect of their greener celebration, from vintage gowns to seasonal flowers, from natural decorations to organic skin care, with gorgeous photographs to show their family and friends. As I have written it, I have included many hints and tips from my years of planning as well as projects to make at home—everything from organic cupcakes to wedding-day bags. It is my ecochic guide to weddings for all couples, regardless of budget. No hairy shirts or mud in sight!

The Natural Wedding is here to dispel the myth that an eco-conscious wedding can't be stylish and look exactly like a "regular" wedding, if that is what you wish for. Similarly, for couples wanting a unique, handmade day, then this is the book to show you how. With just a little effort and forethought, your celebration can be a fabulous and individual event that is a pleasure for you to plan.

So, now you have a copy of this book, I hope that you will enjoy using it and carry it with you to dip into whenever you need a little advice or inspiration. At the end, you will find a comprehensive directory of fabulous ecofriendly suppliers, artisan producers, and generally good people.

Remember, whether dreaming of a formal celebration in a fairy-tale castle or a festival-inspired event with tepees in the woods, planning a natural wedding should be enjoyable, stress free, and about starting your married lives with dainty footprints on Earth.

Have a happy wedding!

Louise
x

Louise Moon
Bath, July 2010

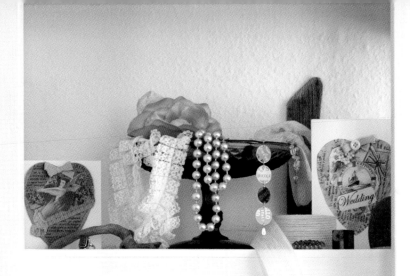
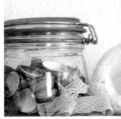
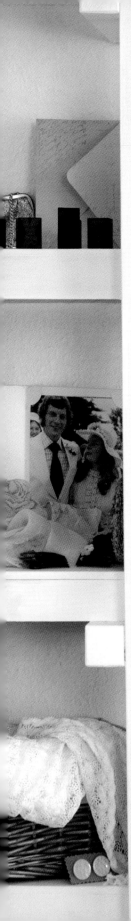
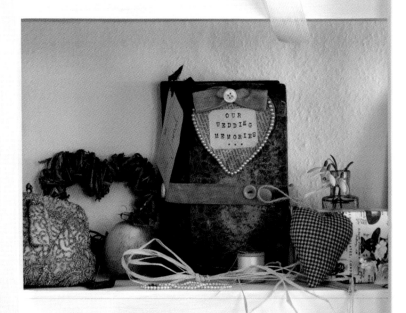

OUR
WEDDING
MEMORIES
★★★

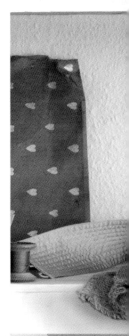
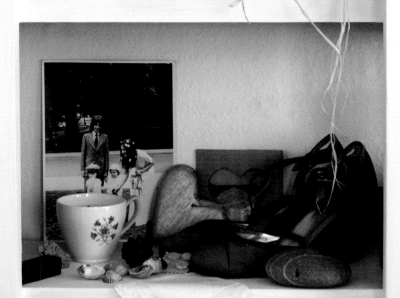
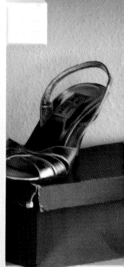

The Style

You've just gotten engaged—congratulations!
And now you're thinking about the kind of wedding
you would like. Maybe you've considered being
greener, or perhaps you're searching for ideas to help
your budget go further or to make your day truly
special and unique. This chapter brings together
themes and inspirations to engage your imagination,
along with practical advice to help you on your way.

Deciding on a natural wedding

The beauty of deciding to have a naturally inspired wedding is the abundance of wonderful possibilities. For me, a natural wedding conjures up images of stunning, locally grown flowers and plants; flavorsome organic menus and artisan treats; gorgeous vintage bridal gowns and jewelry borrowed from friends or relatives; creative, handmade invitations; and relaxing, plant-based facials. And that is just the start.

Given half the chance, most couples would choose a green, natural, and ethical day, but in my experience, many simply do not know where to begin. You may already shop at your local farmers' market and take energy-saving measures at home, use natural cleaning and beauty products and buy fair trade whenever you can; but with so many choices to make when planning a wedding, along with the time pressures and the stress, it can often feel easier to go with the standard options.

The idea of this book is to give you some natural inspiration and to guide you through the information you'll need to make the choices that are best for you—and that are gentler on the environment.

Do just one thing . . .

I always say to couples planning their wedding, "If you can do just one thing. . ." and by this I mean one natural, ecofriendly, or ethical thing. It could be choosing seasonal food, lighting the tables with plant-wax candles, or honeymooning at an ecoboutique hotel. If every couple did this, it would make a real difference to the environmental impact of the wedding industry.

On average, a wedding puts 14.5 tons of carbon dioxide into the atmosphere—or twice your personal yearly carbon footprint. Food flown thousands of miles and travel by guests are the biggest factors. For peace of mind, consider the ethics and chemical content of some wedding products, too (see the Glossary on page 215).

Greener venues

Beaches, arboretums, village halls, charity-owned historic homes, parks, gardens, tepees, and yurts.

Natural inspiration

Being ecoaware doesn't mean a wedding in a scratchy dress and a muddy field (although a field can be an amazing location). You could have a supersoft, hemp-silk couture gown made for your ceremony, then hold a barbecue on a sweeping crescent of beach. Or, imagine brightly colored, people-powered rickshaws, a woodland clearing as your setting, and favor boxes made from wildflower-seed paper.

Choosing your wedding style

Spend time dipping into and choosing elements for your wedding style from the pages that follow. Whichever style you are drawn to, opt for organic and biodynamic food, grown according to ecofriendly guidelines, and fair-trade products that have been ethically made with the welfare of their producers in mind (see the Directory on page 208).

Knowing that your wedding is having a positive effect on the environment is the perfect way for you to start your married lives. So be different, personalize your day, and choose an unusual venue, homemade food, and a stunning ethical dress. You, your family, and your guests will have an unforgettable day.

Wedding planner tip:
As you plan, take pleasure from meeting like-minded people and discover your creative side—and, most important, have fun.

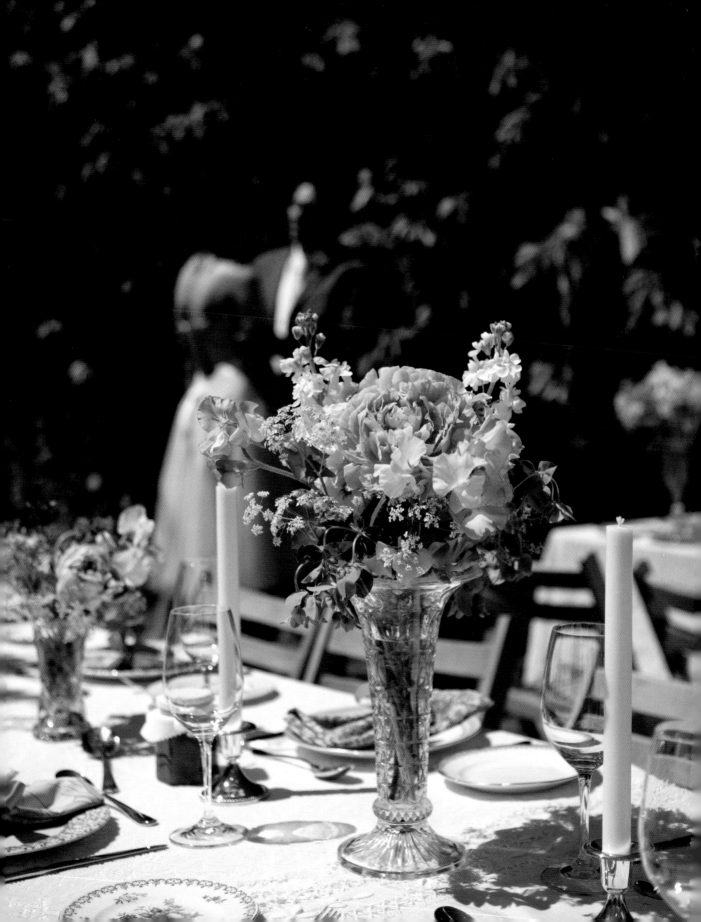

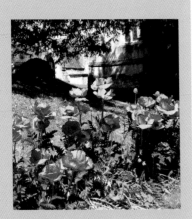

Seasonal weddings

From springtime tulips to brink-of-autumn echinaceas, make the most of seasonal flowers and foliage, and enjoy foods at the peak of their flavor. Fruit, vegetables, and flowers that can be grown naturally outdoors in your region reduce the need for preservatives or artificial climates. Local produce has less distance to travel and helps to reduce your wedding's carbon footprint.

Let the time of the year when you are marrying inspire your choice of wedding location and dress. Tents, tepees, and yurts are perfect for the summer, while ecochic hotels, historic homes, and modern green wedding venues suit cooler winter weather. Often, the surrounding landscape will present the best backdrops to your photographs. Link hands beneath blossoming trees for a natural confetti shot.

Food through the year

Hot comfort food, with rich sauces and deep flavors, will warm up winter-themed weddings. Light, fresh tastes, from tingling fruit sorbets to many-colored salads, are ideal for celebrations in the summer. Organically grown fruit and flowers avoid the synthetic pesticides that are common elsewhere in agriculture. If you find organic produce too expensive to buy, try growing your own (see page 112). Or discover food for free, by foraging for the likes of star-flowered wild garlic on a long country walk.

Making the seasons your wedding style

Any couple can have a celebration that is sensitive to the season, whether you already lead an ecofriendly lifestyle or not. Personalize your day with seasonal elements chosen for the time of year: natural fabrics, such as cool linen or gentle, wool knits; skin-care treats made with local strawberries (see page 180); or a bouquet of cornflowers you have tied yourself (see page 146). For timely themes, think of a country garden, autumn colors, the summer sun, a winter chill, spring blossoms, or a village fête.

All about flowers

Try making flowers—or even a single flower variety—the focus of your wedding design. It's a simple way to create an effortlessly coordinated look.

* Commission an artist to draw your chosen flower, and use the illustration for invitations, menus, and orders of service.
* Use the same kinds of flowers for your table decorations and bouquets.
* Break apart flower heads to make fresh petal confetti (see page 152).
* Ice a floral design onto homemade biscuits for your favors.
* Decorate your cake with fresh flower buds.
* Wear a single bloom in your hair.

Rich pickings

* Fresh-picked strawberries, blueberries, and raspberries
* Brightly colored squashes
* Winter root vegetables
* Homemade elderflower cordial
* Cider made from juicy, local apples
* Locally caught fish or free-range local meat in its prime season
* Homemade seasonal jams
* Home-baked cakes decorated with seasonal fruit or flowers
* Wildflowers grown in your garden
* Berries and seed heads for your decorations

Natural advantages

Locally grown, seasonal food and flowers mean fewer food miles and support local farmers and enterprises.

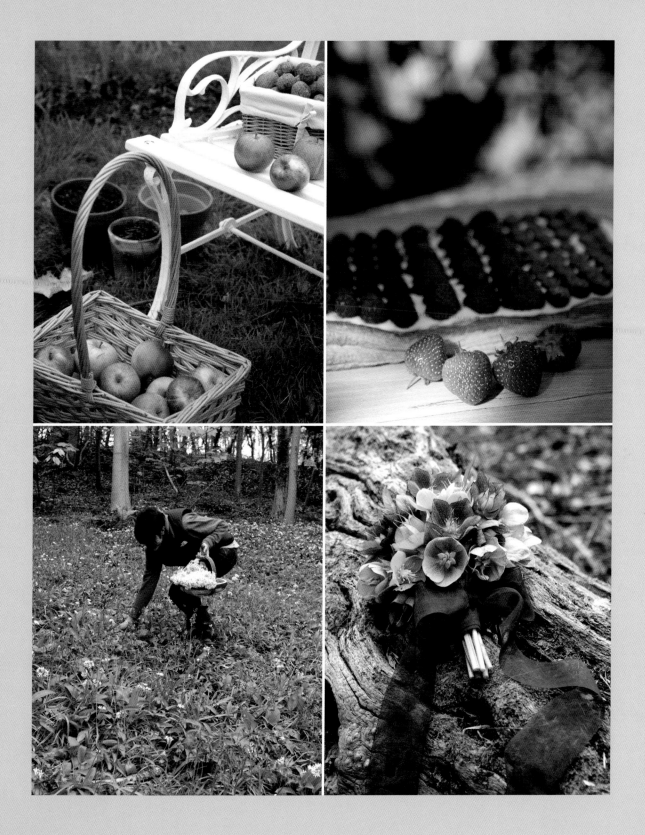

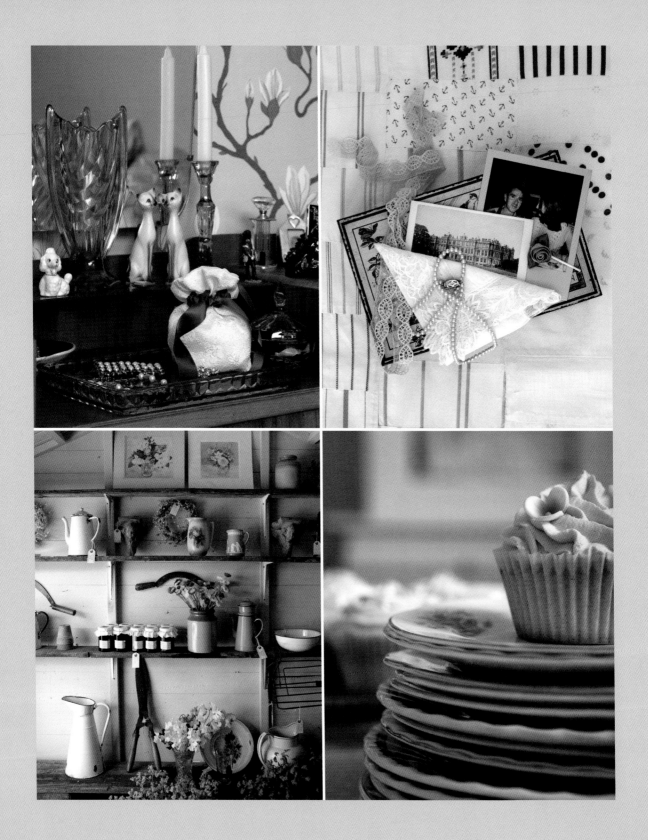

Vintage weddings

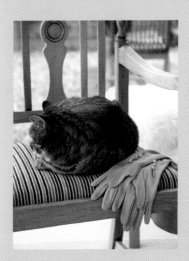

Indulge your vintage side and bring together all those little gems you've collected over the years: the beaded Italian bag; the fabulous 1950s wedding gown; the Edwardian pearl necklace; and the long, elegant gloves. Antique, secondhand, and reused items are great for the environment. They are effectively carbon neutral as they have already been used, and you may well be saving them from being thrown away.

Secondhand stores are a fantastic source of unexpected finds—buying from them will benefit both the good cause and your wallet. Relatives may also have heirloom jewelry, ceramics, or linen to pass down to you. Don't be afraid to use items that do not match—it can create a delightfully eclectic look.

Stylish couples
Take inspiration from these classic, twentieth-century weddings:
* **Grace Kelly and Prince Rainier**
  A fairy-tale wedding in Monaco in 1956, in front of the world's press and the adoring public. She wore a full-skirted gown, crafted from ivory silk taffeta and lace.
* **Edward and Mrs. Simpson**
  They married in 1937 in France, shortly after he renounced the British throne. She wore an elegant, cream-colored, long-sleeved skirt-suit, complete with neat, covered-button detailing, and a stylish hat, and carried a small matching bag.
* **Yoko Ono and John Lennon**
  Sixties fashion at its best. They married in Gibraltar in 1969; Yoko wore a white crêpe minidress, white kneesocks, and a wide-brimmed hat.

Setting up your own garden party
Marry in a local church, then walk to your reception in a friend's flower-filled garden. Decorate a traditional tent with homemade bunting and vintage vases filled with cottage-garden flowers. An elegant string quartet, or friends busking, is the perfect accompaniment. As the sun goes down, light soy candles in recycled jam jars.
* Hired furniture should be delivered the night before and stored under cover.
* Make sure there is enough room for people to walk between rows of chairs.
* Layering vintage tablecloths or spreading lengths of vintage sari fabric over plain white cloths will disguise ordinary tables.
* Arrange flowers the night before, then keep them somewhere cool and dark.

Style from the past
* Eclectic floral china
* Retro, 1960s colored-glass vases
* Antique suitcases
* Beautiful lace dresses
* Original printing stamps
* Chic vanity cases
* Vintage *Vogue* magazines
* Heavy linen tablecloths
* Heirloom veils
* Long white gloves
* Inherited jewelry
* Salvaged dress patterns

Natural advantages
Retro gowns, country-style tea parties, and florals—reusing is effectively carbon neutral and reduces what might otherwise go to waste.

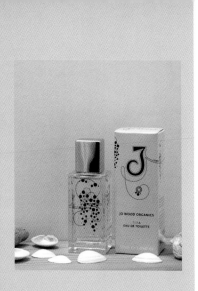

Ecochic weddings

From urban ecoboutique hotels to innovative organic catering, you can have a big day that is contemporary, chic, and green, too. There's no need to compromise your taste. Revel in the growing range of ecodesigner labels and bespoke makers, such as Jessica Charleston, who created the kimono-inspired dress on the opposite page (see the Directory on page 209). If you have a smaller budget, there are ways to create a sleek, modern look for less—take a look at the list on the left.

Ecostores and vendors can provide you with wedding products designed specifically to minimize your carbon impact. Most of these also have outstanding ethics. You can find everything from designer organic cakes to beautiful recycled paper stationery and artisan-made wooden place cards.

Simplicity itself

Fill straight-sided, contemporary glass bowls with organic white roses for minimalist floral displays; choose modern, ethical fabrics such as hemp silk (see page 64); decorate tables with driftwood; and have a clean-lined, white-iced artisan-made cake, decorated with artfully placed fresh flowers and pale green recycled ribbon.

* High-tech organic skin care: luxurious natural brands and makeup free of synthetic chemicals (see page 175).
* City-center ecohotels: minimalist and low impact.
* Biodynamic wines: Some of the world's top vineyards use this approach.
* Peace silk: a light, ethical fabric for a handmade gown.
* Fair-trade artisanal chocolate: for edible favors and cakes.
* Limited editions: Support local artists by choosing handmade decorations.
* Contemporary, ethical jewelry: from certified diamonds to local hardwood rings (see page 79).
* Recycled glass: jewelry made from luminous sea-glass beads, shaped by the ocean (see opposite page and page 80).
* Designer organic cakes: visually stunning, in any shape you can imagine.
* Bespoke bouquets: Use fair-trade flowers to complement your dress, or grow your own flowers and foliage (see page 143).
* Rented topiary: Add elegance with formal box balls or a cloud-pruned olive.
* Ecoregistry: from stylish, green designer names.
* Biofuel wedding cars: Or, go low-tech with bicycles.

Modern for less
* Beachcombed pebbles as place-card holders
* Single flower stems in recycled bottles
* Paperless designer e-vites (www.paperlesspost.com)
* Natural soaps for favors
* A simple, chic color scheme, such as stylish black and white
* White linen tablecloths
* A simple dress with contemporary ecojewelry
* Barbecue on the beach
* White-iced cupcakes on a rented, tiered stand
* Sky lanterns
* Cool camping for your honeymoon

Natural advantages
Green designer services often focus on energy-saving ideas and reusing and recycling, and have strong ethical policies.

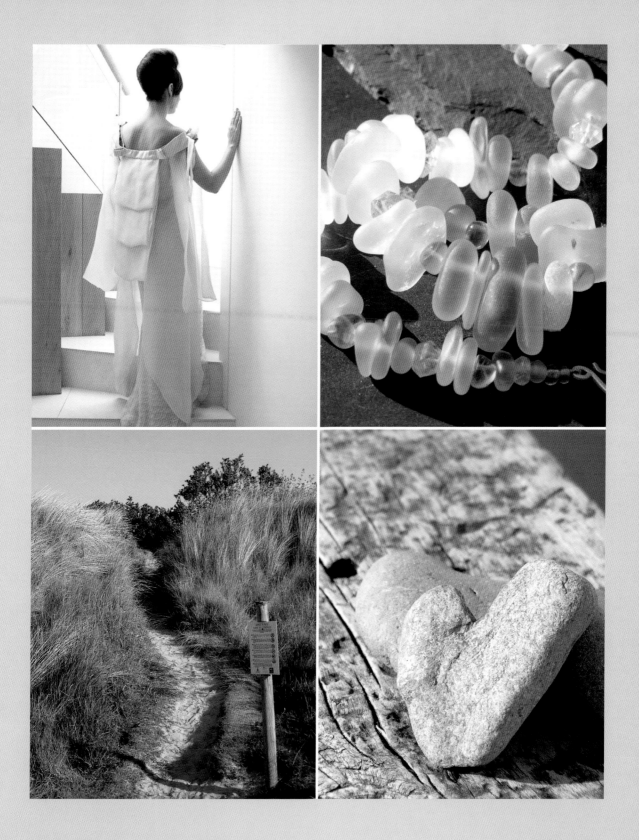

Handmade weddings

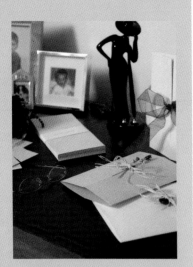

A DIY wedding can be enormous fun to create. Homemade cakes, decorations, invites, and dresses can really personalize your day, while also saving you money. Relax in the knowledge that your wedding will be distinctive and perfectly you.

To ensure your DIY wedding is memorably stylish, coordinate your stationery, match your flowers to your dress details, and choose decorations that complement your venue.

Picture the scene: trees looped with homemade gingham bunting and tables laid with plates of home-cooked food and Grandma's chutney; pretty place cards, showing guests their seats, crafted out of recycled paper and reclaimed lace; a wedding gown made by the bride from a vintage pattern; flowers and herbs, planted into coir pots and small enamel jugs by a friend, and grouped as table displays. Perfect.

Family and friends

Depending on the size of your wedding, you may need an extra pair of hands to craft your day. Ask relatives to help out by making the cake or a plate of food. Or gather bridesmaids together for an evening of jewelry making. Invite a talented friend to take the photographs, and see if an older family member has a gown squirreled away that can be reworked into something wonderful.

Get your groom involved, and persuade him to make the chocolate truffle favors—easy to prepare and delicious. Pack them into biodegradable cellophane bags, tied with natural raffia, for wedding-day gifts. Spend time with friends creating your own recycled fabric corsages, and embellish a guest book using the same materials.

Handmade and bespoke

If hand-crafting isn't for you, or you are not confident of your skills, search out talented local artisans who can make everything from your dress to the bread.

Homemade tips

❉ Borrow books from the library to find out how to make invitations (see page 98).

❉ Find local courses in traditional printing techniques and jewelry making.

❉ Salvage charming old fabrics to make corsages, bunting, and tablecloths.

❉ Adopt "Ladies, a plate," a New Zealand tradition where female guests bring a dish of homemade food—ask all of the cooks among your guests, male and female to join in.

❉ Bake your own cupcakes and decorate them imaginatively (see page 127).

❉ Find a local dressmaker and have a gown made to measure—or, ask a friend or relative to make it for you (see page 62).

❉ Gather flowers from your garden and tie your own bouquet (see page 146).

❉ Make timber signs for the reception with your groom.

Your DIY wedding preparation kit

❉ Salvaged fabrics

❉ Recycled old ribbons and lace

❉ Antique printing kits

❉ Pebbles and beads

❉ Natural raffia

❉ Pinking shears and sharp scissors

❉ Handmade paper

❉ A sewing kit and sewing machine

❉ Plenty of time—and, of course, this book

Natural advantages

Lovingly handmade food, dresses, and decorations can reduce packaging and food miles, and DIY is an excellent thrifty choice.

Pawle and
Kiki,
love, laughter,
and happy times
4 ever ♡
lov,
Rachel + Martin
xx

Budgets and priorities

The budget can be a major influence on your day. But regardless of whether you have been saving for years or are strapped for cash, you can still have a glorious wedding. Don't be tempted to borrow money for your celebration—in my experience, this simply leads to stress and worry. It is better to start your married lives without this burden.

My advice to all couples at the beginning of the planning phase is to make a list of your wedding priorities. You may have your eye on a special designer dress or be desperate to invite two hundred guests, so working out what matters most to you is a good starting point.

Wedding planner tip:
Add up your spending as you go along so you don't go over budget. Simple advice, but surprisingly effective.

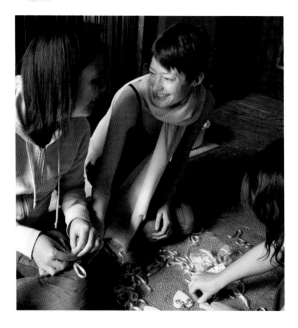

Once you have your list, allocate the sums of money that you are prepared to spend on each item. Some wedding books and magazines suggest percentages for each, from the dress to the music. But if you follow this advice, you may end up spending more than you want on some things. Instead, simply divide up your budget according to your own priorities.

Being inventive

A natural wedding allows you to be resourceful and creative with your spending. If you decide to blow most of the budget on food, see if you can borrow a dress; or, if you simply cannot afford stationery, send out e-vites instead.

Don't be afraid to ask friends and relatives for their help and advice. They will often be happy to make food, provide bunches of flowers from their gardens, or lend pieces of jewelry or even a wedding dress. Make the most of their skills: Ask if they can style your hair, apply your makeup, or even teach you how to lino-cut your own invitations. They will almost certainly love to be involved.

Natural choices

You will probably have ideas about the one aspect of your wedding where it really matters to you to be as green and ethical as possible. Whether it is organic food, vintage collectables, ecofriendly products, or the perfect green venue, put this on your wedding priority list and remember to bear it in mind when searching out vendors.

It is easy to lose direction when planning a wedding and panic-buy things that you don't need and won't use. By re-reading your list and thinking about whether you really need a product, you can stick to your ethical principles and keep a rein on your budget.

For more planning help, see our Wedding Planner on page 202.

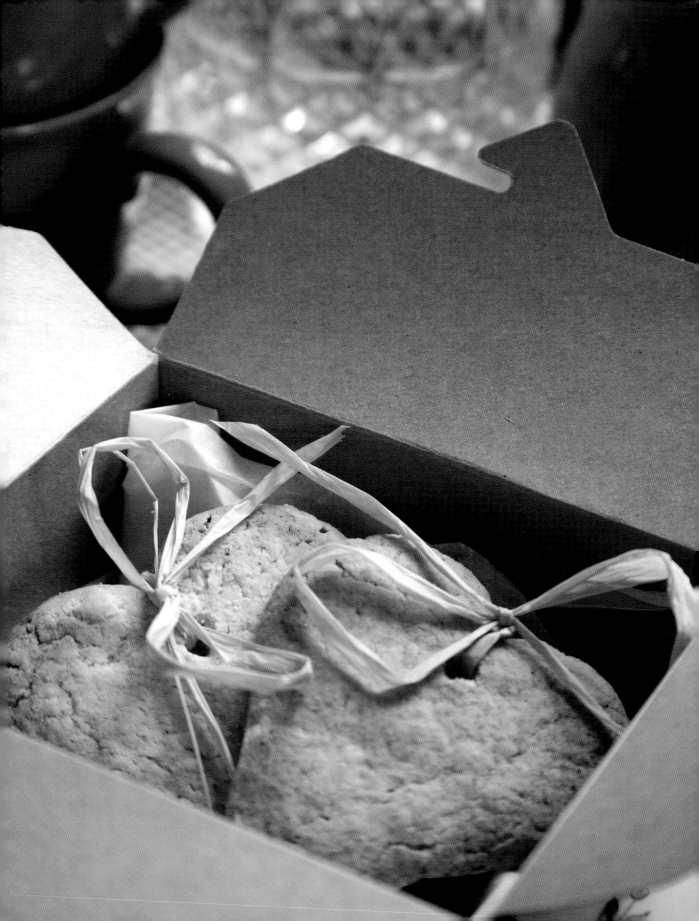

Your ceremony

The ceremony is the keystone of your wedding and will define your day. There are many different ways to wed, whether you dream of a traditional church service or an alternative ritual, prefer a civil route or decide to "marry" without any official, legal ceremony. Rules and regulations differ in every country, so check with your local authority about what constitutes a legal marriage in your area. There are meaningful ceremonies for couples of all faiths; this quick guide will get you started.

Legalities

The requirements for a legal marriage vary from country to country and can be confusing. In the United Kingdom, you can be legally married in a church or other religious building, in a council registry office, or at a registered venue by a registrar. Outdoor marriages are more difficult and are only currently legal for humanists in Scotland. To marry legally outdoors in England, Ireland, or Wales the ceremony must take place under a registered shelter, usually on the grounds of a stately home or hotel.

Humanist weddings

In Scotland, Australia, New Zealand, Canada, Norway, and some states in the United States, humanist weddings are legal. These are nonreligious weddings where couples are encouraged to write their own vows and choose their own music and readings. Ceremonies must be conducted by a registered celebrant but can take place at any location as long as it is "safe and dignified." Whether under a blossoming tree or on a deserted beach, the possibilities for a humanist wedding are truly special.

Gay and lesbian weddings

The laws vary across the globe. In the United Kingdom, civil partnerships (for gay and lesbian couples) are legal in council registry offices and some registered venues. Other countries, such as the United States, allow civil partnerships in certain states, while some do not allow same-sex weddings at all. Any couple can choose to have a nonlegal commitment ceremony—you could even have a friend conduct the wedding.

Hand-fastings

A hand-fasting is an ancient pagan ceremony popular in many countries. During the ceremony, the couple's hands are tied together with a piece of ribbon, fabric, or cord, which when knotted, signifies that the couple's union is permanent. (This is where the saying "tying the knot" originates.) Hand-fastings are usually held in woodland with guests standing in a circle marked with stones. They are beautiful ceremonies and can be combined with a civil wedding for a legal marriage.

It's your day

Unless you are having a formal religious service, generally you can have some input into the design of the ceremony. Personalize your day by writing your own wedding vows and choosing readings, poetry, and music that are special to you both.

Ecophotography

It's simple to be green with your photos—just go digital. Ask your photographer to provide the images on a CD so that you can view and print them as you wish. Traditional photo-printing techniques use synthetic chemicals, so instead, print onto recycled paper using vegetable-based inks—see the Directory for specialist printers.

Wedding albums often have tropical hardwood covers that are sourced from Australia and New Zealand. If you live in the United States, the carbon footprint of the album alone is huge. Choose a company that provides locally produced, handmade paper albums with sustainably sourced timber covers. Old-fashioned, self-adhesive photo corners are preferable to spray glue.

Your wedding notebook—save cuttings, business cards, fabrics, and pictures showing ideas you like into a book to help you design your day.

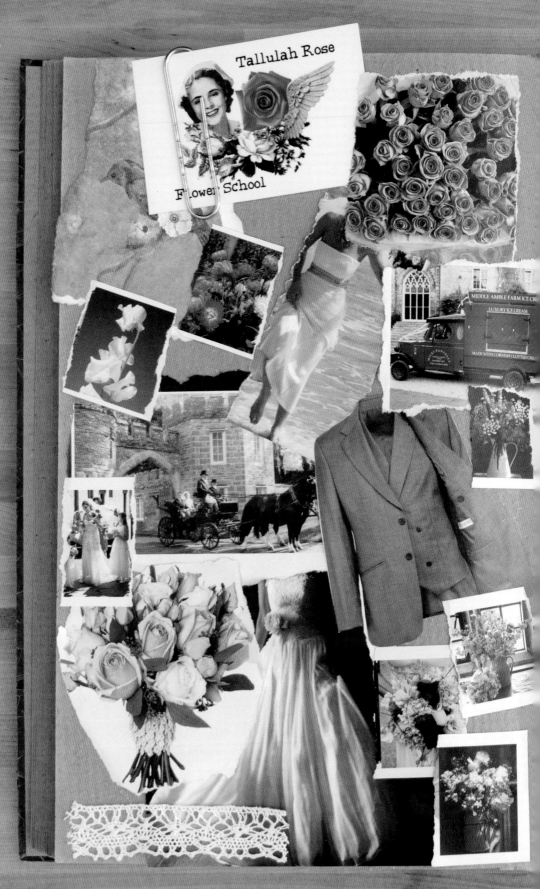

Tallulah Rose

Flower School

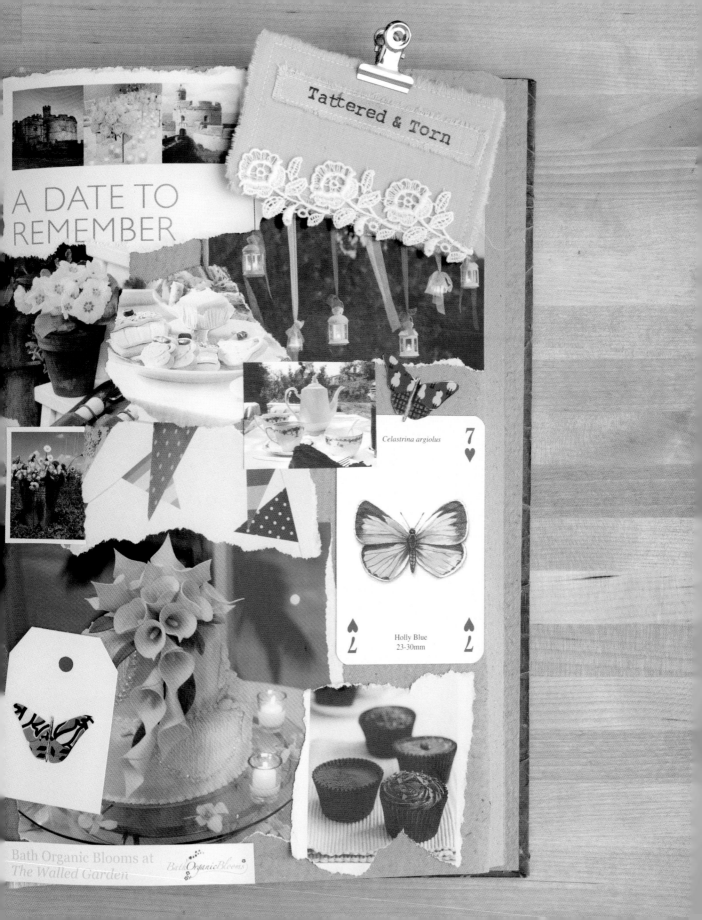

Tattered & Torn

A DATE TO REMEMBER

Celastrina argiolus

7♥

Holly Blue
23-30mm

Bath Organic Blooms at
The Walled Garden   *Bath Organic Blooms*

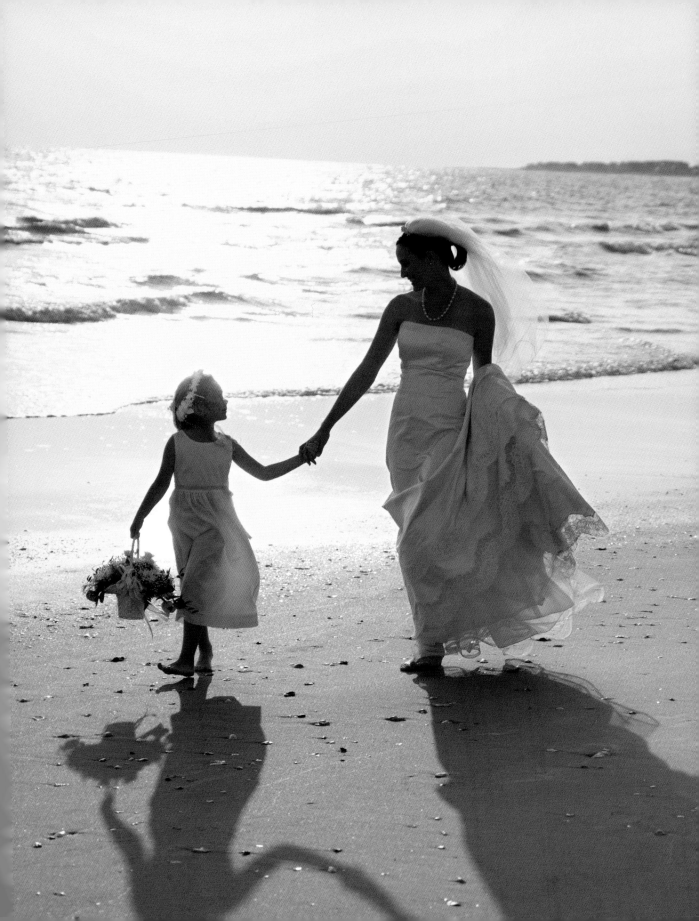

Farther afield and precelebrations

If you plan to marry abroad, with a little thought, it is still possible to have an ecofriendly wedding. A diverse and growing range of ecohotels and lodges across the world use organic food and local suppliers, have recycling strategies and green electricity tariffs, and promote fair trade. For peace of mind, ask the same questions you would of a venue closer to home (see page 38).

Think about how you intend to get there—traveling by train is better for the environment than flying—and consider offsetting your journey through accredited organizations such as www.carbonfootprint.com.

The legalities of marrying abroad vary from country to country. Most will require you to be "resident" for anything from a couple of days to a few weeks. Be prepared to provide a bundle of paperwork, including passports, birth certificates, and sometimes a letter from your consulate. Unless you both speak the local language, an interpreter is essential. Check with the country's consulate for specific requirements and advice.

Dare-to-be-different bachelor parties
❋ Outward Bound weekends
❋ Survival courses
❋ Mountaineering trips
❋ Hiking expeditions

Fashionable bachelorette parties
❋ Crafting weekends
❋ Spa breaks
❋ "Glamping"—or, glamorous camping
❋ Home cocktail parties, complete with a professional mixologist

Alternative bachelor and bachelorette parties

Bachelor and bachelorette parties are a long-standing wedding tradition. But why not try something a little different? Friends of mine held a joint bachelor/bachelorette minifestival in a field. They erected a tent and invited local bands and DJs to play. Guests camped for the whole weekend and brought food to share.

Cheap flights to typical party destinations create large carbon footprints, so stay closer to home and take public transportation or carpool. See the box above for more ideas.

Packing tips for the bride abroad

Transporting a wedding dress can be a challenge. Follow these tips for stress-free packing.

❋ Choose a dress in a fabric that will not crease easily, such as silk.

❋ A shorter dress or skirt-suit is much easier to transport than a long gown.

❋ Place layers of acid-free tissue paper between the folds of your gown to minimize creasing.

❋ Vintage dresses often travel more happily than you would expect, as the beading and lace can disguise wrinkles.

❋ Small, beaded vintage purses make a stylish alternative to a bouquet and take up minimal space.

Wedding planner tip:
Expensive precelebrations can be too costly for some friends. More affordable activities will make it easier for them to join in.

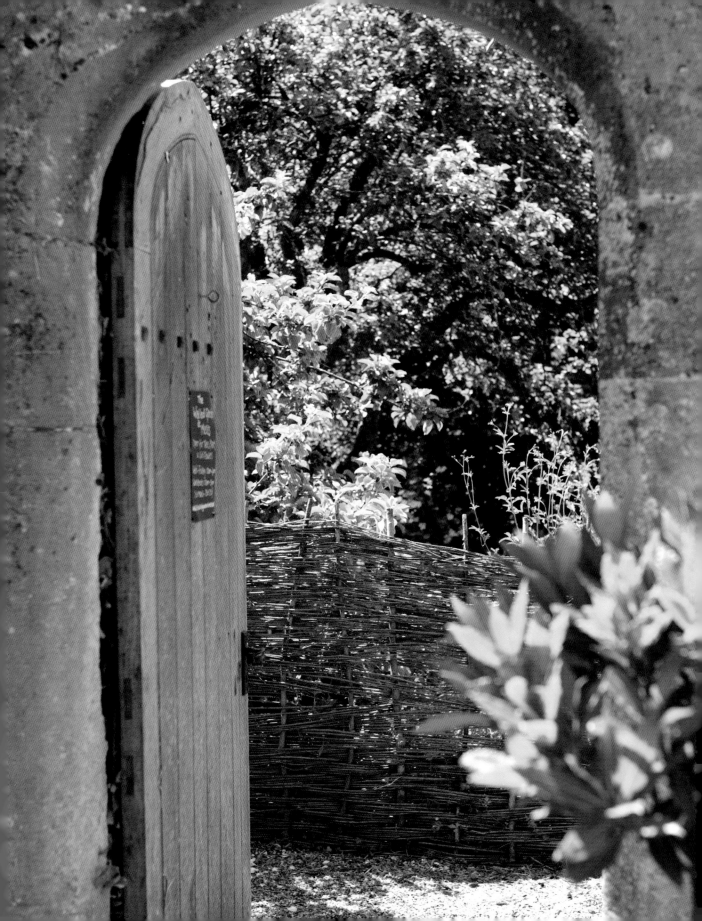

The Venue

Choosing your wedding venue will be one of your
first and biggest decisions, so you'll want it to reflect
your values as a couple. There are plenty of charity,
thrifty, and naturally luxurious alternatives to the
standard hotel wedding package (even though some
chains are trying to be more ecofriendly). You can
hold your reception, and sometimes marry, anywhere
from a yurt in a friend's garden to an ecochic
boutique hotel or sumptuous historic house.

What makes a venue green

There is a stylish green venue for every celebration, whatever your beliefs or religion. The best way to find a venue is by personal recommendation, but guides and Web sites can also help. Some use questionnaires to determine the efforts that venues are making to be ethical and environmentally friendly; others, such as www.ecohotelsoftheworld.com, vet entries.

The questions below will help you to establish a venue's environmental credentials. You may have your eye on a fantastic place that doesn't fulfill all of these criteria, but some effort is better than none. It is up to you to decide what matters most to you.

Questions to ask a venue

❋ Does it have a recycling and waste management strategy?

❋ Does its energy come from a green energy provider, or does the venue generate its own electricity through on-site renewables, such as solar panels?

❋ Do the managers use local suppliers when possible?

❋ Do they choose fair-trade products?

❋ Do they opt for organic food, and is it grown on-site or locally?

❋ Do they clean using products that are free from petroleum-based and synthetic chemicals?

Energy use

Many buildings, from farms to modern hotels, now generate their own electricity. Greener venues may have a biomass boiler or a wind turbine, solar thermal panels, or photovoltaics. If not, they should at least buy their energy from a green provider.

Waste strategy

These days, there is little excuse not to recycle, and food waste is easily composted. However, some venues will go further in reducing, reusing, and recycling. Winkworth Farm in Wiltshire, England, for example, bottles its own water and reuses the glass bottles.

Reducing chemical exposure

Many people are now aware of chemicals such as volatile organic compounds (VOCs) that can affect health. Look for venues that decorate using natural paints and water-based varnishes; use gentle, nonsynthetic cleaning products; and have chosen furnishings that are made using natural materials or meet strict ecostandards, such as the Nordic Swan ecolabel.

Organic food and products

As well as cooking you a delicious organic wedding breakfast, venues can offer many other organic options, such as organic cotton bedding (regular cotton uses a quarter of the world's pesticides), organic bamboo towels, organic plant-wax candles, and organic toiletries. For more about organics and certification, see page 110.

Air-conditioning

Air-handling units (AHUs) use massive amounts of energy and also cause noise pollution. Even in hot and humid conditions, well-designed venues can cool their buildings naturally though windows and roof vents. If there is air-conditioning, make sure it is powered by renewable energy.

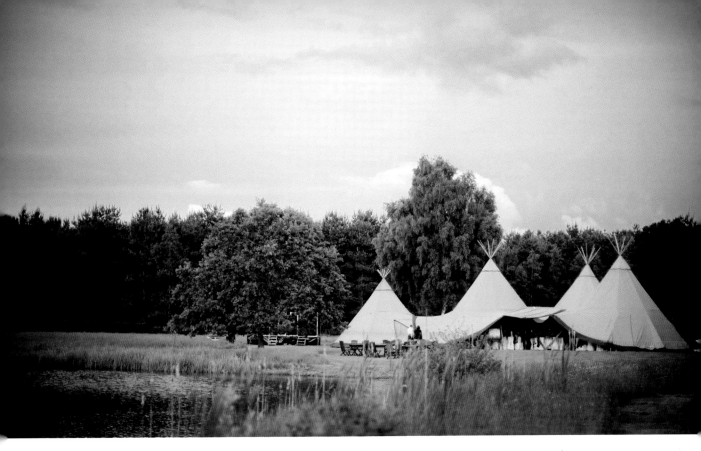

These "giant hat" Kåta tents can be joined in combinations to make different-sized spaces, from www.papakata.co.uk.

Before you start your venue search, it is useful to determine some basic criteria:

❉ Would you like to marry and hold the reception in the same location?

❉ Do you need a venue licensed for marriages? (Not required for hand-fastings or blessings.)

❉ How many guests do you plan to invite?

❉ Do you want the ceremony or reception to be indoors or outdoors?

❉ What time of year do you wish to marry?

Consider how your venue fits with your vision. If you are planning a formal affair with floor-length gowns and a lavish sit-down meal, a grand historic venue would be ideal. With an ecofabric dress, flowers in your hair, and a barbecue, a tepee in a field may be just right.

For more about legalities and licensing, see page 30. If you are marrying abroad, see page 35.

Wedding venue ideas

❉ 10 guests: ceremony in a tiny church, followed by a garden party in a friend's flower-filled garden

❉ 50 guests: civil ceremony and sit-down dinner at an ecoboutique hotel

❉ 100 guests: civil ceremony at a licensed, organic ecocenter, followed by an outdoor cocktail reception

❉ 200 guests: festival-inspired hand-fasting under a tree, followed by a reception in a giant tepee

Wedding planner tip:
To minimize guest miles and keep your wedding carbon footprint low, hold your ceremony and reception at the same venue.

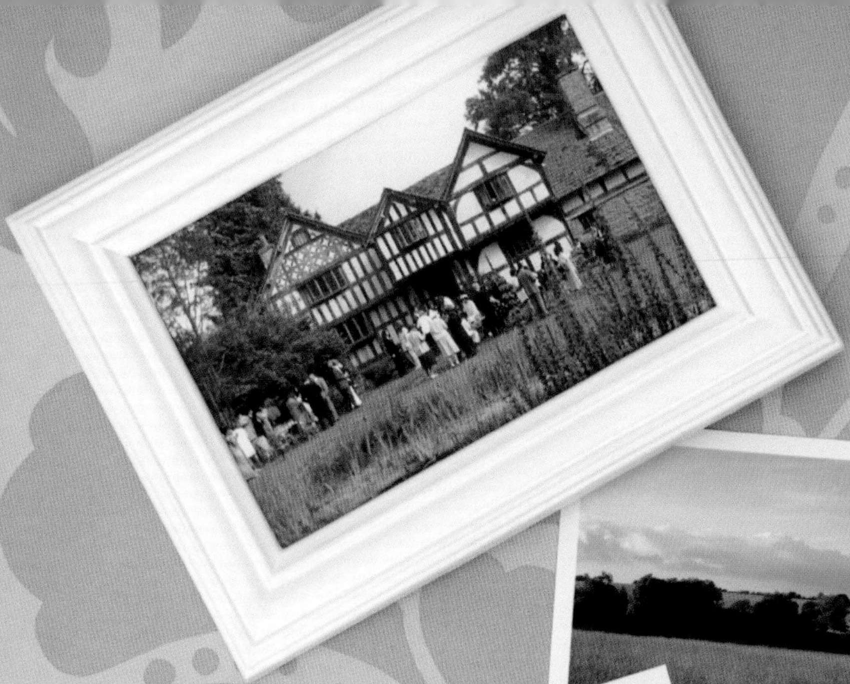

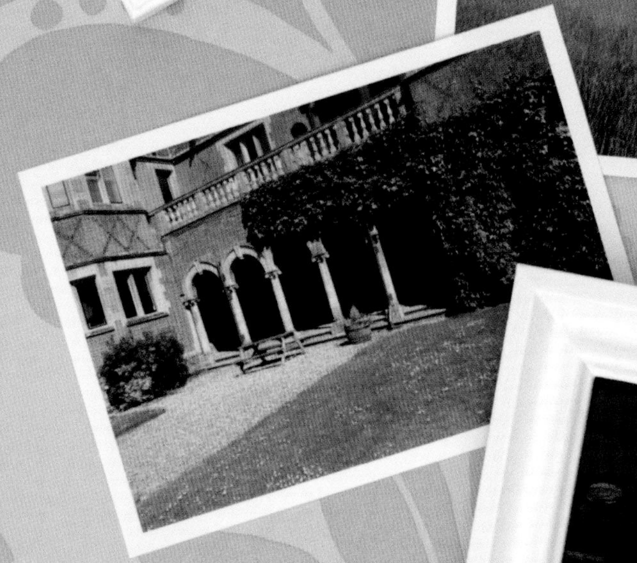

From top: Penrhos Court, views at Winkworth Farm, Dauntsey's School, The Pump Room in Bath, and Forever Green ecocenter.

Ecohotels and centers

Specialist green wedding venues can range from purpose-built ecocenters, constructed using locally sourced materials and sustainable building techniques, to carefully renovated buildings upgraded to the highest environmental standards. Often green venues will also grow their own food and flowers.

Ecovenues usually advertise their credentials, but if there is something specific that you are concerned about, do ask—they are generally happy to help. The Directory on page 208 lists some of our favorites.

Many hotels and ecocenters are licensed for civil ceremonies, while others may have chapels on their grounds, and some are set up to host the perfect hand-fasting (see page 30). Check which type of ceremony they can perform before you book the date.

Ecoboutique hotels

Often elegant town house conversions or innovative new buildings with holistic spas and contemporary interior design, these hotels score highly on the ecocredentials but do not compromise on luxury or comfort. Find ecohotels around the world at Organic Places to Stay (www.organicholidays.co.uk).

Organic hotels and bed-and-breakfasts

These tend to be smaller and more low-key than ecoboutique hotels. They aim to be as green, ethical, and sustainable as possible and use organic products— from soft, unbleached cotton sheets to organic shower gel. Ideal for more intimate weddings, some organic hotels have their own wildflower gardens or private beaches. Moss Grove Organic (www.mossgrove.com) in the Lake District was refurbished using clay paints, wool insulation, and reclaimed stained glass.

Sheepdrove Organic Farm
Berkshire, United Kingdom

Architect designed, with rammed-earth walls and a timber frame, Sheepdrove (www.sheepdrove.com), licensed for civil ceremonies, is a fine example of an ecocenter. The contemporary interior finishes include natural paints and recycled doors. All the food is organic and local, much of it grown on a 2,300-acre organic working farm—they even grow wheat for artisanal bread.

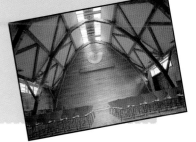

Specialist green wedding venues

Specifically designed or renovated to provide the ideal setting for a natural wedding, venues such as Sheepdrove (above) have the highest environmental standards. Some are entirely wind or solar powered. Most will provide all you need for your day, from locally grown flowers to organic food and their own free-range eggs. Keep an eye out for those that offer something different for your guests, such as a garden maze, a seawater pool, or a stone circle. Many are surrounded by beautiful, organic gardens—a wonderful setting for an idyllic wedding.

Wedding planner tip:
Think about how far your guests will need to travel to your wedding. Long journeys leave large carbon footprints.

Weddings under canvas

Holding a reception under canvas is an exciting prospect and a practical solution for couples with a large guest list but not the budget to match. Marquees, tepees, yurts, and Bedouin tents offer great opportunities for unusual and striking decorations, and an outdoor reception gives a relaxed, informal feeling to the day.

Fields and farms can provide the perfect setting. Often farmers will rent out a field for a day or weekend; some will even provide local produce. Ask if you can borrow straw bales for seating, and whether there are toilets nearby for your guests. Always check with the relevant authorities if you need either a tent or liquor license for the event, and make sure there is access for your tent rental company and any guests with disabilities. You can set up a small kitchen tent and rent catering equipment, although food prepared beforehand will mean less fuss. See page 116 for catering ideas, and the Directory for tent rental companies.

Tepees

Tepees and Kåta tents are hand-crafted timber pole structures covered with natural canvas. The design allows for easy assembly and is intended to include a real fire in the center. "Giant hat" Kåta tents are huge and can be joined together to form beautiful arrangements with enough space for hundreds of guests. Rental companies can provide gorgeously rustic trestle tables and benches, which you can decorate with foliage and candles. During chilly evenings, lay vintage woolen or sheepskin blankets across the benches.

Wedding planner tip:
Ask musical guests to bring instruments with them to play when the band finishes.

Bedouin tents

The traditional, intricate design and colorfully printed canvas of Bedouin tents makes them a stunning backdrop for a wedding. Rental companies can provide hand-painted wall panels, ceiling swags, and embroidered floor cushions, as well as furniture.

Yurts

Curvy and magical, a yurt is a wonderful alternative to a tent. These circular structures can be linked to form yurt villages, which can accommodate the largest wedding party. Separate yurts could have different functions, such as a "bar" or "chill-out" yurt. Choose low tables and floor cushions for a laid-back atmosphere.

Cruck marquees

These are a traditional English timber frame overlaid with natural cotton canvas. Ideal for smaller gatherings, they are usually open at the sides, so are best chosen in months when the risk of rain is low. The attractive structure is simply enhanced by pretty native flowers and flickering candlelight.

Traditional tents

Usually made from natural canvas, with scalloped pelmets and "big top" peaks, these are suited to colorful, homemade bunting and candy-stripe ribbons. I've helped couples keep to a tight budget with a tent by avoiding extras, such as linings and carpets, and renting trestle tables and chairs separately. With all of these tent options, always check what is included in the price.

Guest camping

Some venues offer camping. You could set up a small field of tepees or ask guests to bring their own tents.

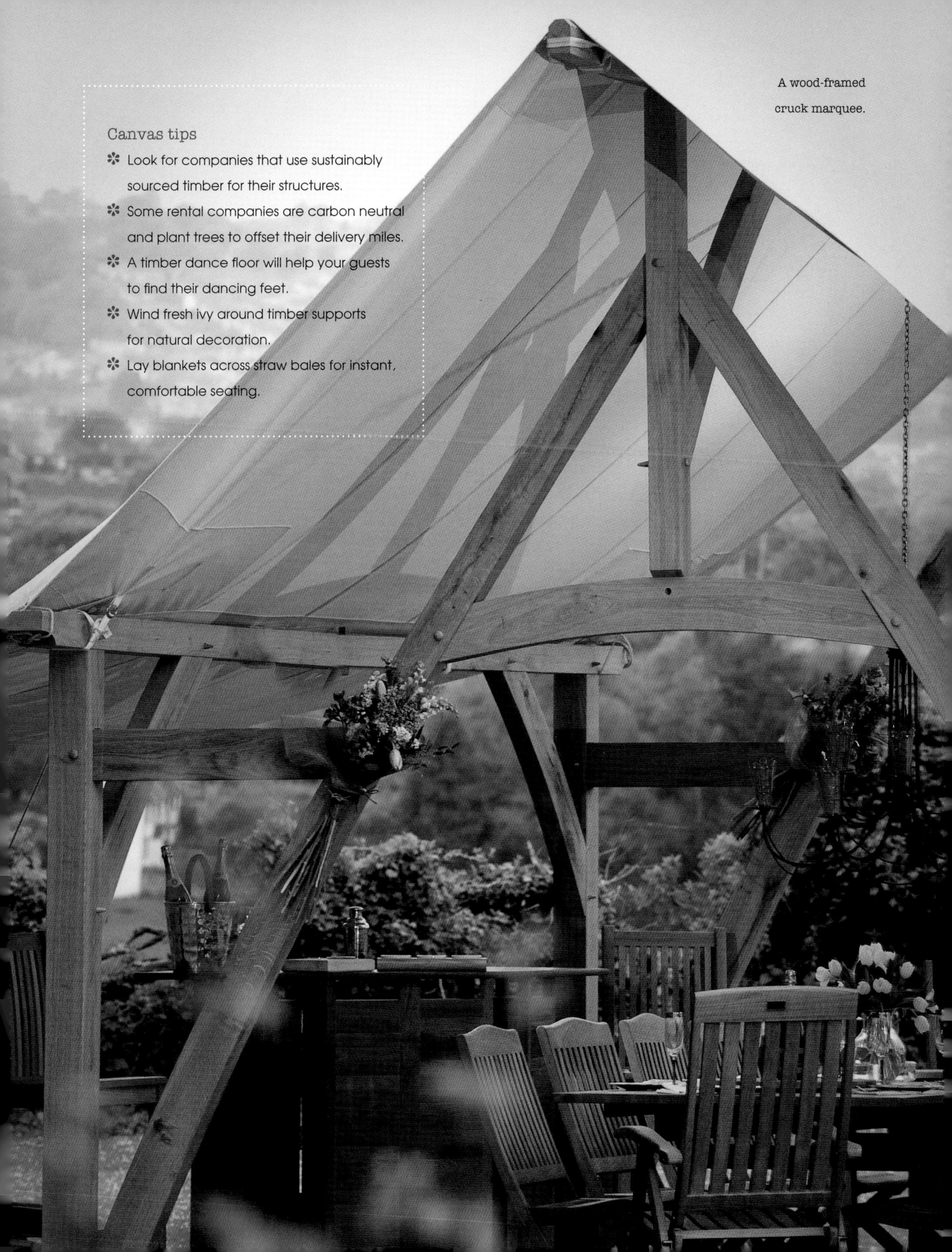

A wood-framed cruck marquee.

Canvas tips

- Look for companies that use sustainably sourced timber for their structures.
- Some rental companies are carbon neutral and plant trees to offset their delivery miles.
- A timber dance floor will help your guests to find their dancing feet.
- Wind fresh ivy around timber supports for natural decoration.
- Lay blankets across straw bales for instant, comfortable seating.

Heritage and historic buildings

It is possible to find remarkable, historic wedding venues that are also ethically sound. Many larger buildings cover their high maintenance costs by hosting weddings and celebrations, so your wedding is helping to preserve them. Old buildings, constructed using traditional techniques, generally contain less-embodied energy than their contemporary counterparts. However, drafty mansions are likely to use more power in their day-to-day running. Venues that have been sympathetically upgraded to high energy-saving standards give the best of both worlds.

Historic homes

Stately homes, and other historic houses, are often licensed for civil ceremonies, and many will oversee all the elements of your day, providing staff and sometimes their own wedding planner. Frequently they have outstanding grounds and gardens. Think about choosing a venue owned by a charity, such as the National Trust (www.nationaltrust.org.uk), which supports architectural conservation. Wakehurst Place in Sussex, managed by the Royal Botanic Gardens at Kew (www.kew.org), includes an arboretum and the Millennium Seed Bank, with all profits going to its plant conservation program.

Country house weddings

Country house parties, where you rent a whole grand house for a day or weekend (rather like renting a vacation cottage), have become highly fashionable. Generally, you will have the place to yourself and are responsible for arranging outside caterers, music, and flowers, but check individual venues to see what is included. Look for those venues that have been carefully restored using environmentally responsible techniques.

Castles and follies

Castles are the ideal backdrop for a fairy-tale wedding. Some can accommodate your guests overnight, which cuts down on travel. Others, such as Thornbury Castle (www.thornburycastle.co.uk), have their own herb gardens and vineyards, so serve their own produce.

Small and intimate, follies range from miniature country houses to classical temples. A few are licensed for civil ceremonies, such as the Red House at Painswick Rococo Garden in Gloucestershire, England (www.rococogarden.org.uk). Team a folly with a traditional tent on nearby grounds.

Mills and barns

Brimming with rustic charm, mills have often been sympathetically converted, and may have fully working waterwheels and flour stones (so you can serve homemade bread using their flour). Winkworth Farm mill (www.winkworthfarm.com) has solar-powered hot water and a cutting garden, too.

Barns can be small and unconverted, with straw on the floor, or grand architectural transformations. There are good examples to fit all budgets and sizes of weddings.

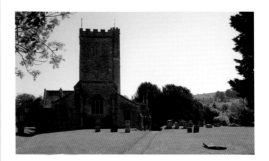

Church weddings

Ancient churches lit by candlelight can be one of the most romantic settings for wedding ceremonies. Fees vary, but all go toward the upkeep and maintenance of these historic buildings. Why not arrange to leave your flowers for the next service?

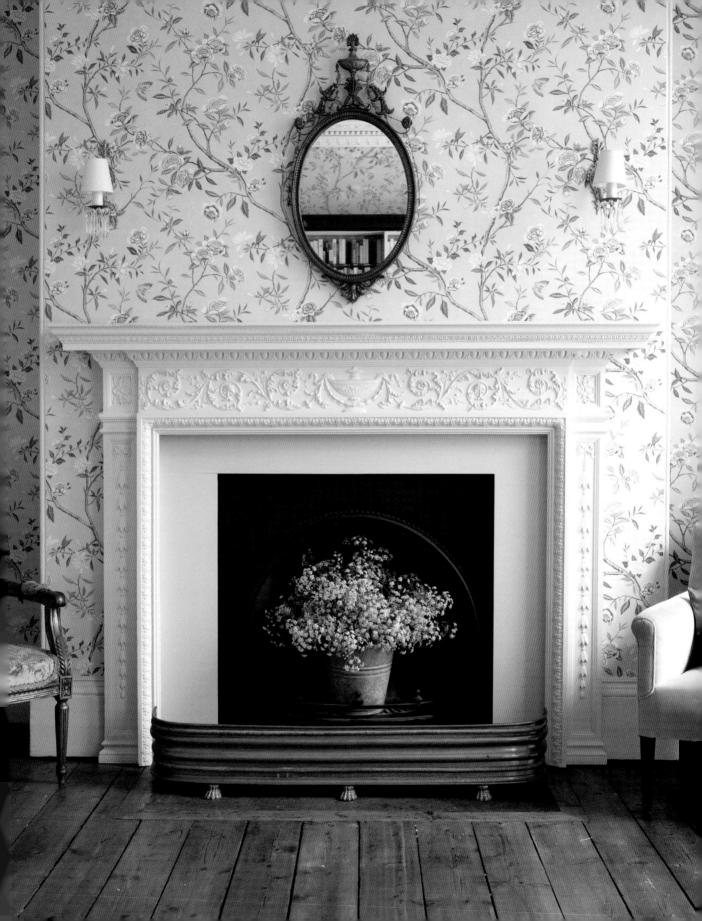

The grounds of Sheepdrove
Organic Farm in Berkshire.

Wedding planner tip:
Ask the owner of a park or garden if
you can pick a few flowers for your hair,
bouquet, or boutonnieres.

The great outdoors

For those who love being outdoors, there can be no better place to marry than in a garden or wood, or on a sandy beach. Riverbanks, arboretums, and lakeshores all make wonderful settings, while marrying under a beautiful, ancient tree is intimate and romantic, with little environmental impact. Inclement weather can pose a problem, so look for a venue with its own shelter, and select appropriate footwear.

For information on the legalities of marrying outdoors, see page 30.

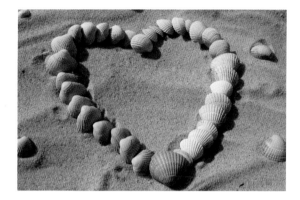

Arboretums

Full of ancient trees, blossoming shrubs, and wildflowers, arboretums, for me, are perfect venues. Many are happy to host weddings and have small buildings available for year-round celebrations, often built using their own timber. Marry in springtime to take advantage of tree blossoms, or in autumn as the leaves change color.

Botanical gardens

What could be better than strolling with your guests through a colorful, wildlife-filled floral garden? Botanical gardens often incorporate streams and boating lakes, and some have their own follies, ideal for a ceremony. Check with the gardens (or the local authority) to find out whether they are licensed and allow weddings.

Local parks

You may have a park near your home that you visit throughout the seasons. Well-maintained and full of champion trees and specimen plants, parks can provide the ideal backdrop—not only for photographs but also for a wedding-party picnic. If you are marrying in a nearby church, why not host drinks in the park? You will need to ask permission from the local authority.

Wildlife conservation centers

These make unusual and inspirational settings. Wildlife charities work hard to protect endangered species and habitats and to rehabilitate animals of all types. You could link your wedding list to your chosen center and ask your guests to make a donation to their valuable work.

Beaches

A beach wedding party can be an ideal low-impact reception. With invigorating scenery, plenty of space for guests, and fabulous photo opportunities, you and your friends will love it. Check for water quality at www.blueflag.org, make sure there are bathrooms nearby, and always clean up thoroughly afterward. Ask the local authority before you plan your event: Some beaches allow campfires, but others have restrictions (on dogs, for example). You should also consider how your guests will travel to the beach, whether there are any hazards, and tide times (so you don't get stranded).

Going local

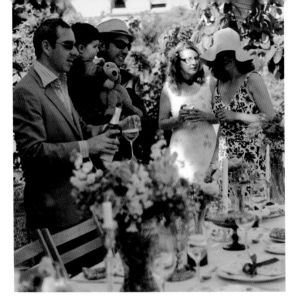

If you live in a house with a beautiful garden, or have friends or relatives who do, why go any farther for your wedding party? It's a thrifty option, and environmentally friendly, as you can recycle as much as you like, and guests may be able to walk there. Encourage those traveling longer distances to use public transportation or to carpool to reduce parking issues. You can easily obtain temporary tent licenses from your local authority—useful in case of rain. Remember to inform neighbors of your plans, to keep them happy, too. For more about setting up a garden party, see pages 23 and 159.

Finding a hall

Village halls and community centers are great for those on a tight budget. Many have on-site catering facilities and provide a blank canvas ready for inventive decoration. Don't worry if you are not keen on the furniture; simply rent different tables, chairs, and linen to personalize your day. Village halls are often positioned next to churches and chapels. At one village hall reception, we strung up floral bunting and laid a single flower on each napkin, and a couple of friends' sons acted as waiters and served the drinks.

Renting what you need

Practically everything you will ever need for a wedding is available to rent. Try to choose natural materials, such as wooden tables and linen tablecloths. Local companies will mean lower transport distances. Appoint a trustworthy friend to unpack deliveries and supervise collection.

Available to rent

Tables, chairs, cushions, blankets, tablecloths and napkins, crockery and glassware, cutlery, bars, candelabras, vases, cake stands, and cake knives.

Quick ways to transform your venue

With some imagination, it is possible to convert the plainest of venues into a wedding wonderland. Work with what is already there—not against it—for the best results. See the Directory for suppliers.

* Rent different furniture—choose trestle tables and benches to make best use of the space.
* Cover unsightly tables with tablecloths made from unbleached cotton, natural linen, or vintage fabrics.
* Use plant-wax candles and lanterns to light the room (check that they are allowed).
* Rent chair covers to disguise old chairs.
* Personalize the bathrooms by providing your own natural soaps and washes.
* Use flowers creatively to divert attention from less attractive elements.
* Put up small handmade signs to direct your guests.
* Use fabric drapes to cover unappealing wall features.
* Choose candles naturally scented with essential oils to make the room smell fresh.
* Bring your iPod for the music.
* Rent mismatched vintage plates for retro chic.
* When choosing flower decorations, complement or incorporate a color that is already in the room.
* Hang homemade bunting outside or inside to brighten up a dull color scheme.

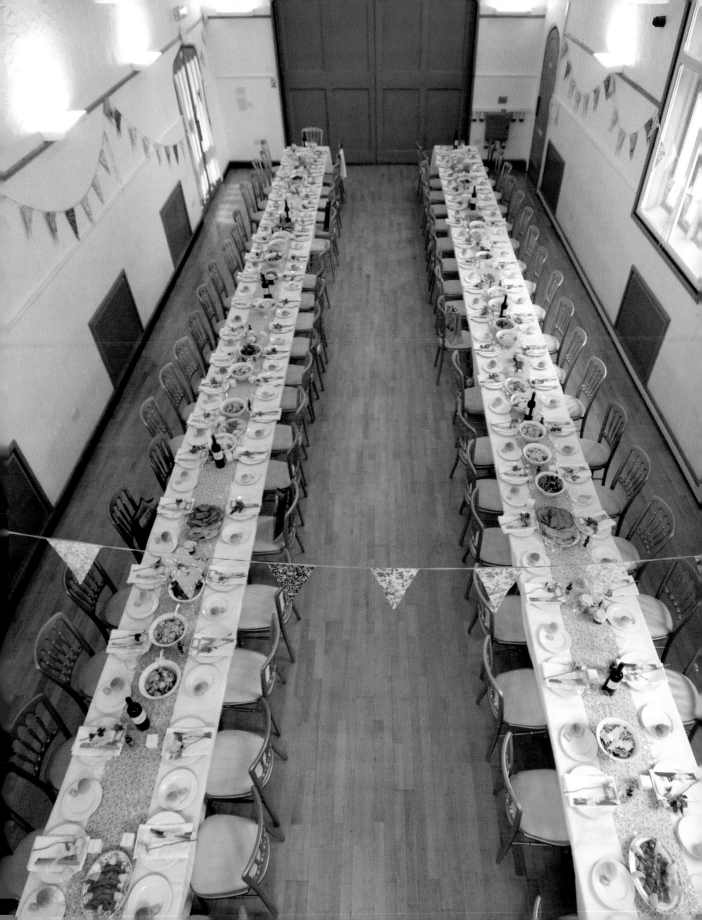

Chair decoration

This decoration was made with fresh lavender, as it was in season at the time, though dried lavender also looks lovely. I find gingham ribbon works particularly well, but you could use whatever suits your style.

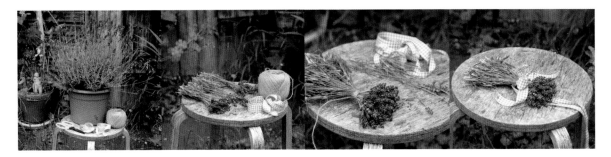

You can use these decorations for the bride and groom's chairs, or to show the seating places for close family. Alternatively, this type of decoration works beautifully for pew ends in a church.

FOR EACH CHAIR YOU WILL NEED:

45 lavender stems

3 ¼ feet of ¾-inch-wide gingham or other ribbon

12 inches of ½-inch-wide matching ribbon

Twine

Florist's shears or garden scissors

Fabric scissors

METHOD:

1. Take two lavender stems and cross one over the other just below the flower.
2. Cross a third stem over the second and repeat until you have fifteen stems, all crossed.
3. Put the bunch aside, and repeat steps 1 and 2 until you have three matching bunches.
4. Take one bunch and carefully add a second to the side. Add the third bunch.
5. Check the symmetry and make sure that all the stems are crossing one another in the same direction.
6. Pull some of the stems lower to create a fuller effect.
7. Tie the bunch together securely under the flowers with a short piece of twine. Knot, and trim the ends off the twine.
8. Checking the size of the decoration against your chosen chair, use the shears to cut the stems off the bunch so that they are level.
9. Place the thinner ribbon vertically behind the bunch and tie it on with the wider ribbon.
10. Wrap the wider ribbon around the bunch a couple of times and fasten into a bow.
11. Trim the ends of the wider ribbon into small Vs with fabric scissors, aligned with the bottoms of the stems.
12. Tie onto your chosen chair.

Wedding planner tip:
Instead of lavender, you could use dried sheaves of wheat for a rural feel or for a harvest-time wedding.

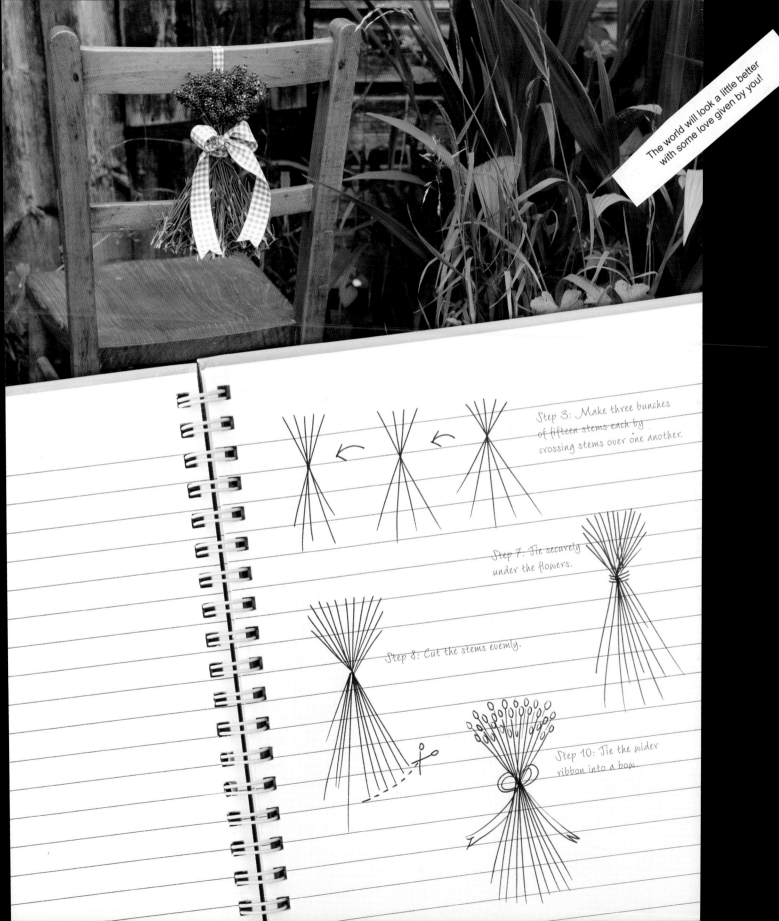

The world will look a little better with some love given by you!

Step 3: Make three bunches of fifteen stems each by crossing stems over one another.

Step 7: Tie securely under the flowers.

Step 8: Cut the stems evenly.

Step 10: Tie the wider ribbon into a bow.

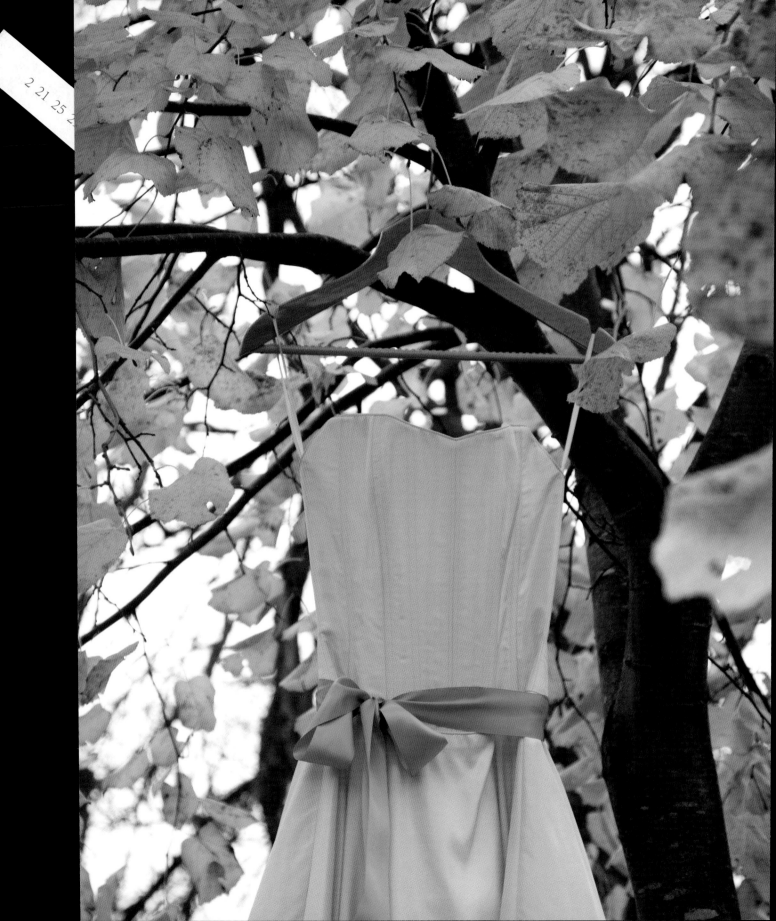

The Dress

The dress is probably the most important and exciting of all your wedding purchases, and what places you center stage. It is essential that you are comfortable in your choice, not only physically (you want to be able to breathe and sit down on your big day, but emotionally, too. This chapter suggests many fabulous, stylish, and unusual options, so relax, take your time, and enjoy finding your perfect gown.

Choosing your style

Step beyond the traditional shop-bought gowns and you'll find many exciting alternatives: svelte 1960s lace-covered shifts won on eBay; froths of chiffon from specialist vintage suppliers; gowns lovingly handmade in peace silk; floaty, organic cotton maxidresses worn with flower-woven hair; an heirloom gown reworked to fit perfectly; or a designer sample donated to a charity. All of them are special and they won't cost the Earth.

Most wedding books will tell you to start shopping with your budget figure in mind, but this may mean you end up spending exactly that amount and discounting other avenues because the dresses are below your budget. The easiest way to begin is by thinking about your wedding style and the season, and how you would like to feel on the day.

What kind of dress do you imagine?

❋ How would you like to feel on the day—elegant, glamorous, dramatic, like a princess?

❋ What style do you imagine for your wedding (see The Style chapter)?

❋ What time of year is your wedding—chilly winter or hot summer?

❋ What type of ceremony are you having—outdoor, church, informal?

❋ How involved would you like to be in the creation of your dress?

❋ Do you want to be able to wear the gown again?

Your wedding notebook

Armed with your answers to the questions on the notepaper (below left), you should be able to focus more closely on your perfect dress type. At this stage, it is useful to keep a small notebook and to clip and paste any pictures, cards, fabric samples, or sketches that you feel could be useful when choosing a dress (see the wedding notebook on pages 32–33). Keep photos of flowers, venues, and accessories, too—they will all help to give you a feeling of your day and to enable you to choose a dress that will fit with your vision.

Starting with your dress

Your dress can influence the whole style of your wedding. So if you dream of an elegant, minimalist reception, look for simple, classic cuts. For an intimate city wedding for two, set off a film-star vintage pencil skirt–suit with a vibrant corsage. Think about colors, textures, fabrics, and shapes.

For a seasonally inspired look, you could choose your dress to complement your flowers—something delicate for cottage garden sweet peas or sumptuous velvet to go with winter blooms and rich foliage.

Natural options

Luckily, there are many different dress avenues open to you, from gorgeous ecofriendly fabrics to vintage dresses to die for. Feel free to mix it up! It's your day and your chance to shine.

Wedding planner tip:
Brilliant, pure white is a difficult color to wear. Ivory, cream, and ecru are generally more flattering.

The dress for your shape

You may have your eye on the perfect dress, but don't be afraid to step out of your comfort zone and try styles that you would usually run a mile from— one of them could surprise you.

A-line

Elegant, with a fitted bodice and a flared but structured skirt. Usually floor-length. Suits most body shapes but may swamp more petite brides. Good if you have larger hips or are pear-shaped, as it flows out from the waist.

Empire line

Classic Jane Austen, fitted under the bust, then falling in soft drapes. Especially lovely in floaty fabrics. Good for small-busted and petite brides, and comfortable with a pregnancy bump.

Prom style

Think 1950s, with a nipped-in waist, strapless or boat-neck bodice, and a full skirt to the knees or floor. Perfect for curvy girls, this style flatters larger hips, bottoms, and thighs.

Bias cut

Glamorous and figure skimming. Look to the 1930s for inspiration. Can be difficult to wear in a slinky fabric but forgiving in a stiffer material. Good for tall brides and those who want to show off their curves.

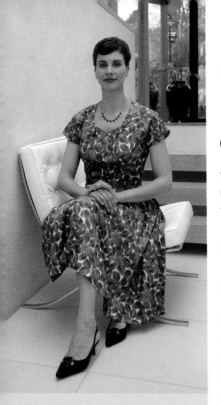

Vintage gowns

Vintage, heirloom, and secondhand dresses (sometimes known as "preloved" or "loved for longer") are perfect for women who, like me, enjoy rummaging in antique and thrift stores. They can be altered or embellished to suit your body shape and personality, and they are often one of a kind. Strictly speaking, vintage covers the 1920s to 1960s, with pre-1920s classed as antique and 1970s onward as retro.

The dress Sophie is wearing in the top picture on page 58 is an early 1960s cream-colored lace shift with an elegant high neck, which I bought a few years ago on eBay, simply because I fell in love with it. The dress cost less than forty dollars, including shipping, and arrived boxed, in perfect condition, complete with details of its happy history.

Where to buy

❋ Specialist vintage clothing shops and fairs in your area
❋ eBay and other online auctions
❋ Markets
❋ Garage and trunk sales (you would be amazed!)
❋ Web sites such as www.freudianslipsvintage.com (see the Directory for more)

Buying a vintage dress

Specialist vintage shops can give invaluable advice. An expert can tell you if a dress will be easy to alter or too fragile to dance in. He or she should also be able to date your find and may even offer insight into its history. Bear in mind that you do pay a premium for this level of service. While it's possible to find good vintage dresses for next to nothing, rare examples can cost the same as, or even more than, a new designer dress.

Get to know the shops you are visiting, as prices will vary. Research your subject so you know what you are looking at and the likely value. It can be helpful to take an honest (but open-minded) friend or relative—and remember that hems can be shortened and embellishments added to cover the odd imperfection. Vintage dress sizes come up about two sizes smaller than modern equivalents. This explains why, although Marilyn Monroe is reported to have been a size 14, her dresses look tiny. Browse the online dress racks at www.londonvintageweddingfair.co.uk for inspiration.

An alternative is secondhand modern dresses, which can be cheaper and in better condition. We found Lisa's pink dress on page 187 at the Frock Exchange in Bath.

Online tips

Good measuring is the secret to buying when you can't try on. Check the waist, hips, bust, shoulder width, overall length, and sleeve length. Then compare these with a dress that fits you well.

Ask questions of the seller: Does the zipper work? Are there any visible marks or moth holes? Does the dress have any odors? You can always ask for extra photographs.

Opting for certified delivery will help to ensure your gown arrives as promised.

Wedding planner tip:
Look online for wonderful vintage designer dress patterns—they cost a fraction of the price of a designer-label gown.

Decades of style

1920s: The flapper dress

Skirt lengths rose daringly high (for the time) and bodices were short sleeved or sleeveless. This was an age of elaborate decoration and fine fabrics: tiny glass beads and metallic threads combined with crepe de chine, satin, and taffeta.

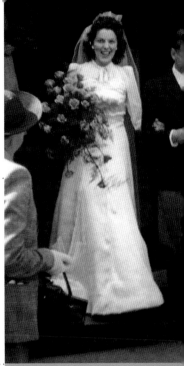

1930s: Age of glamour

Slender waistlines, long skirts, and long sleeves, often in satin. The backless, bias-cut evening gown created a silhouette favoring slim hips and wider shoulders. Accessorized with boleros and small capes.

1940s: Wartime utility

Dresses were well proportioned and made to last. Silk was banned during the war, as it was needed for parachutes. Embellishments included covered buttons and sequins, which were readily available.

1950s: Prom queens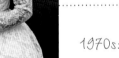

A nipped-in waist and big, circular skirt, preferably with a full underskirt. Bodices were usually strapless and worn with elegant, elbow-length gloves and strings of pearls.

1960s: The mini

This style was boyish, with straight-cut minishift dresses teamed with block heels and glossy patent leather. Decoration was minimal for the modern look.

1970s: Boho style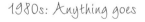

After the geometric tailoring of the 1960s came the long, flowing lines of the maxidress, with extended angel or bell sleeves. A fluid, romantic look decorated with strings of beads and daisy appliqué.

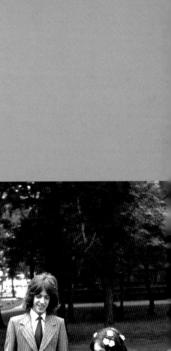

1980s: Anything goes

Many different styles emerged, from punk to Victoriana, with wedding dress styles following high-street fashion. The quintessential 1980s dress had a full skirt and was heavily decorated with frills, ruffles, puff sleeves, and lace.

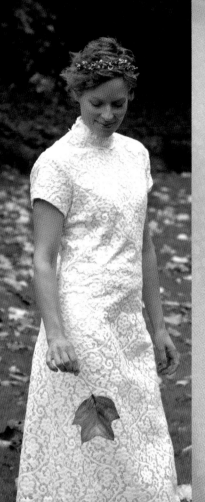

Charity chic

Charity shops have become increasingly popular in recent years, as fashionable celebrities frequent their local branches, looking for treasures. This new awareness has brought more competition for bargains, but it also means there is a wider choice of donations, including higher-priced items. Most thrift stores will stock wedding dresses from time to time, but it's worth visiting often, as stock may change daily. Ask friendly sales assistants if they can let you know when a wedding dress has come in.

Designer samples

The same rules apply to charity shopping as to vintage shopping, but if you have qualms about a secondhand dress, you'll be pleased to hear that many gowns donated to larger charities are either unworn, end-of-season stock, or runway samples given by designers. The dress pictured on the bottom left of this page still had its tags, and it was a fraction of the price it would have been in a designer shop. Reusing a dress or accessory is the ultimate in recycling, and it will help your budget, too.

Charity shops are also an Aladdin's cave of affordable accessories: everything from sparkly brooches and beaded tiaras to pretty vintage wraps and shoes. After the wedding, you can always donate items back to the shop.

Oxfam Bridal

Oxfam has a number of specialist bridal departments in the United Kingdom, stocking hundreds of fabulous dresses. Their prices will please the thriftiest of brides-to-be, and with the proceeds going to charity, it really is the most ethical choice. These bridal departments also stock jewelry, shoes, veils, bridesmaids' dresses, ring bearers' suits and flower girls' dresses, and menswear. With huge mirrors, generous fitting rooms, and a relaxed, friendly staff, you will not only have fun but likely also find a dress to impress.

My charity shopping tips

* Try to be open-minded and prepared to wait. You may discover the dress of your dreams on your first visit, but you may have to return several times to spot new arrivals.
* If you find a dress that seems perfect but is too big, don't despair. Most dresses can be altered to fit. If in doubt, ask the assistant to reserve the dress for you, and go back with an experienced seamstress to advise on alterations.
* Chances are there will only be one of each dress style, so if you fall in love with a gown, either buy or reserve it straightaway.
* Charity shopping, like vintage shopping, is all about being unique. So dare to be different, accessorize with flair, and be yourself.

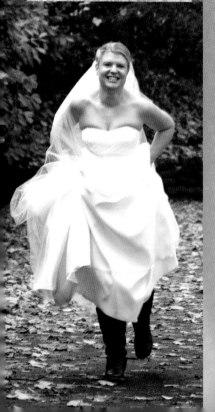

All of these dresses
came from eBay and
our local Oxfam Bridal.
We took them to the
park, and had some fun
trying them on.

This hand-finished dress
by Jessica Charleston
is made from fine
natural silk.

New dresses

When buying new, there are, fortunately, now many designer brands that take ethics and the environment seriously. We love these labels and have listed some in the Directory. You could also try www.greenunion.co.uk or www.ethicaljunction.org. Garments made in good, humanitarian conditions tend to cost more, but you can find beautiful fair-trade silk and cotton gowns you will love.

Tammam, for example, uses organic and fair-trade materials, peace silks, and vintage trimmings, and sells off-the-rack as well as custom-made gowns. Alternatively, find a maxidress or a suit from an ethical designer, through ethical shopping sites such as www.ascensiononline.com, and add wedding touches with your accessories. Or try the amazing, deconstructed garments at www.junkystyling.co.uk, where you can take your old dresses to be reworked into something unique. Also check the guide to ecofriendly fabrics on page 64.

Shopping ethically

Not all bridal shops advertise where their dresses are made or the conditions for workers there. Some mainstream brands are manufactured in China and left chunky carbon footprints.

Many companies understand it is not acceptable to use child labor or pay below a minimum wage, and are making efforts to source their clothes more ethically, but unfortunately bad practices still exist. It is sometimes argued that developing countries need the employment provided by Western economies, but some employees are expected to endure unacceptable conditions, and communities may be exposed to toxic substances, such as the pesticides used to grow fiber crops, as a result.

My advice would be to ask where a garment has been manufactured. If you are keen on a particular brand, ask to see their ethics statement.

Wedding fairs

People often dismiss wedding fairs, but they can be a great place to discover small, family-run companies that manufacture locally, and up-and-coming designers of dresses, accessories, and wedding decorations who use natural and vintage materials. Many designers will sell their samples or discontinued stock and may offer a special exhibition discount. If you are prepared to decide on the spot, you could save a small fortune. Go wearing neutral underwear, pack your notebook, and take your mom or a friend. It can be a bit of a madhouse, so try not to impulse buy because you feel pressured.

Bridal shops

Some bridal shops are wonderful, will expertly fit a sample dress to your frame, and help you to choose the perfect accessories and bridal underwear to complete the picture. Others, however, will dictate which dresses you are "allowed" to try, tut under their breath, and generally make you feel uncomfortable. If you are looking for an ethical dress or natural fabrics such as silk, do ask questions, and feel free to visit and try on a dress more than once. Ask how many fittings are required and say when you would like the final one. There may be charges for delivery and storage.

Wedding planner tip: I always recommend that brides sit down in a dress they are trying. Is it still comfortable?

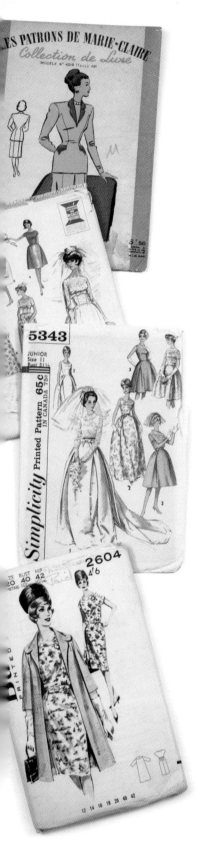

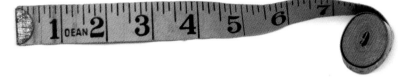

Handmade and homemade

A handmade dress is a wonderful luxury when it's thoughtfully designed and made to fit you perfectly. Think about choosing an eco- or vintage fabric (see page 64). Handmade doesn't have to be expensive. Making your own wedding gown is completely possible if you have good sewing skills and the time. A reasonably simple pattern will be less stressful. Or you could ask a friend or relative—although, remember that you may have to request alterations if there are details you don't like, and you may find this awkward. The main cost will be the fabric, which can prove to be expensive.

If your ideal dress is elaborate, then a specialist dressmaker may be the wisest choice. Whichever route you decide on, have your wedding notebook on hand, with pictures, samples of fabric and other inspirations, to make sure that everyone understands your vision of the dream dress.

Home sewing

Before buying your pattern, it helps to try on ready-made dresses in differing styles so that you know what suits you. With your pattern, first make up a model in a cheaper fabric, such as natural calico (or an old bed sheet), so that you can adjust the fit and details.

Alternatively, use a dress that you love from your closet as a template. You will have to cut your own pattern, but this is not difficult, and most sewing classes can teach you how. Alternatively, a good dressmaker could do this for you. For hints and tips on all things sewing, www.burdastyle.com is the Web site to visit.

Vintage patterns

These are available through the same outlets as vintage dresses (see the Directory); patterns are inexpensive and easily customized.

Before you buy a vintage pattern:
❈ Check that all parts of the pattern are included.
❈ If the pattern has already been cut (not necessarily a problem), make sure it has been cut to your size or larger.
❈ Double-check measurements, not just the dress size, as vintage sizes are smaller.

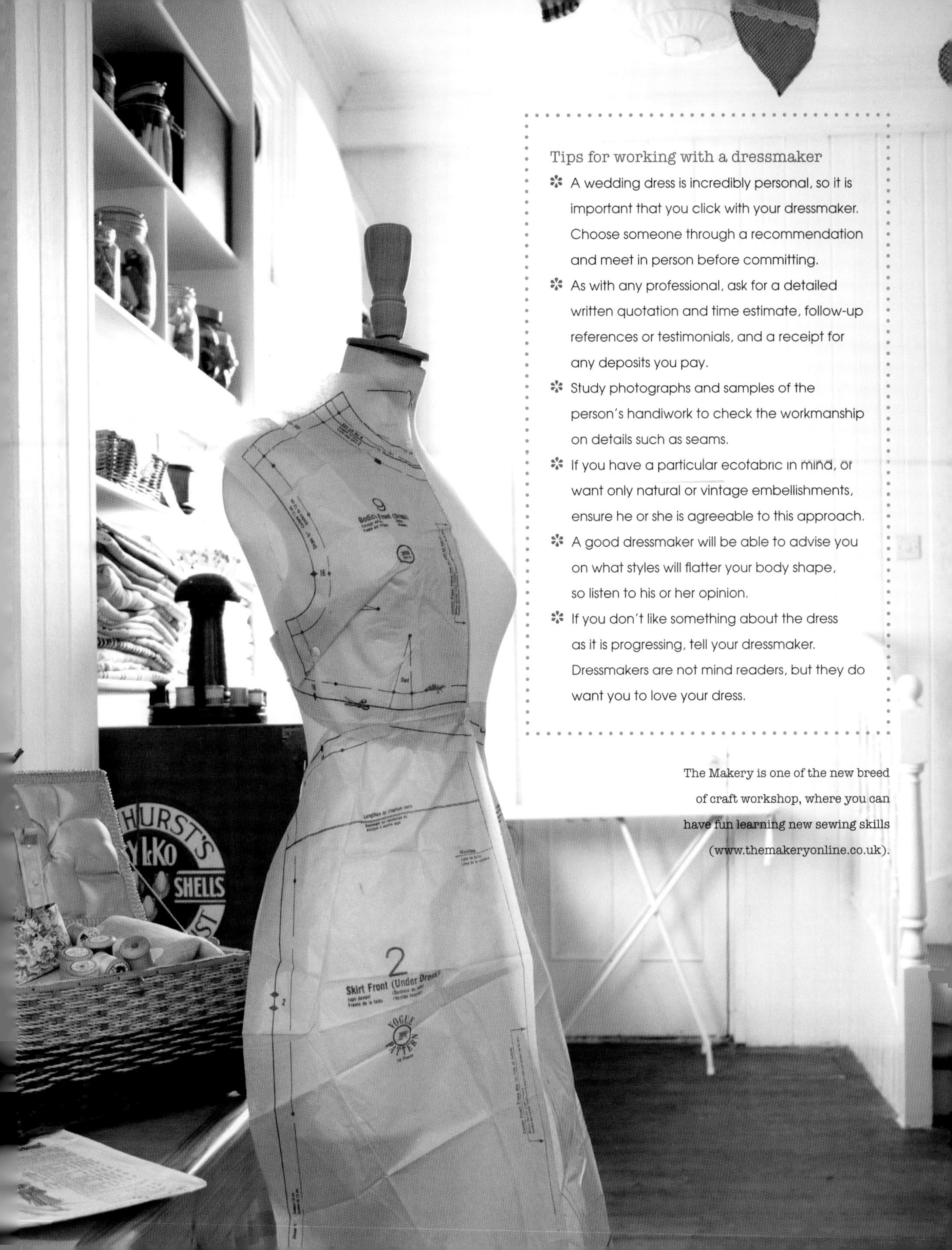

Tips for working with a dressmaker

�֍ A wedding dress is incredibly personal, so it is important that you click with your dressmaker. Choose someone through a recommendation and meet in person before committing.

�֍ As with any professional, ask for a detailed written quotation and time estimate, follow-up references or testimonials, and a receipt for any deposits you pay.

�֍ Study photographs and samples of the person's handiwork to check the workmanship on details such as seams.

�֍ If you have a particular ecofabric in mind, or want only natural or vintage embellishments, ensure he or she is agreeable to this approach.

�֍ A good dressmaker will be able to advise you on what styles will flatter your body shape, so listen to his or her opinion.

�֍ If you don't like something about the dress as it is progressing, tell your dressmaker. Dressmakers are not mind readers, but they do want you to love your dress.

The Makery is one of the new breed of craft workshop, where you can have fun learning new sewing skills (www.themakeryonline.co.uk).

Ecofabrics

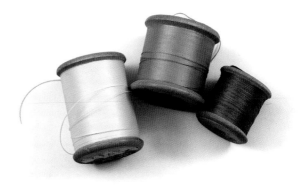

*D*esigners and producers are bringing us a growing range of gorgeous fabrics that are gentler on our skin and on the environment. Many of these ecofabrics are a fresh twist on long-loved natural fibers. For suppliers see the Directory on page 208.

Peace silk (vegetarian or wild-crafted silk)

Silk is a completely natural product made from the cocoon of the silkworm. It is wonderfully light and breathable. However, traditional silk is harvested by boiling the cocoons and killing the worms before they hatch, which may offend some people.

When a silkworm hatches, it makes a hole in the end of the cocoon, breaking the continuous silk thread. With peace silk, the worms are allowed to hatch, and the fabric is made with the cocoon remnants. The resulting material is slightly rougher than regular silk but still beautiful. It is rarer and more expensive.

Hemp and hemp silk

Hemp is a relatively new material for wedding dresses, although it has been used in everyday clothing for many years. Environmentally friendly, hemp cloth is soft to the touch, although it has a slightly grainy appearance. It is often blended with silk to make a soft-sheen, satiny fabric that is lovely for special lingerie. Hemp grows quickly and easily, even in wet climates, and doesn't require fertilizers or spraying with insecticides.

Bamboo

Bamboo is a soft and smooth natural fabric that drapes well, almost like silk. Bamboo grass doesn't require fertilizers, grows quickly, and absorbs vast amounts of carbon dioxide. The fabric does not wrinkle easily, has natural antibacterial properties, and is a safer option for sensitive skins. Natural organic, unbleached bamboo is a flattering creamy color.

Organic cotton

Cotton is often overlooked as a celebration dress fabric, but it can be gorgeous when stitched with lace, and it is light and cool in summer. Most cotton is heavily sprayed with pesticides, so choose organic and fair trade when possible. For pure whites, look for ecobleached cotton.

Linen

You probably already have some linen in your wardrobe. Made from the flax plant, it is fairly labor-intensive to process, hence its high price. Linen is a great choice for summer, as it is so cool to wear, but beware of the dreaded linen wrinkles.

Nettle

Some may balk at the thought of using stinging nettles for their wedding dress, but they make a fabulous fabric with a slightly silky feeling. The fiber is often blended with organic cotton. Nettles are environmentally friendly plants, growing abundantly in damp, temperate climates.

Natural dyes

Modern, natural vegetable dyes, and instructions on getting the best results from them, are available online. You can transform any of the ecofabrics mentioned here to a color of your choice: Either dye the whole dress or just one element of it, such as a sash or corsage. Vegetable dyes come in an exciting range of colors, but if you feel unsure about dying the fabric yourself, buy it already dyed. For more information, look at www.greenfibres.com.

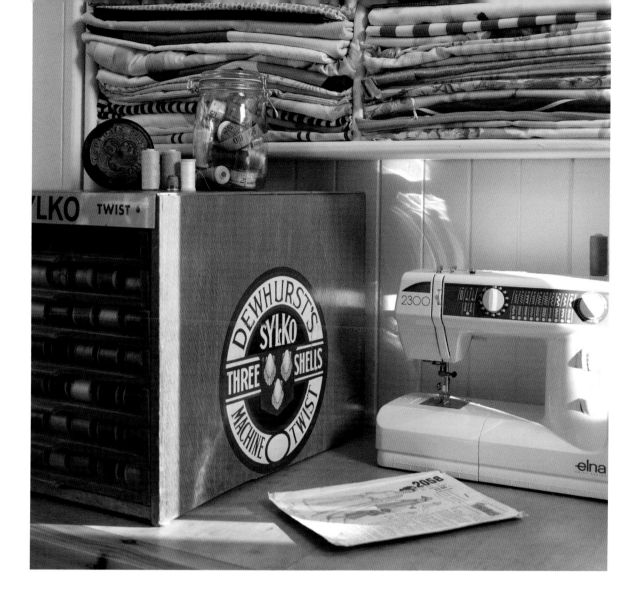

Vintage and reclaimed materials

A handmade dress in a vintage fabric will give you a gown that's unique and with a low carbon footprint, as the material has already been used once. You may have a trunk of fabrics and trimmings in your attic, but if not, you can find these in thrift stores, vintage costume stores, and online. You could also use material from an existing wedding dress—great if you have an heirloom or eBay dress and adore the fabric but not the style.

Think about remnants from fabric stores, too: There is minimal expenditure, and you're making use of a resource that might otherwise have been thrown away.

But remember that a wedding gown uses considerably more material than a regular dress. Embellishments such as ribbons, buttons, and bows can all be given a fresh lease on life as part of a new gown.

Wedding planner tip:
Use a vintage dress pattern with a contemporary ecofabric for a chic, individual look.

Dresses for free and cleaning

A free wedding dress? The idea will probably come as a surprise to most brides, but searching for a free dress can turn into an exciting challenge. Freecycle is a free-to-join online community where members post notices about unwanted items or ask for things they need. Do a search to find your local Freecycle or a similar community. You may get lucky and find an "OFFER: Wedding Dress," but you will almost certainly have to put up a "Wanted" post. Personalize this request, as the potential giver will want to know her special dress is destined for a good home. Freecycle is full of wonderful people, but like all online resources, it can be victim to the occasional bad penny, so be sensible when going to collect.

Something borrowed

"Swishing" parties have become something of a craze. Essentially, they are clothes-swapping events, to which you take your lovely-but-no-longer-worn items to give away in hopes of bagging a few choice pieces to revive your wardrobe. You are unlikely to find the wedding dress of your dreams, but may discover the perfect accessory, or even a white day dress or beaded evening gown.

How about borrowing from a friend? Most brides keep their dress for a couple of years at least. Don't let age fool you, either: Your mom's best friend may have the perfect vintage dress hiding in her closet. Check that it fits and that the owner doesn't mind if you make alterations.

Heirloom gowns

You may be the lucky inheritor of an heirloom wedding dress, passed down from your mother or even your grandmother. Don't discount it because it is not your style. Most dresses, even 1980s meringues, can be reworked, although you may need a seamstress. Alternatively, just reclaim the fabric and trimmings.

To rent or not to rent

New gowns that would cost thousands of dollars can be rented for a fraction of the price, and the fact that a rented dress is worn a number of times makes it a potentially ecofriendly option. However, the dresses will be dry-cleaned each time they are worn. If you have sensitive skin or are worried about the chemicals used, ask exactly how the shop cleans the dresses and if they use a more environmentally friendly cleaning process.

Cleaning and storage

Dresses should always be cleaned immediately after wearing and before being stored, as any perspiration on a dress discolors over time. While some modern dresses are machine or hand washable, others are dry-clean only, especially if they have beading or decorative elements. If a vintage gown looks clean but smells musty, hang it in a steamy bathroom for a couple of days. The steam will remove odors and help any creases to drop out.

Some specialists can dry-clean your dress without the toxic chemicals used in regular dry-cleaning. One option is called the GreenEarth process (www.greenearthcleaning.com). This is becoming increasingly widespread. These dry-cleaners are also the best places to buy an acid-free box and tissue in which to store your precious gown (remember to pad out the bodice with tissue if it is boned).

Covering stains

If stains refuse to disappear, you can always cover them up. First try a little chalk. This is a good emergency trick for marks discovered on the big day, and it will cover a blemish on most shades of white. Or hide the mark with an accessory, such as a corsage or brooch. No one will ever know! See the box on the opposite page for more ideas to add a fresh spark or personalize your dress.

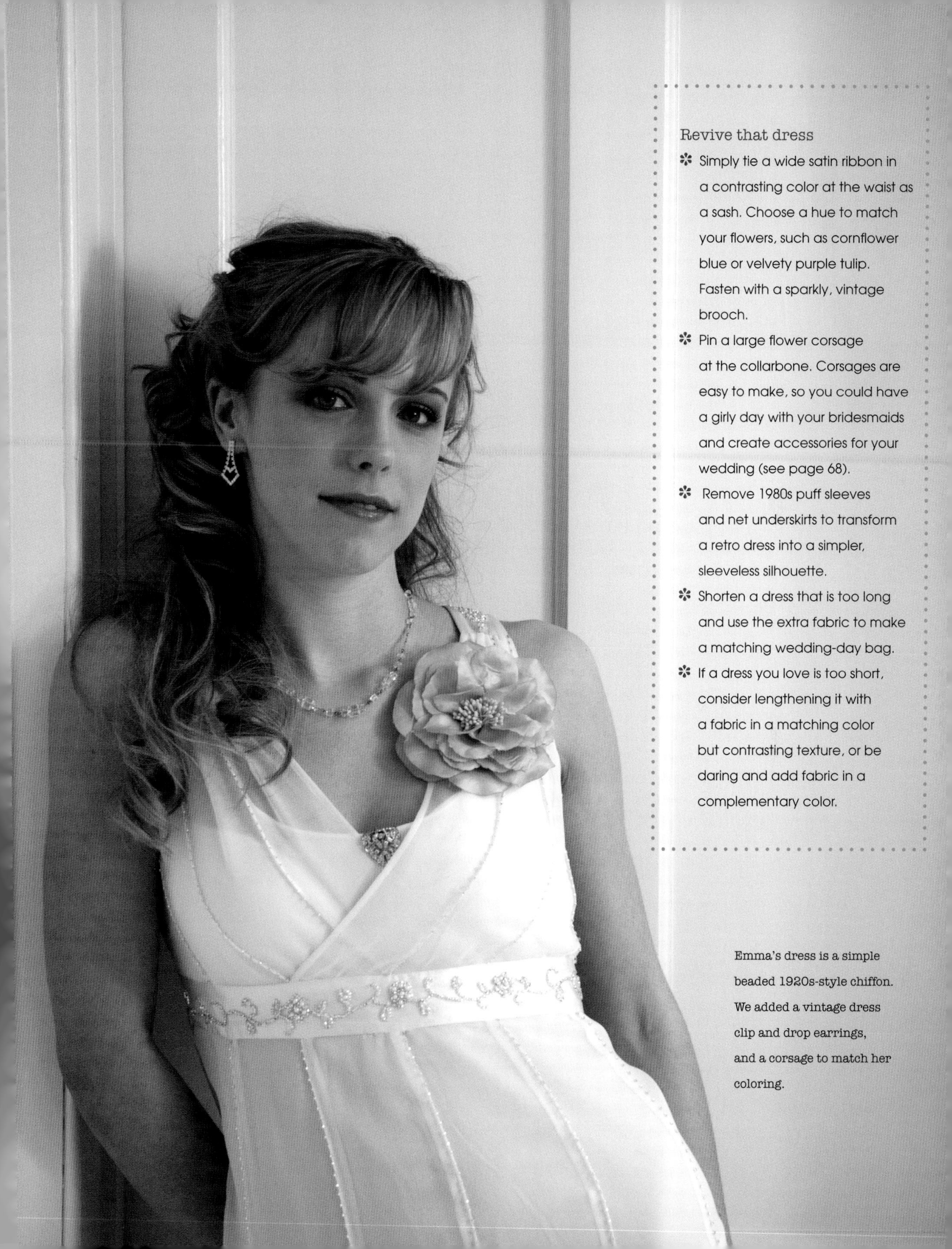

Revive that dress

- Simply tie a wide satin ribbon in a contrasting color at the waist as a sash. Choose a hue to match your flowers, such as cornflower blue or velvety purple tulip. Fasten with a sparkly, vintage brooch.
- Pin a large flower corsage at the collarbone. Corsages are easy to make, so you could have a girly day with your bridesmaids and create accessories for your wedding (see page 68).
- Remove 1980s puff sleeves and net underskirts to transform a retro dress into a simpler, sleeveless silhouette.
- Shorten a dress that is too long and use the extra fabric to make a matching wedding-day bag.
- If a dress you love is too short, consider lengthening it with a fabric in a matching color but contrasting texture, or be daring and add fabric in a complementary color.

Emma's dress is a simple beaded 1920s-style chiffon. We added a vintage dress clip and drop earrings, and a corsage to match her coloring.

Fabric flower corsage

This corsage is easy to make in about an hour. You can use as many layers of fabric as you wish—the more layers, the more elaborate the finished corsage will be. For those shown in the photograph on the opposite page, I used a vintage silk slip combined with organic cotton.

YOU WILL NEED:

Natural fabrics such as silk, hemp, or organic cotton

Reclaimed netting from underskirts

Fabric scissors

Needle, pins, and matching thread

Piece of paper

Vintage buttons or a vintage brooch

Brooch backing

METHOD:

1. Cut a circle of fabric 4 inches in diameter, another in a different fabric 3½ inches in diameter, and a third 2½ inches in diameter. Cut two circles of netting, one 3½ inches in diameter and one 2½ inches in diameter.

2. Take the larger of the two fabric circles and place the larger netting circle on top of it. Secure together with a small stitch in the center.

3. On a paper measuring 4 x 2 inches, draw the shape shown on the opposite page, and cut out.

4. Cut out a rectangle of fabric 4 x 4 inches, and fold in half. Pin on the paper template and cut it out of the fabric. If using silk, after cutting, gently pull the edges at a diagonal, for a fluted effect. Make four more of these shapes.

5. Fold each fabric shape diagonally across once, then again, to make a "quarter." The edges should *not* line up.

6. Take two of the quarters and overlap them slightly, securing them with three small stitches. Overlap the other two quarters similarly; stitch to secure.

7. Place your "circle" of quarters in the center of your circle from step 2, then layer the remaining two fabric and net circles on top.

8. Position your button or brooch in the center and sew everything together.

9. Cut one final circle of fabric 1 inch in diameter. Take a brooch backing and sew this securely, through the tiny circle, onto the corsage.

10. Fluff up the petals, and enjoy.

Wedding planner tip:
These measurements are for the smaller corsage shown. To make a larger one, simply increase the sizes of fabric circles.

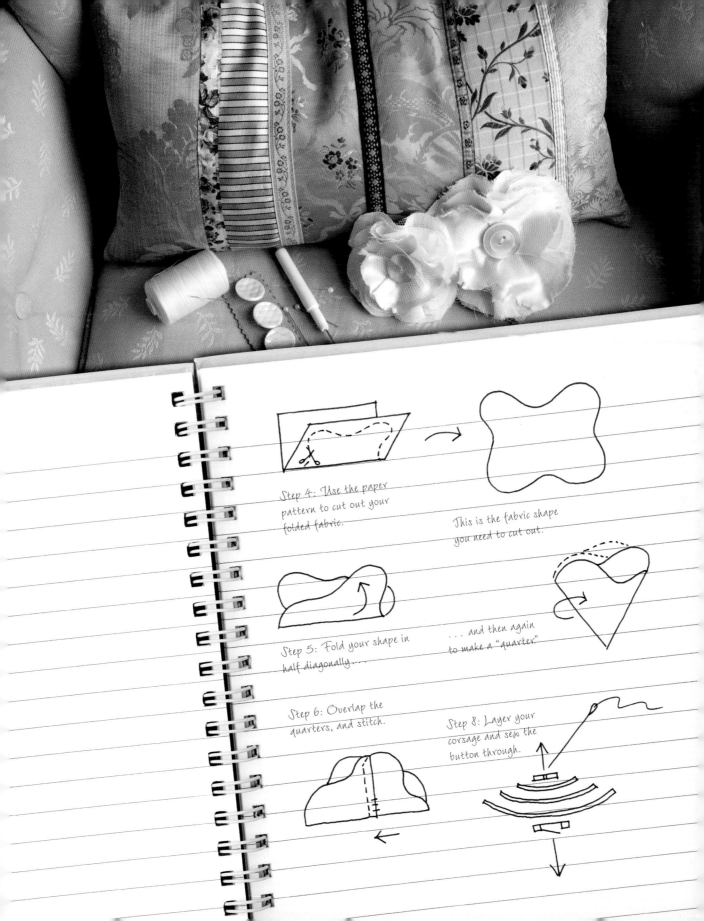

Step 4: Use the paper pattern to cut out your folded fabric.

This is the fabric shape you need to cut out.

Step 5: Fold your shape in half diagonally....

... and then again to make a "quarter"

Step 6: Overlap the quarters, and stitch.

Step 8: Layer your corsage and sew the button through.

Shoes, veils, and trains

It's often assumed that brides will wear white satin heels, but most of us don't have any use for this kind of shoe after the big day. How about silver or gold sparkly sandals, or even flip-flops, instead? Or invest in two pairs (affordable if they come from a thrift store): the killer heels for the ceremony and a comfortable alternative for dancing. If you choose something you really like—not just to go with the dress—you'll be more likely to wear them again.

Embellishing shoes can be surprisingly enjoyable: Pin on corsages or brooches, or glue on beads and sequins to give a wedding lift (but remember that less is more with decorations). I once worked with a bride who wore a formal floor-length gown, but glimpsed beneath, when she lifted her skirt, were a pair of pretty white shoes with crisscrossing blue ribbons. She had carefully stitched on the ribbons to mimic ballet slippers, and tied them in a decorative bow. The ribbon was vintage, so it was her something old as well as her something blue—and it added an element of surprise to her traditional outfit.

Depending on the time of year and where you are marrying, I would also recommend taking along a pair of Wellies. You can then go striding around the lake for amazing photographs with your new husband.

Veils

Some brides cannot imagine their wedding outfit without a veil, while others dread the thought. It also depends on your dress—a gold, sparkly cocktail dress wouldn't take a veil, for example. The usual guideline is that veils look best with white, ivory, or cream. The question of veil length is a minefield, but a good rule of thumb is the longer the dress, the longer the veil.

If you are lucky enough to have inherited a veil from a family member, it would be lovely to include this heirloom in your day. You can also find vintage veils, and with a little patience, you can make your own. Veils that are too long can be easily shortened with a few basic sewing

skills (or by a seamstress). Similarly, you can buy a plain veil and add panache by sewing on small glass beads or ribbons. This could take a few hours but it will save you a small fortune. Look at embroidery books—the older, the better—for unusual patterns; search on Amazon for ideas.

Tips for choosing a veil
* Consider your dress color, style, and length.
* Do you want to be able to remove the veil after the ceremony, or would you like to keep it on for the reception and dancing?
* Think about contrasting fabrics, such as lace.
* Are you going to be wearing your hair up or down?
* What time of year are you marrying? A veil can be quite a handful in gusty winds!

A quick word on trains

Generally speaking, the more formal the wedding, the longer the train—although, if you yearn to wear a gown with a ten-foot-long train on the beach, why not?

Make sure that you or a friend know how to bustle up the train (wedding speak for tying it up under the gown so you can dance without tripping over it). Long trains can be held off the floor with a thumb loop that hooks around your thumb or middle finger, allowing you to swish around elegantly.

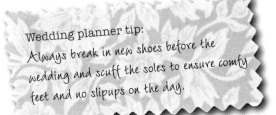

Wedding planner tip:
Always break in new shoes before the wedding and scuff the soles to ensure comfy feet and no slipups on the day.

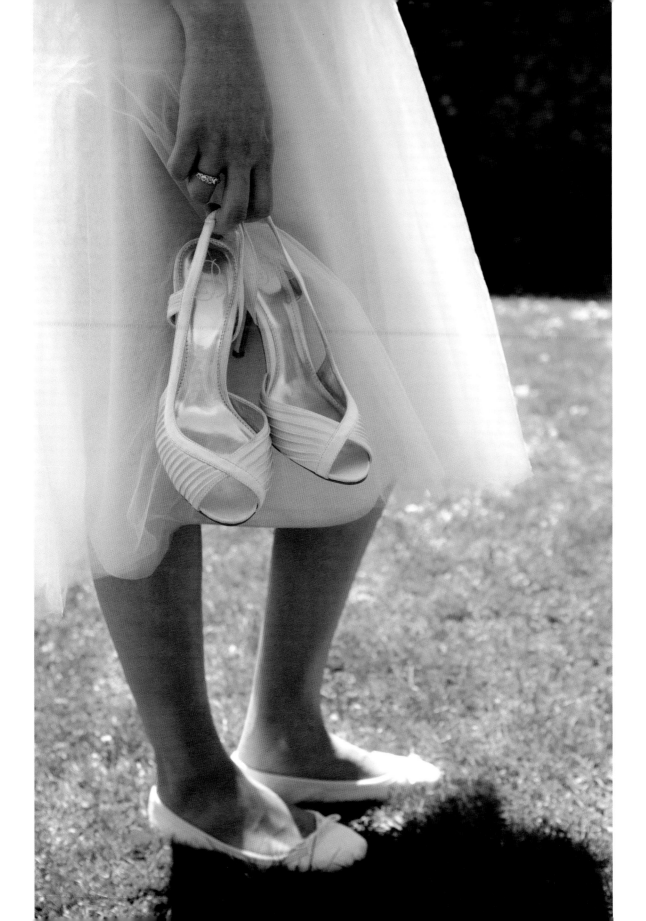

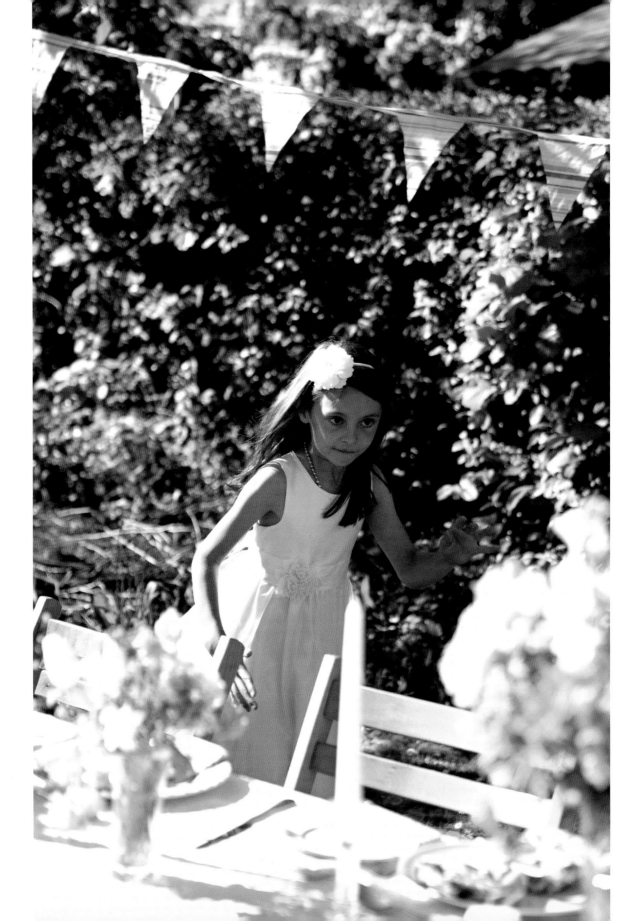

Grooms and bridesmaids

A groom can be adventurous, ethical, and ecochic—and enjoy being in the spotlight alongside his bride. It helps if your bride and groom outfits are in sync. With a groom in top hat and tails, the bride really needs a fabulous floor-length gown; but if you are wearing a short, silk shift dress, then he should be in a suit and tie. Think about coordinating the color of your bouquet or sash to his tie, cravat, or suit lining. You could even have fabrics or handkerchiefs dyed with natural vegetable dyes to match.

Natural fabrics

In summer, there's nothing more comfortable than a linen suit. Linen allows the skin to breathe, keeping the wearer cool. Remember it can crease, and looks better in a lighter color. Men's shirts can also be found in the natural fabrics listed on page 64. Hemp and organic cotton both look and feel great, and they are readily available.

Vintage groom

Your fiancé may have an heirloom suit hidden away, but if not, men's vintage shops are starting to spring up. Vintage or retro styles—think 1950s pinstripes and wide shoulders, or Sean Connery, slim-line 1960s suits—have become fashionable for grooms. As well as secondhand, you could also look at vintage-inspired styles, such as floral-patterned shirts.

Wedding planner tip:
Find ties, shoes, and cuff links in charity shops. Or, translate the tradition of wearing something borrowed to the groom.

Rented groomswear

Renting a suit is popular with grooms, as it's easy and costs less—especially with formal options such as morning dress. For a large wedding, with many ushers and groomsmen, renting is the perfect way to make sure the bridal party matches. If the groom wants to stand out, he could buy a colorful cravat, tie, or shirt to personalize his outfit. Pedro's outfit on page 187 is from www.mossbros.co.uk.

Splurging

Once in a while, a groom will have a suit custom-tailored for his big day. A lovely idea—and green, too—if the suit can be worn again. He could choose a lining in a bright color, perhaps one to match your sash or corsage. Why not opt for an ecofabric, such as linen, or an organic or vintage wool weave, and complement it with an unusual vintage lining.

Bridesmaids

Most of the advice in this chapter also applies to bridesmaids' outfits. For a formal wedding, the usual "rule" is that the bridesmaids should match the bride in some way, or, at least, one another. But if you are a free spirit, why not let your bridesmaids choose their own dresses?

I attended a wedding where the bridesmaids wore bright, floral, 1970s-style frocks not at all in keeping with the bride. But the overall look was amazing. If bridesmaids make their own choices, chances are they will wear their outfits again, making it more environmentally friendly.

With ring bearers and flower girls, the advice is simple: Make sure they are comfortable. For girls, ballet slippers are the best footwear. Flower girls like to have accessories, such as baskets of fresh flower petals, to make them feel special. Little boys are typically not fussy!

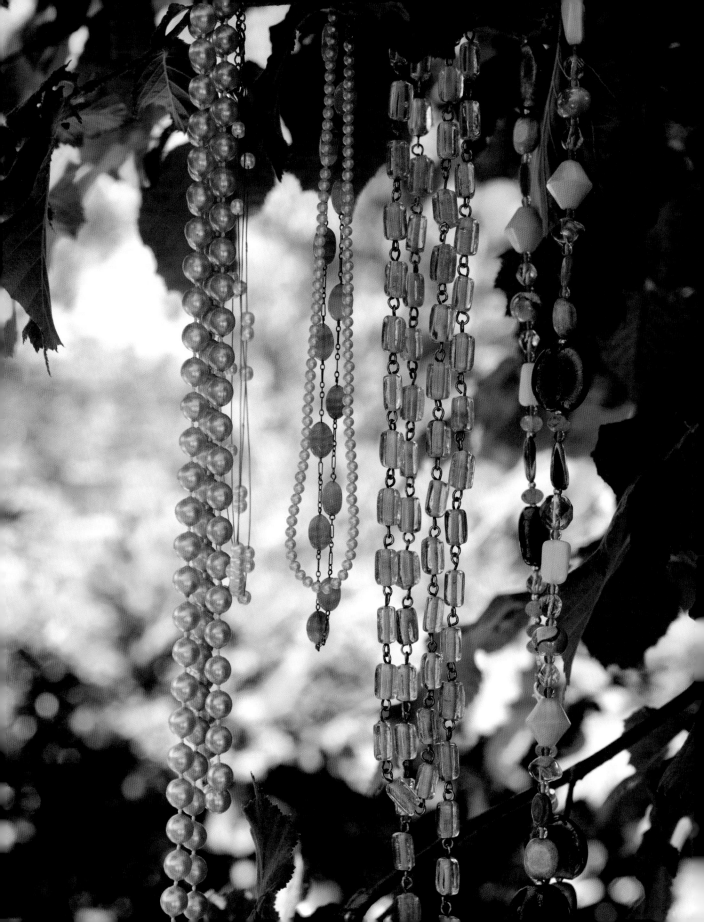

The Accessories

Choosing all the little bits and pieces to go with your dress—the bags and earrings and bracelets—can be such fun. Rummaging in vintage shops and antique markets with your friends; discovering artisan craftspeople and modern ecodesigners who'll craft something special. Personally, I can't resist searching for something unusual, and this chapter has plenty of ideas so you can find your dream accessories, too.

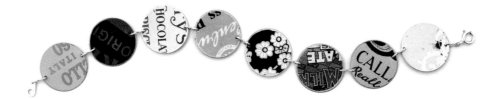

Creative places to find your jewelry

Shimmering sea-glass beads and intricate Victoriana earrings; heirloom gold bands; or sleek, modern minimalism—it's surprisingly easy to find a wealth of ecochic accessories, whatever your budget and personal style. There are plenty of alternatives, from online ethical stores to charity shops, recycling, borrowing, or making your own (see the Directory).

Take a picture of your dress or a cutting of the fabric with you to markets and shops, and remember Coco Chanel's advice: "When accessorizing, always take off the last thing you put on."

Heirloom finds

You may be lucky enough to have an heirloom piece from a relative. If it is faultless, you could wear it conventionally or think about imaginative ways to show it off. Pin a brooch onto a waistband, or use it as a hair accessory or to decorate a bag. Dress clips make fabulous shoe embellishments, and long necklaces can be wound around several times for a more modern feel.

If an item is damaged, don't rule out having it mended by your local jeweler or asking him or her to rework it into something more wearable. Stones can be salvaged and reused to make a completely different piece.

Antique gems

High-quality antique jewelry is an investment, but it often costs only a fraction of the price of a new piece and, being secondhand, is effectively carbon neutral.

You'll find geometric Art Deco rings, Edwardian marcasite brooches, Victoriana hat pins, and Georgian glass necklaces in specialist antique jewelry shops and markets, or at auctions by www.christies.com or www.bonhams.com—and they won't all cost a fortune. Online, browse www.alfiesantiques.com and www.steptoesantiques.co.uk. Pre-1940 jewelry is classed as antique, later as vintage.

Hallmarks on precious metals will tell you the quality of the piece, its age, and where it was made. The Miller's antiques guides are helpful if you want to learn more.

Vintage costume jewelry

Vintage jewelry is one of my favorite things and is easily found in flea markets, antique fairs, and thrift stores. Try www.vintagefair.co.uk, www.manhattanvintage.com, or www.lovevintage.com.au, depending on where you live. Raid your grandmother's or mother's jewelry boxes (with their permission, of course); they may have beautiful necklaces or brooches squirreled away that will look fresh and modern when teamed with the right dress.

Charity shops

These can be a rich source of inexpensive accessories, especially if you are happy to revisit regularly to check for new donations. Styles range from long, wooden-bead necklaces to delicate silver chains, lucite bangles, 1950s clip-on earrings, and 1980s cocktail rings. Frequently, they will be in immaculate, unworn condition. But even if a piece is broken or dusty, you can have it cleaned and repaired for minimal cost—so if you love it, take it home. Buying from charity shops is ecofriendly and ethical, too.

Markets and trunk sales

These are good places to find more modern secondhand designs. Go early to catch the bargains, and remember that they will only have one of each item.

This vintage-inspired, handmade pendant is by Jessie Chorley (www.jessiechorley.com). The bracelet on the opposite page is artisan-made from recycled tins.

Be different with jewelry

❇ Use oversized vintage earrings as brooches.

❇ Antique charm bracelets can look really pretty.

❇ Marcasite is inexpensive and sparkly—perfect for a glamorous wedding.

❇ Use broken jewelry to make something new, such as a tiara.

❇ Embellish fabric corsages with small brooches for a touch of sparkle.

STOCKMAN

38

once upon a time

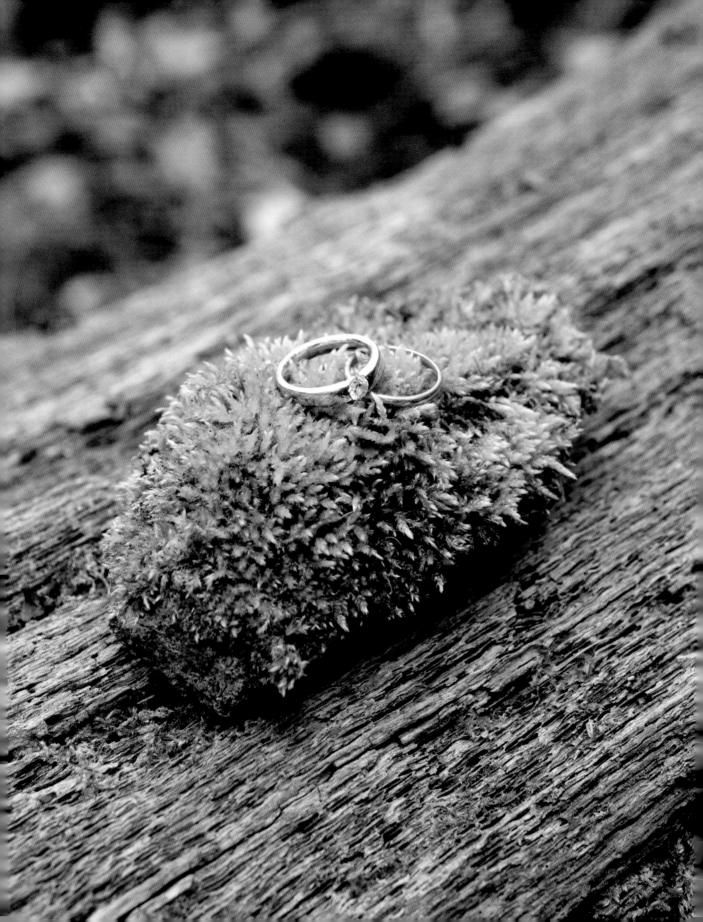

Ethical rings

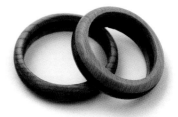

The production of new gemstones can be damaging to the environment and sometimes the well-being of local communities, due to invasive and chemical-laden extraction techniques. Unethical working practices are commonplace. Responsible jewelry designers are now realizing that this is unacceptable and are reusing and recycling stones and metals when possible. You can also find beautiful fair-trade designs. See the Directory for jewelers we recommend.

Ethical diamonds

The issue of conflict (or blood) diamonds is now widely documented. Diamonds are still the preferred gem for engagement, wedding, and eternity rings, so it is important to do your research and buy with care. Nonconflict diamonds that have been mined and exported under fair-trade and ethical conditions are widely available. But the only way to be certain of where yours come from is to buy from a reputable dealer and check that he or she has certification. The Kimberley Process runs an international certification program for rough diamonds, helping to prevent the trade in conflict gems.

The Diamond Council also has a System of Warranties, whereby buyers and sellers of both rough and polished diamonds have to confirm that they are conflict-free and in compliance with United Nations' resolutions. See www .greenkarat.com and www.diamondfacts.org.

Unfortunately, all diamond mining—even ethical production in countries such as Canada—causes environmental damage, simply due to the process. Synthetic diamonds are becoming more popular as an alternative and are said to be indistinguishable from mined diamonds. Whether they are a suitable replacement for a naturally occurring mineral comes down to personal choice, although they are now considered to be the most ethically and environmentally conscious option. Browse online at www.greenkarat.com.

Cleaner gold and platinum

Gold and platinum extraction carries a high environmental price, since it uses chemicals such as mercury and cyanide. You can find cleaner gold and platinum, mined under better environmental and fair-trade conditions, although supply is currently limited. Ask your jeweler if he or she uses these cleaner metals.

Both gold and platinum are highly recyclable and can be reused to make rings and jewelry that appear new, with no further environmental impact. Look for artisans using postconsumer, recycled gold and platinum.

You may have a piece of jewelry at home that could be melted down and made into a new ring. Some jewelers will happily do this for you and encourage you to be involved in its design. A number of innovative companies hold workshops at their studios so that you can come in and help with the process of making the rings yourselves (see the Directory).

Wooden rings

These are a delightful, ethical alternative to metal rings and are skillfully crafted from native nontropical hardwoods, such as yew, oak, and cherry. Completely natural, and warm to wear, wooden rings will last for years with the correct care. They often come presented in a matching wooden box. The rings pictured above are from www.wooden.co.uk, or see www.etsy.com.

Wedding planner tip:
Clean gemstones using an old, soft toothbrush and eco-dishwashing liquid for sparkling results.

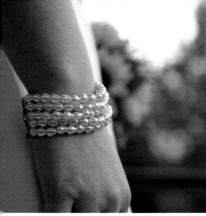

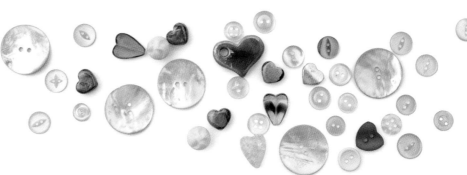

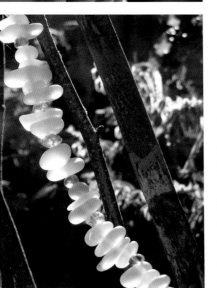

Beads for all occasions

Beads are always in fashion, whatever the season, and come in all manner of sizes, lengths, shapes, and styles (see the tips on the opposite page for ideas). They are easy to string yourself: Look for courses to learn beading techniques and to gather inspiration. Try salvaging broken necklaces and using the beads to create something new.

Sea glass

Fragments of glass are naturally polished by the sea into smooth pebbles in shades of blue and aqua, foamy white, rich green and amber, and, occasionally, rare pink. Sea glass can be hundreds of years old, and each piece is unique. Gina Cowen (www.seaglass.co.uk) makes magically beautiful sea jewels (see left and page 25).

Recycled beads

Look in galleries and online for inspiring artisan-designed, ecofriendly necklaces and bracelets made from recycled glass beads. Brilliantly reflective and found in countless colors, they make stunning jewelry (see www.juzionline.com).

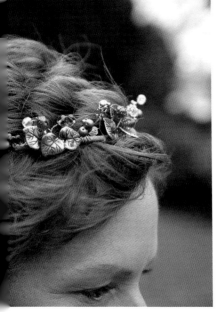

Buttons

Pretty vintage and antique buttons with intricate designs can be used in the same ways as beads. Simply thread them onto fine beading string (available from craft suppliers) so the buttons lie flat. Search out antique mother-of-pearl buttons, which gently reflect the light. Find vintage buttons at charity shops (they are often cut off of damaged garments that are going to be recycled as textiles), online, and at specialist antique market stalls.

Beaded tiaras

These are easy to make—and a workshop can be a fantastic alternative bachelorette party. Use salvaged beads and recycled fine wire for a perfect ecoaccessory. It's worth checking frequently in a mirror to make sure that your design suits your face shape.

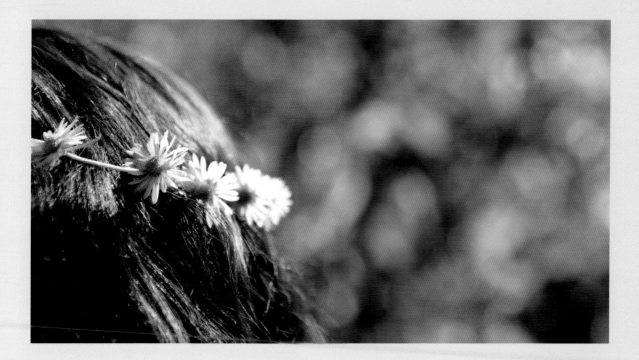

Hair bands and daisy chains

Hair bands add interest with minimal effort, whether your hair is long or short. Simple to make from elastic or wire, they can be wound with fine ribbons and decorated with vintage corsages, bows and brooches, or fresh flowers.

Narrow, fabric hair bands are especially chic worn across the forehead with loose, flowing hair—perfect for a laid-back beach wedding. Decorate with small, fabric blooms and tiny beads for natural summer style.

We made impromptu daisy chains for our bride, Lisa, above, and our flower girls—simple, beautifully effective, and ideal for an informal country or garden wedding. Remember to make them at the last moment so that they stay fresh.

Tips for wearing your beads

❋ Wooden beads are an environmentally sound choice if they are vintage or FSC accredited, and they look fabulous with 1970s flowing gowns. Choose pale woods to suit a light-colored dress.

❋ For a 1950s-themed wedding, accessorize with vintage, chunky-beaded necklaces in bold, primary colors.

❋ Delicate glass and crystal beads catch the light beautifully. Look out for antique strings for romantic simplicity.

❋ Antique pearls are timeless and will suit almost any outfit. Colors vary so choose carefully to complement both your dress and your skin tone.

Wedding planner tip:
The current trend is to wear either earrings or a necklace, but not both together.

Boleros and corsages

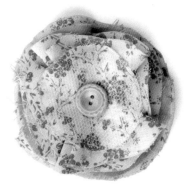

The accessories you choose can lift a plain dress or tie an outfit together. Try unusual combinations of color, textures, and layering, as we have in the photograph on the opposite page. Boleros and wraps can be useful whether your wedding is in deep winter or high summer.

Boleros, which are cropped, midsleeved jackets, are smart and stylish as part of a skirt-suit, or keep cold at bay when worn over a dress in the winter months.

Fine silk wraps will shield bare arms from hot sunshine or add a layer of warmth in early spring and autumn. Knitted ballet-wrap cardigans in creamy whites and soft pinks, finished with wide, satin ribbon ties, add a twist to a traditional strapless dress.

Scarves

I always feel that scarves are an underused wedding accessory, whether vintage silk or heavy knit. If your photographs are being taken in snow, a chunky, white bobble scarf will add fashion-shoot glamour.

Gorgeous old silk scarves from vintage shops come in all sorts of patterns, colors, and sizes. Larger ones can be used as a wrap, while the smaller ones look fabulous simply tied asymmetrically around the neck. This look is especially chic with a 1950s dress. You can even use men's brightly colored, silk hankies as scarves—vintage handkerchiefs are usually well made.

If you are having a dress made in an ecofabric such as hemp silk or raw peace silk, you could use the offcuts to make delicate scarves to match.

> **Wedding planner tip:**
> Update an existing wrap cardigan by swapping knitted ties for beautiful, reclaimed satin ribbons.

Ribbons

Vintage ribbons in unusual colors and textures can make strikingly simple accessories. For an almost instant choker, hem the ends and attach a small piece of Velcro or a button fastening to them. A friend made a contrasting black-and-white choker as a last-minute necklace alternative before heading out as a wedding guest. You could try layering ribbons in different widths and tones, or sewing on a corsage, beads, or buttons.

Corsages

Fresh-flower and fabric corsages are in vogue, worn with jeans as well as wedding dresses. You could make your own from cream-toned ecofabrics, handmade felt, or brightly colored offcuts of material (see page 68 for my simple method) or scout out vintage gems. If you find a fabric corsage that you adore but is in poor condition, give it a new lease on life by carefully taking it apart and reworking it, adding extra fabrics and ribbons.

Using fresh flowers

Floral accessories have a minimal carbon footprint if the flowers have been grown locally.

❋ Fresh-flower wrist corsages are the ultimate retro-prom accessory. They can look wonderful, especially for an outdoor wedding—and you could give your bridesmaids smaller matching versions.

❋ Try attaching a single fresh flower to one side of a ribbon sash. Ask advice from your florist as you will need a relatively hardy species.

❋ Floral headdresses have recently come back into fashion. They work best with tiny seasonal blooms that complement your skin tone and dress.

Ways with corsages

❋ Fasten a beautiful, antique corsage to a length of ribbon as a vintage-inspired choker.

❋ Wear a large fresh-flower corsage in your hair.

❋ Oversized, soft, ecofabric corsages look fabulous attached to matching wide belts for urban ecochic.

❋ Ask your dress designer for extra fabric to make your own corsage.

❋ Give your bridesmaids individual style with matching dresses but contrasting corsages.

This simple dress, shot at the Makery, is lifted by a matching 1940s corsage and ballet wrap, and a play-in-the-snow, chunky knit scarf.

Hemp-silk camisole from
Jenny Ambrose at Enamore.

Camisoles and pretty underwear

Beautiful underwear made from hemp silk and vintage ribbons are a fabulous indulgence for a bride. Ecogirls will love the soft, organic bamboo or natural cotton ranges that are now available, complete with pretty lace trimmings. Look online at makers such as www.enamore.co.uk. Choose fair trade for maximum ethical score, or make your own using vintage fabrics. Find easy patterns at www.burdastyle.com.

Perfect underwear

❁ Try your chosen underwear on with your dress, as sheer fabrics may reveal more than you bargained for.

❁ Ivory or nude-colored underwear is best under white, ivory, and champagne dresses. With a strong-colored dress, such as red, you could team your underwear accordingly.

❁ Splurge on some beautiful wedding-night lingerie in a light, ecofriendly hemp-silk mix.

❁ Lingerie workshops, where you can learn to make your own, are a new craze. Use organic, skin-friendly ecofabrics and vintage ribbons and lace to fashion something unique.

❁ Embellish your own favorite underwear with vintage, blue ribbons for your "something old" and "something blue."

Corsets

Amazing handcrafted corsets in modern ecofabrics will help to define your shape on the big day. These can be an extravagant purchase, but they are tailored to fit and will last for years if well made. Corset making is a skilled art with a finished piece taking many hours to complete. A design decorated with ribbons and lace will add a feminine touch. You will need to take details of your dress with you so the corsetiere can work to its shape.

Garters

Garters are a frivolous accessory that most brides will only wear on their big day but a traditional part of any wedding outfit. You can find handmade garters fashioned from salvaged lace and natural silk—and finished with a blue ribbon bow.

Having a Hepburn moment

Gloves can add a chic dimension to any wedding outfit—think of cult screen-icon Audrey Hepburn. They come in many lengths, from wrist to above the elbow, in a variety of fabrics to match or contrast with your dress. Pretty lace gloves work well with a delicate dress, heavier fabrics with more structured gowns.

Vintage gloves are usually beautifully made, readily available, and often cost only a few dollars from eBay and vintage specialists. Ensure that they are scrupulously clean, and remember that you will need to remove the left-hand glove during the exchange of rings, so make sure you can easily undo any buttons.

Think about dainty, knitted fingerless gloves, hand-embellished with tiny beads, for a winter wedding. You could team them with a delicate matching wrap or knitted choker. Gloves can also be useful for early spring or late autumn weddings. If you are wearing a cape, or a bolero or jacket with three-quarters-length sleeves, they will keep your arms warm.

Wedding planner tip:
Always hand wash silk and hemp-silk underwear to keep it looking its best, using a mild, plant-based detergent.

Bags of ideas

It is now perfectly acceptable for a bride (and her bridesmaids) to carry a small bag on the big day, sometimes in place of a bouquet. It can hold any items you may need, such as a hankie for those emotional moments or a lipstick for touch-ups. If you are making a speech, it's the perfect place to stash your notes.

You will find bags in the most unlikely places. I was browsing a stall that sold old tools at my favorite outdoor antiques market when I caught a glimpse of something sparkly—it turned out to be an apricot 1930s beaded bag, complete with an original vanity mirror. The stallholder told me that I could buy it for £5, and I still have it to this day.

You could also ask mothers and grandmothers, or try antique shops and trunk sales. Charity shops offer thrifty bags, some in as-new condition, from delicate satin clutches to modern, patent-leather purses.

Crafting your own

For those brides (or mothers) who are keen to make their own, try the instructions on page 88. This bag is quick and easy to make, and you can use pretty fabric remnants you may have at home or a new ecofabric (see page 64).

Embellish a bag

Even easier is to embellish a bag you already own. Adding a piece of vintage lace, a satin corsage, or a sparkly brooch can instantly transform a plain bag.

Top bag tips

* Enliven a simple dress with a decorative bag.
* Gold and silver bags double as jewelry.
* A vintage purse can become your "something old."
* Decorate with an extra-long ribbon for a bow, for minimal expenditure but maximum impact.
* Try a reversible bag for daytime-to-evening contrast.
* Be ecochic and have a go at making your own.

The two bags on the opposite page came from charity shops and were simply embellished with lace and ribbons in minutes.

Wedding planner tip:
If you are having a wedding dress made, ask the seamstress for a little extra fabric to make your own matching bag.

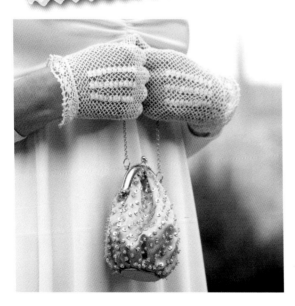

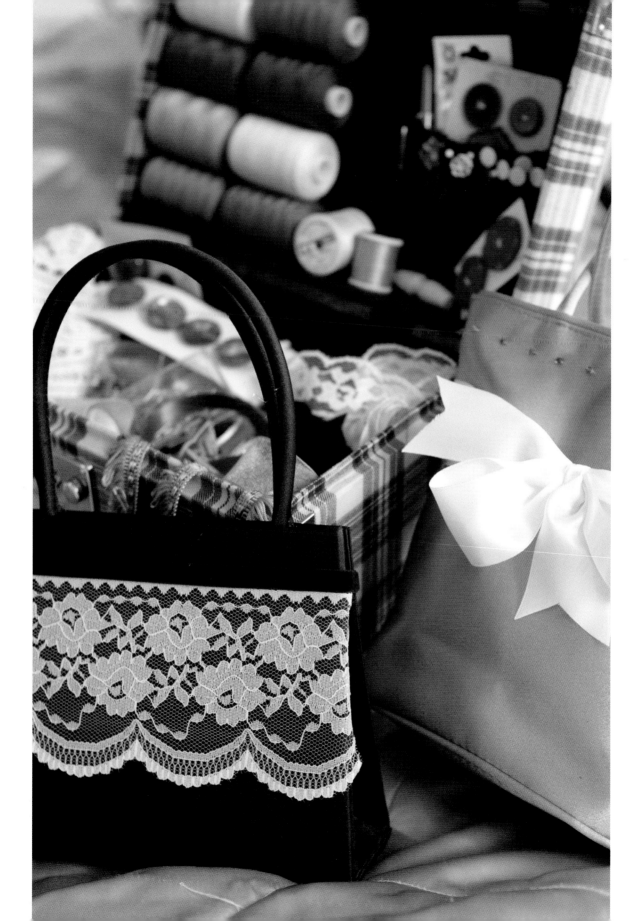

Wedding-day bag

This neat bag is the perfect accessory to have with you on the big day. It also works well for bridesmaids. This method is great if you come across a garment you love but that has marks that make it unwearable—and you don't need a sewing machine. I used both the lacy outer fabric and lining of a top I discovered in a thrift store.

YOU WILL NEED:

A piece of rough paper, 8½ x 11 inches

An old top or blouse in a pretty fabric—
    preferably lined

A piece of plainer fabric if the top is not lined

3¼ feet of ¾-inch-wide ribbon

5 feet of narrower ribbon in the
    same color

Short length of even narrower ribbon

Cotton thread in matching colors

Needle, scissors, and pins

An embellishment, such as a button or brooch

METHOD:

1. Place the paper on the garment, with the short side aligned with the bottom edge of the fabric, so any pattern runs in the right direction. Pin in place and cut around it, then repeat with the lining fabric.

2. Fold the outer piece in half, with the right side of the fabric inward and short edges together at the top. Seam neatly down each side, about 2 inches in.

3. Repeat the above two steps for the lining, but leave a gap on one side of about 2¾ inches at the top.

4. On the outer layer, with the right side still inward, open up the bag and pinch out the bottom two corners. Stitch horizontally across each corner to form equal triangles (see opposite page). Repeat the above step for the lining material. Turn through the outer layer so the right side now faces outward.

5. Take a piece of ¾-inch-wide ribbon and pin all the way around the neck of the outer layer, until the ends just touch. Cut the ribbon to this length and unpin. Hem the ends of the ribbon by ¼ inch.

6. Pin the ribbon back onto the outside of the bag, about 2 inches from the top, making sure that the gap in the ribbon is centered. Sew on with two rows of stitching, close to each edge, to make a casing.

7. Now, the tricky bit: Place the lining bag inside the outer bag so the good sides are facing each other. Stitch together at the top edge all the way around, about ½ inch in.

8. Pull the lining bag up, and pull all of the fabric through the hole in the lining. Sew up the hole, push the lining back down into the outer bag, and shake into place.

9. Sew a small, wrist-sized loop of ribbon to the lining, 2 inches down from the edge, on the opposite inner side to the gap in the ribbon casing.

10. Cover the loop ends with a vintage button, small corsage, or brooch.

11. Thread the thinner ribbon through the ribbon casing and gather as a drawstring. Tie in a bow and voilà!

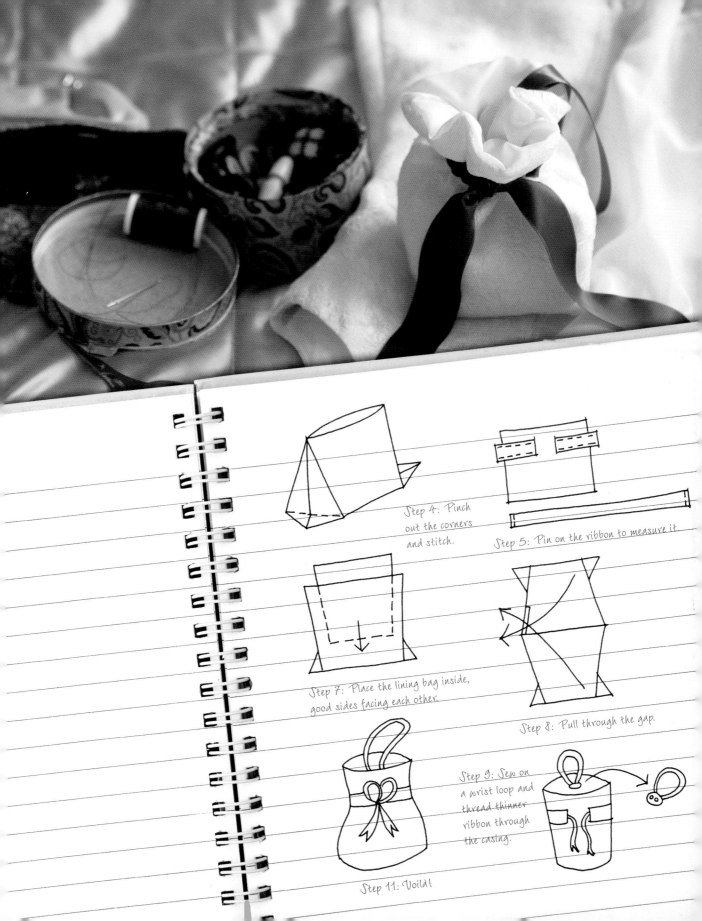

Step 4: Pinch out the corners and stitch.

Step 5: Pin on the ribbon to measure it.

Step 7: Place the lining bag inside, good sides facing each other.

Step 8: Pull through the gap.

Step 9: Sew on a wrist loop and thread thinner ribbon through the casing.

Step 11: Voilà!

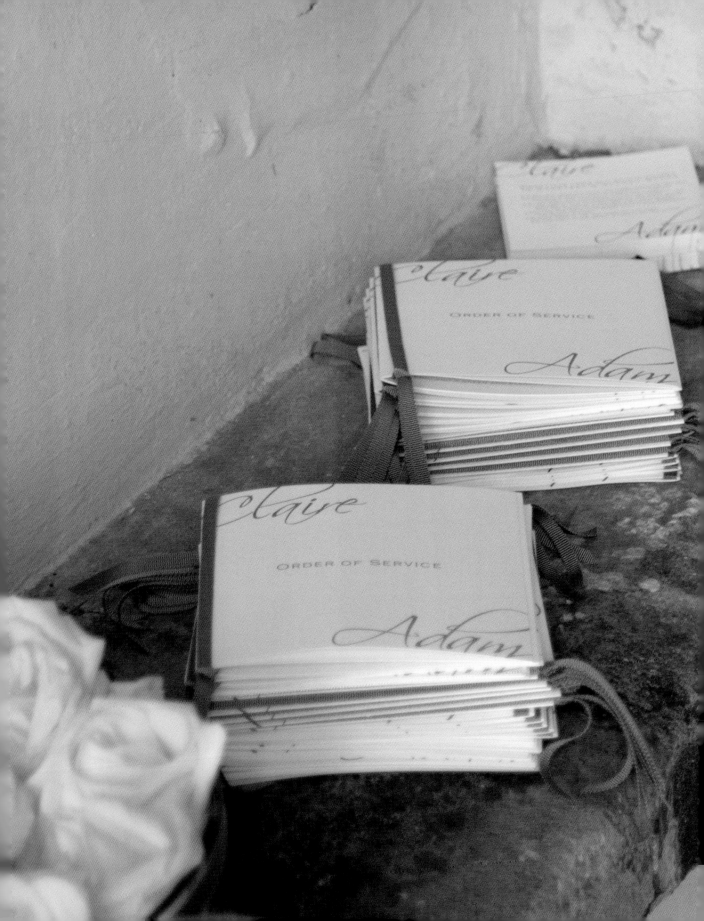

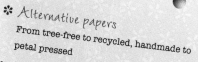

* *Alternative papers*
  From tree-free to recycled, handmade to petal pressed

* *Wildflower-seed paper*
  An easy-to-master method to make your own gorgeous recycled paper

* *Fashionable printing*
  Old-fashioned letterpress to modern waterless techniques

* *Making your own*
  Ideas to get you started and where to learn craft and art skills

* *E-weddings*
  Virtual invitations and wedding Web sites

* *Greener registries*
  One-of-a-kind presents, charity registries, and rainforest-friendly guest books

The Invites

The invitations are the first hint guests will have of your wedding style. I find it helps to let your choice of venue inspire the design: intimate or formal, high glam or laid-back. Ecofriendly invites can be some of the most beautiful you'll find, as old-fashioned art and craft techniques become newly desirable. Letterpress printing, for example, can give you crisp formality, or you could choose a quirky design from an ecocard designer—or learn how to do it yourself.

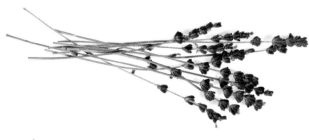

Alternative papers

*C*hoosing an environmentally friendly paper is a simple way to instantly turn your invites a shade greener. Handmade papers and creatively produced, recycled cards will make your wedding stationery distinctive, too.

Recycled paper
This is widely available in a range of colors and finishes. A 100 percent–recycled paper has a slightly rougher texture than virgin fiber, so for that "brand-new" paper sheen, opt for a blend of recycled content and virgin Forest Stewardship Council (FSC) paper. You can now find pure-white recycled paper, too, although you may want to choose an obviously recycled "fleck" finish as a design statement. The most eco-conscious option is postconsumer recycled, which has already had one use as a newspaper or magazine. See the Directory on page 208 for paper suppliers.

Forest Stewardship Council (FSC)
FSC-certified paper (www.fsc.org) is made from sustainably sourced timber. It is produced using virgin fiber so trees are felled, but new trees are replanted and protected rainforests are never destroyed. When talking to your printer, ask if the paper he or she is using is FSC accredited, and check for the logo.

Map paper
This is made by cutting old or out-of-date maps into sheets and envelopes. Each piece is unique. This is a great option for a couple who likes to travel.

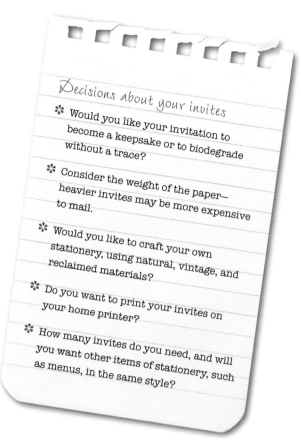

Decisions about your invites

❉ Would you like your invitation to become a keepsake or to biodegrade without a trace?

❉ Consider the weight of the paper—heavier invites may be more expensive to mail.

❉ Would you like to craft your own stationery, using natural, vintage, and reclaimed materials?

❉ Do you want to print your invites on your home printer?

❉ How many invites do you need, and will you want other items of stationery, such as menus, in the same style?

Tree-free papers
These are produced using other naturally occurring fibers, such as coffee and banana skins. They are available in either plain sheet form or as ready-made cards you decorate yourself. Some of the papers mentioned may be made in developing countries. As long as the paper is fair trade, this is a great way to ethically support a country; however, because of the transport distances, they will leave a larger carbon footprint than papers made locally.

Ellie Poo paper
Handmade from elephant dung, this paper carries no odor and is perfectly safe to use. Made using the fiber that passes naturally through the elephant from its wild diet (usually grasses), it is washed a number of times. The resulting paper is cream colored with an attractive natural flecking. Another alternative is Rhino Poo paper, while locally made Sheep Poo paper offers fewer "paper miles" in sheep-rearing nations.

Banana paper

This is made using the waste fibers from banana plantations. Mixed with postconsumer, recycled content, the resulting paper is naturally speckled and incredibly strong, with good environmental credentials. Try using it to make paper decorations and flowers (see page 162), as well as invitations.

Handmade paper

Handmade paper can be plain or include different natural materials, such as petals, grasses, seeds, and leaves. Try coordinating your paper with the table decorations, or even with your flowers. Pink rose petals are gorgeous in paper and can be scattered on wedding party tables to continue the theme.

Seed paper

Perfect for the natural wedding, seed paper can be planted by guests as a reminder of the day. It is available ready-made, or try making it yourself (see my method on the page 94).

Recycled and homemade envelopes

You can buy recycled envelopes, but to craft your own, take a square piece of paper that fits around your invite and draw faint pencil lines across the diagonals. Take any corner and fold across to half an inch past where the lines cross. Repeat with the opposite side, then fold and glue the bottom point in place. Fold over the top triangle to form a neat, square envelope.

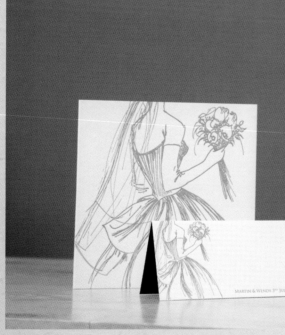

These letterpress cards were printed on recycled paper by Noble Fine Art. This family company can also print a hand-drawn picture of your wedding venue.

Wedding planner tip:
Design your wedding invitatation as a postcard—as well as being original, it will reduce the amount of paper you need.

Wildflower-seed paper

The measurements for this recipe depend on how much paper you would like to make. Try it out with a few sheets of scrap paper first, to get a feel for the technique. It can be messy, so you might want to work outside. I like to add wildflower seeds, but you could also use petals or foliage.

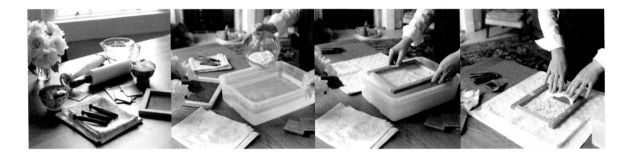

YOU WILL NEED:

At least 2 dry tea towels

A stash of scrap-paper offcuts

Deep bowl for blending

Electric hand mixer

Mesh tray (available at artists' supply stores)

Large, waterproof, flat container (larger than your mesh tray and at least 4 inches deep)

1 packet small wildflower seeds

1 damp tea towel

METHOD:

1. Lay your clean, dry tea towels to one side of your waterproof container.

2. Shred your scrap paper into small pieces and place them in a deep bowl. Cover with water.

3. Using your hand mixer, carefully pulse to purée the paper and water into a pulp.

4. Fill your large, waterproof container with water up to about 3½ inches, and stir in the paper pulp.

5. Scatter in the wildflower seeds, mixing thoroughly (alternatively, you can scatter the seeds over the damp paper in the tray, after step 7).

6. In one, quick movement, slide your mesh tray into the pulpy water and lift it up, so that you have a fine, even covering of pulp on the mesh. If it is too thick or uneven, plunge the tray back into the water.

7. Scrape the excess water from the underside of the mesh tray with your hand, and place the tray on a dry tea towel, mesh-side down.

8. Roll the damp tea towel into a smooth, flat wad, and use this to press carefully all over the new paper while it is still in the tray, to squeeze out excess water. Wring out the tea towel between presses.

9. Turn the tray upside down and pat gently to allow the paper to release onto the other dry tea towel. Make sure that the paper is as flat as possible before leaving it to dry.

10. Dry for at least twenty-four hours, then use it to make invites, place cards, favor boxes, and other stationery.

Wedding planner tip:
If you find your paper is sticking around the edges of the mesh tray when you flip it over, try using the underside of the tray instead.

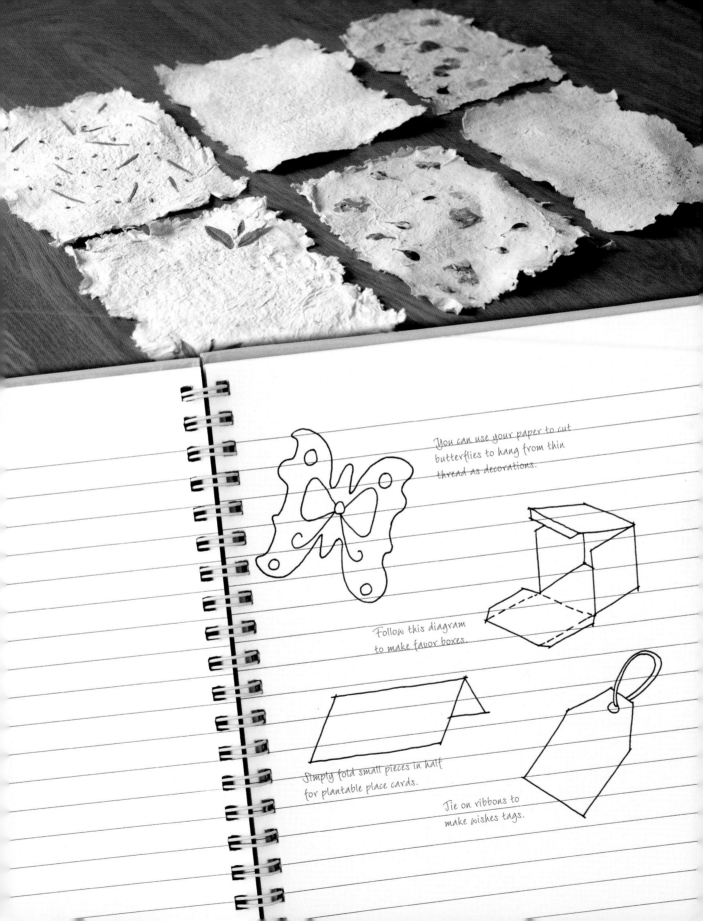

You can use your paper to cut butterflies to hang from thin thread as decorations.

Follow this diagram to make favor boxes.

Simply fold small pieces in half for plantable place cards.

Tie on ribbons to make wishes tags.

Fashionable printing

Whether you prefer the smart, traditional look of letterpress or the rustic individuality of hand-carved wood blocks, there are plenty of printing styles to explore. Ecoprinting methods have developed rapidly, so you don't have to compromise on style or ethics.

Be bold with color and explore motifs that fit with your theme. A winter wedding I attended had a striking black-and-white color scheme, and the bride had designed the invitations to match, embellishing them with fine ribbon. The wedding was held at the elegant eighteenth-century Assembly Rooms in Bath, where Jane Austen would have danced, and the invite decoration was a chandelier in silhouette.

Vegetable-based inks

Inks made from natural vegetable oils are much kinder to the environment than regular petroleum-based inks. Many ecoprinters specialize in "veggie inks," and other printers now offer them as an alternative. The color choice and print quality are just as good as standard inks.

Waterless printing

Conventional printing emits thousands of tons of volatile organic compounds (VOCs) into the atmosphere every year and uses vast quantities of water. Waterless offset printing is a revolutionary method that uses no water in its process and has the added benefit of wasting less paper.

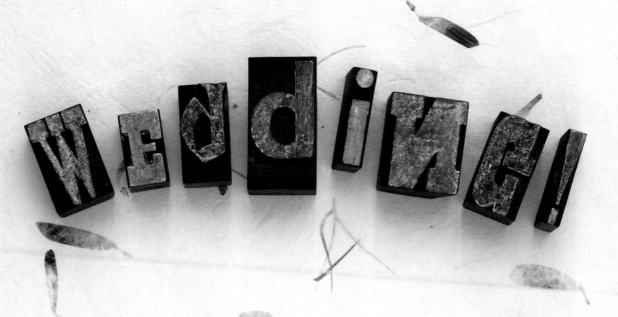

The print quality is thought to be better than conventional printing, with a full range of colors. A selection of printers offering this method is listed in the Directory.

Letterpress

This elegant, old-fashioned method of printing is enjoying a reviva and lends a touch of old-school glamour to an event. Many letterpress companies still use the original hand-operated antique machines, so their energy consumption is minimal. With an amazing range of typefaces, and the ability to print onto heavy paper stock, it is a fantastic choice for wedding stationery.

DIY

For smaller numbers of invites, using your household printer can be a thrifty option. Larger quantities may use many ink cartridges, which can be expensive, so it may be cheaper to have them printed professionally. Always recycle your empty cartridges—often charities will collect them or, alternatively, have them refilled to reuse.

Designer ecostationery

Many companies can both design and print your invites. If you would like to find an artisan craft printer, research local art colleges, check press and local Web sites for open studios, and try the crafters' Web sites such as www .etsy.com. Some will design a custom invite especially for your big day. Others offer an off-the-rack range of stationery that you can personalize with your own wording. Choose designers using recycled, handmade, or tree-free paper, embellished with natural and reclaimed materials.

Always ask for a written quotation listing the items and quantities, and overorder slightly, as you may make mistakes or have last-minute guests.

> Wedding planner tip:
> Order or make some blank place cards, in case you want to invite more guests just before the wedding.

Making your own

Hand-crafting your own invitations is fulfilling and can give stunning results. You could design and create a card from scratch or embellish a plain, ready-made ecocard. Collage and simple printing techniques are easy to master, and there are some quick-fix decoration tips below. Spend a lazy Sunday afternoon playing with ideas to see what works for you both.

Printing stamps and natural prints

This is perhaps the simplest way to craft cards. For a vintage-themed wedding you could invest in some antique wooden printing stamps, like those on page 97. Use letters of varying sizes and typefaces to create a simple but fashionable design.

You can find stamps online or at flea markets and antique fairs. Keep an eye out for unusual patterns, such as lovebirds or flowers.

One of my favorite ways to print natural designs is to use fresh leaves. Choose a leaf with a prominent vein pattern, brush ecopaint onto its back, and press it onto a card or paper. Use a single color with a variety of leaf shapes for a contemporary effect. For more ideas and methods, *Printing by Hand* by Lena Corwin has lots of lovely techniques, including stencilling.

Collage

Cutting, sticking, and layering materials can produce a wow-factor card, even if you are a relative craft novice. Plan your pattern first, and draw around a template for regular shapes. Use recycled and reused papers or magazine pages, vintage fabrics, and antique buttons.

Calligraphy

If you are having an intimate wedding, a beautifully handwritten invitation is a delightful indulgence. If you feel your own handwriting isn't up to the task, you could ask a friend or find a professional calligrapher.

Tips for home-crafted cards

✣ Design your invitations to minimize paper wastage.

✣ Consider how your embellishments will fare in the mail. If you are worried, mail a trial invite to yourself to check that it survives.

✣ If you don't have the skills to make the invites you would love, why not learn them? Workshops are available for techniques such as screen printing and letterpress.

✣ Bear in mind the number of cards you will be making, and keep to a process that you feel comfortable repeating.

✣ Find ecocraft supplies online (see the Directory on page 208 for details).

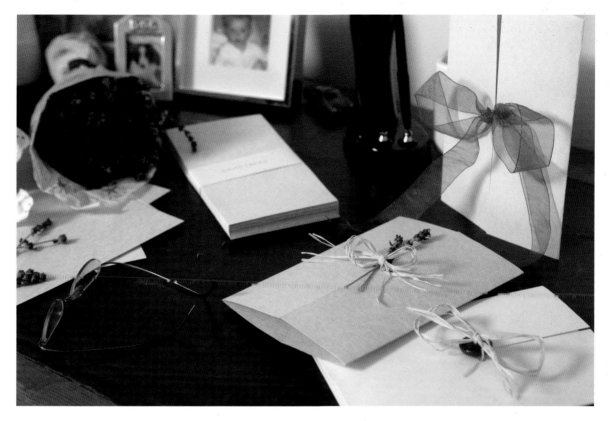

Linocuts

Linocutting involves carving a design into a small offcut of linoleum (supplies are available from art stores and aren't expensive). You can easily create letters and intricate designs and then print them onto your chosen paper. The block is re-inked between each print, so every card has a charming one-off quality. Check local art colleges for courses, or learn the skills and get expert advice at a craft studio (see the Directory on page 208). If you don't feel artistic, it's easy to trace an existing design onto the lino.

Woodcuts

Woodcutting is a more skilled method, where you carve the design into a block of wood with chisels. For this, you will definitely need to invest some time mastering the techniques, but the finished woodblock will make an amazing ornament and memento of your day.

These invites show three easy homemade styles. Use a hole punch, and tie with raffia or vintage or re-used ribbon, looping in vintage buttons or other decorations.

Screen printing

The ink is squeezed through a stencil onto the paper or card below. You can design and cut stencils yourself or buy them ready-made. It's possible to screen print onto a variety of media, from handmade paper to vintage textiles. For instructions and inspiration, see *Simple Screenprinting* by Annie Stromquist.

Wedding planner tip:
Try framing one of your invitations as a lasting reminder of your special day.

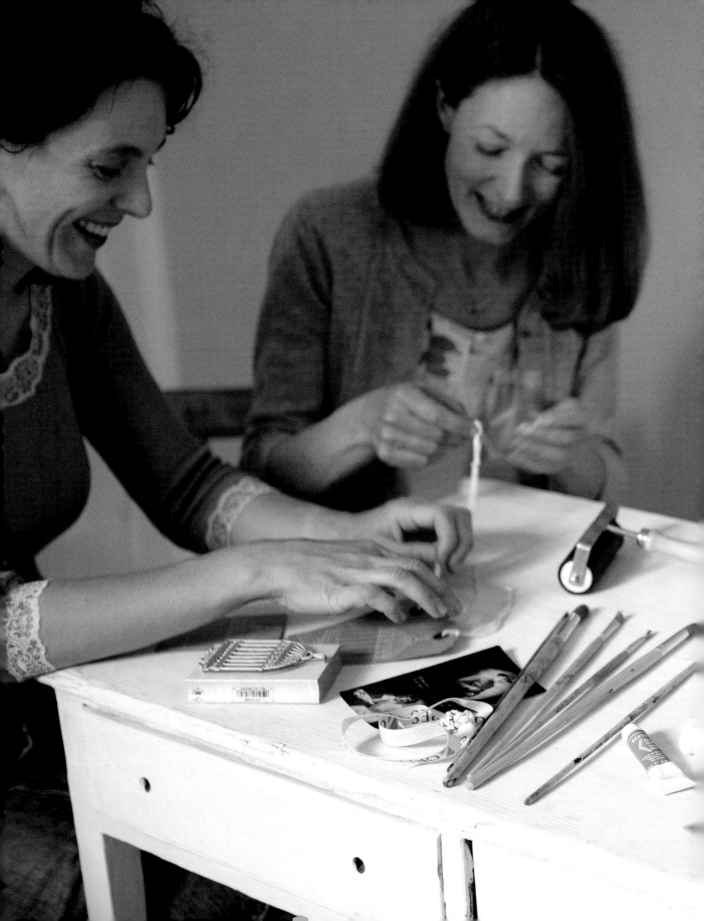

DIY invite inspirations

Decadent ribbons and fabrics, paper butterflies, and watercolor paints—they all add that extra wedding sparkle. Delight in selecting from the range of natural and vintage ornaments at your fingertips. Browse vintage origami books for inspiration—there are some beautiful folded patterns that you can use on cards. I also recommend *Nature Printing* by Laura Donnelly Bethmann; *Good Mail Day: A Primer for Making Eye-Popping Postal Art* by Jennie Hinchcliff and Carolee Gilligan Whoolor; and the stationery section at www .allthisismine.com.

Simple embellishments

Ribbons are a fantastic and quick way to give cards a professional finish.

❋ Tie together a paper insert and an outer card using a wide ribbon for elegant simplicity.

❋ Use three strands of thin ribbon in contrasting colors for a candy-stripe theme.

❋ Fashion sumptuous ribbon bows for a decadent look.

❋ Layer heavy vintage ribbon and delicate lace for perfect winter style.

Quick ways to add your personal touch

Find ready-made, tree-free cards and decorate them with natural and reclaimed materials.

❋ Salvage fine wire and shape it into simple shapes such as butterflies or flowers. Fix to the cards using small sewing stitches.

❋ Hand-color one or two elements of a black-and-white card with watercolor paint or colored inks.

❋ Print an insert for a bought card on your home printer; assemble the invite by tying it with natural raffia.

❋ Gather ribbons around a card and fix them in place by threading them through an antique button.

❋ Glue dried petals in a pretty pattern.

Vintage stationery

❋ Search out antique postcards or photo cards. Use them as they are (if not already written on) or mount them onto recycled card stock. Stamp with your chosen text, and embellish with white ribbon and buttons for an individual twist.

❋ Collage an invite using vintage magazines—fashion titles work especially well. Choose a stylish era such as the 1950s—perfect if you will be wearing a 1950s-style dress.

❋ Cut squares of reclaimed fabrics and mount them onto card stock, then decorate with paper butterflies and brightly colored ribbons for a summery look.

❋ Trace a 1960s fabric pattern to make your own linoleum stamp, and print this onto handmade paper for a touch of retro style.

Your raw materials

❋ Natural raffia
❋ Vintage buttons
❋ Dried flowers
❋ Lavender stems
❋ Vintage lace
❋ Salvaged wire
❋ Antique beads
❋ Velvet ribbon
❋ Shells (sustainably sourced)
❋ Hemp twine
❋ Organic cotton string

Wedding planner tip:
Tint the paper, fabric, and trimmings for your invites naturally with strong tea or beetroot juice.

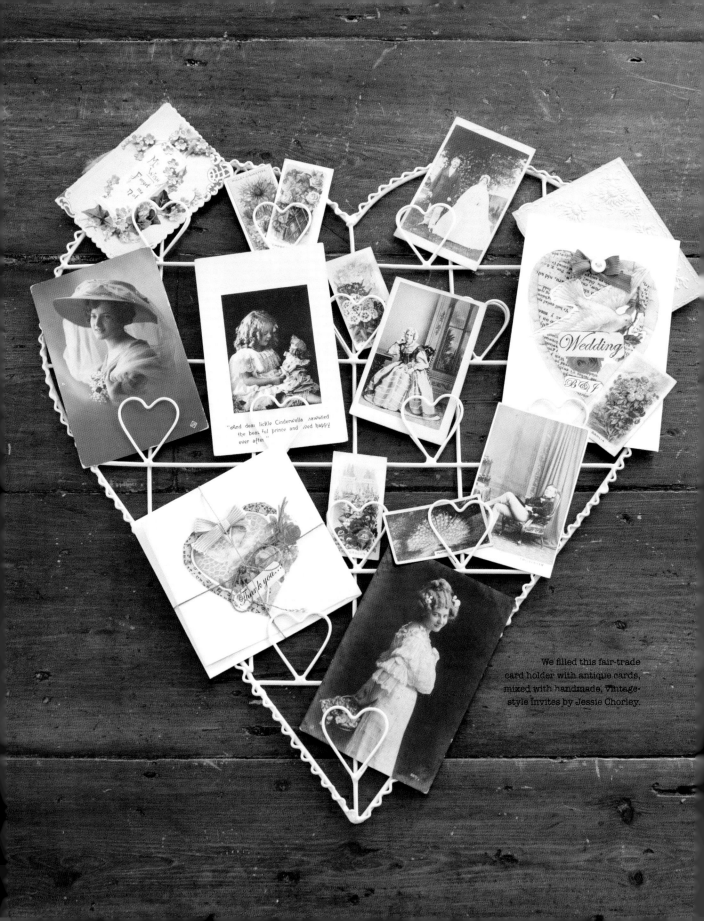

We filled this fair-trade card holder with antique cards, mixed with handmade, vintage-style invites by Jessie Chorley.

Escort cards and wedding Web sites

Not all items on the usual list of additional stationery are necessary, and you may prefer to opt for invites only. Think about combining elements when possible, such as having the wine list on the menu, to keep your "paper footprint" smaller.

Escort cards

This American tradition has become popular worldwide and is a novel way to help people to find their seats. Guests' names are written on small cards (with the table number on the back or inside) and then showcased in a variety of ways, to fit your theme.

Fair-trade, wire card holders come in an array of shapes and sizes. A cream or white heart with scalloped name cards gives a romantic look. The card holder can be hung on a wall or placed in the garden and reused after the wedding. Suspend your escort cards from an antique birdcage for a striking display, or use rustic wooden vegetable crates or vintage mirrors to create a fabulous backdrop. For travel enthusiasts, tie named brown-paper luggage tags onto an antique leather suitcase.

Thank-you cards

Photo thank-yous are popular and can be prepared by your photographer, or you can print them at home on recycled cards. Alternatively:

❋ Send all the guests small packets of seeds, wrapped in personalized paper sleeves and tied with vintage ribbon.
❋ Be kitschy and send each guest a postcard from your honeymoon location, complete with a "Wish You Were Here" motif.
❋ Save cardboard food or drink boxes from the reception to craft into pop art–style cards.
❋ Keep the petals from your bouquet and use them in handmade paper thank-yous.

E-vites and paperless weddings

E-vites, or virtual invitations, are the greenest option, and if you are a whiz on a computer, you can create something delightful. Alternatively, there are nifty design companies that will design a fabulous e-vite for you, complete with a sumptuous, addressed e-envelope. Designs range from minimalist chic to lavish traditional, and you can send thank-yous by e-mail afterward.

Include a link to your wedding Web site for guests to RSVP and find event information, such as directions, accommodations, and the registry. With no paper costs or postage to pay, e-vites are a thrifty option. But remember to make a small batch of paper invitations for those guests without Internet access or who will treasure an invitation for years to come.

Wedding Web sites

These are still a fairly new phenomenon but are growing in popularity. You can give Web links to local places to stay; ask for guests' special needs, such as dietary requirements; and add fun, personalized information, such as photos of the bridal party. Think about including a song request page for the DJ or band and a link to your online wedding registry.

After the wedding, the site can be updated with highlights, photos, and thank-you messages, and you can ask guests to upload their own photos from the day. See the Directory for wedding Web site providers.

> Wedding planner tip:
> Build your own wedding Web site and have it hosted by a solar-powered Web host for a truly eco-online experience.

Greener registries

With more people marrying later in life and setting up house before the big day, there is less need for the traditional kettles and ironing boards. Wedding registries today can be for anything and everything, and they should reflect your values and style as a couple. If you want to include details on your Web site, remember that you will need to decide on the list beforehand.

Ecohoneymoon fund

Ask family and friends to contribute to your honeymoon fund, perhaps for two weeks in an ecolodge in Botswana or five days in a tepee at the Glastonbury music festival. There are some fabulously romantic honeymoon options close to home, from cool camping to ecochic boutique hotels; for more inspiration see page 192.

Ecofriendly guest books

Guest books capture the memories and sentiments of the day. Look for recycled, FSC-accredited or tree-free papers, and covers made from locally sourced, salvaged wood. Or try embellishing the cover of a plain book with your own design of pressed leaves, shell buttons, and fine wire. Guests could be asked to sign a special item, such as a photograph, or a piece of handmade paper that can be framed for posterity.

One idea I've seen work beautifully is for each guest to bring a leaf, then have the collection fused in glass to produce a lasting artwork.

A wedding list with a difference.

Ethical stores

Register with an online ecostore (see the Directory for suggestions). They stock an amazing array of brilliant, energy-saving gadgets, from solar panels to windup radios, as well as natural beauty and home wares. Most supply truly fair-trade products, so you can shop safe in the knowledge that your ethics are in good hands.

Other ecopresents

❊ Charity registries such as www.oxfamunwrapped.com offer fantastic selections of "gifts" that help countries around the world requiring aid.

❊ Set up a donation Web site, such as www.justgiving .com, to give to a charity close to your heart.

❊ For one-of-a kind gifts, ask your guests to make you something themselves, from jam to cushions, sculptures to renovated furniture.

❊ If you want truly one-of-a-kind presents, make a request for "anything secondhand," from retro children's board games to a French antique chest.

❊ Perhaps you've always dreamed of owning a patch of native woodland. A wedding fund means your favorite people can contribute to something that you will appreciate for years to come.

Wishes trees

These are charming. Plant a small tree or branching shrub—perhaps a blossoming fruit tree—into a decorative pot. Place it somewhere guests will have space to sit and write, and provide a stack of paper luggage tags or cards with ribbon or raffia ties.

Guests note down their message, tie it onto the tree, and make a wish. After the wedding, you can collect the tags into a book or special box for safekeeping.

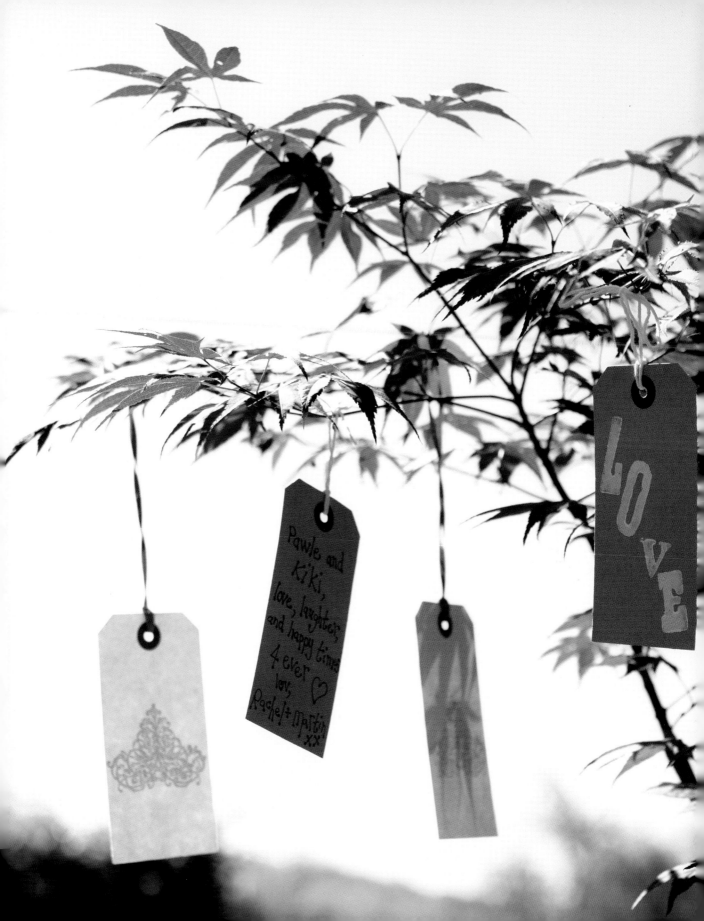

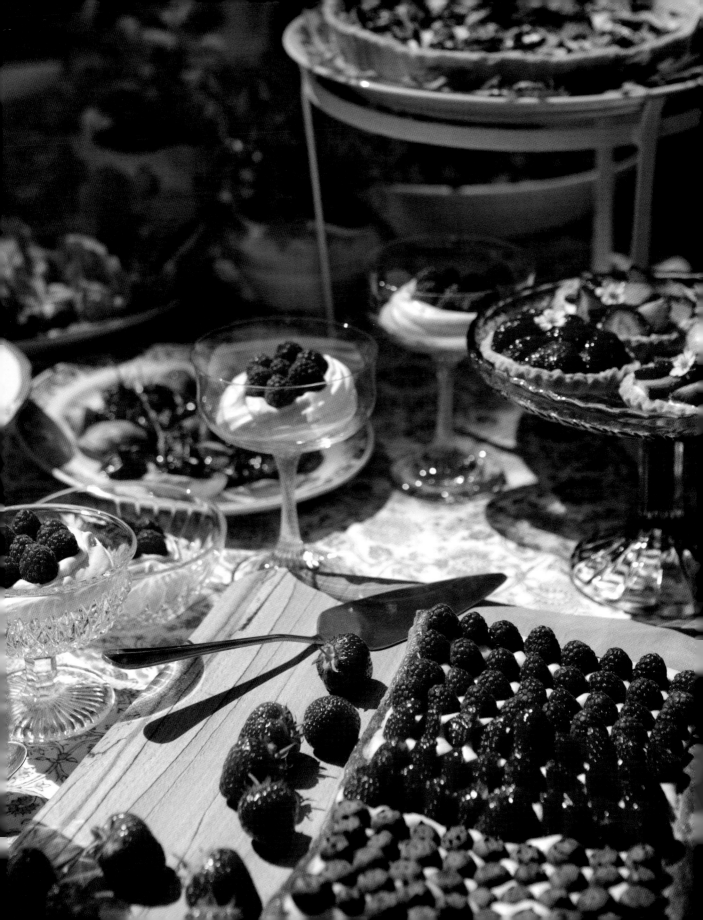

* **Food for all seasons**
  Sourcing your food and choosing a caterer
* **Finding produce you can trust**
  Organic and biodynamic, plus foraging tips and edible flowers for the adventurous
* **DIY catering**
  Recipe ideas and growing your own fruit and vegetables
* **Lou's homemade chutney**
  Easy to make from windfall apples
* **Eating outdoors**
  Barbecues, picnics, and campfires
* **Drinks for your celebration**
  From local wines and organic cocktails to homemade lemonade

The Menu

Food to share with friends and family; a meal to celebrate the beginning of your marriage—that's the essence of a wedding reception. You can make it a formal occasion with the best organic, local, and seasonal caterers or try picnicking in summer fields, barbecuing on the beach, or hosting a fashionable tea party. Some of the most enjoyable meals are those to which guests each bring a dish, so everyone can join in.

Food for all seasons

Planning your menu around seasonal food is the most environmentally friendly choice, as the wedding meal is usually the element of the day with the largest carbon footprint. Often, fruit and vegetables are flown thousands of miles so that we can enjoy them out of season, and most people have lost track of whether products are locally made or grown, or imported.

Try to buy direct from local greengrocers, orchards, dairies, and farmers' markets, and ask where the produce comes from. Seasonal foods usually taste better, and they are cheaper, too. See our Seasonal Fruit and Vegetables calendar on page 216.

What to ask a caterer

These simple questions will help you judge a caterer's environmental credentials.

❋ Do they source their food locally?

❋ Can they provide an organic, seasonal menu?

❋ Do they use free-range meat, poultry, and eggs?

❋ Do they choose Marine Stewardship Council–accredited fish?

❋ Do they choose fair-trade products for staples such as sugar, tea, and coffee?

❋ Can they compost the food waste, and do they buy produce with less packaging?

❋ Do they make their own bread?

Farmers' markets and artisan producers

Farmers' markets are brilliant places to buy directly from local growers and suppliers, and everything from wonderfully flavored organic vegetables to handmade macaroons, local cream to free-range chicken is available. Make a beeline for small, artisan makers who take pride in the food they create. The bread on page 116 is from the United Kingdom's Thoughtful Bread Company (www.thethoughtfulbreadcompany.com), which uses traditional methods and foraged herbs. Find other artisan producers through our Directory.

Meat and poultry

While organic is the most sustainable farming method, all meat is considered to have a high environmental impact. To reduce your wedding's carbon footprint, why not choose recipes that combine a little free-range meat with a delicious variety of vegetables and other ingredients? This will also be more economical.

Catering choices

Your choice of menu will depend on your wedding style, together with your budget. If your venue is an ecohotel, then you will probably be tied to using its in-house caterers. But if not, specialist caterers can prepare the freshest organic meals, using ethical and local produce. Similarly, you can find dedicated vegan and vegetarian caterers. Look in the Directory for our favorites.

The most expensive option is a three-course, sit-down, plated meal, served at individual tables by a waitstaff. If you have a large guest list, or are on a budget, a buffet or tea party will be more manageable.

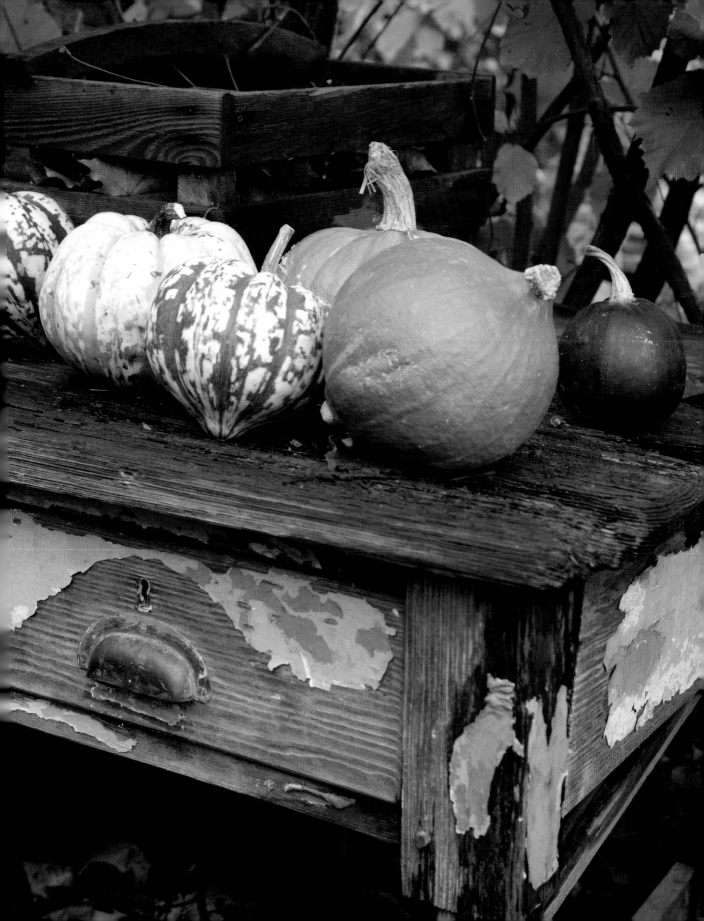

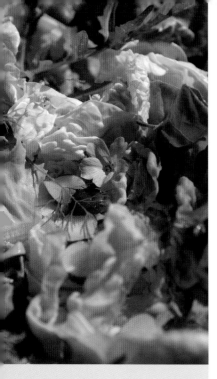

Finding produce you can trust

*C*hoosing ethical, organic, and sustainable produce is good for farm workers, the environment, and your health. Whether you are using a caterer or buying your own, free-range poultry, sustainable fish, fair-trade staples, and pesticide-free vegetables are all now widely available. For a real hands-on experience, try foraging wild foods.

Organic

Produce labeled as organic is grown without the use of synthetic pesticides, fertilizers, drugs, antibiotics, or wormers, and it is subject to strict regulation. Farmers are encouraged to control pests with natural predators and companion planting, and genetically modified crops are banned. Land that is used to grow food or rear animals must be "chemical free" for a minimum of two years before organic certification is awarded.

Biodynamic

This established method follows the astronomical calendar to determine when to harvest, plant, and cultivate crops. It is based on a self-sufficient farming system, producing natural animal feeds, manures, and fertilizers on-site. Herbs and special natural preparations (some of which contain animal products) are also used to achieve healthy, strong plants. Demeter (www.demeter.net) is the international certification body.

Fair trade

Many staple foods are grown in developing countries, where farmers rely on exporting cash crops to earn a living. Unfortunately, child labor, low wages, and dangerous working environments are all too common. The Fairtrade Foundation was set up to stop this. Look for the international FAIRTRADE certification mark.

Marine Stewardship Council

The MSC (www.msc.org) promotes sustainable fishing practices and protects the marine environment around the world, and its blue logo guarantees traceability back to a certified source. It helps to ensure that resources are not overfished and that destructive fishing methods are banned. The MSC can also tell you where to buy certified fish.

Edible flowers

Many varieties can be used in salads and as edible decorations. As with foraging (see opposite page), ensure that flowers are picked at their freshest, grown without the use of pesticides, washed thoroughly, and used quickly. Research your subject and get to know what is safe to eat. Nasturtiums, calendula, geraniums, elder, and rosemary flowers can all be used in recipes and make delectable garnishes.

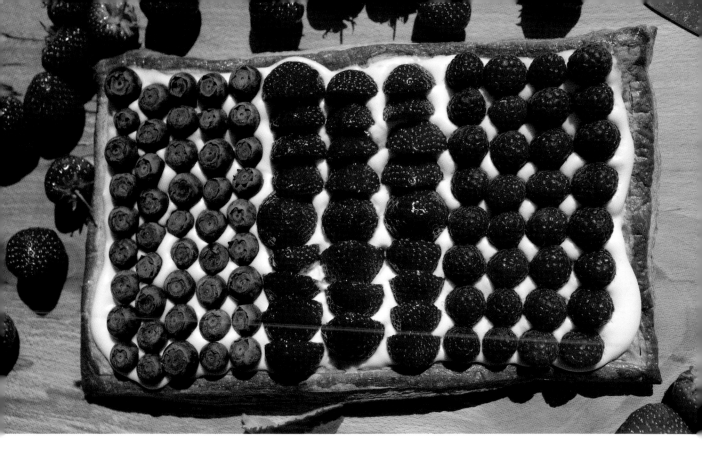

Slow Food

The Slow Food movement, which began in Italy, is winning worldwide supporters as it says no to fast foods, plastic bags, unethical produce, pesticides, and food that has traveled thousands of miles. Instead, it promotes traditional and artisan foods that taste wonderful and that are produced sustainably and ethically, with pride and passion (see www.slowfood.com). Grow your own vegetables, bake bread at home, ask your grandma to write down her favorite recipes for you, and try regional products crafted from ingredients grown close to home. Slow your pace of life and enjoy food you have taken time to prepare for your wedding feast.

Foraging

Consumers are beginning to realize the foragers' feast available to them on country walks and in their gardens. Some ingredients, such as wild garlic, are easy to spot—just follow your nose. Mushrooms, on the other hand, take a practiced eye. Read a good foraging book before you start, to ensure that what you are picking is safe to eat, and never dig up plants. (My top tip is to avoid picking anything around the base of trees, which may have been popular with dogs.)

Wedding planner tip:
Check that caterers can provide sauces and condiments made with free-range and organic ingredients, too.

DIY catering

Preparing your own food is a wonderful way to put your personal stamp on the day and to keep your spending down. You can be sure of the origin of your ingredients and lavish lots of care and attention on each dish.

A meal for sharing

Do things a little differently with your catering, and ask family and friends to bring something delicious for all to share, perhaps suggesting either sweet or savory, to keep a balance. Noncooks can bring a bottle of something fizzy instead. If you feel uncomfortable asking, propose this as your wedding gift—much more useful than another toaster. Not only will guests enjoy a wonderful range of flavors, but those with special diets will be able to bring a dish that suits them.

Easy recipes for homemade menus
Wild-rice salad ❖ spiced, toasted seeds and nuts ❖ potato salad with baby onions ❖ honey-roasted ham ❖ poached fish ❖ homegrown leaf salads brimming with radishes and tomatoes ❖ spinach and wild garlic ❖ char-grilled peppers and mushrooms ❖ homemade rolls with tasty herb spreads ❖ free-range mayonnaise

For winter
Root-vegetable stews ❖ spicy curries ❖ tasty soups ❖ hot flatbreads ❖ bowls of ratatouille

Follow with simple desserts
Huge pavlovas filled with organic whipped cream and homegrown berries ❖ homemade ice creams or sorbets.

Big platters

Vintage platters are easy to find in thrift stores and markets. Seat guests at long trestle tables, and place your large platters of different dishes down the middle.

Growing your own

If you have a garden or yard, then it's possible to grow some of your own organic produce for your wedding. There is nothing more satisfying than seeing vegetables spring up from a packet of seeds, or fruit from an unpromising twig in the ground. You can buy organic seeds and plants at nurseries or online. Remember to choose sustainable, peat-free, organic compost so that natural peat bogs are not depleted.

You will need to plan ahead and allow sufficient time to grow the ingredients that you would love to have on your menu. Some, such as broccoli, need many months to mature, while salad leaves can be raised from seeds in a couple of weeks. Soft fruit, such as strawberries, raspberries, and blueberries, take little effort and are ideal for summer weddings; serve them in meringues or on your cake (see page 124) or use them to make jam.

Windowsill herbs

Herbs such as oregano, coriander, and sage are easy to grow, and even if you don't have a garden, you can keep them in small pots on your kitchen windowsill. Raise them organically, and they will instantly add another dimension to your wedding salads. You could also try fiery chili plants.

Wedding planner tip:
Serving bowls, platters, and large dishes can all be rented if you don't have enough.

Drinks for your celebration

Wines produced by exciting local vineyards will keep down your wine miles; go to a tasting at the vineyard or a nearby supplier so you can try before you buy. The wines on the opposite page come from the award-winning Avonleigh organic vineyard in north Somerset, England, and Wickham Vineyards in Hampshire, England.

High-quality organic wines and champagne-style sparkling wines are now widely available, and biodynamic vineyards produce some of the world's finest bottles. Check labels for low or zero sulphur content if you have dietary sensitivities.

Organic fruit wines have a long history but are generally not drunk as often as grape wines. Choose from varieties such as elderberry, plum, ginger, or tayberry. See the Directory on page 211 for suppliers.

Artisan cider and perry

Specialist ciders and perry (pear cider) are becoming popular alternatives to wine. There are some delicious, light, champagne-method varieties that rival sparkling wines in taste; I particularly like Ashridge from Devon. Serve in tall, elegant, stemmed glasses. If you have an orchard and cider press nearby, you could even have a go at making your own cider.

Mulled wine and mulled cider

Rich with the taste of cinnamon, orange, and spices, these mixes bring a glow to a winter wedding and are simple to prepare at home. Try adding a glug or two of brandy before serving for extra warmth.

Homemade cordials and lemonade

Fragrant elderflower cordial and zesty lemonade are superb nonalcoholic alternatives that are easy and cost-effective to make yourself. Buy organic, unwaxed lemons and scrub thoroughly before use. Pick your elderflowers from traffic-free spots, and wash thoroughly. Use fair-trade, unrefined sugar and store in recycled bottles. In the winter, offer guests your own mulled elderberry cordial made from dried elderberries and spices—delicious and great to keep colds at bay.

Mineral water

Ideally, serve tap water in pretty glass jugs to reduce water miles and waste. If you do opt for bottled, choose a nearby supplier who sources from a local spring and buy in large containers. Recycle bottles and see if you can buy on sale or return.

Organic cocktails

Bramley & Gage produces delicious liqueurs from homegrown soft fruit using traditional French methods. For an elegant, summery drink, mix sparkling wine or water with raspberry liqueur and serve with a raspberry in the bottom of the glass. Delicious.

HEDGEROW SLING

¼ cup organic sloe gin

2 tablespoons fresh lemon juice

2½ teaspoons Bramley & Gage blackberry liqueur

Soda water, or naturally sparkling water

Shake the sloe gin and lemon juice with ice and strain over fresh ice into a Collins glass. Top with soda water and float the blackberry liqueur. Garnish with fresh blackberries.

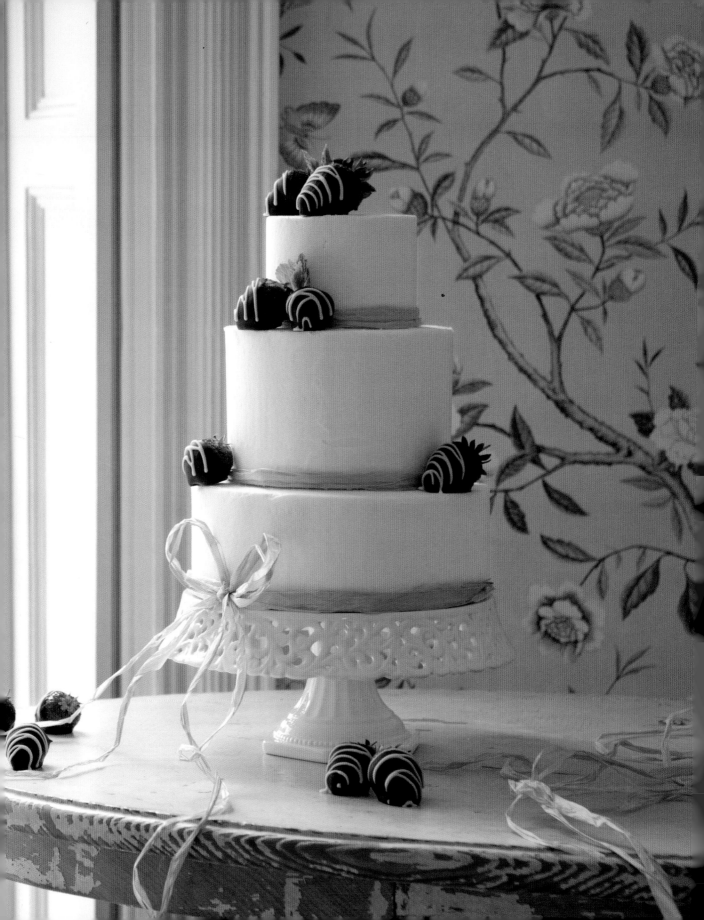

The Cake

The wedding cake has to be the most delicious
element of the day. You can really have fun with it,
regardless of how formal the wedding. There are all
kinds of exciting possibilities, from brightly colored
cupcakes to classic elegance or a modern sculpture in
chocolate. Some of the prettiest cakes I've seen have
been iced plainly, then decorated with soft-petaled
roses, or had each tier topped with close-packed
raspberries. The only limit is your imagination.

Choosing your perfect cake

Everyone loves a wedding cake, and you can find styles to suit the most unusual of celebrations. Some cakes sit happily as part of an afternoon tea at a relaxed summer garden party, while others can take center stage in the grandest country house. You can be greener with your cake by choosing local, seasonal, and ethically sourced ingredients and save pennies by having the cake double as your favors or dessert.

Your cake personality

Your choices of venue, dress, and flowers can help you find your cake "personality." Look for inspiration in your wedding-day notebook (see page 32) and books such as *Cakes for Romantic Occasions* by May Clee-Cadman, which is lovely, and *Cake Chic* by Peggy Porschen. The www.thecaketress.ca Web site has some amazing designs, too. Save offcuts of dress fabrics and ribbon to help when selecting decorations.

At one outdoor wedding, with playful ribbons in the trees and the groom arriving in a decorated camper van, the bride chose a birdcage cake by the Utterly Sexy Café (www.utterlysexycafe.co.uk), iced in pastel blue with ornamental garlands of magenta icing flowers. But if your own dream wedding is more formal and Grace Kelly in style, with a floor-length gown and hundreds of guests, an elegant and traditional white, tiered cake, with fresh white roses, is gorgeous.

Colors and decorations

Cakes can be created in any color imaginable, from bright turquoise to shocking pink. You could even have each tier be a different color. With combinations of icing, ribbons, and flowers, it is easy to match your cake to your wedding color scheme.

For a dramatic look, team a base of black icing with delicate, white, filigree-piped icing (see page 125). This is easy to do at home yet gives a professional result.

If you are not keen on icing, simply stack light sponge cakes. Add a generous dusting of icing sugar and decorate with plump, seasonal berries.

Baking your own cake can be an enjoyable challenge and help your budget, too. You may be surprised at what you or your family can achieve. Alternatives, such as tarts and mousse cakes, can be served as part of a meal.

Remember that your cake needs to feed all of your guests, so calculate quantities carefully. Bear in mind the time of year you are getting married, as the availability of seasonal ingredients will vary.

Professional cake bakers

An online search or asking locally will turn up a host of cake bakers. Prices and ethics vary, so shop around and always check references. Book a tasting session before you order, to try different types of cake and icing, and don't be afraid to ask it they use organic and local ingredients. To reduce your food miles, try to choose a baker who is closer to the venue; some venues will even bake the cake on-site.

If you would like to do the decorating yourself, many bakers will provide a plain iced cake: This keeps costs down, and you can exercise your artistic flair. Alternatively, you can have a homemade cake professionally iced and decorated—ideal if you love your mom's fruit cake but don't want her to worry about her icing skills.

Your ingredients

Maybe you can barter with neighbors for fresh eggs or make your own fruit preserves. Local magazines and Web guides will lead you to nearby farms, mills, and farmers' markets. See the Directory for Web sites listing producers in your area. By taking the time to choose your ingredients carefully, you will rest easy knowing your cake does not have a large carbon footprint or contain synthetic additives—and it will taste great.

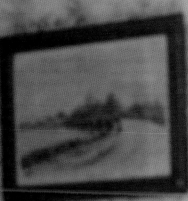

Rachel at Planet Cake (www.planet-cake.com) uses eggs from her own hens. She crafted the flowers from sugar paste, so it's all edible.

Wedding planner tip:
Cover plain cake boards with a layer of white icing to give your display a professional finish.

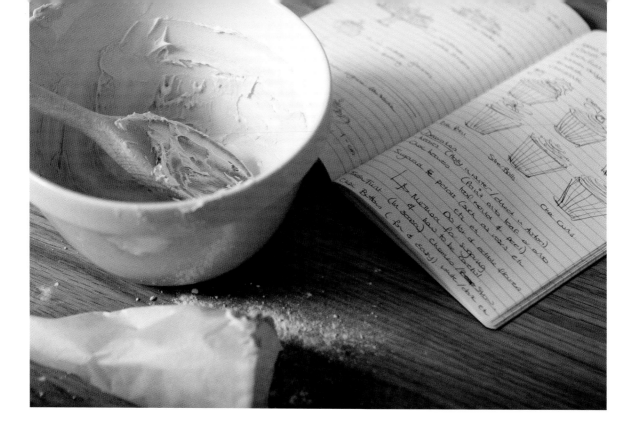

Baking your own cake

Making your own wedding cake needn't be daunting. It means you know exactly what it contains, and you can choose your own favorite recipe. Plan ahead and have a trial run if possible, especially for the decorations. Take photographs of the finished cake, make an equipment and ingredients list, and time the whole procedure. By estimating how long it will take to decorate your final cake, you can calculate when it needs to be baked.

Fruitcake can be kept in an airtight container for weeks but sponge cake only has a shelf life of a few days. If you are planning on keeping a top tier for a christening, always choose fruitcake, as it will freeze easily. For recipes, *Delia's Complete Cookery Course* is my must-have bible. You can make your own decorations (see page 132) or buy them ready-made; with either it's possible to create beautiful designs with minimal effort. The Planet Cake

(www.planet-cake.com) buttercream stack on page 120 shows how simple you can go. Dip strawberries in slightly cooled, melted dark chocolate; leave them to set on wax paper; then zigzag them with melted white chocolate using a piping bag.

Mom's finest

Family members and close friends will be thrilled to be involved and might even make the cake their wedding gift to you. Have a discussion beforehand and show them photos and sketches so that they understand the cake you are envisioning. Renting the baking tins or stands and buying ingredients will help them out. Remember transportation on the day of the wedding: Check if they are happy to deliver the cake to the venue, and provide sturdy boxes or an extra pair of hands if required.

Which style of cake?

Tiered cakes

This formal design usually has three or more tiers of different sizes, suspended above one another on pillars. Always ask for white plaster or timber pillars and timber dowels to keep things natural. Unless you are experienced with tiered cakes, my advice is to leave this style to the professionals. An easy way to create an elegant tiered effect, without the worry, is to use a tiered cake stand. You can rent one of these and then simply place a cake, on its board, on each level.

Stacked

This is a more modern style—most of the tiered cakes shown in this chapter are stacked. Here, the tiers are placed directly one upon the other. When kept simple, this can be a beautiful option, and it can be decorated with elegant trimmings, such as ribbons and vintage jewelry. You still need dowels and boards, but the home cook can easily achieve a two-tier, stacked cake.

Contemporary designs

Many bakers now offer extraordinary contemporary cake designs, from striking sculpted chocolate to edible rice-paper creations. Whether you dream of a breathtaking, long and low, ice-white winter scene or a tall tower of dark chocolate curls, the only limit is your budget.

If baking your own, search in specialist shops for unusual cake-tin shapes, and see page 135 for instructions on making chocolate curls.

Maya made her own wedding cake. Here she is showing filigree icing, using her own design. The dots make it an easy technique to master.

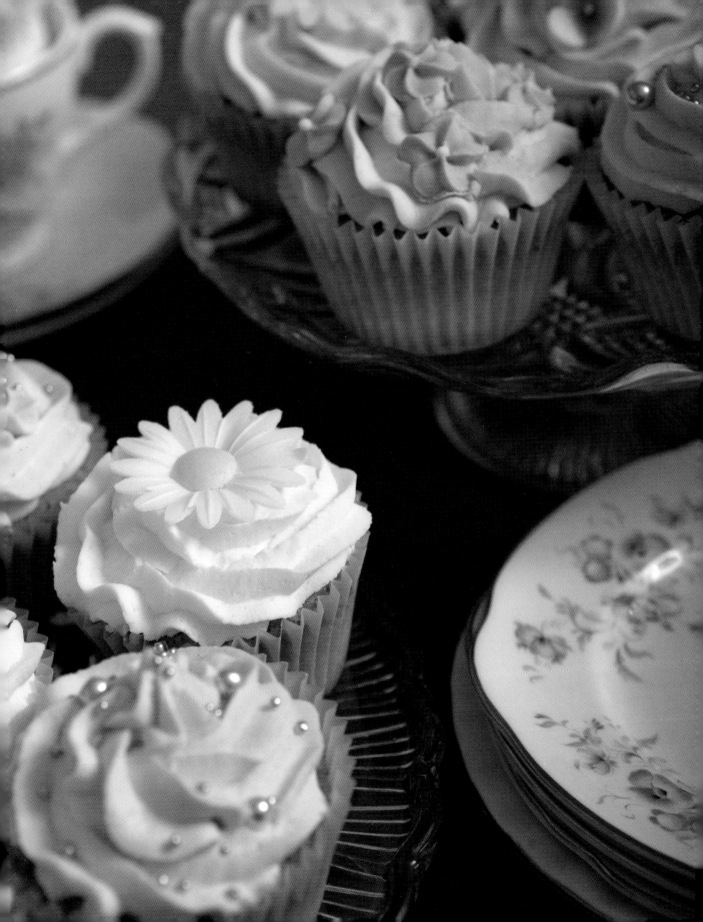

Versatile cupcakes

These colorful cakes have become extremely popular. They can be served as a cake course or pudding, or even used as favors. Recipes range from traditional sponge cakes to minifruitcakes, gluten free to spiced carrot. All can be baked and decorated by the most inexperienced of home cooks, and there will be a flavor to suit each of your guests, regardless of taste or dietary preference. For display ideas, see page 136.

Vintage
Decorate the edge of the paper liners with lace and ribbons, neatly secured with a small dot of icing. Serve on floral vintage crockery with miniature, antique cake forks.

Traditional
Use pure-white icing and select only white decorations, such as small sugar flowers or delicate dots of filigree icing. Try icing and decorating the cakes in three different styles and then mixing them up. White cupcakes on a tiered cake stand can give the impression of a traditional, tiered cake.

Contemporary
Choose bright shades of icing, or even glossy dark chocolate, and combine with fresh flowers in vibrant shades for a dramatic effect. Try placing a fresh flower between each cupcake on a tiered cupcake stand. Arrange the blooms just before serving so that they don't wilt, and check that they are safe to be in contact with food.

Natural
Match vanilla icing with unbleached paper liners and sugared petals made from edible garden flowers that are in season (see page 135). Decorate the stand with raffia for a naturally beautiful display.

Delicious cupcake tips

* Use muffin tins and muffin liners, and fill only halfway. This means you will have room for piped icing.

* Why not gather your bridesmaids and friends for an evening of baking/ Make sure to bake a few extras to "test"!

* Pipe butter icing onto the tops— a star-shaped nozzle is best. Ice from the edge of the paper liners inward.

* Alternatively, "flat ice" the cakes with a small palette knife dipped in hot water.

* You could also pipe on whipped cream and decorate with fresh seasonal fruit— but prepare these cakes at the last minute, and be sure to refrigerate them.

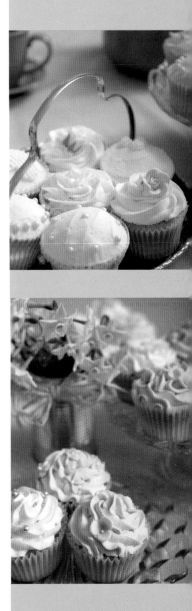

Top: Elegant white from www.countrycupcakes.com.
Above: Sugar flowers are easy to find and quick to apply.

Lou's gluten-free lemon cupcakes

You can find all sorts of options for regular sponge cakes — the classic formula is to weigh three eggs and use the same amount of flour, butter, and sugar. Below, I've given you my favorite gluten-free recipe, as these can be more difficult to track down. This recipe can also be baked in one large tin.

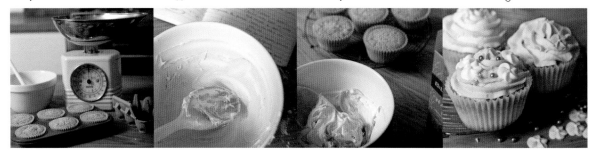

MAKES 12

INGREDIENTS:

Paper muffin liners

1½ stick of unsalted butter

¾ cup superfine sugar

2 beaten eggs

½ cup ground almonds

Finely grated zest and juice of 1 unwaxed lemon

¼ cup gluten-free plain flour

½ teaspoon gluten-free baking powder

5 tablespoons polenta flour

METHOD:

1. Preheat your oven to 350°F.
2. Line a muffin tin with grease-proof muffin liners in a color of your choice (remember, they are going to be on display).
3. Beat the butter and sugar together until pale and creamy, then stir in the eggs and almonds, and then the lemon zest and juice.
4. Sift the gluten-free flour and baking powder into this mixture; add the polenta flour, and stir gently until combined.
5. Carefully spoon the mixture into the muffin liners, being careful not to spill any on the sides. Only fill them halfway (to allow room for the icing).
6. Bake for 20 minutes or until the cupcakes are firm to the touch. If in doubt, gently test with a skewer: if it comes out clean, they are done. (The cakes will have risen but will still be below the tops of the muffin liners.)
7. Transfer to a wire rack and allow to cool completely.

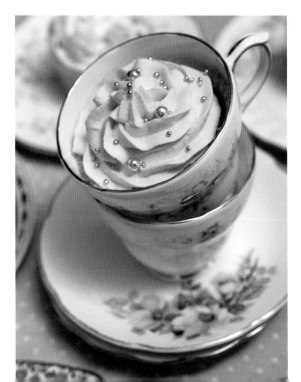

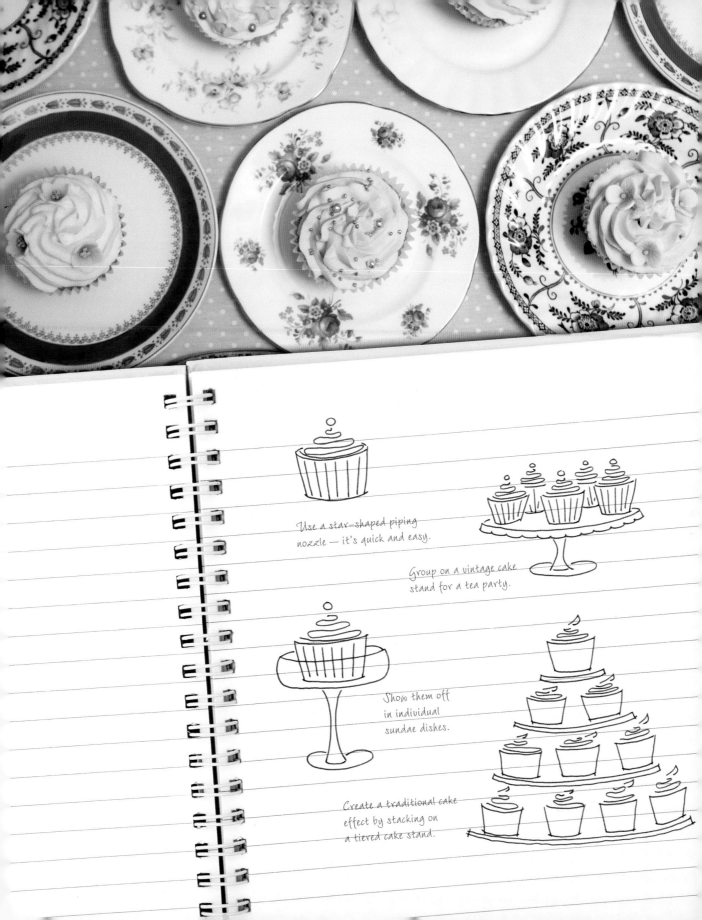

Use a star-shaped piping nozzle — it's quick and easy.

Group on a vintage cake stand for a tea party.

Show them off in individual sundae dishes.

Create a traditional cake effect by stacking on a tiered cake stand.

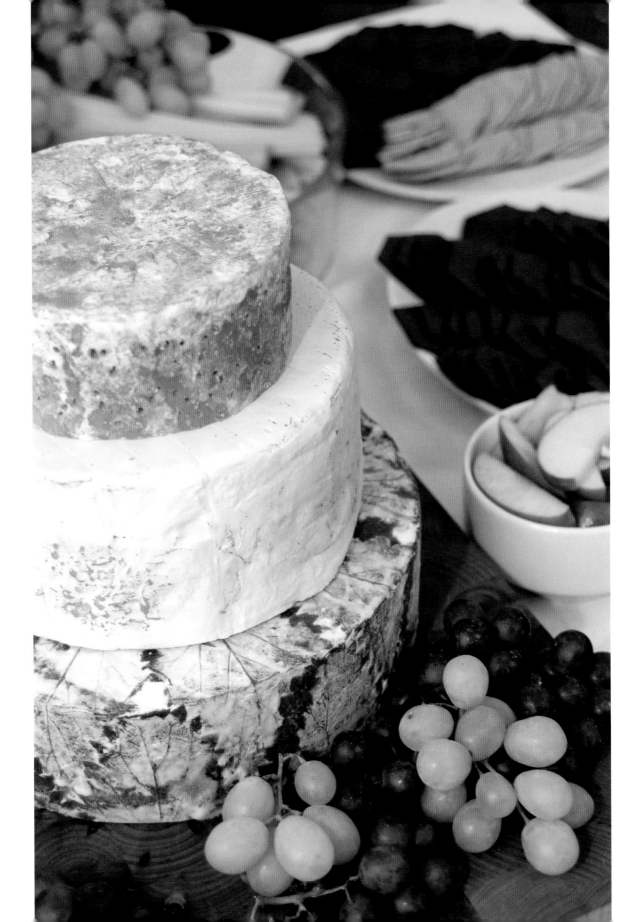

Alternative cakes

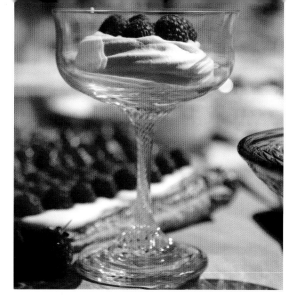

Of course, you don't have to serve cake at all—your wedding is an opportunity to be original. Many of these alternatives can be made by home cooks, although some do require skill. If you would like your tiered wedding cake to double as dessert, choose a sponge recipe and serve with homemade fruit coulis or local ice cream.

The cheese "cake"

Wheels of your favorite local cheeses can be stacked as you would a traditional cake and decorated with fresh flowers or fruits—ideal if you don't have a sweet tooth. Cut in the usual way, and serve to your guests after the meal with homemade crackers and seasonal fruit. (Bear in mind that blue and soft cheeses can have a distinctive scent and are not recommended for pregnant women.)

Fruit tartlets

Tiny mouthfuls of buttery pastry, delicious patisserie cream, and fresh fruit are delightful and easily made at home. Fruit tartlets can be displayed as you would cupcakes (see page 136); include a slightly larger tart for the bride and groom to cut and share.

Minimeringues

These are light and sculptural—and a perfect, thrifty choice. Topped with fresh cream and berries or sugared edible flowers, they can also be your dessert.

Little mousse cakes

These perfectly formed stacks of vanilla sponge, whipped cream, and fresh fruit or chocolate mousse can be assembled with a small, removable patisserie ring (found in cookware shops and online). Dust with powdered sugar and top with chocolate leaves or marzipan fruits for a light and delicious cake substitute, and serve with tea on dainty china. Vary the mousse flavorings to give different colors, such as strawberry pink or blueberry lilac.

Sweet individual cheesecakes

These can look completely at home at a wedding if they are carefully baked and decorated. Mixing dark and white chocolate in your fillings gives a contemporary, marbled effect. If serving as a pudding, add a fruit coulis to cut through the richness and to add a touch of elegance.

Mini wedding cakes

These are literally miniature versions of a full-size cake, with perfectly smooth icing and sumptuous decorations (see page 137). They look elegant stacked on a tall stand and are ideal as favors—but you're best off asking a local cake specialist to make them for you.

A note about chocolate

Cocoa beans come to us from countries with a favorable growing climate, such as Venezuela, so they will always have a larger carbon footprint than local produce. But there are plenty of organic and ethical brands; ideally, check for fair-trade accreditation marks.

If you are feeling adventurous, you could try making your own raw chocolate—it's surprisingly easy. You'll find courses, instructions, and cocoa beans to order online (see www.chocolatealchemy.com or www.williescacao.com). The results are delicious, and you can make them sugar free, too. Plain, raw chocolate is also stocked in health-food shops.

Decorations for your wedding style

From velvety roses to delicate gypsophila, fresh flowers and foliage will give your cake a seasonal, natural charm. There are also many inventive vintage and homemade possibilities. Nonedible decorations will need to be removed before the cake is sliced, so let your caterer know that you want to save them as a memento.

Flowers and fruit

Make the most of seasonal blooms. The cake on the opposite page has been dressed with flowers that can easily be found in the late spring: early roses, and white lilac and bluebells from a friend's garden. If you are on a budget, you could choose a small posy for your bouquet and transfer it to the top of the cake after the ceremony. Some flowers, such as nasturtiums, are edible, but make sure that any flowers you use have been grown without pesticides.

Colorful fruit can turn a plain cake into a culinary masterpiece. Heap seasonal, ripe berries onto each tier of a stacked cake and dust with powdered sugar for a mouthwatering, professional display.

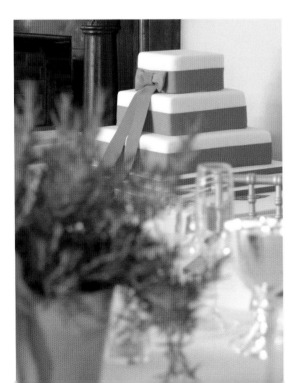

Raffia

One of the natural products I like best, raffia can be used to great effect on cakes of all types. For simple country chic, take about twenty long strands and tie them in a big bow around the waist of a white, iced cake.

Vintage jewelry

If you are wearing vintage jewelry with your wedding outfit, you could incorporate a matching brooch into the design of your cake. Marcasite and anything sparkly works well, particularly antique dress clips and buckles. Tie a long satin ribbon around the top tier of your cake and fix your find to the center of the bow for instant glamour.

Ribbons and trims

Search online shops and visit vintage fairs for all manner of trimmings, from ribbons and tassels to Christmas bells. A large, blousy antique silk flower looks fabulous on the top tier of a cake, teamed with vintage ribbons in a matching color. Or make your own sugar-paste ribbons and bows, as seen on the cake pictured on the left (see page 134 for how to do it).

Tea lights

These are stunning for a late-evening wedding. Place the tea lights in small, clear glass holders; site them on the top tier of a royal, iced cake; and surround with small, fresh flowers. Be sure to choose unscented, plant-wax candles, and check that other decorations are not flammable.

Paper flowers

If you love trying new crafts, try making beautiful paper flowers for your cake (see the paper-flower bouquet on page 163). There are courses and many books on the subject that include patterns. You could even fold origami flowers from edible rice paper.

A beginner's guide to icing types

Royal icing

Traditional, hard sugar icing, usually bright white.
Fairly easy to make and use if you have a steady
hand and the right equipment, but it sets like rock.
Royal icing can only be used with fruitcakes, which
must be covered with marzipan first.

Sugar paste (regal ice)

A soft, roll-out icing. Popular and easier to use than
royal icing, it gives a rounded edge to the cake
tiers. You can decorate the cake by crimping:
making small, decorative pinches with a tool
found in sugar-craft supply shops.

Pastillage

Absolutely beautiful. An advanced technique
in which sugar dough is formed into intricate
sculptures. I would advise you to take a course if
you want to learn the skills.

Butter icing

Delicious and easy to whip up. Usually used for
small cakes or large sponge cakes, it can give
a sharp edge to the tiers. The UK version is ivory
colored and has a short shelf life due to the
butter content. US buttercream often uses white
vegetable shortening for a purer white icing.

Recognize this cake? It's the same basic,
butter-iced stack shown on page 120. Rachel
from Planet Cake has made a space with two cake
boards for florist Tallulah Rose to fill with flowers.

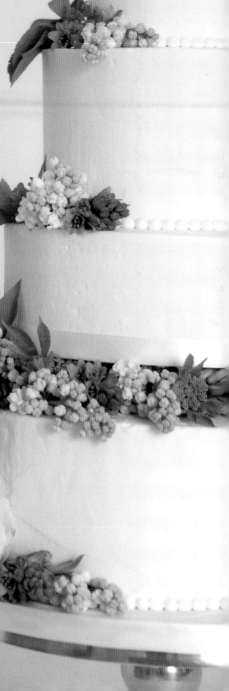

Sugar paste, glitter, and chocolate curls

Edible decorations are ideal for a natural wedding—at the end of the big day, whatever is not eaten will biodegrade. It is easy to make your own, but if you are not sure of your sugar-crafting skills, you can also buy ready-made sugar flowers and decorations.

Edible cake toppers
Sugar-paste figurines of the happy couple are available ready-made in a range of styles to match your theme, or you could have a go at making your own. You can also buy sugar flowers of many kinds (the roses on this page came from a local shop).

Glitter you can eat
Edible glitter is a relatively new concept in cake decorating but is proving popular as a dusting for cupcakes and to give a sparkle when added to the icing of larger cakes. You can find glitter made from natural gum arabic as well as from sugar.

How to make sugar-paste bows
A simple yet extremely elegant way to decorate a plain cake with the minimum of fuss. Tint some sugar-paste icing to match your wedding accent color and roll out to about ¼ inch thick.

Cut long, straight ribbon strips of matching width (1 inch works well) and secure them around the bottom of your cake tiers with a little sieved apricot jam. Make a bow using the same width strips and allow it to dry and harden before fixing it to the cake. Cut the ends of the bow into little Vs for a professional finish. These work particularly well on square, tiered cakes.

Edible decoration ideas

* Giant chocolate buttons—choose organic fair-trade chocolate in white, milk, or dark

* Seasonal fresh fruit

* Chocolate shapes and leaves—make your own or buy from online stores that promote fair trade

* Sugared edible flowers

* Rice-paper flowers—easy to make (or buy) and highly decorative

* Sugar-paste ribbons and bows

* Edible glitter

Make your own chocolate curls

YOU WILL NEED:

Fair-trade organic chocolate (dark should be 70 percent cocoa solids)

A cold, hard surface, such as a granite countertop or a chilled baking sheet

A sharp knife and flexible palette knife

Wax paper for the finished curls

METHOD:

1. Melt the chocolate slowly in a double boiler (or in a bowl over a pan of just-simmering water), stirring gently with a wooden spoon.

2. Take off the heat and spread the chocolate onto the cold surface in a thin layer using the palette knife. Allow to cool.

3. Once cooled and solid—but not rock hard—use a sharp knife or cheese shaver to scrape up into individual curls. Place on wax paper to set in a cool place or in the fridge for a couple of hours.

Make your own edible sugared petals

YOU WILL NEED:

Wax paper

Superfine sugar

1 egg white and a few drops of water

Three handfuls of fresh, edible flower petals, washed and patted dry

Small artist's paintbrush

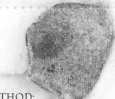

Wedding planner tip:

For a professional touch, marble the chocolate for decorations such as leaves or curls by partially mixing white and dark.

METHOD:

1. Put a sheet of wax paper on a baking tray and dust with sugar.

2. Lightly whisk the egg white and water in a bowl until just frothing, then paint the mixture onto the petals in a thin layer. Hold the bottom tip of the petal carefully in your fingers or with a pair of tweezers. Be careful to cover the whole petal surface with egg white, or your flowers will brown.

3. Dust the petals with sugar, and place them on the wax paper. Repeat, then allow to dry completely in a warm, dry place. They keep for a few days in a dry, airtight container but will go soggy in the fridge.

Showing off your cake

A wedding cake can make a wonderful centerpiece for your celebration. Elaborate icing deserves to be fully appreciated, so try placing your cake in front of a vintage mirror to allow your guests to see all angles. For a relaxed outdoor reception, you can achieve a more rustic look by setting your cake on a tree stump or upturned antique vegetable crate. Make sure that it is level and out of the way of inquisitive children and pets.

If you are having a small wedding with one long trestle table of friends and relatives, position the cake in the middle as a focal point, and surround it with flowers, foliage, and candles. This works particularly well for winter and Christmas-themed weddings, and it means the cake will be center stage in photos.

Imaginative touches

Flowers, foliage, clean driftwood and shells, leaves, petals, and fruit will all create beautiful and unusual displays around the base of your cake. Save magazine pictures and look at www.devondriftwooddesigns.com for inspiration. Ivy cascading down the length of a table makes for a magical effect.

Any individual cake, whether it's a cupcake, tartlet, minimeringue, or pastry, can be presented as a favor for a guest. If the cake is delicate, or you are worried about flying insects, place it in a clear cellophane bag tied with a ribbon or raffia. Cellophane is made from plant cellulose and is fully biodegradable.

For unusual and theatrical table settings, serve cupcakes in vintage teacups, or group perfect minicakes on vintage shelves or in an apothecary's chest.

I always enjoy hunting around flea markets and antique centers, and collecting Victorian tiered wire and wrought-iron plant stands. These work beautifully as alternative cake stands. Clean thoroughly and revive with a coat or two of natural paint; afterward, you can reuse the stand for your plants.

Displaying cupcakes

❋ Show them on vintage, glass cake stands or plates gathered from thrift stores or flea markets—keep an eye out for rare colored glass. Group the stands together in threes for a stylish effect.

❋ Rent a professional, tiered cupcake stand. These are available in anything from three tiers to eight. You can decorate the edge of each level with a thin ribbon in a complementary color.

❋ Use a Wilton stand. This is a professional wire stand that holds each individual cupcake at a slight angle, like branches on a tree. It is a good option if you are only having a small number of cakes, but make sure the stand you order is for the correct number.

❋ Be bold and line your cakes up along a narrow table. Interweave them with flowers, petals, leaves, ivy, and raffia.

❋ Place a small flag or sail in each cake with the name of the guest. Alternatively, have the names iced directly onto the cakes as edible place "cards."

❋ Serve in pretty 1950s glass sundae dishes as a thrifty dessert.

❋ Add interest with gorgeous cupcake wrappers. Available in recycled paper in pretty and intricate designs, such as butterflies, you wrap them around the plain liners to add a professional finish. Try making your own from real petal paper for a thrifty cake upgrade; find templates and instructions online. You can scallop the edges with craft scissors.

Rachel made several variations of these
Planet Cake blossom minicakes, and
we displayed them in a set of vintage
champagne saucers.

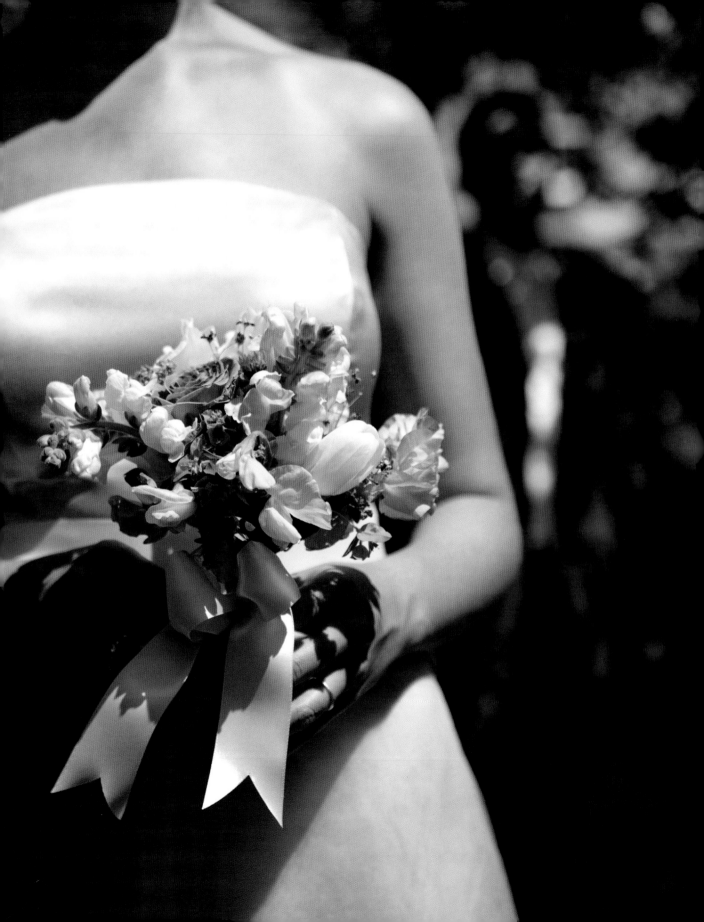

* **Seasonal blooms**
  Local and organic flowers, working with a florist, and DIY workshops

* **Growing and sourcing flowers**
  From delicate wildflowers to elegant lilies

* **The perfect bouquet**
  Styles for all dress shapes, and how to tie your own gorgeous bouquet

* **Individual displays**
  Unusual and inventive ways to "dress" your wedding with flowers

* **Herbs, pots, and foliage**
  Delicious table herbs and decorative ideas for foliage

* **Petal confetti and giving flowers away**
  What could be more natural than petals? Presenting your confetti with style.

The Flowers

Local and seasonal flowers, and cottage garden and prairie blooms, are in vogue—and not just at green weddings. The beauty of seasonal flowers is that the variety and color palette change throughout the year. I love the seasonality of flowers, and choosing a species associated with a particular time—early spring anemones or midsummer poppies—means that the bloom will always remind you of your wedding date.

Seasonal blooms

Seasonal flowers are the best choice for a natural wedding, especially when grown locally. There are gorgeous natural options in every season (take a look at the Seasonal Flowers calendar on page 217 for inspiration). The hellebores used as hair decorations on page 183 bloom from late winter, while evergreen foliage and fruits can be used to make stunning displays.

Themes throughout the year
- ❋ Spring: early flowering bulb plants in unusual pots, such as brightly colored hyacinths
- ❋ Summer: vintage vases filled with roses, peonies, and sweet peas
- ❋ Autumn: big bunches of golden sunflowers or late-season rich colors and seed heads
- ❋ Winter: festive wreaths with rosehips, crab apples, fir cones, and cinnamon sticks, or hand-crafted paper flowers (see page 163)

Most store-bought cut flowers travel hundreds, if not thousands, of miles by air or sea, creating an enormous carbon footprint. Instead, buy local flowers from farmers' markets and smaller, cottage-garden growers. Seasonal blooms are less expensive and often fresher, too.

Organic, fair-trade, and biodynamic flowers
Look for flowers certified by organizations such as the Soil Association or USDA, or grown biodynamically under the Demeter mark, which have not been sprayed with pesticides. If you have your heart set on a flower that isn't in season at the time of your wedding, try buying fair-trade blooms. There are many other ethical and ecocertification systems worldwide, so check for their marks (see pages 110 and 217 for more information).

Floral workshops
Why not create your own wedding flowers? Once you know the basics, you can easily make arrangements, boutonnieres, and posies. Floristry workshops are a great place to find out tricks of the trade, the equipment required, and which flowers complement one another. My friend and talented florist Rachel, from Tallulah Rose Flower School in Bath, England, taught me how to make the hand-tied bouquet shown on pages 146–147.

Jane Packer's *Flower Course* is an excellent book full of hints and tips, and among Paula Pryke's titles, I particularly recommend *Wreaths and Bouquets*.

Planning with a florist
You may wish to employ a professional florist, especially for a large celebration. Good florists are worth their weight in gold and can create breathtaking arrangements to suit your wedding style and budget. Choose one who can provide you with seasonal flowers, preferably from a local source, and follow-up references. Flowers can be one of the most expensive wedding services, so ensure that you have a budget in mind before you meet. And take along a picture of your wedding gown and proposed hairstyle to help determine the design of your bouquet.

Wedding flowers
- ❋ Bridal bouquet
- ❋ Bridesmaids' bouquets and men's boutonnieres
- ❋ Flower-girl posy or willow wand
- ❋ Church arrangements
- ❋ Pew ends or chair decorations
- ❋ Table centerpieces and mantelpiece displays

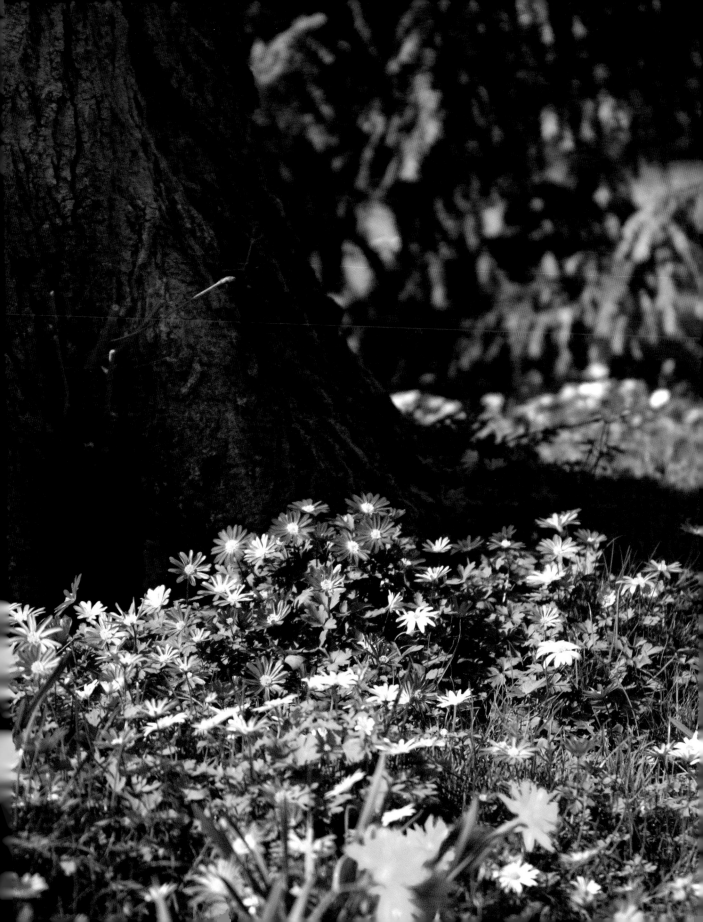

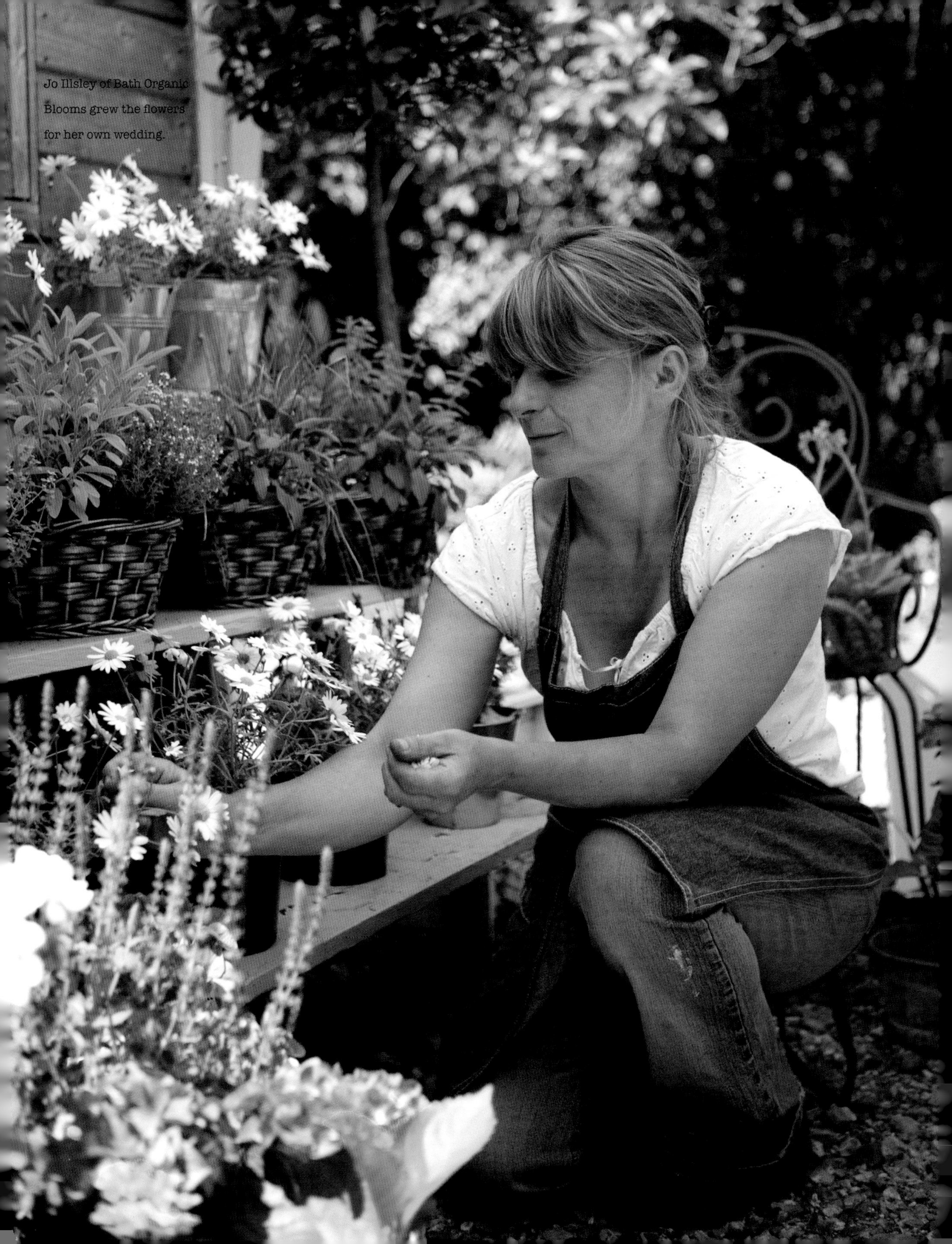

Jo Ilsley of Bath Organic Blooms grew the flowers for her own wedding.

Growing and sourcing flowers

Even if you are a novice gardener, it is relatively easy to grow your own flowers to cut and arrange in vases, or to raise plants and herbs to display in their pots. You can glean ideas from open gardens and plant nurseries and borrow books such as Sarah Raven's *The Cutting Garden*. If you are planning your wedding a year in advance, see what is in bloom in the month you are marrying. Friends may have established plants already in their gardens or be happy to plant some for you. Join an organic gardening organization to get advice and referrals.

If you are lucky enough to have a yard or a good-sized kitchen garden, set aside one bed for your wedding flowers in the weeks leading up to the big day. Saving seeds or joining a local seed swap, where you swap spare seeds with like-minded people, are thrifty options.

Wildflowers

Although it is tempting, never pick wildflowers while out on country walks. Take photographs instead. Wildflowers, such as cow parsley, are an enormous benefit to local wildlife and support natural ecosystems. If you would like to display wildflowers at your celebration, grow your own at home for harvesting before the big day. Seeds are available from garden centers or online sources such as www.organiccatalog.com and can be grown with little effort. Or, buy them from cottage-garden growers.

Wildflowers are extremely delicate and can wilt shortly after cutting, so grow them in unusual pots and containers and, instead, display the flowers as growing plants.

Farmers' markets

These are wonderful places to buy local flowers directly from the growers. Imagine galvanized buckets full of wide-open anemones or bunches of vibrant cornflowers tied with raffia. Take a camera and ask questions about the flowers' origins and longevity. Many growers will be able

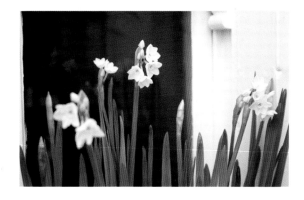

to take orders for collection the day before the wedding. When buying local, seasonal flowers, bear in mind that weather conditions may affect what is available.

Cottage-garden flowers

In colors from pure white through to sugar pinks and pale lilacs, on to deep purples, I love fragrant sweetpeas. Try using a single color for an elegant but informal bridal bouquet. Cut the stems quite short, and tie them with wide, satin ribbons for a professional finish.

Dried flowers and wheat sheaves

Naturally dried wheat sheaves, barley sheaves, poppy heads, and teasels can be bunched together, as you would a hand-tied bouquet, and secured with raffia or ribbon as a centerpiece. For a more elaborate display, mix in fresh blooms such as roses or lavender. A mini version makes a lovely, country-style bridal posy.

Wedding planner tip:
Calla lilies are easy to grow at home and make a striking bridal bouquet, suitable for the most glamorous of weddings.

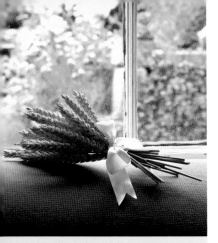

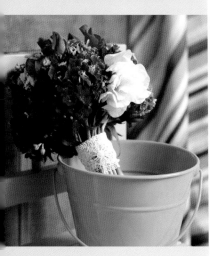

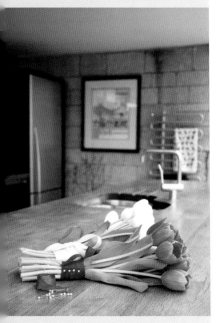

Your bouquet style

The shape and color of your bridal bouquet or posy will be guided by your dress. Have you chosen a formal gown, which will be best complemented by an elegant bouquet filled with structured flowers and foliage? Usually, these bouquets feature a single color theme. Or, will you be wearing a cocktail, prom-style, or flowing empire-line dress, which will be enhanced by a gentle, delicate posy? For these styles, you could try wildflowers or cottage garden blooms in a mix of colors, loosely tied together.

Bouquets for dress styles
* Formal: hand-tied bouquets
* Prom style: spherical posies or pomanders
* Empire: single flower

More petite brides benefit from teardrop-shaped bouquets to lengthen their frame, while taller brides can carry off spherical arrangements with ease.

Don't forget that bouquets, like dresses, can be embellished to match your theme. You could include vintage lace (which has been used to wrap the sweet william bouquet to the left), antique brooches, or an heirloom silk flower.

Bridesmaids
Usually bridesmaids will carry a smaller version of the bridal bouquet. As an alternative, think about pomanders, corsages, or posies, and keep to the same color scheme but vary your choice of flowers.

Flower girls
Small posies or pomanders, or even decorated willow wands, make perfect floral accessories for children. Make sure that they are reasonably robust, as they will inevitably be thrown around with exuberance on the day.

Boutonnieres for the seasonal groom
Boutonnieres can add a special touch to a groom's outfit. Traditionally, boutonnieres are worn on the left, and the groom has a more elaborate design than his best man, ushers, and groomsmen.

Herbs make fabulous boutonnieres, whether teamed with a flower head or on their own. Rosemary signifies remembrance, so if there are family or friends who cannot be there, this is a nice way to remember them. Avoid using large, open blooms as these can

Wellington boots

Clean Wellington boots filled with flowers make a humorous and charming display. Although waterproof, the boots can be unstable when filled with water. To steady them, first fill the bottoms with heavy stones. Choose cottage-garden colors, arrange the flowers in a loose style, and set the Wellies on your tables. If you love this idea but are not keen on having boots on your tables, stand them in doorways and in corners to catch guests' eyes.

Jam jars

For an outdoor wedding, a wonderful way to denote an "aisle" is to hang recycled jam jars, filled with flowers, on wooden stakes or poles. To create a hook for the jar, tie floristry or recycled wire around the neck and twist it into a hook or handle. Short-stemmed sweet peas, cornflowers, and peonies look amazing displayed in this way. For a fairy-woodland theme, use minijars and single blooms hung on willow branches.

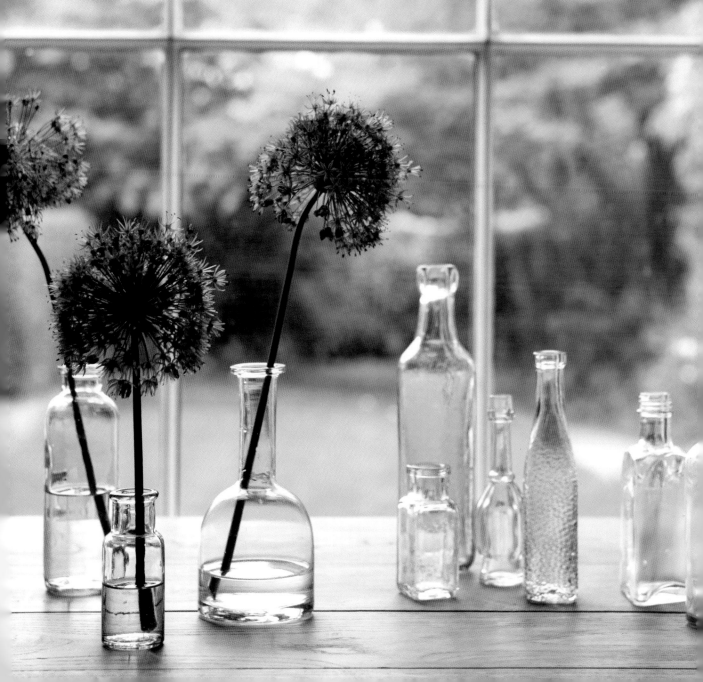

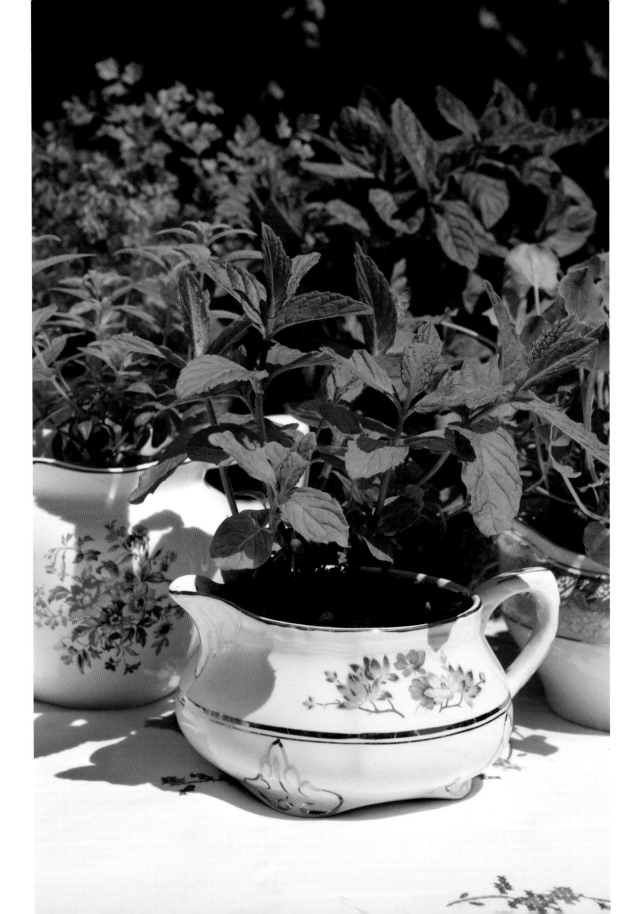

Herbs, pots, and foliage

One of the most ecofriendly ways to incorporate flowers into your celebration is by using potted plants and herbs. This allows them to go on living after the wedding and leaves no waste. At the end of the day, give your decorations to guests as lasting keepsakes.

Herbs as flowers and to eat

Herbs are some of my favorite wedding flowers, as they are so incredibly versatile. Sweet-scented herbs, such as lavender and rosemary, make gorgeous displays, while others, such as thyme and basil, can be eaten as part of the meal: Encourage guests to pick off the fresh leaves to accompany their food. (A zingy, home-grown tomato tart is enhanced by a few tender basil leaves, while rock hyssop is delicious on risottos.)

For table centers, you could plant herbs in antique terra-cotta pots tied with vintage ribbons, or choose herbs that come in natural coir pots. Decorate these biodegradable containers with natural raffia for a fully plantable decoration. You can also buy your own natural coir pots online from ecogarden suppliers: Choose minipots for small herb varieties or large ones for centerpieces. Try unusual containers, too, such as food tins with the labels removed, or vintage teapots.

Branches and blossoms

All year round, you will find interesting foliage in the garden, both evergreen and deciduous. If you are marrying in the spring, take advantage of the abundant blossoms on trees and bushes, from bright yellow forsythia to pale pink cherry.

Bare winter twigs and branches pruned from garden trees can be decorated with lanterns or with fresh flowers hung in minijars, for a fashionable room display. Boughs of catkins, soft leaf buds, or tiny blossoms look fabulous in tall enamel jugs or old milk churns.

Unusual pot plantings

From brightly colored daisies to tall, waving sunflowers, mini rose bushes to deep purple hyacinths, you can present growing flowers in interesting pots and containers.

❊ Group pots of small plants in odd numbers on tables. For a modern feel, use pots of the same size lined up in rows; for a country look, use different sizes grouped more loosely.

❊ For an outdoor wedding, plant small flower varieties in vintage wooden seed trays. Place these on the centers of the tables, and decorate them with matching ribbons.

❊ Use vintage ceramic vases as pots, and plant with wildflowers to bloom in time for your wedding.

❊ Daffodils, hyacinths, and snowdrops make an uplifting springtime display. Plant them into unusual containers, such as vintage tins and wooden bowls.

Evergreen ivy

Whatever the time of year, ivy can be found scrambling up walls and covering the ground, and it is easy to cultivate at home. Team it with large blooms, such as roses, for an elegant look, or with wildflowers for a more rustic feel. One couple on a tight budget was holding their reception on a barge. I draped the cabin with muslin and ivy bunches, transforming it from a plain, utilitarian interior into a mini wedding marquee.

Wind ivy around staircases and along tea light–dotted mantelpieces for a winter theme, or use it as the base for a wreath with pine cones and cinnamon sticks. (Check beforehand that you are not allergic to ivy.)

Petal confetti and giving flowers away

Biodegradable confetti is the only choice for a natural wedding. Don't be tempted to ask the guests to throw rice after the ceremony. Wild birds tend to eat it, and then it swells in their stomachs. Instead, choose natural petal confetti, either fresh or dried. It can be found in every color imaginable, to match any wedding theme. Some dried petal confetti will stain if it becomes wet, so if you are worried about rain, choose white petals to avoid accidents.

Dried petal confetti

As dried petals are much lighter than fresh, they take longer to fall through the air, giving more opportunity to catch that confetti photograph. The beautiful confetti on the opposite page came from British company Shropshire Petals. Here is a guide to the different colors available:

❁ Pinks: roses, peonies, hydrangeas, heather
❁ Blues: hydrangeas, delphiniums
❁ Yellows: sunflowers, roses, jasmine
❁ Oranges: marigolds, roses
❁ Whites: delphiniums, roses, hydrangeas
❁ Lilacs: hydrangeas, lavender
❁ Reds: roses, hydrangeas
❁ Greens: roses, hydrangeas

Fresh petals

The best flowers for fresh confetti are roses of any type—even the small, tight ones—as they have lots of petals. About twelve roses should be enough for a large basketful. You could ask local flower stalls for blooms past their best at the end of the day, which would otherwise be disposed of. Florists can also provide fresh petal confetti, as they may have flowers that are not good enough quality for displays, but are fine for use as confetti.

How to make fresh confetti

❁ Take two bunches of garden, local, or fair-trade roses.
❁ Wrap your hand around the whole flower head.
❁ Pull gently, in a twisting motion.
❁ The petals should come off in one bunch, leaving behind the center part of the bloom.
❁ Gently separate the petals into a bowl, basket, or paper cones.

Displaying and distributing your confetti

To minimize paper wastage, place your petals in one big glass bowl or basket, and ask guests to help themselves. Or give your flower girl a pretty basket of confetti that she can hand out to guests as they leave the ceremony. For an outdoor wedding, she could scatter petals down the "aisle."

Alternatively, you could make your own confetti cones out of recycled or handmade petal paper and arrange them in a basket, box, or bowl. A nice touch is to make the cones from seed paper containing the seeds of your confetti flowers (see page 94). Guests can then take home the cones and plant their own confetti.

After the big day

You may have decided to give all of your flower displays to guests, but if not, you could ask one of your bridesmaids to take them to a local retirement home. Displays will often last for a good week after the wedding. Floral arrangements made for churches and chapels may be left at the venue for other congregations to enjoy; check that the church is happy for you to do this. Table confetti, cake flowers, and displays that have been out of water for some time should be composted, but remember to keep any trimmings, such as ribbons, for reuse.

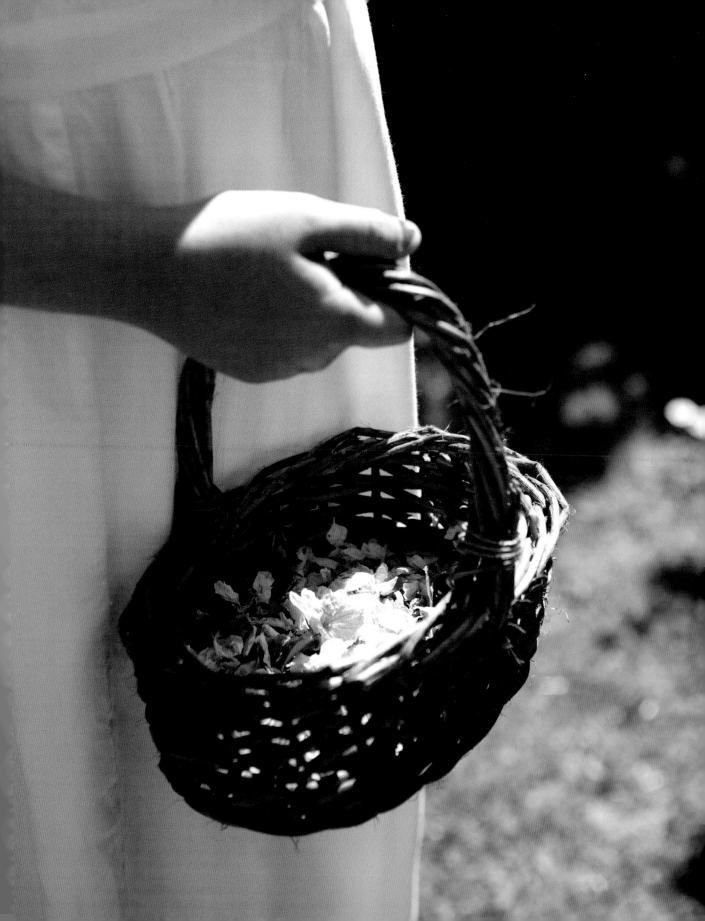

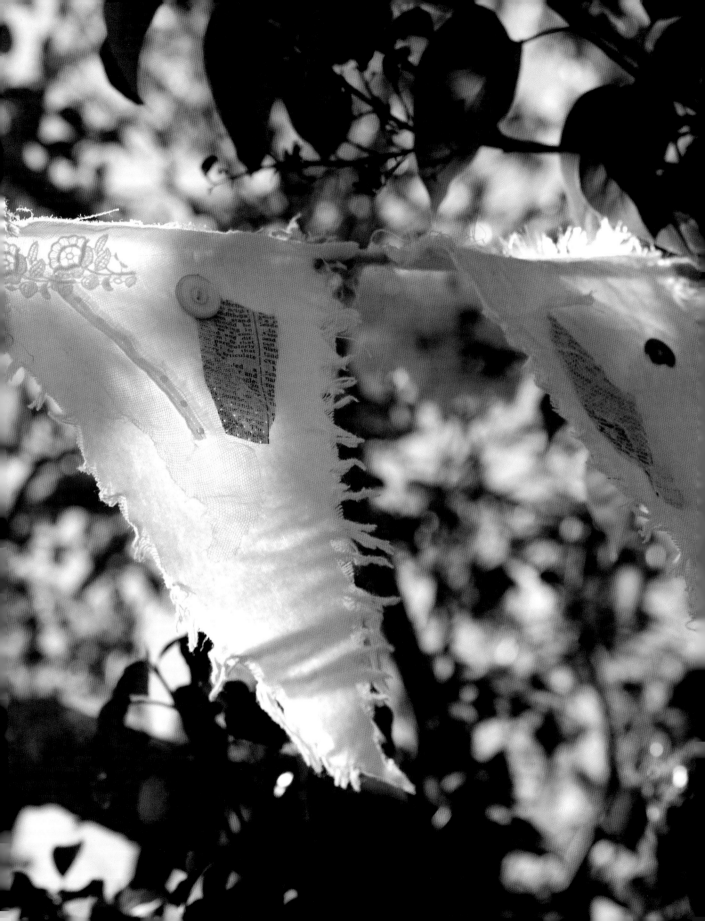

The Decorations

Choosing a seasonal or vintage theme will make your decorations eye-catching without costing a fortune. Search out the best green suppliers and products hand-crafted by artisans, or try making your own. Decorating your wedding, whether a simple ceremony or a lavish celebration, with flair, will wow your guests and give your day its own unique atmosphere. And it is simpler than you might think to achieve a beautiful, natural wedding setting.

Natural decorations

Fruits, flowers, and foliage can all be used to style a wedding day (for more about flower displays, see page 148). Collect and beachcomb driftwood, pebbles, leaves, and twigs. By using objects from nature, sourced locally, you can be sure that your trimmings will have a minimal carbon footprint and will biodegrade or that they can be returned to their environment.

Ways with fruits, flowers, and foliage

❋ Fruit: Use as place holders by tying miniature luggage tags onto the stems. Guests can eat the fruit as part of the meal.

❋ Driftwood: Place clean, pale driftwood down the center of a long table and intersperse it with plant-wax tea lights.

❋ Leaves: Scatter russet or golden dried leaves on the tables, or wrap fresh leaves around candles.

❋ Blossoms: Gather blossoms and scatter them on tables and in gardens.

❋ Pebbles: Use as place holders by either painting on the name of the guest or tying on a small tag with rustic twine.

Beach weddings

Let your imagination fly with what is naturally available. Build sand castles with intricately molded buckets and jewel them with collected shells; they could outline an "aisle" or standing area. Draw patterns in the sand, gather pebbles to make heart shapes, and tie reclaimed fabric onto willow twigs to make gently swaying flags or wind catchers. Group together flowers and beachcombed driftwood in tin cans.

Seasonal ideas

❋ Spring: dainty wildflowers, spring bulbs, and pots of grasses and herbs. Choose from sweet-scented jasmine; exotic-looking hellebores; magnificent magnolia blossoms; and fresh, green foliage.

❋ Summer: bunting in the trees, antique galvanized watering cans bursting with local flowers, and potted strawberry plants from which guests may help themselves.

❋ Autumn: rich, red leaves and glossy berries; deep-colored blooms and willow twigs; teasels and other dried seed heads; pumpkins; decorative squashes; and rosy apples.

❋ Winter: plant-wax candles; log fires; storm lanterns; holly; winter-white flowers; natural ivy; fir cones; cinnamon sticks; and rich, sumptuous ribbons.

Trees and herb favors

Tiny trees in plantable coir pots make fabulous favors that will last a lifetime. Choose a native species, or try raising your own baby saplings from acorns and collected seeds. Baby herb plants are wonderful gifts, too; grow them in small, antique terra-cotta pots or present the plants in burlap bags. To make the bag, cut a square of natural burlap four times the width of the root ball, pop the herb roots into the center, and gather up the corners. Tie a piece of string, ribbon, or twine around the neck and fasten in a bow. See *Jekka's Complete Herb Book* and www.jekkasherbfarm.com for varieties and advice.

6

5

Wedding planner tip:
Recycle Christmas decorations for a festive
theme—place delicate glass baubles in tall,
clear vases for a striking centerpiece.

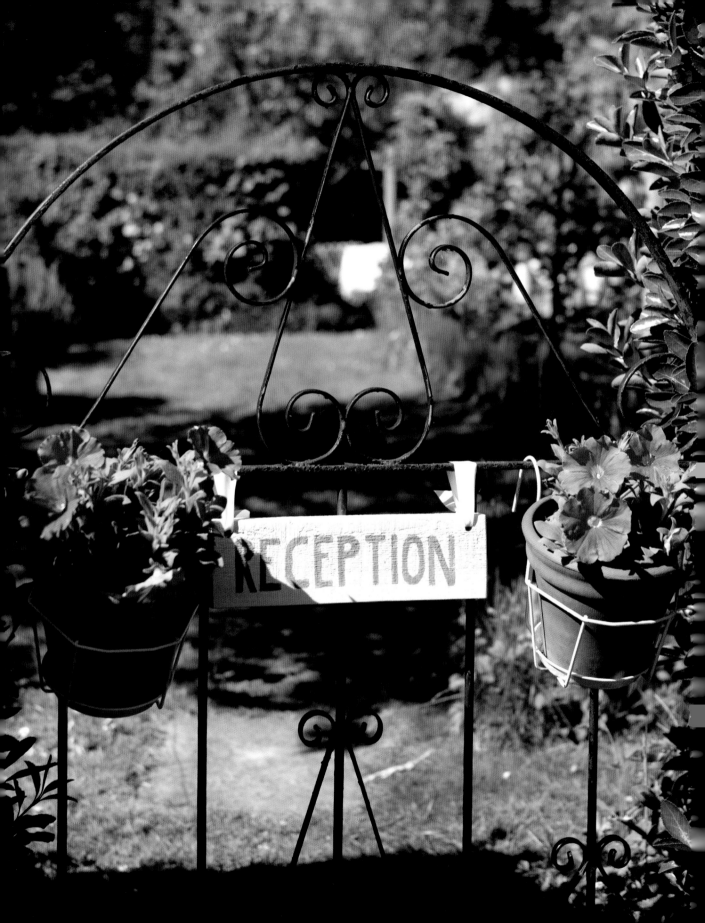

Original and unusual

Stage a wonderful display with antique planters, old jam jars, and even bicycles—see if salvaged and recycled bits and pieces can be given new leases on life. We created the wedding notice on the left with two flea market–bought French wire plant holders and a handmade wooden sign, painted with natural paints.

For the garden-party wedding that you see throughout the book, I covered wooden trestle tables with plain white tablecloths, then laid beautiful vintage and secondhand lace cloths over the top. Cut-glass vases and jugs, collected over the years, were filled with country-style flowers, from blousy pink peonies to fragrant white stocks. In between these, I arranged old glass and silver candlesticks holding plant-wax candles.

The places were set with mismatched vintage crockery, and the look was completed by my homemade napkins, in different fabrics, tied with offcuts of ribbon. The result is something you could create yourself—add your own original elements and personality.

Sky lanterns

Drifting skyward on a summer evening, sky lanterns are a magical, romantic decoration. Made from paper, with a beeswax disk that you light to send them into the air, they are silent and completely biodegradable. They are much more environmentally friendly than fireworks, which will scare wildlife. Visit www.skylanterns.com, who delivers worldwide.

Ribbons in trees

For a seaside wedding, I decorated the branches of the surrounding trees with vintage and recycled ribbons and pretty glass lanterns. It worked for both daytime and evening. So quick and easy to put up, ribbons are a cost-effective decoration and look fabulous if cut long so that they can catch the breeze. Choose colors to complement your theme.

Bicycles

If your style of dress allows it, arrive at your wedding on a bike, with veil flying, for an amazing photo opportunity. Embellish your cycle to make it the perfect wedding transportation.

- ❋ Baskets: Fill the front basket with armfuls of seasonal blooms.
- ❋ Panniers: Secure the bridal bouquet onto the rear pannier.
- ❋ Signs: Direct guests to the reception with your bike. Hang a sign from the crossbar and decorate it with flowers and foliage.

Handmade wooden signs

If you need signs for your event, why not make your own from timber? Salvage wood—preferably planks with the bark still on the edges—and use a soldering iron to "write" onto the surface for a rustic effect. You could also use large printing stamps with waterproof inks or paints.

Mirrors

Prop antique or vintage mirrors from thrift stores and online auctions behind displays of flowers to create an illusion of depth. Or lay them flat and arrange pillar candles on top to reflect the light and, more practically, catch any wax drips. You can always change the color of the frames by repainting them.

Wedding planner tip:
Place jam-jar lanterns next to marquee tent pegs to help guests avoid tripping over the ropes at night.

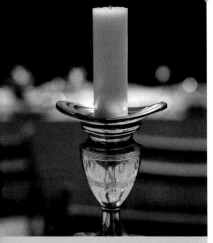

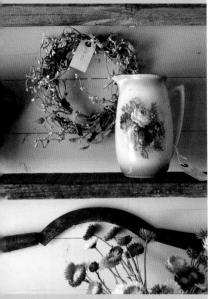

Vintage themes

From 1970s flower power to 1950s chic to delicate Victoriana—vintage elements can fit both traditional and alternative weddings. If you are not sure where to start, find a vintage object that you adore, such as a teacup or candlestick, and build your decoration style around it.

Crockery

I love vintage—especially crockery. Everything from tea sets to cake stands, glassware to milk jugs. I started collecting years ago and now have a huge chest filled with my finds, which I rent to couples for their wedding or party (you can see a few of these pieces pictured on the opposite page and on page 171).

For your own, look in junk shops, at trunk sales, and in thrift stores to deck out your wedding at minimal cost. Don't forget that you can always sell crockery afterward. Once friends and family know that you are collecting for your big day, you will probably be showered with their collections to borrow or keep. Mix and match designs for a deliciously eclectic look, and place vintage teacup candles (see page 164) on shelves and tables, and in gardens. See the Directory for vintage rental companies.

Ornaments

Antique and vintage ornaments can all be used to great effect on tables and mantelpieces, and outdoors. Glass candlesticks, pretty ceramic birds, candelabras, and strings of beads are an easy way to theme your day. Pick them up at charity shops and flea markets for a small outlay, and donate them back to charity afterward.

Jewel favors

For female guests, buy small vintage brooches and pin them onto their napkins. This can be inexpensive, and it will create both a lasting favor and a fabulous decoration.

Bunting for all occasions

Bunting is ideal for weddings, silently dancing in the breeze, tied onto trees or around marquees. Debbie Coutts (www.tatteredandtorn.co.uk) made the gorgeous bunting on page 154. She uses only reclaimed and vintage fabrics and trimmings, tints them with tea and plant dyes, and sews the flags by hand. Try making your own, perhaps in different shapes, such as hearts or stars, and embellish it, with vintage buttons and ribbons.

Retro details
* 1950s teacups in single colors
* 1960s brightly colored art-glass vases
* 1970s floral tablecloths
* Victorian glass candlesticks
* Antique lace
* Vintage teacup candles (see page 164)
* Salvaged vintage newspapers
* Retro magazines

Delightful place cards

✳ Try vintage playing cards, traditional postcards, or antique photo cards. Write the names by hand in large letters in a contrasting color.

✳ Salvage retro magazines and cut out quirky ads or pictures to paste onto recycled cards.

✳ Secure vintage newspapers (sepia tones work well) onto recycled paper as a backing for a hand-printed name.

Handmade and DIY

Embellish your wedding with delightful decorations skillfully handmade by local artisans, or make your own with natural, recycled, and biodegradable materials.

Paper and fabric flowers

Gorgeous and available in a rainbow of colors, these can be arranged in the same way as fresh flowers. Look for handmade paper blooms or choose fabric blossoms sewn with vintage materials; a bouquet fashioned from salvaged lace and silks can be just as beautiful as a fresh posy—and it will last a lifetime.

The paper roses on the opposite page were created by skilled maker Wendy Morray-Jones, who bases her designs on a vintage pattern book and cuts each petal individually. Search on the craft site www.etsy.com for techniques and inspiration.

Recycled sculptures

Artists and designers can craft unusual decorations out of reclaimed wire, wood, and metal, from tiny birds to delicate snowflakes. Group them together as a centerpiece or set them individually at each place setting.

Glass hanging ornaments

These catch the light beautifully and are usually handmade from recycled glass. Tie them onto willow branches or hang them from trees for an outdoor celebration.

Wooden name tags

These are great for decorations and also guest favors. Buy tags with a small hole in one end so that you can thread them with a ribbon, and tie them onto napkins or favors. Or else, make your own tags by salvaging offcuts of reclaimed wood and printing words or names onto them with old printing blocks.

Seating plans

If you are opting for a traditional, large, written seating plan, try displaying it on a timber easel, decorated with seasonal blooms and foliage, for a secret garden feel. Enclose it in a gilt picture frame so that you won't need to mount it onto card stock. Outside a marquee, use a blackboard on an easel for guests to write messages or to chalk up the menu.

For a striking display, suspend place cards from an antique birdcage. Alternatively, old rustic wooden vegetable crates or pretty vintage mirrors create a fabulous backdrop. Travel enthusiasts will appreciate named brown-paper luggage tags hung inside an antique leather suitcase, and for an outdoor wedding, simply tie them onto tree branches with natural raffia.

Soaps

Natural soaps make fantastic decorations and favors. Either buy them from a local, natural skin-care company or try making your own—look for soap-making workshops online or at the craft spaces in the Directory on page 208. Choose small soaps decorated with dried rosebuds or lavender, wrap in brown wrapping paper, and tie with ribbons and twine. Add a recycled paper name tag, and place on napkins for a gift and place card in one.

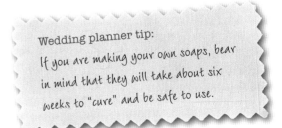

Wedding planner tip:
If you are making your own soaps, bear in mind that they will take about six weeks to "cure" and be safe to use.

Paper roses by Wendy

(www.wendymakesroses.com)

formed into a bouquet by

Rachel of Tallulah Rose Flower School.

Teacup candles

These are simple to make yet incredibly beautiful. Find your plant waxes and natural wicks from reputable suppliers to ensure that they are clean burning and ecofriendly, and buy teacups from thrift stores. After the wedding, clean the cups and either make more candles or use them for tea.

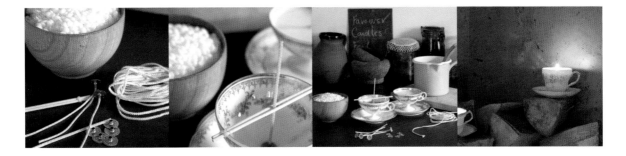

YOU WILL NEED:

Tiny rubber bands

Wooden cocktail sticks

A selection of pretty teacups and saucers

Natural wax, such as soy or rapeseed

Double-boiler pan or a heat-proof bowl and saucepan it can sit in

Natural wicks with metal sustainers attached

Wooden spoon

Scissors

METHOD:

1. Hold two cocktail sticks together and secure each end with rubber bands. Repeat until you have the same number of these as cups.

2. Heat the teacups by placing them in a warm oven for 5 minutes.

3. Melt a spoonful of wax in the double boiler or in the heat-proof bowl over simmering water. Gently dab onto the bottom of the metal wick sustainers.

4. Quickly center the sustainers in the bottoms of the cups. (If you prefer, you can use glue dots instead of wax.)

5. Place the cocktail-stick "wick holders" across each cup, threading the wicks between the sticks until they are secure and upright.

6. Pour the wax into the double boiler and heat until it melts and reaches the temperature recommended on the packet. Stir at all times and be careful not to overheat.

7. Carefully pour the melted wax into each teacup, making sure that the wick holders do not move. Fill to ½ inch below the tops of the cups.

8. Leave until completely set—do not move or shake the cups during this time.

9. Trim the wicks to ¼ inch long with sharp scissors.

10. Arrange at your wedding and enjoy.

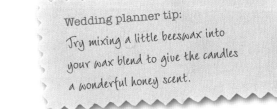

Wedding planner tip:
Try mixing a little beeswax into your wax blend to give the candles a wonderful honey scent.

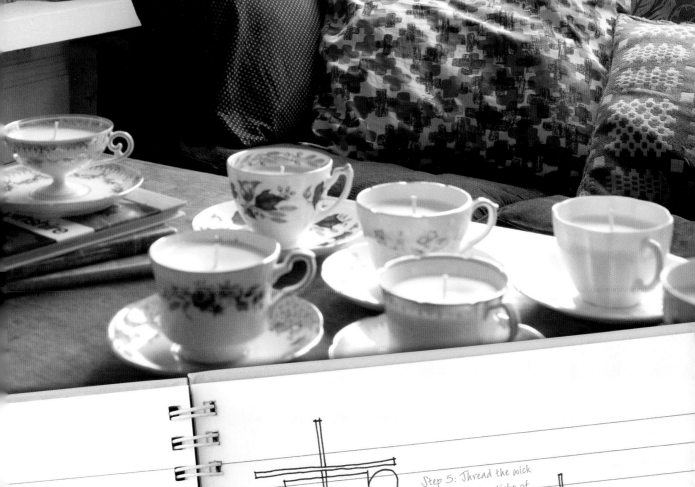

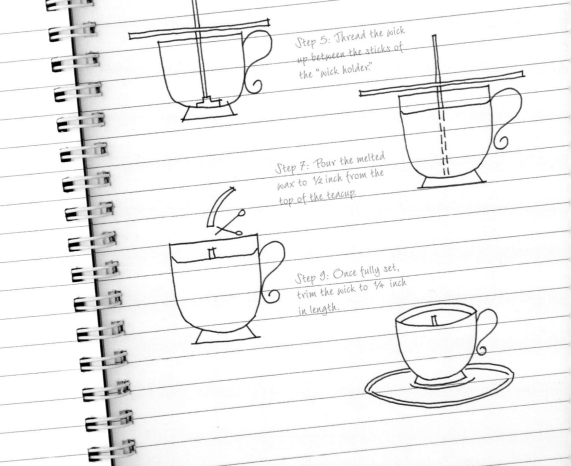

Step 5: Thread the wick up between the sticks of the "wick holder."

Step 7: Pour the melted wax to ½ inch from the top of the teacup.

Step 9: Once fully set, trim the wick to ¼ inch in length.

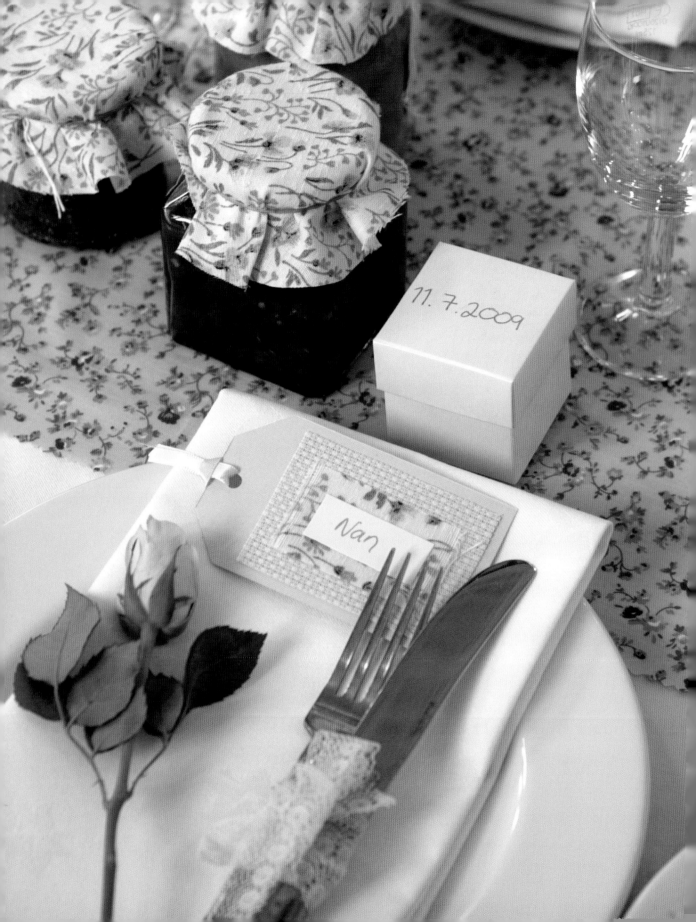

Decorations on a shoestring

For those on a tight budget, simply beg, borrow, and make everything you need. Freecycle is a great resource for finding items for free. After the wedding, recycle them back into the system or give them to charity (www.freecycle.org). Or, why not borrow eye-catching decorations from friends and family?

My money-saving tips include using timber picnic tables so that you don't need tablecloths and making your own bunting from pretty, secondhand bedsheets. Cut the sheets into rough triangles of the same size, and stitch them onto "ribbon" from the same fabric. Candy stripes or florals give different looks, or else, mix them up. Don't worry about frayed edges—they are part of the charm. Arranging your own flowers is also good for the budget: Garden varieties, such as hydrangeas, in simple, contemporary glass can look stunning. And for the ultimate fuss-free reception, host a picnic or barbecue—either of which needs little adornment other than the bride and groom, some friends, and food to share.

Glass bottles

Reuse wine bottles to hold dinner candles or hand-dipped tapered candles or to display single flowers. Keep the labels on if they are interesting; soak the bottles with black tea to make them appear aged. Fill wide-necked bottles with bunches of flowers, either fresh or paper. Decorate with ribbons, strings of secondhand beads, or raffia. Raffia is inexpensive, and it can be used to decorate everything from chairs to candlesticks.

Pots, jars, and tins

Large, clear-glass pots or jars filled with fir cones, fruit, pebbles, leaves, or sand can make interesting bases for either candles or flower displays. Some items can quite happily be immersed in water but others, such as fir cones, are best left dry.

Fill other containers with small plants or sweets. Flowers look charming arranged in tins or jam jars, and remember that the smaller the jar or vase and the narrower its neck, the fewer flowers you will need—which can also help to keep costs down.

Renting

Renting is often a more affordable alternative to buying. You can even rent smaller finishing touches, such as butterfly decorations and table numbers (see the Directory).

Fair-trade decorations

If you need to buy anything from farther afield, look for products bearing the FAIRTRADE mark, from paper flowers to hand-printed fabrics, festive baubles to storm lanterns. Search online ethical stores or fair-trade shops; you'll find our favorites in the Directory.

Inexpensive and gorgeous

Raw materials
- Vintage buttons
- Homemade wildflower paper
- Bunting made from scraps of fabric
- Secondhand tablecloths
- Recycled ribbons
- Big bunches of natural raffia

Pots and jars
- Vintage terra-cotta
- Coir pots
- Tin cans
- Glass jam jars
- Wooden bowls
- Vintage cocktail glasses
- Sundae dishes
- Wide-necked bottles

Fair-trade ideas
- Wire card holders
- Tea-light holders
- Hand-printed napkins
- Strings of paper flowers
- Hand-sculpted ornaments
- Plant-wax candles
- Handmade paper cards

Creative lighting

Lighting is important as it helps to establish a special atmosphere. Candlelight and lanterns are warm and flattering, and both create a romantic ambience perfect for weddings.

Jam jars and hand-blown lanterns

Jam-jar lanterns are a thrifty yet pretty adornment. Collect jam or chutney jars in the weeks leading up to your wedding and wrap salvaged wire around the necks. Bend a hoop of wire over the tops and either leave them as they are or decorate them with a ribbon. They look magical hung from trees or on beaches.

Hand-blown, fine, recycled-glass lanterns can be used to decorate tables and to line pathways. Or, try filling them with water and using them as vases for a pretty, hanging flower display.

Tin-can candles

Following the method on page 164, fill an old food tin halfway with plant wax and leave it to cool completely. To create a lantern effect, punch a few holes in the sides of the tin, above the level of the candle, using a bradawl and small hammer. Add a wire hook if needed.

Pumpkin lanterns

For a memorable and quirky seasonal decoration, carve pumpkins into intricate butterfly- or flower-pattern lanterns, and place them in the centers of tthe ables or in hidden corners indoors or outside.

Vintage candlesticks

From Victoriana glass to antique silver, candlesticks can dress any table or display. Collect clear-glass candlesticks in different sizes, and arrange them in groups of odd numbers, such as threes or fives, in the centers of the tables. Or, try alternating short and tall candlesticks between vases of flowers. Use dinner candles made from plant-based waxes fragranced with essential oils, but be careful not to place candlesticks near open windows or drafts, as the breeze will make the candles drip and burn more quickly.

Candelabras

Stylish and graceful, candelabras always suit formal weddings. Decorate them with flowers, as shown on the opposite page, or leave them unadorned and light cream-colored, plant-wax candles for elegant simplicity. Look for antique or vintage candelabras, perhaps borrowed from friends, or rent them from a good rental company.

Ecofriendly candles

Regular candles are petroleum based and usually have synthetic fragrances. They can give off smoke and toxic chemicals as they burn. Instead, choose clean-burning candles made entirely from plant wax. Candles that are naturally fragranced with pure essential oils smell wonderful and can have therapeutic benefits, too.

Beeswax candles

Long-burning beeswax candles smell divine. They are available as either poured, container candles or hand rolled from sheets; try to buy those made from organic beeswax, and look for kits containing everything you need to create your own rolled dinner candles. (Remember that beeswax is not a vegan product.)

Tea lights

Plant-wax tea lights are delightful, creamy little candles. They tend to burn for considerably longer than regular tea lights and are often made from soy wax. Soya is a cash crop, and sometimes protected rain forest is destroyed in order to plant it. So look for candles made from sustainably farmed soy, produced without such deforestation.

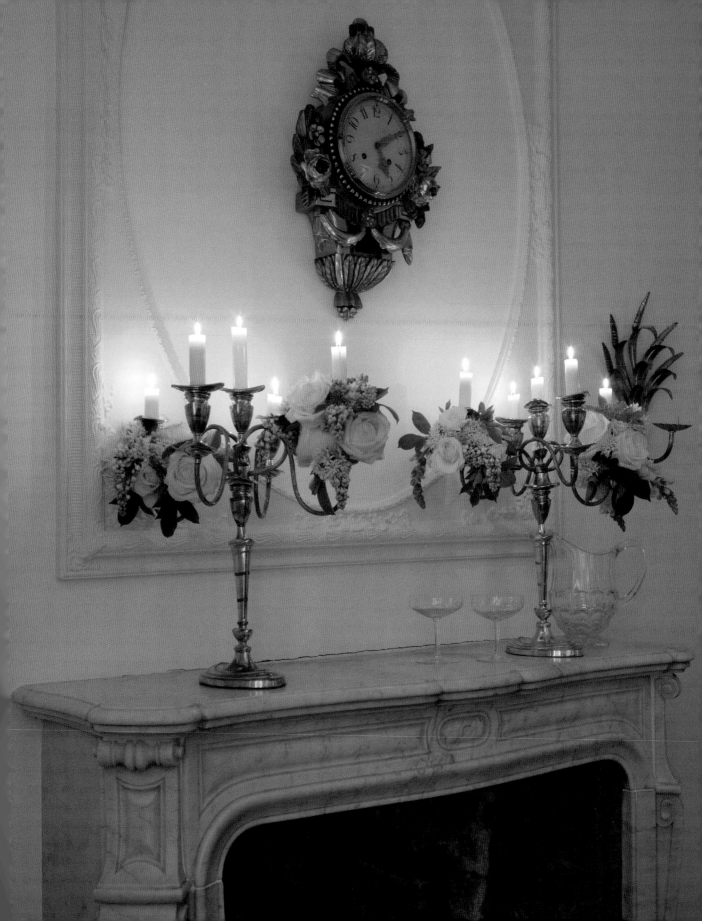

A feast of homemade favors

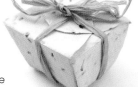

avors are traditionally given as thank-you tokens to guests for attending your wedding. From heavenly chocolates to personalized cards, you can make all manner of gifts that will please your family and friends, young and old. Think of unusual options that say something about you as a couple. I recently attended a wedding in Wales where they gave minipackets of Welsh cakes (a traditional type of fruit drop scone).

Truffles

Decadent little rounds of soft chocolate, dusted with fine, fair-trade cocoa powder, melt-in-the-mouth truffles are simple to make at home. Prepare them just a few days beforehand, and keep them cool.

Homemade sugared almonds

Five sugared almonds is the original favor given to symbolize wealth, happiness, health, long life, and fertility. But rather than buying preservative-laden store varieties, try cooking your own caramel-scented sweets with fair-trade organic almonds.

Heart biscuits

Delicious butter biscuits are a cost-effective treat. Use a heart-shaped cookie cutter, and pack the cookies into biodegradable cellophane bags tied with a natural raffia bow. For extra decoration, add colored icing and a dusting of edible sparkle. For a Christmas wedding, choose a holly- or tree-shaped cookie cutter, and pierce holes at the tops of the biscuits before baking. Once cooled, thread with ribbons so they double as tree decorations.

Favor boxes

Tiny decorative boxes are extremely popular to hold gifts, from trinkets to flower bulbs. Mass-produced boxes may have traveled many miles, so make your own, or buy boxes made from recycled or handmade paper and

those bearing the FAIRTRADE mark. The most ecofriendly favor boxes are plantable ones made from wildflower-seed paper (see page 94), which can be planted in guests' gardens after the wedding. Look online for templates, and opt for a design in one piece, like the box above, rather than with a separate lid. These require less paper and are easier to make.

Seeds

Wrap organic seed packets in paper sleeves, hand-printed with details of your wedding. For a surprise, decant the seeds into handmade paper envelopes decorated with a vintage card and tied with a plush ribbon (remember to include planting instructions).

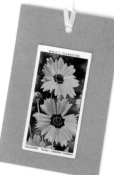

Lavender bags

Gorgeous, scented lavender bags are easy to sew and thrifty. For each bag, cut two heart shapes from a reclaimed fabric, preferably one with a small pattern. With right sides facing out, fill the center with dried, organic lavender flowers and topstitch neatly all the way around, three-quarters of inch in from the edge, by machine or hand. Carefully trim the edges with pinking shears; finish with a ribbon loop, fixed in place with a vintage button.

Paper scrolls

Combine place cards and favors by writing the table names or numbers, together with personal messages, on small pieces of handmade paper. Roll them into scrolls and display in alphabetical groups in terra-cotta pots or glass vases.

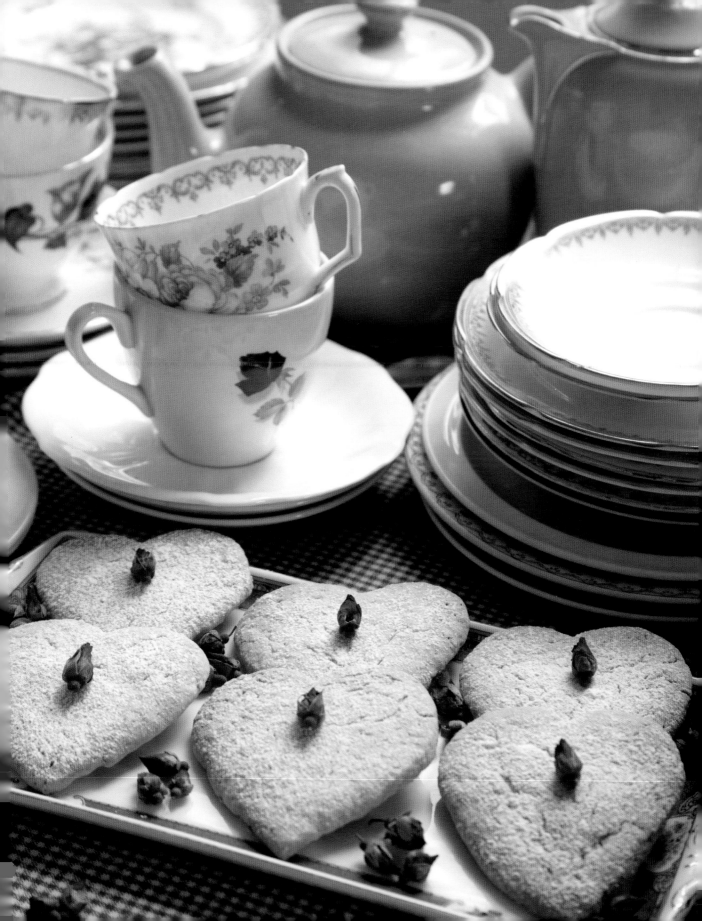

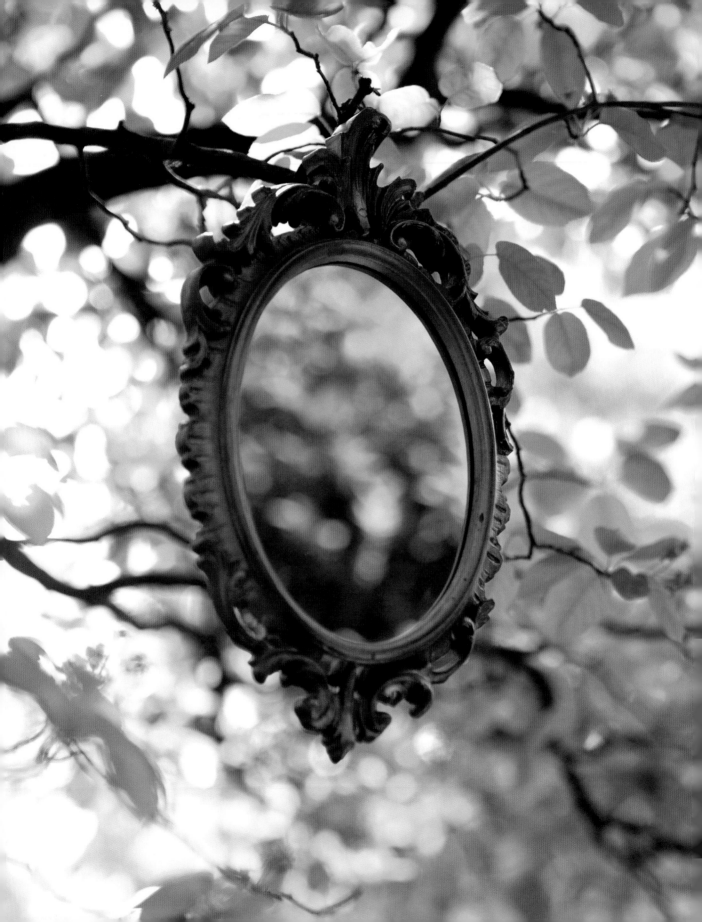

Natural Beauty

The best beauty preparations for a bride-to-be are a good skin-care regime and plenty of relaxation. I've been using and learning about natural products for many years now and am delighted whenever I can pass on what I've discovered to my friends and brides. As well as delicious skin-care brands and secrets, I've included some simple relaxation techniques and pampering treats. Enjoy them as you get ready for your big day and as part of your future lifestyle.

Ingredients to avoid

Parabens, mineral oils, synthetics, sulphates, SLS, silicones, nano particles, GMOs, phthalates, carbomers, DEAs, artificial colors, and animal-tested ingredients. See the Glossary on page 215.

Organic skin care

Natural and organic skin care is increasingly popular, and a regimen based on plant products will contain fewer man-made chemicals, a number of which can trigger allergies. From the simplest range for sensitive skin to cutting-edge, plant-based brands, there is a solution for every bride (and groom). If you are changing from a synthetic product, give your skin a few weeks to adjust. You may get some blemishes at first, but drink lots of water and persevere—your skin will thank you for it.

Creams made from vegetable oils, fruit and nut oils, nut butters, and beeswax, fragranced only with pure essential oils, are good for the planet as well as your skin. You can find out more, including skin-care recipes, from *The Green Beauty Bible* by Sarah Stacey and Josephine Fairley, and *Natural Health and Body Care* and *Recipes for Natural Beauty*, both from Neal's Yard Remedies.

Why choose nonsynthetic?

The skin is the largest organ of the human body, and a significant percentage of what you apply to it is absorbed into your bloodstream. Most standard skin-care products contain chemicals that are either synthetic or petroleum based, and studies have shown that a number of these ingredients can have a detrimental effect on skin health.

Some mainstream companies have realized that consumers are examining labels more closely and have removed parabens and SLS (sodium lauryl sulphate, a harsh degreasing detergent). Nonetheless, labeling can be deceptive: Some products marked "natural" or "plant-based" only contain a small proportion of ingredients derived from nature. The way to tell if a cream or lotion is really natural is by checking the ingredients list and looking for logos, such as the Soil Association, BDIH, Ecocert, OFC, and USDA. A few products in our Directory may contain tiny amounts of food-grade preservatives, but these have been included because of their otherwise outstanding environmental credentials.

Your natural essentials

Cleansers
Cream or oil-based cleansers, especially those with sesame or jojoba oil, are great for dry skin. Coconut-derived rinse-off cleansers suit normal to combination skin.

Toners
Try rose for sensitive skin, neroli for dry skin, and lavender for problematic skin. Atomizers will minimize cotton-wool waste.

Serums and elixirs
These advanced antiaging products, designed to plump fine lines and add radiance, use beneficial plant extracts that firm and tighten skin. Apply them sparingly under moisturizer.

Facial oils
A great alternative to day or night cream, these pure botanical oils leave skin nourished, not greasy.

Moisturizers
Fragranced only with essential oils, these protect against atmospheric pollution as well as hydrate the skin. Neroli and shea butter are good for dry skin and rose for dehydrated; frankincense has amazing antiaging effects.

Face masks
Apply once a week; clay based will unblock pores and cream based will enrich parched skin.

Exfoliators
Choose a fine-grained product with ingredients such as ground oats and seeds. Use twice a week to reveal healthy new skin.

Organic muslin cloths
These can be used to remove cleansers and masks and to gently exfoliate.

A naturally healthy glow

Makeup, like skin-care products, can also contain undesirable ingredients. Fortunately, natural cosmetic companies now offer us the same standard of color and coverage without the unnecessary chemicals. Formulations have improved, and products are available for all skin types and tones, from sparkly eye shadows to creamy organic lipsticks.

Look for brands that are pushing the boundaries, using recycled packaging and renewable energy in their production. We chose Elysambre (www.elysambre.com) for most of the bridal looks in this book. It offers refillable containers for all its cosmetics, which are both ecofriendly and superstylish. For more ideas, visit www.naturisimo.com or www.futurenatural.com, and see the Directory.

Getting the best from ecomakeup

❖ Apply an organic moisturizer to prime the skin for a natural mineral-based foundation.
❖ When using a matte lipstick, apply organic lip balm afterward to help it set and to minimize dry patches. Apply lip balm before lipstick for a sheer look.
❖ Natural mascara is not waterproof but will suit contact-lens wearers and is easy to remove.
❖ Curl eyelashes before applying mascara to make your eyes appear bigger and your lashes longer.
❖ Check your makeup from the side using a handheld mirror in daylight, to see the photographer's view.

Animal testing

It is widely acknowledged that it is not ethically acceptable to test either products or ingredients on animals, but unfortunately it still happens. Truly natural skin care companies only test their ranges on human volunteers. Vegan brides should check if products contain beeswax.

Blemishes

If you develop a pimple the night before the wedding, cleanse your face, pat it dry with a clean towel, and apply tea tree essential oil to the blemish with a cotton ball. Before bed, change your pillowcase for a clean one, as the used one could harbor blemish-creating bacteria. To reduce the chance of pimples before the big day, take these small steps:

❖ Drink plenty of water in the preceding months.
❖ Follow a balanced organic diet.
❖ Keep stress levels low.
❖ Change your pillowcases twice a week.
❖ Find a natural skin-care regimen that suits you and follow it religiously.
❖ Always remove makeup before bed.

Puffy eyes

If you wake up on your wedding day with puffy eyes, place either a slice of fresh organic cucumber or a cool, wet chamomile tea bag on each eye for five minutes.

Miracle creams

Fruit-acid face masks or oil-rich balms are the perfect prewedding skin savers (never use clay-based masks on the day). Simply apply on the morning of the wedding, following the instructions, for smooth, photo-ready skin. Follow with an antiwrinkle cream to help minimize the appearance of fine lines and to prep your face for makeup. My favorites are as follows:

❋ Logona Wrinkle Therapy Fluid: a miracle cream that erases lines before your very eyes

❋ Nude Skincare's Miracle Mask: so simple to use, with fantastic line-reducing results

❋ REN Glycolactic Skin Renewal Peel Mask: an exfoliating mask to improve skin tone and firmness

❋ Neal's Yard Remedies Wild Rose Beauty Balm: a fragrant balm that reduces fine lines, boosts radiance, and softens dry skin

Karen and Lee, of
Lee Matthews Studio,
have created striking
hair and makeup styles
for this book.

Be stress free

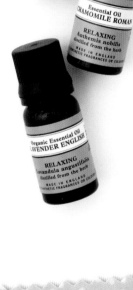

Wedding planning can be stressful, however organized you are. I've included these relaxing tips to help keep your stress levels down and your energy high. Allow yourself an hour a week to unwind and to pamper your body and soul. Play soothing music and light candles to create a warm, calming atmosphere.

Aromatherapy oils

Essential oils extracted from plants and flowers can balance, relax, or energize. You can use them in an oil burner, in the bath, or for massage. All these methods can have positive effects on the senses and the skin. Never apply them directly to the skin (except for tea tree oil on pimples, see page 176); always dilute them first in a carrier such as almond oil. Pregnant women should consult an aromatherapist before using any essential oils.

Flower remedies

These are useful for emotional upset and stress. Bach Remedies are made from British flowers and Bush Remedies from Australian plants. The best known is Bach Rescue Remedy, a multipurpose remedy that is valuable after an accident, shock, or upset, and also for nerves. Carry it with you during the planning stage and on the wedding day, just in case. My favorite individual remedy is White Chestnut. This helps to quiet an active mind at night, when your thoughts are swimming with invitations and color schemes.

DIY spa treats

You can easily replicate many therapeutic spa treatments at home with a few simple ingredients. Look for oils, dried flowers, and herbs in natural beauty stores such as Neal's Yard Remedies. Try the ideas below with your groom, mom, or bridesmaids.

Facials

A monthly facial will improve the health of your skin and help it glow. First, apply cleanser and slowly massage it into the skin using small circular motions. Finish each circuit of the face with a gentle press on the temples. Once rinsed, apply a face mask, avoiding the eye area. Pop fresh slices of cooled cucumber over your eyes, sit back, and relax for ten minutes—enjoy a warm herbal tea for maximum therapeutic effect.

Remove the mask with a warm muslin cloth, and splash your face ten times with fresh, cold water to close the pores. Then, using a few drops of organic facial oil, gently massage, following the contours of the face. Finally, apply a small amount of eye gel or cream to the eye area using small patting motions with your ring finger.

Wedding planner tip:
To help essential oils to disperse in bath water, mix a few drops into a tablespoon of milk first.

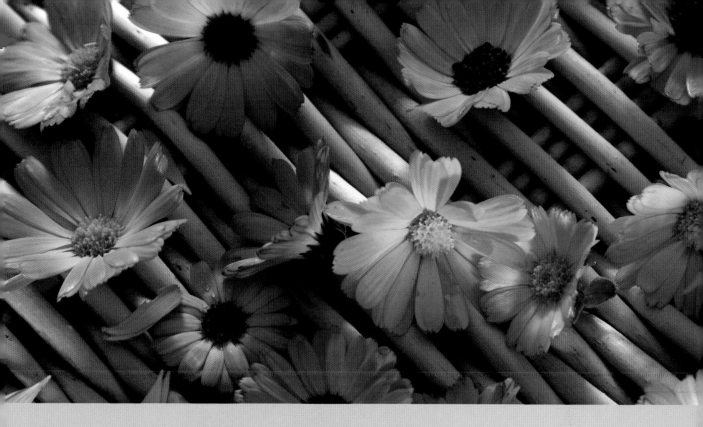

Body scrub

For baby-soft skin, make a paste from three tablespoons of olive oil, a couple of drops of essential oil, a teaspoon of runny honey, and a handful of either sugar, salt, or coarse oats (avoid salt if you have sensitive skin). Rub the mixture lightly onto dry skin, paying attention to elbows but avoiding the face. Rinse off with warm water and pat your skin dry. Follow with a rich organic body cream or oil.

Bath soak

For a relaxing and skin-softening bath, place a handful each of oats, dried marigolds, and lavender or rose petals in a muslin cloth. Tie the cloth into a ball and plac it e under the hot tap while you run the bath. Let the herbs infuse in the water and add a tablespoon of shea butter.

And breathe . . .

If you are about to make a speech or walk down the aisle and are feeling a little anxious, take three deep breaths. This will help you to relax and give you a confidence boost. Similarly, if you are having difficulty sleeping and switching off, concentrate and breathe in gently for a count of seven, then breathe out for a count of eleven. Repeat until you feel more relaxed.

Stress-busting essential oils

❋ Chamomile: a heavenly scent, and deeply relaxing. Blend with lavender and rose in a bath before bedtime for a good night's sleep.

❋ Geranium: a balancing oil, useful when you feel out of sorts. Blend with rose to enhance your mood.

❋ Jasmine: When things get tough, choose sweet-smelling jasmine to bring a sense of renewed optimism.

❋ Rose: If you feel weepy from emotional stress, the scent of rose can help keep tears at bay. Plus, it smells divine.

Edible face masks

These face and hand treatments are all made using ingredients found in your fridge, garden, or greengrocery. Choose organic fruits to minimize exposure to pesticides. Afterward, relax with a lavender eye mask.

STRAWBERRY EXFOLIATING MASK

1 tomato

3 strawberries

1 teaspoon of manuka honey

Chop the tomato finely and mash with the strawberries and honey. Apply to damp skin, avoiding the eye area, and leave for 5 minutes. Rinse well and moisturize for silky-smooth, decongested skin.

AVOCADO, HONEY, AND OATMEAL
NOURISHING MASK

1 ripe avocado

1 teaspoon of manuka honey

1 teaspoon of fine ground oatmeal

Mash all the ingredients together and apply to clean, dry skin. Leave on for 10 minutes and rinse off with plenty of water. Follow with a good natural moisturizer for soft, nourished skin.

TOMATO AND YOGURT HAND MASK

1 ripe tomato

1 small container of natural yogurt

Mash the tomato and mix with the yogurt. Smooth the mixture onto dry, clean hands and leave on for 30 minutes. Rinse well and apply hand cream.

LAVENDER EYE MASKS

These are perfect for soothing a stressed mind and also help to de-puff eyes. Take a piece of fabric and fold it in half. Draw the outline of an eye mask and cut it out so that you have two identical pieces. With right sides facing inward, carefully stitch all the way around the edges, leaving a small hole about three-quarters of an inch long. Turn the bag inside out and fill it with dried lavender flowers. Sew up the hole and stitch a wide ribbon onto each side seam as a tie. Lie back, place the mask over your eyes, and relax.

Hair and finishing touches

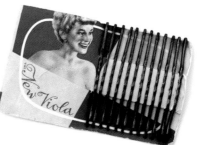

Organic natural shampoos, conditioners, hair masks, and styling products now rival mainstream brands and keep your hair and scalp healthy without synthetic chemicals. Choose your wedding-day hairstyle with your dress in mind. With a floaty 1970s chiffon dress, flowing locks and a simple hair band around the forehead are perfect, or try a daisy chain with long dresses that have simple lines. Structured modern gowns favor an amazing updo, while vintage skirt-suits look stunning with short hair. Pretty antique tiaras and homemade flower corsages complement almost every style and can lift a look with minimal effort.

For shiny, conditioned hair, work in a tablespoon of pure coconut oil, wrap your hair up in a towel, and leave for an hour. Then massage unscented shampoo into the hair before adding water to create a lather. Rinse with plenty of warm water, and dry as normal.

Teeth and tans

Book a dental checkup at least a month before the wedding, to allow enough time for any work you may need. Rather than having teeth chemically whitened, make a "clean and polish" appointment with a hygienist three days before your wedding.

Fake tans have become a popular preparation for the big day. You can now find natural fake tans in both cream and spray applications. Exfoliating thoroughly beforehand and moisturizing well afterward will help them last.

Nails

Most nail polishes contain toxic chemicals such as formaldehyde. A few companies have developed kinder alternatives, in fabulous colors such as vintage rose and hot pink. Either choose a brand such as Zoya or Butter London—which are toluene, formaldehyde, and DBP free—or, alternatively, shine your nails with a buffing board for an elegant look without polish.

Natural perfumes

Scents are notorious for containing many synthetic chemicals. Happily, companies such as Jo Wood Organics are producing organic eaux de toilette, while Florascent uses natural essences. Robert Tisserand's *The Art of Aromatherapy* tells you how to make flower waters (my tip is to put flower water in an atomizer with a drop of essential oil from the same flower to accentuate the scent).

Time out for the two of you

It is important that you and your groom have time for each other in the weeks leading up to the big day. In the final weeks, a wedding can become time-consuming, so my advice is that you take at least a day off each week to relax and enjoy each other's company, with no mention of the wedding. This ensures that you remain focused on why you are marrying and don't exhaust yourselves.

Beauty must-haves for the big day

❋ DIY mineral-water spray—decant local mineral water into a small bottle with an atomizer top. Use during the day to refresh skin; it also helps to "set" makeup.

❋ Small makeup kit containing natural lipstick, lip balm, and powder.

❋ Organic blotting tissues to keep shine under control.

❋ A small deodorant stone (available from health-food stores and natural pharmacies). These leave no stains and are completely natural.

❋ Aloe vera gel. In summer, arm yourself with a parasol to keep shaded, but if your skin is exposed to the sun, aloe will soothe it and reduce redness.

Top DIY hair tips

❋ Make your own salt spray by dissolving sea salt in boiled water. Spray onto damp hair and style for a tousled, fashionable matte finish. Ideal for a beach wedding.

❋ Decorate your hair with small fresh flowers (your florist can provide these on clips). Alternatively, try tiny vintage corsages and fine hair bands for 1950s chic.

❋ Be comfortable on the day. If you usually wear your hair loose, don't feel pressured to have it up.

❋ If you are home-styling your hair, have a couple of trial runs and take photographs from the front, side, and back to remind you of what works.

❋ Choose a natural, nonaerosol hairspray to set your updo.

Lee has used hellebores to dress Karen's hair. Hand-finished couture silk gown by Jessica Charleston.

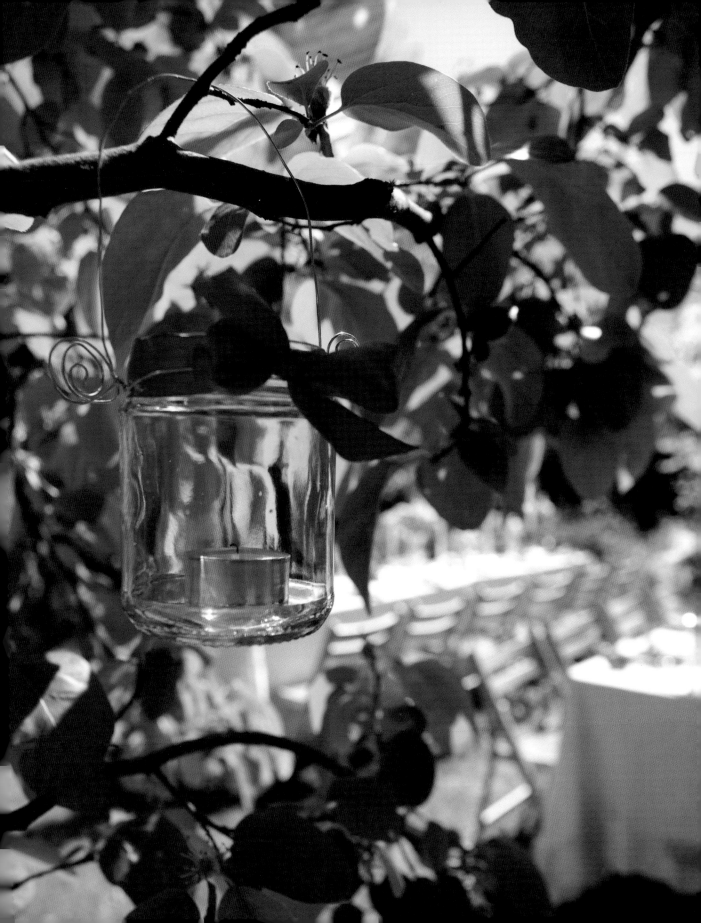

* **Enjoying your day**
  My essential wedding kit and tips for an enjoyable day, including the art of delegation

* **Bridesmaid tote**
  An easy-to-sew pattern that can be a thank-you gift and hold all their little essentials

* **After the wedding**
  Making memories, recycling waste, gifting flowers, and composting

* **Your honeymoon**
  Adventures for the bride and groom, from luxury ecohotels to volunteering

The Big Day

You've searched out the best in eco- and organic suppliers; hand-made your invites, cake, or favors; chosen gorgeous seasonal flowers and local food; and revived an exquisite vintage dress. And now, the big day has finally arrived. In this chapter, you'll find tips on how to enjoy your wedding, as well as essential information on fabulous Earth-friendly honeymoons.

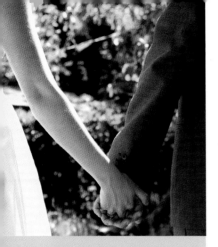

Enjoying your day

Planning a wedding is time-consuming and requires considerable effort. You may have spent months, even years, preparing for your perfect big day and carefully choosing your green products and services. And the bulk of this work usually falls on the bride. The result is a day to which a great deal of expectation is attached.

The anticipation of a wedding can be delightful but can also bring stress and worry. In my experience, the best advice I can give to brides is to relax on the day and go with the flow. Small things may go wrong—a guest might be late or you may stain your dress—but these tiny annoyances are unimportant. The reason you are holding a wedding is to be married; the party is a nice aside. So be happy, smile, relax into your day, and enjoy every minute, as it will fly by in no time.

Keep your sense of humor

A bride once called me the day before her wedding in an absolute panic. She was beside herself: Something terrible had happened, and she had no idea what to do. "Louise, you have to help me," she pleaded.

It turned out that her dog had eaten all her artisanal chocolate favors, handmade boxes and all. This bride was a lifelong friend, so I instantly knew what to do: I laughed. And the minute I laughed, so did she. In that moment, she realized that it wasn't the end of the world; it wouldn't stop the wedding. New favors were made, the guests loved the story, and we still laugh about it to this day.

Delegation

On-the-day delegation is an important part of wedding planning. If you are employing the services of an ecowedding planner, you won't need to do this, but if not, it helps to have friends on standby for specific tasks. Write each person a list so that he or she understands what is required. If responsible for checking that vendors have arrived, make sure that the person has the correct contact details.

Husband and wife

After the ceremony, try to have at least ten minutes alone together, away from the hustle and bustle of the party. You will be entertaining your guests for the rest of the day so pencil in time that is just for the two of you.

Inclement weather

Be prepared and take a golfing umbrella and Wellies. Wind and rain can, however, make for dramatic outdoor photos—bride and groom under an umbrella with veil flying in the breeze. If you laugh about it, you will feel much better.

My essential, natural wedding-day kit

I would recommend that you pack a little bag, well in advance of the day, containing these essentials. It is surprising how useful they can be!

* Bach Rescue Remedy or Bush Flower SOS remedy
* A natural headache remedy
* Traveler's first-aid kit, including bandages
* Safety pins
* Pocket sewing kit, including thread that matches your dress
* Chalk to cover marks on your dress
* Small ball of natural string or twine
* Scissors
* Organic flannel
* Matches
* Some essential items of natural makeup—lip balm, mascara, powder
* Packet of FSC or recycled tissues, or a handkerchief
* Hair pins that match your hair color
* A golfing umbrella, preferably a white one, or a paper parasol in high summer, to protect you from rain or sun

Wedding planner tip:
Remember to talk to your groom! It is easy
to spend all of your time speaking with your
guests instead, but remember it is your day.

Bridesmaid tote

This tote is a great thank-you gift and can be made with any fabrics you have on hand. It looks pretty with a complementary, paler lining. Fill with on-the-day essentials to make bridesmaids feel appreciated.

YOU WILL NEED:

2 pieces of fabric, at least 1¼ x 3 feet each

A piece of fabric 3¼ feet x 6¼ inches, for the handle

Measuring tape, tailor's chalk, and fabric scissors

Ribbons and lace

Vintage buttons

Needle, pins, and matching thread

Sewing machine (not essential)

METHOD:

1. Draw 4 rectangles measuring 1¼ x 1½ feet on your material—2 on each pattern of fabric, if you are using a different lining material. Cut them out.

2. Take the piece that will be the outside front and stitch ribbons and lace on top to make a design (see the photograph on the opposite page).

3. Pin the front and back outside pieces together, right sides facing inward, and stitch along three sides to form a bag shape.

4. Repeat with the two lining pieces, this time leaving a 2-inch gap in the seam.

5. Pinch out the bottom two corners of the outer bag, and stitch horizontally across each corner to form an equal triangle. Repeat with the lining bag.

6. Cut 2 more pieces of fabric, 3¼ feet long and 3 inch wide, for the handle. Pin them together, right sides inward, and stitch down each long side. Turn the handle right side out.

7. Turn the outer layer of the bag right side out, and place it inside the lining so that the right sides of the fabric face each other.

8. Tuck the handle in between the bags so it falls in a loop at the bottom, and line up the edges of the handle between the raw seams on each side.

9. Stitch together at the top edge, all the way around.

10. Turn the bag right side out by pulling all the fabric, including the handle, through the hole in the lining.

11. Sew up the hole, pushing the lining back down into the outer bag, and shake.

12. Embellish with a pin-on corsage (see page 68).

Wedding planner tip:
Press the seams as you go along for a crisp, professional finish, then lightly press the whole bag at the end.

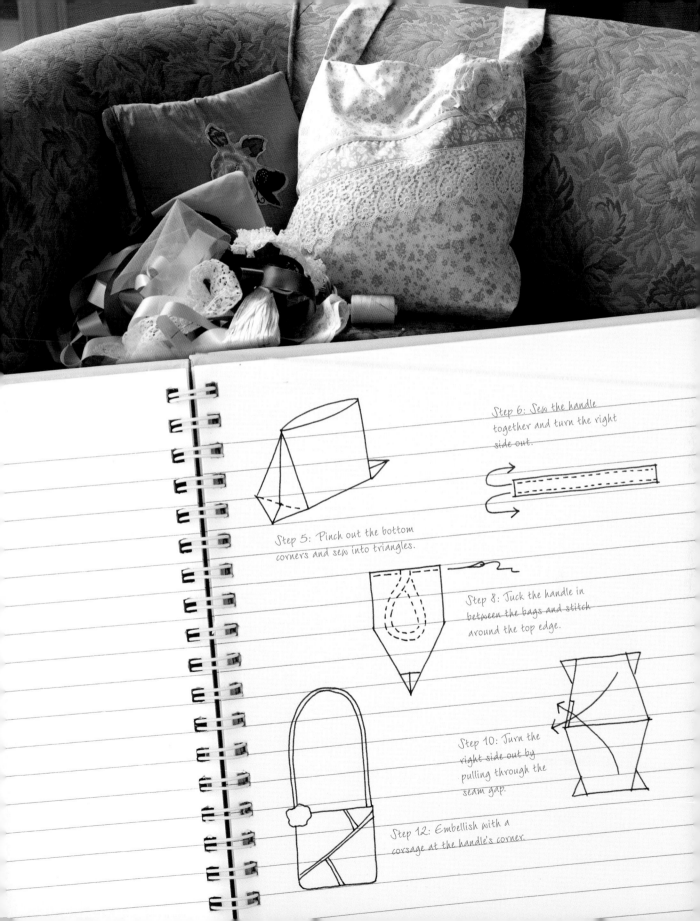

Step 6: Sew the handle together and turn the right side out.

Step 5: Pinch out the bottom corners and sew into triangles.

Step 8: Tuck the handle in between the bags and stitch around the top edge.

Step 10: Turn the right side out by pulling through the seam gap.

Step 12: Embellish with a corsage at the handle's corner.

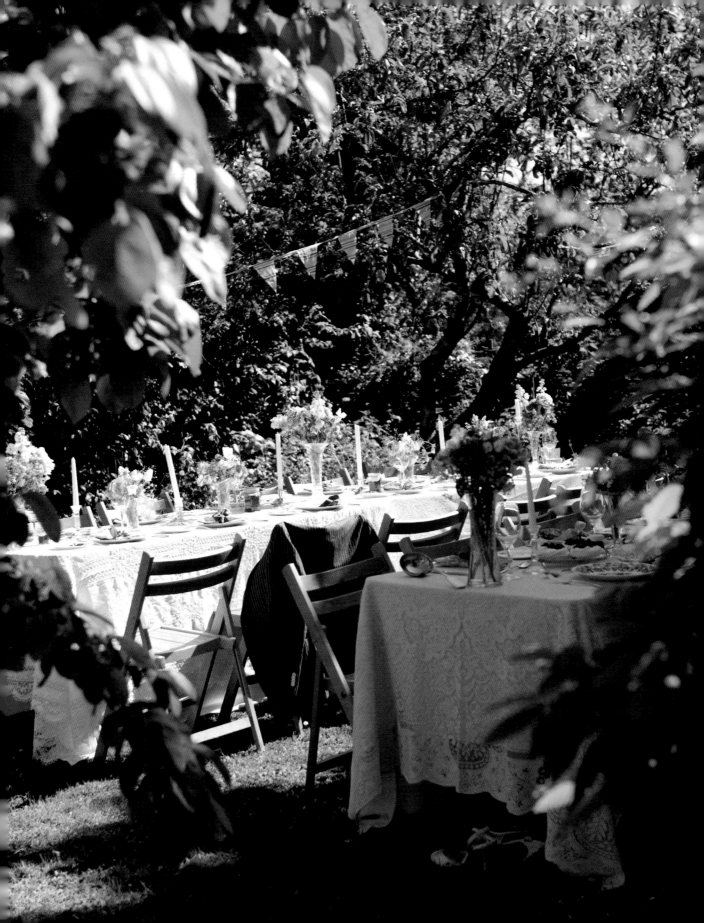

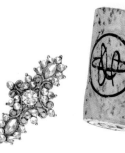

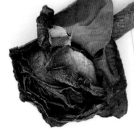

After the wedding

It is a fashionable custom to leave your reception before it ends and go straight to the honeymoon. Whether it's a snug bed-and-breakfast a mile down the road or a train ride to somewhere you've never explored, it is fun to dress for the occasion. If you love vintage, why not invest in an original 1950s frock and vanity case for your trip, and enjoy filling the case with natural and organic treats?

Wedding memories

Keep tokens from your day as mementos and gather them into an antique box or handmade album. A pressed flower from your bouquet, place card, bottle label or cork, pebble, dried leaf, program, handful of confetti, and speeches can all be saved and enjoyed for years to come.

The postparty cleanup

Delegate post-party tasks to your good friends, so that you don't have to worry. Here are a few tips to get them started:

❋ Provide marked recycling bins for paper, cans, food waste, and plastics.

❋ Try to use cardboard boxes or biodegradable cornstarch bags to collect waste.

❋ Collect any spare toys, games, and nonperishable favors, and take them to a local thrift store.

❋ To make distribution of floral displays easy, write notes on the place cards of the guests you would like them to go to, so that they can take them home. Alternatively, hold a raffle using the place cards.

❋ Ask the venue managers if there is a compost bin for food and floral waste.

❋ If you are having a beach, park, or garden wedding, ask a few friends to pick up litter to ensure that you don't leave any trace.

❋ Allocate one person to oversee the return of rented items, such as furniture and suits, the following day.

Maya & Marc

ARE
TYING THE KNOT
-
CEREMONY AT
3.00PM
(PLEASE ARRIVE AT 2.30)
IN THE OCTAGON
THE ASSEMBLY ROOMS
-
CELEBRATIONS COMMENCE
WITH DRINKS IN THE CARD ROOM
FOLLOWED BY
AN EVENING RECEPTION
IN THE TEA ROOM
WITH
FOOD, MUSIC, DANCING
&
LOTS OF CAKE

SATURDAY 7TH FEBRUARY 20
at the *Assembly Rooms*
BENNETT ST
BATH
BA1 2QH

UNTIL MIDNIGHT

Good morning!

If you and your guests are staying the night, continue the celebrations the following morning with a big, organic breakfast. Make the most of a Kåta tepee or yurt by eating together inside before the tent is dismantled.

Your honeymoon

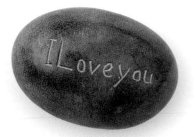

The choice of eco-aware honeymoon possibilities is endless, whether volunteering in Eastern Europe or luxuriating at an ecospa. Consider "slow" travel and ethical options to minimize your impact.

Organic bed-and-breakfasts and ecohotels

Think about staying close to home. You can find environmentally aware and organic bed-and-breakfast retreats for many countries in *Alastair Sawday's Green Places to Stay* (www.sawdays.co.uk). Spend a day beachcombing, then head back for dinner in front of a log fire. Sample delicious local breakfasts and natural toiletries while wrapped in an organic cotton bathrobe.

For luxurious organic spa days and Michelin-starred food, try an ecohotel from one of the sites listed in the Directory, with gorgeous natural furnishings and modern green gadgets.

Honeymooning on a shoestring

Backpacking, hiking, house-swapping, camping—you can have a dream holiday and spend very little. If you crave luxury, book a weekend in an ecoboutique hotel. Alternatively, many organic farms now have permanent yurt fields, with proper beds and warm blankets. Zac and I spent a fabulous shoestring break in Venice, camping at Marina de Venezia, next to miles of sandy private beach. By day, we took the boat across to Venice; in the evenings, we barbecued at the campsite and watched the sun go down together.

Festivals

These can offer distinctive accommodation as well as music and atmosphere. Glastonbury, for example, has private tepees in the festival fields or luxurious shikar tents on the outskirts, complete with butlers and a private bar. Festivals are held across the globe; choosing one local to you will help to reduce your carbon footprint.

Ecotourism

You may have been dreaming about and saving for your honeymoon for years, and looking forward to relaxing and exploring somewhere different. There are many ecofriendly options worldwide, from safari lodges in Africa to snorkeling in tropical blue seas. Avoid large chain hotels and, instead, choose local independents who work hard to protect the environment and benefit their neighboring society. Visit www.ecotourism.org for more information.

Slow travel

Go slow and choose more sustainable transport, such as bus, train, and passenger boat. Not only will you use less carbon, you will see more of the country. If you have to go by air, then offset your flight through a reputable carbon-offset program.

Volunteering holidays

Adventurous couples could go on a volunteering holiday. Companies offer expeditions across the globe to carry out important conservation work. Whether restoring forests in Cameroon, repairing mountain trails in Iceland, or building nesting sites for wild birds in Bulgaria, you will have fun while helping the environment.

Wedding planner tip:
Pack lavender essential oil to treat mosquito bites, citronella oil to repel insects, and aloe vera gel to soothe sun-exposed skin.

Easy ecopacking

A friend once told me that the golden rule with packing is to lay everything you plan to take on your bed and then half it.

❉ Pack items that have more than one use. Linen caftans are the perfect beach cover-up, make a pretty top with jeans, or can be teamed with a belt for an evening dress.

❉ Tie a square, vintage silk scarf at the neck, use it as a bikini top, or wrap it around your head in hot sun.

❉ Always pack an ecobag such as an Onya (www.onyabags.com). It's ideal for shopping, the beach, or even sitting on.

❉ Vintage clothing can be a pleasure to pack, as it is often made with fabrics that don't crease easily.

❉ Take a vacuum flask or mug to minimize paper cup and bottle waste.

❉ Remember a natural SPF sunscreen.

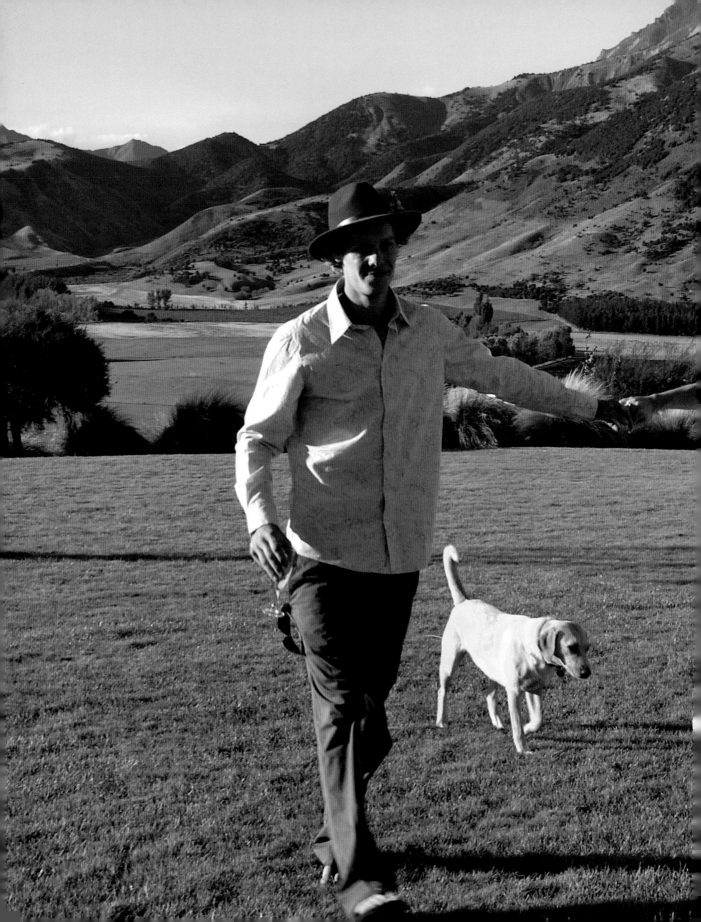

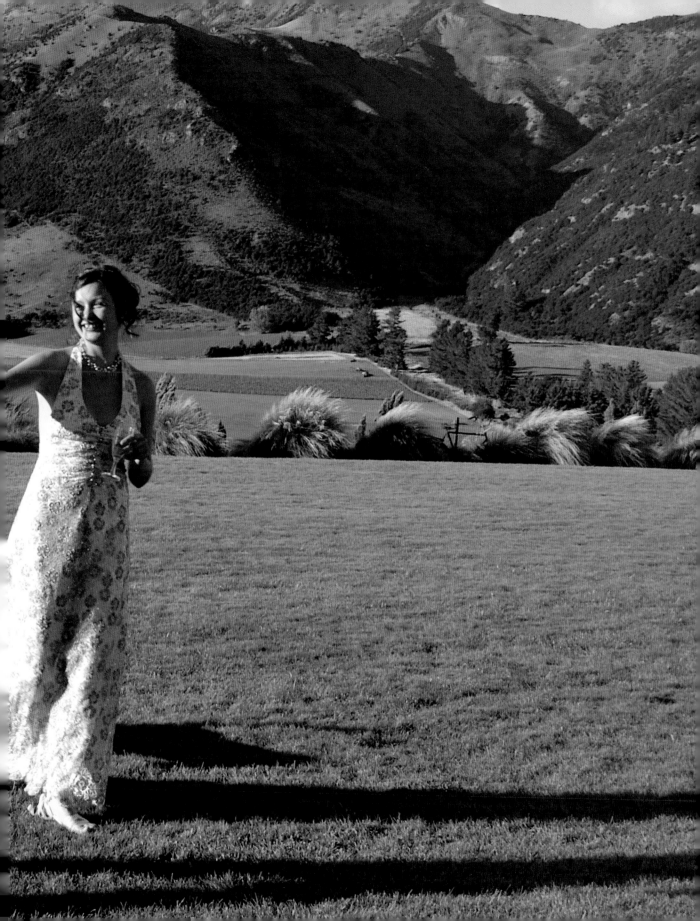

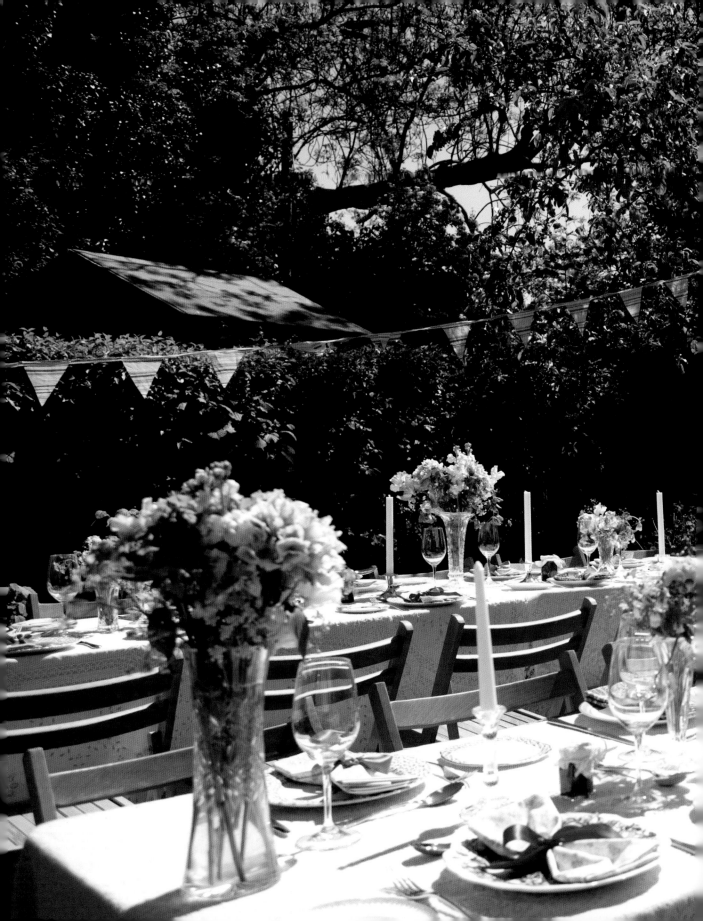

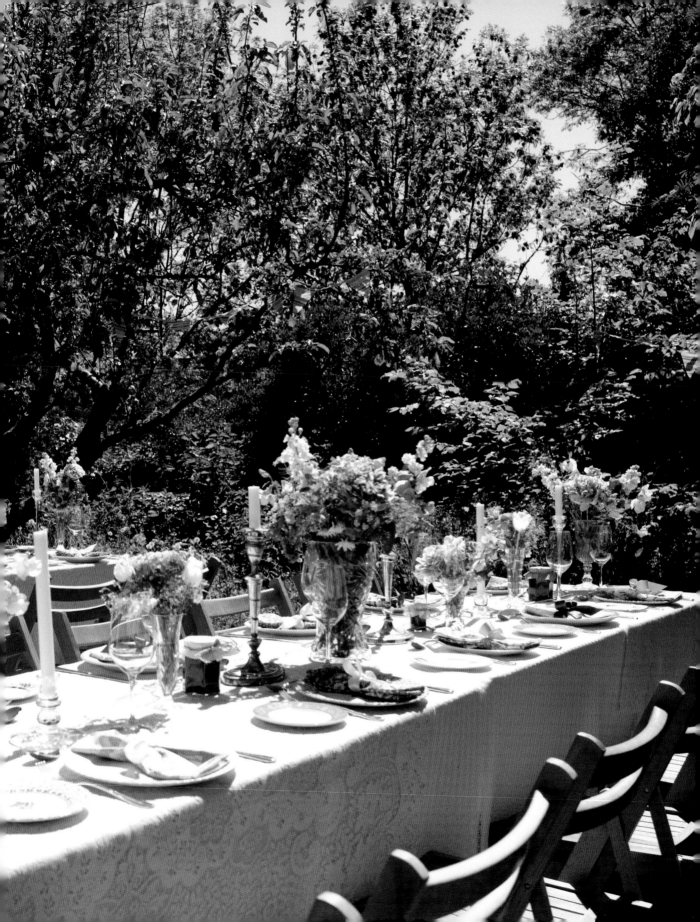

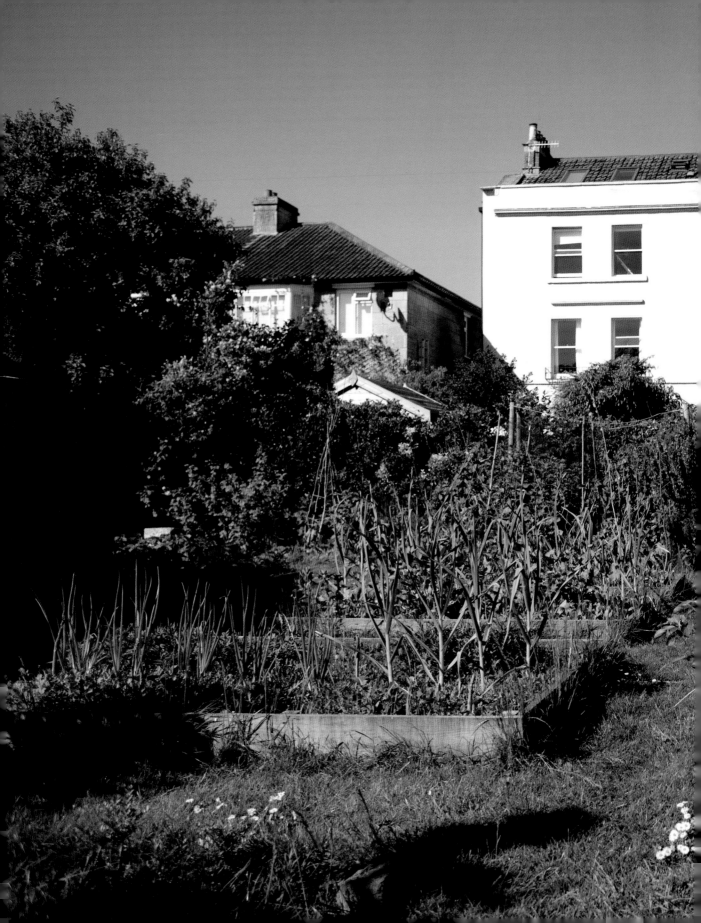

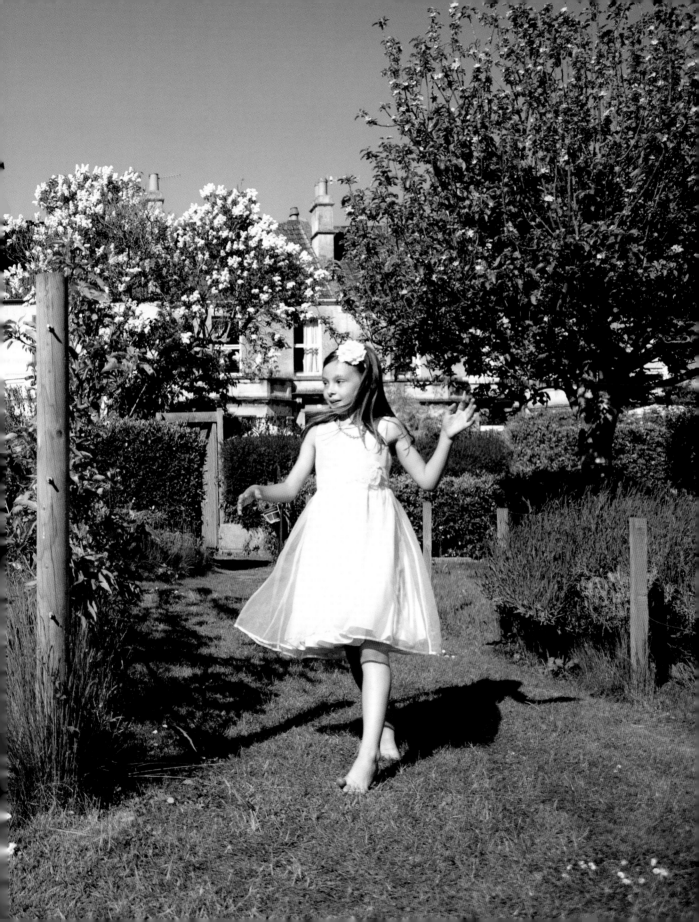

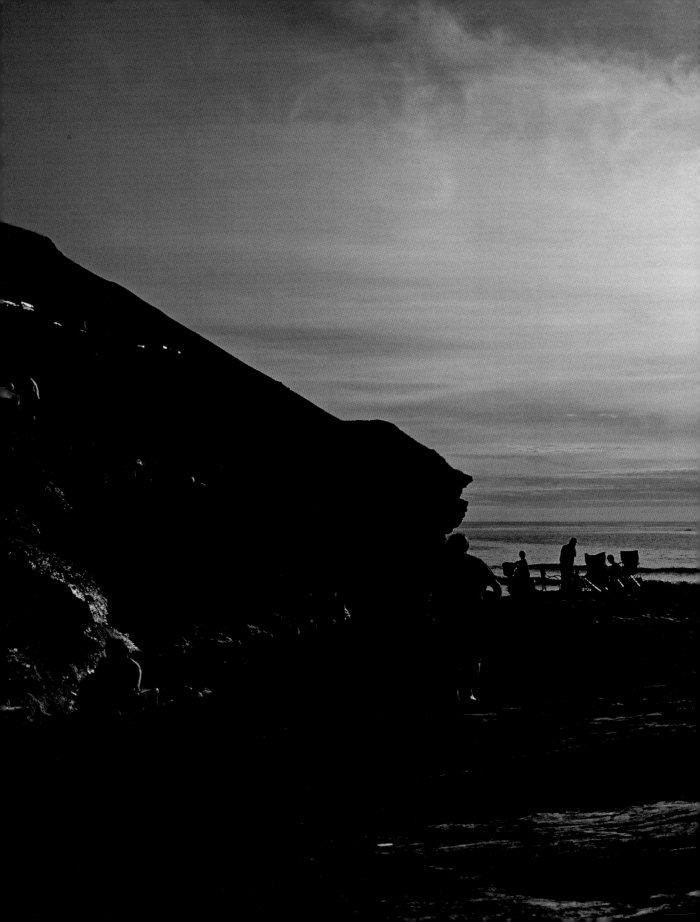

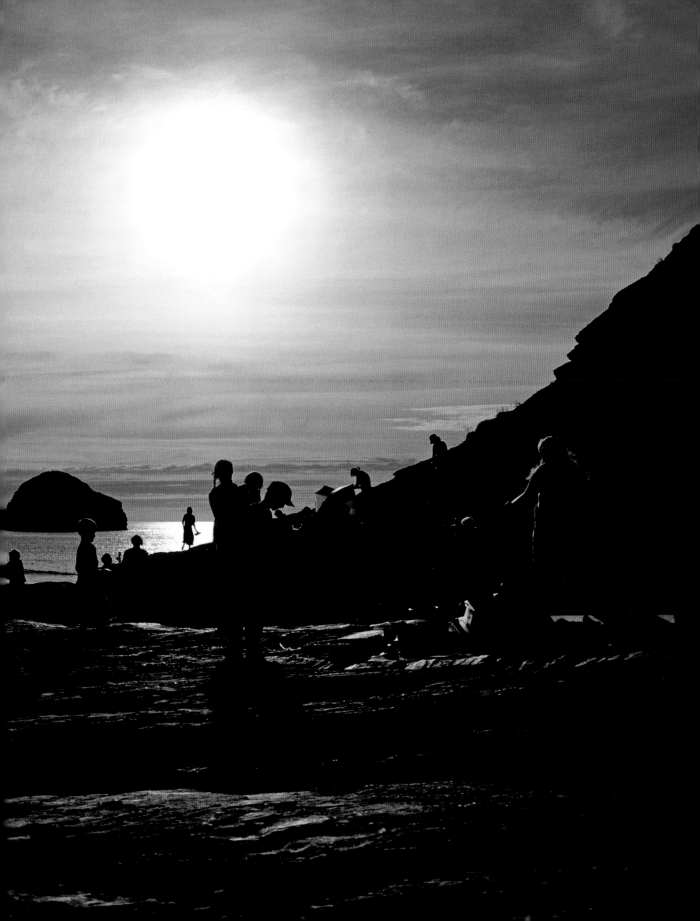

Natural Wedding Planner

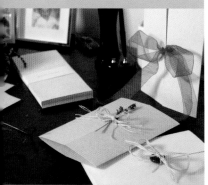

This planner is based on the main stages of organizing your wedding, rather than on a specific timeline. Some couples may have years to plan their wedding, while others may only have a few weeks. You may not need all of the elements below—many will only apply to larger weddings—so simply choose those which are relevant, and check them off as they are done.

Stage 1: The exciting bit

This stage can take as long as you want it to. But remember that some popular venues and churches need to be booked well in advance.

Start compiling your wedding notebook (never too early) with ideas for your natural day (see page 32). ☐

Choose your wedding date. ☐

Decide the type of ceremony you would like to have (see page 30). ☐

Consider how many guests will attend. ☐

Research seasonal flowers and produce available at the time of your wedding (see the seasonal calendars on pages 216 and 217). ☐

Select and book the venue for your ceremony (if required, meet with the rabbi, vicar, priest, or minister). ☐

Select and book the venue for your reception (after visiting different options). ☐

Choose your best man and maid of honor, if appropriate. ☐

Rent a tepee or tent and furniture. ☐

Buy wedding insurance, if it will be a large wedding. ☐

Decide on your wedding registry. ☐

Make wildflower-seed paper for invites, decorations, and favor boxes (see page 94). ☐

Order or make your invitations. ☐

Launch your wedding Web site. ☐

Send out invitations or e-vites. ☐

Start your natural skin-care regimen. ☐

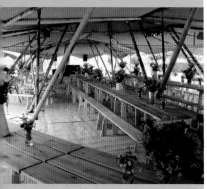

Stage 2: Bride and groom

Enjoy spending time with your groom on these elements—they are all the personal aspects of your day.

Shop for or make your dress. ☐

Find your bridal accessories and make your dress corsage (see page 68). ☐

Book your honeymoon (if you need your passports, make sure they are valid). ☐

Book first-night accommodation (if you are not going straight to your honeymoon or staying at the venue). ☐

Choose your groom's outfit. ☐

Find accessories for the groom. ☐

Shop for wedding rings, or have an existing ring reworked (see page 74). ☐

Sew your wedding-day bag (see page 88). ☐

Choose your first dance song. ☐

Discuss the ceremony music, hymns, vows, poetry, and readings. ☐

Stage 3: Vendors

Some vendors get booked up quickly, especially photographers. If you are planning on a handmade or DIY day, this stage might take a little longer.

Book a photographer and discuss the shots you would like. ☐

Book a DJ or compile your iPod playlist and/or hire musicians. ☐

Book hair and makeup appointments or decide on a style to do yourself. ☐

Book a caterer or decide on your own homemade menu. ☐

Make chutneys a few weeks beforehand, so that they can mature (see page 114). ☐

Rent crockery, cutlery, and serving dishes, if required. ☐

Collect baskets and crates to transport food, if required. ☐

Book a florist or attend a floristry workshop. ☐

Book transport—rickshaws, buses, or tandems—if required. ☐

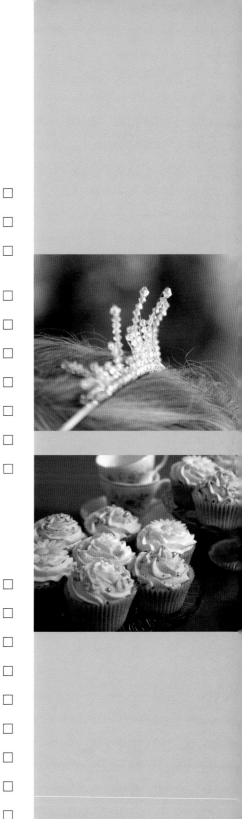

Stage 4: Guests

Bear in mind that set seating plans can take a long time to finalize.

Find bridesmaids' outfits. ☐

Draw up the final guest list. ☐

Design the seating layout, if required. ☐

Finalize guest numbers with caterers or calculate food requirements
if making your own food. ☐

Arrange guests' camping fields or other accommodation. ☐

Sew bridesmaids' tote bags and fill with handmade gifts (see page 188). ☐

Make gifts for family and friends. ☐

Stage 5: Decor and details

The length of time to allow for this stage depends on whether you are buying eco-,
vintage, and fair-trade decorations, or making your own.

Create or find chair or pew decorations (see page 50),
bunting, and other venue decorations. ☐

Make teacup candles, if required (see page 164). ☐

Make favors for each guest. ☐

Make or order place cards (plus a few extras, just in case). ☐

Order the cake from a baker or ask a friend or relative (if you are making
your own, have a trial run). ☐

Enjoy your bachelor and bachelorette celebrations, whether separate or joint. ☐

Have a dental checkup. ☐

Write down a list of friends' duties for recycling after the reception. ☐

Choose one or two friends to supervise the cleanup, and book necessary rental
company collections after the day. ☐

Give the best man and maid of honor the telephone numbers of all vendors. ☐

Have a makeup and hair trial, whether professional or at home. ☐

Make or have printed the menus and other on-the-day stationery (see page 103). ☐

Put all your decorations into boxes or crates labeled with the contents. ☐

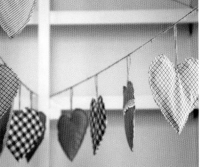
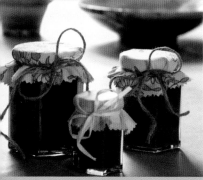

Stage 6: The week before

It's important to set aside time to relax during this stage, so that you don't burn out.

Haircuts for bride and groom. ☐

Write speeches. ☐

Final dress fitting, if necessary. ☐

Break in your shoes. ☐

Order your flowers, if not using a florist. ☐

Check that you have something, old, new, borrowed, and blue. ☐

Bake your own cake or cupcakes (see pages 124 and 128). ☐

Prepare your own food with family and friends. ☐

Pack your wedding-day kit (see page 186). ☐

Pack your honeymoon bags (remember your passport). ☐

Confirm all vendors by telephone. ☐

Tell the best man which vendors need to be paid in cash on the day,
and give him the correct amount of money in labeled envelopes. ☐

Stage 7: The day before

If it is a hot day, remember to keep out of the sun to avoid tan lines or burning.

Decorate the tent or venue with friends and family. ☐

Tie your bridal bouquet, if you are making it yourself—keep it somewhere
cool and dark. ☐

Ask a friend to transport your cake, if homemade, to the venue. ☐

Give yourself a home manicure. ☐

Enjoy a relaxed dinner with friends. ☐

Wash your hair. ☐

Add any extras to your wedding-day kit, such as your speech or family gifts. ☐

Give your bridesmaids their thank-you tote bags filled with
little handmade gifts and treats. ☐

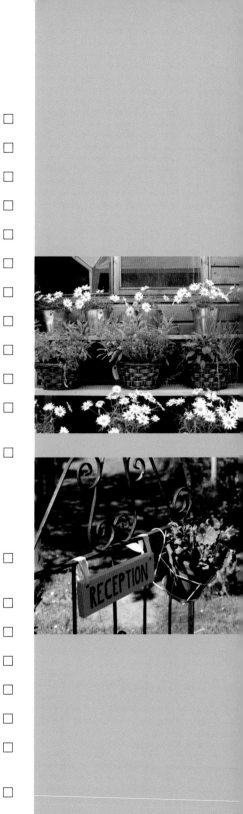

Stage 8: On the day

This really is the best part—enjoy every minute. Smile, whatever the weather—
it's your wedding day!

Enjoy a relaxing bath or shower with aromatic, natural bath products. ☐

Eat a little breakfast, even if you don't feel like it. ☐

Arrange to have a gift or note delivered to your groom as a surprise. ☐

Have your hair and makeup done, or do it yourself. ☐

Enjoy spending time with your bridesmaids. ☐

Ask a bridesmaid to make fresh petal confetti from roses
(this takes minutes—see page 152). ☐

Get dressed an hour before you are due to leave, to allow time for fabulous photos. ☐

Take your bouquet out of water thirty minutes before you leave for the ceremony
and pat the stems dry. ☐

Have a happy wedding and enjoy your day! ☐

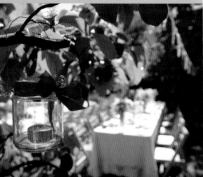

Stage 9: After the wedding

Enjoy your ecohoneymoon with your husband!

Send out thank-you cards or e-mails. ☐

Dry your bouquet as a memento of the day. ☐

Look forward to seeing the beautiful photos. ☐

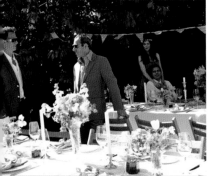

Important for all weddings

Obtain written quotations for any vendors or services.

Book everything in writing and keep the letters or e-mails together somewhere safe.

Pay deposits to vendors on time.

Keep receipts for any payments made.

Remember to take time off from the wedding planning—at least one day a week should
be wedding free. Go out, fly a kite, walk the dog, and relax.

This is a selection of my favorite books for natural-wedding reading. Some of them relate to weddings and honeymoons and some do not, but all are useful and interesting to leaf through, look at, and keep by for tips.

Venue and travel guides

The Alastair Sawday guides:
Eat Slow Britain
Go Slow England
Green Places to Stay
Special Places: Venues in Britain

Eco Hotels of the World, Alex Conti
Ecoescape: Responsible Escapism in the UK,
    Laura Burgess
The Guardian Green Travel Guide, edited by Liane Katz
Organic Places to Stay, Linda Moss

Cooking, growing, and picking your own

Cake Chic, Peggy Porschen
Cakes for Romantic Occasions,
    May Clee-Cadman
The Complete Gardener, Monty Don
The Dairy Book of Family Cookery, Alexandra Artley
Encyclopedia of Organic Gardening, HDRA
Favourite Country Preserves: Traditional Home-made
    Jam, Chutney and Pickle Recipes, Carol Wilson
Flower Course, Jane Packer
The Forager Handbook: A Guide to the Edible Plants
    of Britain, Miles Irving
How to Store Your Garden Produce: The Key to
    Self-Sufficiency, Piers Warren and Tessa Pettingell
The International Book of Sugarcraft (books 1 and 2),
    Nicholas Lodge and Janice Murfitt
Jekka's Complete Herb Book, Jekka McVicar
The Little Book of Organic Farming,
    The Soil Association
Seasonal Preserves, Joanna Farrow
Seasonal Wreaths and Bouquets, Paula Pryke
Sugar Flowers for Cake Decorating, Alan Dunn
Your Organic Allotment, Pauline Pears and Ian Spence

Handmade and DIY

Creative Handmade Paper, David Watson
Knitting in No Time, Melody Griffiths
Loop Pretty Knits, Susan Cropper
Papermaking with Garden Plants and Common Weeds,
    Helen Heibert

Printing by Hand: A Modern Guide to Printing with
    Handmade Stamps, Stencils, and Silk Screens,
    Lena Corwin
Sew It Up: A Modern Manual of Practical and Decorative
    Sewing Techniques, Ruth Singer
Wedding Invitations, Jennifer Cegielski

Vintage and shopping

Alligators, Old Mink and New Money:
    One Woman's Adventures in Vintage Clothing,
    Alison Houtte and Melissa Houtte
It's Vintage, Darling!: How to Be a Clothes Connoisseur,
    Christa Weil
The Little Guide to Vintage Shopping: Insider Tips,
    Helpful Hints, Hip Shops, Melody Fortier
Making Vintage Bags: 20 Original Sewing Patterns for
    Vintage Bags and Purses, Emma Brennan
The Rough Guide to Ethical Shopping,
    Duncan Clark
Secondhand Chic: Finding Fabulous Fashion at
    Consignment, Vintage, and Thrift Stores, Christa Weil
Shopping for Vintage: The Definitive
    Guide to Vintage Fashion, Funmi Odulate
Vintage Fashion: Collecting and Wearing Designer
    Classics, Carlton Books
Vintage Handbags, Marnie Fogg
Vintage Shoes, Caroline Cox

Natural beauty

The Art of Aromatherapy, Robert B. Tisserand
The Green Beauty Bible, Sarah Stacey and
    Josephine Fairley
Natural Health and Body Care,
    Neal's Yard Remedies
The Practice of Aromatherapy, Dr. Jean Valnet
Recipes for Natural Beauty, Neal's Yard Remedies
Vogue Natural Health and Beauty, Bronwen Meredith

Eco, ethical, and thrifty

Ms. Harris's Book of Green Household Management,
    Caroline Harris
The Thrift Book, India Knight
What's in This Stuff?, Pat Thomas

Natural Wedding Directory

Officiants

www.weddingceremony.org
Find an officiant in your state.

Venues

www.audubonnaturalist.org
Marry in one of the society's properties and support its education and conservation programs.

www.barndiva.com
Weddings in the barn or vineyards in California, with local and organic food.

www.business-services.upenn.edu
The Morris Arboretum is part of the University of Pennsylvania.

www.dinegreen.com
Find green restaurants near you.

www.duckfarm.org
Langetree Duck Farm ecocenter, Texas.

www.elmontesagrado.com
Luxurious ecohotel and spa in Taos, New Mexico, with its own natural water recycling and sacred circle.

www.environmentallyfriendlyhotels.com
Rated listings of green hotels by city and state, showing the efforts they are making, from renewable energy to organic food.

www.greenalpacayurts.com
Yurt set in secluded woodland in the New Hampshire countryside.

www.greenhotels.com
Web site of the Green Hotels Association.

www.gwinnettehc.org
Environmental and heritage center available for weddings and celebrations in Georgia.

www.hawaiiislandretreat.com
Green boutique hotel, spa, and yurt village on Big Island, with ocean-view wedding locations and organic catering.

www.heardmuseum.org
The Heard Natural Science Museum and Wildlife Sanctuary, Texas, with native plant garden and a striking amphitheater.

www.herecomestheguide.com
Search for venues, including farms, ranches, and beachside locations, in California; Washington, DC; and Chicago (check with individual venues about their green credentials).

www.hotelhelix.com
Ecoboutique hotel in Washington, DC.

www.lfy.ca
Sale and rental of hand-built yurts made from coppice wood in Nova Scotia.

www.littlestsimonsisland.com
Conservation is key on Little St. Simons Island, Georgia, which is ideal for small weddings.

www.museumca.org/usa
Museums offer a different kind of venue.

www.nps.gov
The National Park Service Web site—Yellowstone, Yosemite, and more all over the United States.

www.nypl.org/spacerental
The New York Public Library is a beautiful reception space.

www.stanfordinn.com
Including weddings in the organic herb garden, with award-winning vegetarian and vegan food, in Mendocino, California.

www.tpforganics.com
Traders Point Creamery is an organic dairy farm and restaurant near Indianapolis, with contemporary rustic interiors and gardens.

www.freewebs.com/wedsea
Mary Crook's selections of wedding locations along the Oregon coast.

Green wedding Web sites

www.greenweddingshowcase.com
Mid-Atlantic green wedding show.

www.green-wedding.net
Site with green wedding products available to buy online.

www.thenaturalweddingbook.com
The Web site of this book.

www.thenaturalweddingcompany.co.uk
Site with advice and directory, including US and Canadian suppliers.

Event planners and photographers

www.engagingaffairs.com
Eco-aware wedding planners in Washington, DC.

www.gorgeousandgreenevents.com
San Francisco–based green event planner; also has a boutique with recycled cards, upcycled jewelry, and more.

www.greenerphotography.org
Find green photographers in your area.

Wedding gowns

www.bridesagainstbreastcancer.org
Find gown sales across the country and support the Making Memories charity.

www.consciouselegance.com
Established, award-wining ecowedding gowns, based in Pennsylvania.

www.ebay.com
One-stop online auction site.

www.etsy.com/shop/lillipopsdesigns
Perfect ecofriendly outfits for flower girls.

www.fashion-era.com
Information site featuring vintage clothing and patterns.

www.freecycle.org
Source of dresses and accessories completely for free.

www.little-flowers.com
Environmentally friendly bridal gowns, bridesmaids' and flower girls' dresses.

www.lorimarsha.com
Unusual bridal gowns made from recycled fabrics and trimmings.

www.naturalbridals.com
Beautiful gowns made with sustainable fabrics, from Atlanta, Georgia.

www.preownedweddingdresses.com
Find your dream dress at this online boutique.

www.punkrockbride.com
Alternative wedding dresses made to order.

www.puridee.com
Gowns crafted using natural and ethical fabrics.

www.recapturedesigns.com
Restyled vintage gowns from a Berkeley, California, studio, and online accessories boutique.

www.recycledbride.com
Gently worn dresses and vintage jewelry online.

www.ruffleswap.com
Dress-swapping marketplace for lovers of fashion.

www.thecottonbride.com
Beautiful handmade dresses in cotton, linen, and silk.

www.thefrock.com
Online boutique of exquisite vintage bridal gowns.

www.thegartergirl.com
Gorgeous ecofriendly garters for your big day.

www.voguepatterns.com
Fabulous vintage *Vogue* patterns to buy online.

Accessories and groomswear

www.beyondskin.co.uk
Cruelty-free, vegan, handmade footwear, delivered worldwide.

www.junkystyling.co.uk
Fabulous menswear created by reworking vintage pieces, available in New York City.

www.magpievintage.co.uk
Vintage bags and accessories, delivered worldwide.

www.recapturedesigns.com
Vintage bridal accessories.

www.terraplana.com
Fabulous ethical shoes for any occasion.

www.urbanfoxeco.com
Ecofriendly lingerie company based in the Midwest.

www.vintagevixen.com
Camisoles, gloves, purses, and more from the twentieth century.

Rings and other jewelry

www.bario-neal.com
Hand-crafted jewelry with reclaimed materials and ethically sourced stones.

www.brilliantearth.com
Canadian diamond rings made with recycled gold and platinum.

www.greendivabridal.com
Ecofriendly, vintage, and fair-trade products.

www.happymangobeads.com
Recycled and hand-crafted beads,
many fair trade.

www.kylerdesigns.com
Stylish, sustainable jewelry.

www.leblas.com
Jewelry made from recycled metals
and conflict-free gems.

www.newyorkweddingring.com
Spend a day making your own
wedding rings.

www.nodirtygold.org
Information on gold and unsustainable
mining practices.

www.queensofvintage.com
Online zine for lovers of vintage
everywhere, including shops,
exhibitions, and fair locations.

www.ruffandcut.com
Ethical rough-cut Canadian diamond
rings made using recycled metals.

www.simplywoodrings.com
Eco-conscious wooden wedding and
engagement rings.

www.touchwoodrings.com
Gorgeous, sustainable wooden
wedding rings.

www.vintagebeadslaramiestudios
.com
Wonderful selection of vintage,
costume-jewelry beads.

www.wood-rings.com
Unusual and ethical composite
wooden rings.

Jewelry and other craft workshops

These can be great places to
learn skills or host alternative
bachelorette parties.

www.craftzine.com
Projects, forums, and news about
classes and events nationwide.

www.makeworkshop.com
From earrings to crochet, soap to
screen printing, based in Manhattan.

www.etsy.com
Enjoy Etsy Labs craft nights in Brooklyn
and San Francisco, or find beautiful
things from other makers.

www.homeecshop.com
Craft shop and classes in Silverlake,
Los Angeles.

www.themakesite.com
Boutique and contemporary craft
classes in Dallas, Texas.

www.theurbancraftcenter.com
Sociable crafting and parties in
Santa Monica, California.

Invites

www.bellafigura.com
Classic and contemporary letterpress
invites printed on cotton paper made
from reclaimed fibers.

www.dauphinepress.com
Elegant designs printed by
ecofriendly letterpress.

www.earthlyaffair.com
Pretty, modern invites responsibly
printed on recycled paper.

www.earthinvitations.com
Handmade paper invitations, paper,
and DIY kits.

www.botanicalpaperworks.com
Handmade "plantable" paper invites
and stationery.

www.charlotterice.com
Fabulous contemporary recycled and
ecofriendly invites.

www.green-wedding.net
Tree-free and recycled invites online.

www.invitesite.com
DIY wedding stationery on recycled,
tree-free, and handmade papers.

www.oblationpapers.com
Simple and stylish letterpress invites
and other stationery.

www.pagestationery.com
Letterpress invites with
stylish typography.

www.spilledinkpress.com
Ecochic stationery made using FSC
and recycled paper.

Paper and printing

www.conservatree.org
Information on environmentally friendly
papers, including photo paper.

www.ecofont.com
New software allowing you to print text
using 25 percent less ink.

www.environmentalpaper.org
Information on sustainable paper.

www.greenpaperstudio.com
Environmentally friendly papers.

www.sgppartnership.org
Web site of the Sustainable Green Printing Partnership, including details of member printers.

www.waterless.org
Web site of the Waterless Printing Association, with printers around the country.

E-weddings

www.paperlesspost.com
The coolest e-vites available.

www.greenvelope.com
Classic e-vite designs.

www.weddingwebsites.com
A guide to choosing your wedding Web site, with a listing of providers.

Catering and local food

Find your local artisan producers through the listings sites here or your local publications. Many caterers will offer local, seasonal menus if you ask.

www.ams.usda.gov
Home of the USA's National Organic Program.

www.atlanticbrewing.com
Microbrewery crafting special and seasonal ales and beers.

www.breadalone.com
Artisan-baked bread in New York.

www.eco-bar.net
Mouthwatering organic, mobile cocktail bar.

www.edf.org
Check out their seafood selector for the most sustainable fish.

www.honesttea.com
Organic, fair-trade tea bags and bottled beverages.

www.localharvest.org
Find farmers' markets, farms, and sustainable food in your area.

www.maineventcaterers.com
Carbon-neutral event-catering business based in Arlington, Virginia.

www.montereybayaquarium.org
Useful Web site to help you choose sustainable fish in your region.

www.occasionscaterers.com
Washington, DC–based sustainable caterer using organic, local, and seasonal produce.

www.pickyourown.org
Find pick-your-own fruit farms near you.

www.threetwinsicecream.com
Organic ice cream available in bulk for weddings and events.

www.transfairusa.org
International fair-trade certification.

Cakes

www.cmnycakes.com
New York–based cake baker.

www.edithmeyer.com
Organic cakes from Santa Cruz, California.

www.hellocupcakeonline.com
Cupcakes made using local, seasonal

ingredients, delivered throughout Washington, DC.

www.lusciousorganicdesserts.com
All-natural, organic cakes and desserts, based in California.

www.mallowdrama.com
Organic wedding cakes and truffles, and special diets catering in Reston, Virginia.

www.stickyfingersbakery.com
Delicious vegan cakes and treats.

www.tallanthouse.com
Seattle-based cake baker using organic and seasonal ingredients.

www.whole-cakes.com
Mouthwatering cakes—100 percent organic—in the Bay Area.

Favors

www.botanicalpaperworks.com
"Plantable" seed favors and favor boxes.

www.divinechocolateusa.com
Fair-trade chocolate favors.

www.green-wedding.net
Gorgeous favors, all earth friendly and fair trade.

Flowers

www.ams.usda.gov
The USA's National Organic Program.

www.bohemianbouquets.com
Locally grown flowers and gorgeous bouquets.

www.goodolddaysflorist.com
Organic, locally grown flowers.

www.gorgeousandgreenevents.com
Local and organic bridal flowers.

www.harmonyhillgardens.com
Organic home-grown flowers.

www.locoflo.com
Local, sustainable florist based
in Baltimore.

www.lovenfreshflowers.com
Gorgeous home-grown cut-flower
florist in Philadelphia.

www.organicstyle.com
Certified organic and VeriFlora flowers.

www.robinhollowfarm.com
Locally grown cut flowers.

www.soulflowersf.com
Supporting local and organic
flower farms, based in San Francisco.

www.tiarefloraldesign.com
Fair-trade, organic, and sustainable
floral design, Tacoma, Washington.

www.transfairusa.org
International fair-trade
certification organization.

www.veriflora.com
Sustainable flowers and horticulture.

www.wisterialaneflowershop.com
Elegant organic arrangements.

Decorations

www.allsopgarden.com
Pretty hanging solar lanterns.

www.beeswaxcandles.com
Beeswax and soy-wax
natural candles.

www.branchingoutt.com
Recovered tree-branch decorations.

www.ecolecticevents.com
Ecofriendly decorations.

www.eluckyme.com
Wedding Web site with ideas and
templates for DIY decorations
and favors.

www.etsy.com/shop/KristinaMarie
Recycled garlands made from maps
and old paper.

www.green-wedding.net
Site of green wedding products
available to buy online.

www.nimli.com
Ecohomewares, candles, and
decorations.

www.skylanterns.com
Biodegradable flying lanterns.

www.westelm.com
This online store has a green section
with storm lanterns.

Natural beauty

www.barefoot-botanicals.com
Try their rose-scented body-sculpt
body cream for defined curves.

www.comvitahuni.com
Delicious Huni skin care, which uses
manuka honey.

www.decadentbeauty.com
Natural and organic beauty brands.

www.drhauschka.com
Established natural skin-care brand.

www.futurenatural.com
Online shop selling organic and
natural beauty products.

www.jowoodorganics.com
Gorgeous perfumes for organic girls.

www.jurlique.com
Australian beauty products and the
best body scrub available.

www.lavera.com
Fabulous, affordable natural makeup
and skin care; Touch of Sun is a
beauty- bag must.

www.lavere.co.uk
Ethical skin care designed for
thirtysomethings-plus.

www.livingnature.com
Pure skin care from New Zealand.

www.logona.co.uk
Makeup and skin care—they produce
the iconic wrinkle-therapy cream.

www.luzernlabs.com
Luxury natural skin care that
delivers results.

www.naturisimo.com
Online natural beauty store.

www.nealsyardremedies.com
Organic skin care with online store.

www.nudeskincare.com
The best natural makeup remover
available; try their night oil, too.

www.purist.com
Bath and body products for bride and
groom from A'kin.

www.skinbotanica.com
Gorgeous natural beauty.

www.theorganicpharmacy.com
Home of organic skin care and
makeup.

www.weleda.com
Established superethical
skin-care brand.

Registries

www.changingthepresent.org
Select from charities benefiting
causes from animal protection to
human rights.

www.giveincelebration.org
Cancer Research Web site for gift
donations and favors.

www.idofoundation.org
Charity-linked registries.

www.justgive.org
Charitable wedding registries.

www.justgiving.com
Charity donation Web site.

www.oxfamamericaunwrapped.com
Many alternative gifts that benefit less
developed countries.

www.rainforestconcern.org
Sponsor an acre of rainforest.

www.rowemountain.com
Fabulous fair-trade gifts
and homewares.

Honeymoon

Also see the hotel resources listed
under Venues.

www.ecofriendlyhotels.co.uk
Ecofriendly hotels all over the world.

www.ecotourism.org
Home of the International
Ecotourism Society.

www.elevatedestinations.com
Responsible travel destinations.

www.energystar.gov
Find energy-efficient hotels.

www.greentraveller.co.uk
This Web site is all you need to plan
your green break.

www.organicholidays.co.uk
Fabulous organic hotels, farm, and
self-catering accommodation
across the world.

www.responsibletravel.co.uk
The world's leading travel agent for
responsible holidays.

www.seat61.com
How to travel the world by train
and ship.

www.uplandescapes.com
Ecofriendly walking holidays.

Carbon offsetting

www.carbonfund.org
Offset your carbon footprint here.

www.climatecare.org
Credible carbon-offset company.

Green Web sites

www.ecofashionworld.com
Information and directory of
ecobrands and ecostores.

www.eere.energy.gov
US Department of Energy's information
Web site on green energy.

www.epa.gov/greenvehicles
Look up your wedding vehicle online
to check its emissions.

www.gengreenlife.com
Search the green business directory.

www.greenyour.com
How to make many areas of your life
more ecofriendly—including travel
and weddings.

www.sierraclubgreenhome.com
General green-information Web site.

www.treehugger.com
From environment and ecodesign
news to buyers' guides.

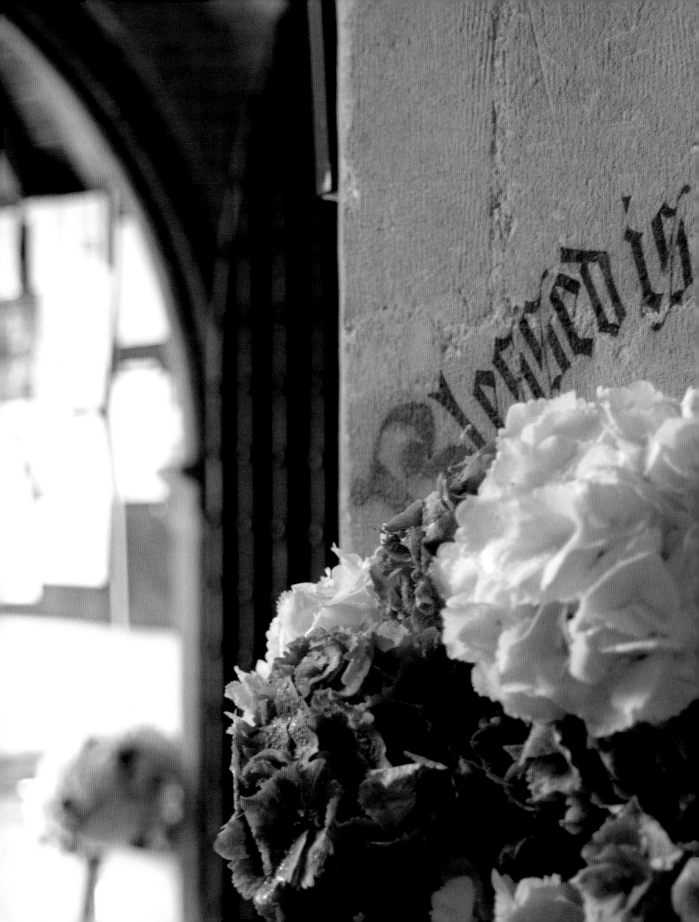

Glossary

BDIH
The European organization that certifies beauty products as being natural (www.kontrollierte-naturkosmetik.de).

Biomass boiler
A boiler powered by wood chips or pellets that can be used to heat water or as part of a central-heating system.

Carbomers
Synthetic polymers, or plasticlike substances, used to thicken cosmetics and stop them from separating.

DEAs
Compounds of diethanolamine, which have a range of uses in cosmetics and skin-care products. Also look for TEA, or triethanolamine. There are concerns that these can react with certain other ingredients to form cancer-causing chemicals, which have led to restrictions on how they can be used.

DBP
A type of phthalate.

Ecocert
French organic and sustainability certification body for food, cosmetics, and textiles (www.ecocert.com).

Embodied energy
The total energy required to make a product, from extraction and manufacture to transport. Some analyses also include the energy required to disassemble and dispose of the product after use.

GMOs
Genetically modified organisms.

Mineral oil
Also listed as paraffinum liquidum. Clear, odorless oil derived from petroleum. Believed to interfere with the body's own protective oily barrier.

OFC
Organic Food Chain, an Australian certification body (www.organicfoodchain.com.au).

Parabens
Widely used as artificial preservatives in cosmetics. There is concern that some may be carcinogenic.

Phthalates
Used as softeners in plastics but found widely in products such as hairspray and perfumes.

SLS
Sodium lauryl sulfate is a harsh and potentially skin-irritating detergent used as a foaming agent in shampoos and toothpaste. Some natural products use sodium laureth sulfate as an alternative, but there are questions about this compound, too.

Sulfates
A catchall term employed to mean detergents such as sodium lauryl and laureth sulfates and other similar compounds. Not all chemicals listed on labels as a sulfate are detergents.

USDA
The US Department of Agriculture, which oversees and sets the regulations for organic certification in the United States (www.usda.gov).

Note:
The use of all chemicals in cosmetics is under constant review and regulation by organizations such as the US Food and Drug Administration (www.fda.gov).

Seasonal Fruit and Vegetables

Note that January includes some produce that comes into season late in the year but continues to be available through winter.

January

Vegetables
Cabbages
Cauliflower
Cavolo nero
Jerusalem artichokes
Kale
Purple sprouting broccoli

Fruit
Champagne rhubarb
Late pears, such as
    Conference
Seville oranges for
    marmalade and other
    citrus fruits

February

Vegetables
Greenhouse lettuces

March

Vegetables
Chives
Nettles
Watercress

April

Vegetables
Early baby salad leaves and
    winter lettuce
Radishes
Sorrel
Spinach
Wild garlic

May

Vegetables
Asparagus
New potatoes
New season carrots
Wild rocket

June

Vegetables
Autumn-planted onions
Broad beans
Lettuces
Peas and mangetout
Tomatoes from greenhouses

Fruit (and flowers)
Cherries
Elder flowers
Gooseberries
Red currants
Strawberries

July

Vegetables
Artichokes
Beetroot
Cauliflower
Chanterelle mushrooms
French and runner beans
Garlic
Onions
Tomatoes grown outdoors
Zucchini

Fruit
Black currants
Blueberries
Raspberries

August

Vegetables
Broccoli
Chard
Cucumbers
Eggplants
Fennel
Oyster mushrooms
Porcini mushrooms
Sweet corn

Fruit
Apples (early varieties)
Apricots
Autumn raspberries
Blackberries
Damsons
Plums

September

Vegetables
Borlotti beans and other
    pulses for drying
Cabbages
Chilies
Kale
Peppers
Squashes and pumpkins

Fruit
Apples
Elderberries
Greengages
Pears

Nuts
Hazelnuts

October

Vegetables
Celeriac

Fruit
Apples for storing over
    the winter
Crab apples
Grapes
Quinces
Sloes

Nuts
Walnuts

November

Vegetables
Brussels sprout tops
Cavolo nero
Chicory and radicchio
Jerusalem artichokes
Parsnips
Swedes

Nuts
Chestnuts

December

Vegetables
Brussels sprouts
Spring greens

Fruit
Champagne rhubarb
    (forced)
Citrus fruits

Seasonal Flowers

January

Dogwood stems
Hellebores
Hyacinths grown indoors
Snowdrops
Winter cherry blossom
Witch hazel stems in flower

February

Camellias
Dwarf irises
Narcissi (early)
Ornamental quince blossom

March

Catkins and
   willow branches
Cherry blossom
Daffodils
Forsythia
Hyacinths
Tulips
Wood anemones

April

Forget-me-nots
Fritillaries
Lily of the valley
Magnolia
Plum and apple blossom
Violets in pots and for
   edible blossoms

May

Alliums
Bluebells
Bupleurums
Calendula
Calla lilies
Campanulas
Cornflowers
Cow parsley and
   other umbellifers
Foxgloves
Irises
Lady's mantle
Lilac
Oriental poppies
Peonies
Roses
Snapdragons
Stocks
Sweet peas

June

Astrantias
Lavender
Monardas
Nigella
Sweet williams

July

Bells of Ireland
Cosmos
Delphiniums
Hydrangeas
Lilies
Phlox
Scabious
Zinnias

August

Echinaceas
Fresh hops
Grasses
Love-lies-bleeding
Sunflowers

September

Agapanthus
Asters
Dahlias
Eryngiums
Japanese anemones
Sedums

October

Hips and crab apples
Maples and other
   autumn foliage
Nerines

November

Chrysanthemums
Pansies
Winter-flowering
   honeysuckle stems

December

Amaryllis grown indoors
Cyclamen in pots
Holly
Ivy
Paperwhite narcissi
   grown indoors
Viburnum blossom stems

If you do buy imported flowers, look for the following accreditations to make sure they are grown in a socially and environmentally responsible way:

EcoBlooms
VeriFlora
FAIRTRADE
Transitional
Florverde
Ecocert
Rainforest Alliance
Fair Labor Practices
FlorEcuador

Index

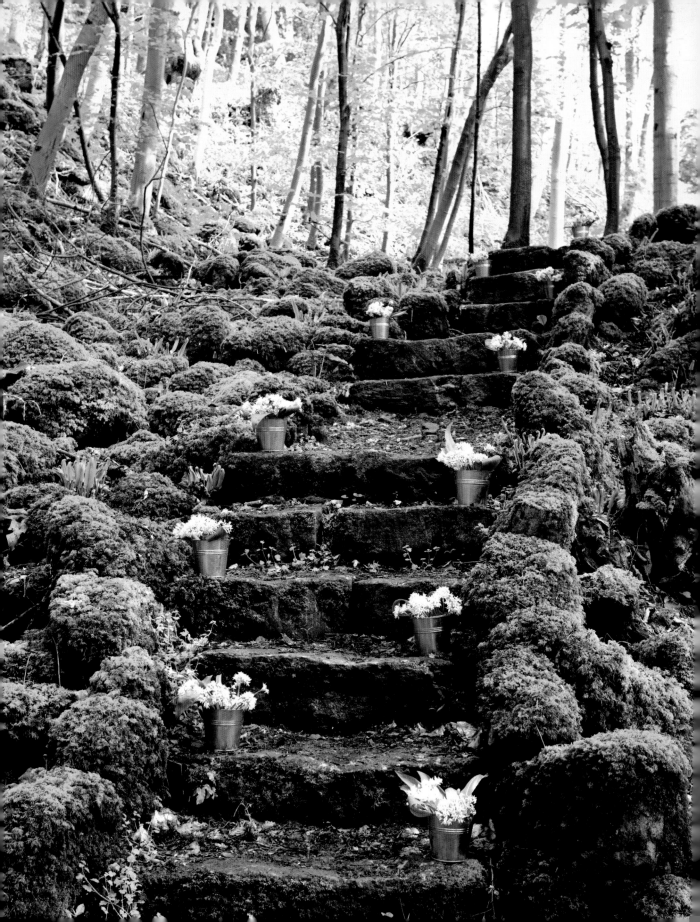

Acknowledgments

I would like to express my thanks to everyone who has been involved in this book, right from the start; my sincere appreciation goes out to them all.

Firstly, to my gorgeous friends who agreed to model for us: Lauren Bunclark, Emma Savage, Karen Matthews, Esther Lincoln, Sophie Shenstone, Vicky Millar, Maya Cavin, Jo Illsley, and Rachel Wardley, along with newlyweds Lisa and Pedro, and Tom and Clare; flower girls Sadie and Angelica; and the garden-party wedding guests. You were all stars, even in the rain.

Secondly, to our professional team of wedding specialists who all so kindly gave their time: Karen and Lee Matthews from Lee Matthews Hair Studio Ltd., Rachel Hill from Planet Cake, Joanna Sinska from Josi, and Rachel Wardley from Tallulah Rose Flowers.

Thirdly, a huge thank-you to my best friend, Justyn Turnbull, who let us invade his house, lent us numerous props from his collection, and cooked us the most delicious food, which can be seen in the Menu chapter.

A big, big thank-you also goes to Caroline Harris, my editor and friend, who has held my hand and guided me through this whole process with patience, sound advice, and many cups of peppermint tea. I would also like to thank Marc Wilson for taking such beautiful photographs, Shelley Doyle for her inspired designs, and editorial assistant Harriet Steeds, who helped enormously.

Finally, I would like to thank my fiancé, Zac. This book really would not have been possible without his constant support, love, serenity, and belief in me and my idea.

Many people and companies have also donated their time or products, or allowed us to use their spaces for the photo shoots. Special thanks go to Jessica Charleston, Jo Illsley at Bath Organic Blooms, Sue Harper at Sweet Loving Flowers, Kate Smith at The Makery, Marylyn and Philip at Rocks East Woodland, Kate Robinson, Janet Meadowcroft and Jill Martin for use of their lovely homes, Adam and Claire Scott-Bardwell, Jessica and Ben Eyers, Louise McGraw, Di Francis of Avonleigh Organic Vineyard, Debbie Coutts from Tattered and Torn, Danaë Duthy of Country Roses, Oxfam Bridal, Nikki from Country Cupcakes, Wendy Morray-Jones, Shropshire Petals, Bramley and Gage, Neal's Yard Remedies, Great Elm Physick Garden, Lavera, Logona, Sante, Elysambre, Peachy Keen Organics, Trevarno, Jonathan Ward, Jo Wood Organics, Mandara, Living Nature, Luzern, A'kin, Nude, Jurlique, Organic Blue, Organic Pharmacy, REN, Butter London, Kimia, and Barefoot Botanicals.

Additional photography: page 25 (sea-glass beads, heart pebbles, beach track) and page 98, Caroline Harris; page 34, © iofoto/Fotolia.com; pages 39 and 202, PapaKåta; pages 41 and 46, Sheepdrove Organic Farm; page 43, Cruck Marquees; page 47, © Marcus Kleppe/Fotolia.com; page 75, family photographs, with thanks to Jackie Carr, Joan and Austen, and Joy and Barry; page 193, © MN Studio/Fotolia.com; page 194, Ruth Brown; page 200, © Marc Wilson/Getty Images.

First published in the United States of America in 2010 by
UNIVERSE PUBLISHING
A Division of Rizzoli International Publications, Inc.
300 Park Avenue South
New York, NY 10010
www.rizzoliusa.com

This book was created by
Harris + Wilson ltd
18 Larkhall Place
Bath BA1 6SF
England
www.harrisandwilson.co.uk

Designed by 20 Twenty Design, www.20twentydesign.co.uk
Edited by Caroline Harris

2010 2011 2012 2013 / 10 9 8 7 6 5 4 3 2 1

ISBN: 978-0-7893-2087-2

Library of Congress Control Number: 2010923744

Printed in China